Drugs
for the
Heart

Provided as a service to medicine by Servier

Drugs for the Heart

REVISED SIXTH EDITION

Lionel H. Opie, M.D., D.Phil., D.Sc., F.R.C.P.
Director, Hatter Institute for Cardiology Research,
Chris Barnard Building;
Professor of Medicine Emeritus,
University of Cape Town,
Cape Town, South Africa
Visiting Professor (1984–1998),
Division of Cardiovascular Medicine,
Stanford University Medical Center,
Stanford, California, USA

CO-EDITOR

Bernard J. Gersh, M.B., Ch.B., D.Phil., F.A.C.C., F.R.C.P.
Professor of Medicine,
Mayo College of Medicine;
Consultant, Cardiovascular Diseases,
Mayo Clinic,
Rochester, Minnesota, USA

WITH THE COLLABORATION OF

- John P. DiMarco, M.D., Ph.D.
- Antonio M. Gotto, Jr., M.D., D.Phil.
- Norman M. Kaplan, M.D.
- Marc A. Pfeffer, M.D., Ph.D.
- Philip A. Poole-Wilson, M.D., F.R.C.P.
- Harvey D. White, D.Sc.

FOREWORD BY

Eugene Braunwald, M.D.

ELSEVIER
SAUNDERS

ELSEVIER
SAUNDERS

The Curtis Center
170 S Independence Mall W 300E
Philadelphia, Pennsylvania 19106

Previous editions copyrighted 2001, 1995, 1991, 1987, 1984
Illustrations copyright © 2001, 1995, 1991, 1987, 1984 by Lionel H. Opie.
Adapted from *Drugs and the Heart*, copyright © 1980 by Lionel H. Opie.

Library of Congress Cataloging-in-Publication Data

Opie, Lionel H.
   Drugs for the heart / Lionel H. Opie, Bernard J. Gersh—6th ed.
      p.   ;   cm.
   Includes bibliographical references and index.
   ISBN 0-7216-2839-7
   1. Cardiovascular agents.   I. Gersh, Bernard J.   II. Title.
   [DNLM: 1. Cardiovascular Agents—pharmacology.   2. Cardiovascular
Agents—therapeutic use.   3. Cardiovascular Diseases—drug therapy.
QV 150 O61d2005]
RM345.D784 2005
615'.71—dc22   2004050810

Publishing Director: Anne Lenehan
Editorial Assistant: Vera Ginsburgs

Last digit is the print number: 9   8   7   6   5   4   3   2   1

Disclaimer

Every effort has been made to check generic and trade names and to verify drug doses as correct according to the standards accepted at the time of publication. The ultimate responsibility lies with prescribing physicians, based on their professional experience and knowledge of the patient, to determine dosages and the best course of treatment for the patient. The reader is advised to check the product information currently provided by the manufacturer of each drug to be administered to ascertain any change in drug dosage, method of administration, or contraindications. In no case can the institutions with which the authors are affiliated or the publisher be held responsible for the views expressed in this book, which reflect the combined opinions of several authors. Please call any errors to the attention of the authors.

"When an approved treatment is considered for an unapproved indication, the physician must evaluate the safety of the medication, its value in related conditions, and the individual patient. What is asked is that he make a prudent decision based upon full knowledge of the available evidence."

JUDGE'S INSTRUCTION TO JURY

Contributors

John P. DiMarco, M.D., Ph.D.
Professor of Medicine,
Cardiovascular Division, and
Director, Clinical Electrophysiology Laboratory,
Cardiovascular Division,
University of Virginia Health System,
Charlottesville, Virginia, USA

Antonio M. Gotto, Jr., M.D., D.Phil.
The Stephen and Suzanne Weiss Dean, and
Professor of Medicine,
Weill Medical College of Cornell University,
New York, New York;
Provost for Medical Affairs,
Cornell University,
Ithaca, New York, USA

Norman M. Kaplan, M.D.
Clinical Professor of Internal Medicine,
Department of Internal Medicine,
University of Texas Southwestern Medical School,
Dallas, Texas, USA

Marc A. Pfeffer, M.D., Ph.D.
Professor of Medicine,
Harvard Medical School;
Interim Chairman,
Department of Medicine,
Brigham and Women's Hospital,
Boston, Massachusetts, USA

Philip A. Poole-Wilson, M.D., F.R.C.P.
Professor,
Department of Cardiac Medicine,
National Heart and Lung Institute, and
Faculty of Medicine,
Imperial College,
London, England, United Kingdom

Harvey D. White, D.Sc.
Honorary Clinical Professor,
Department of Medicine,
Auckland University;
Director of Coronary Care and Cardiovascular Research,
Green Lane Cardiology,
Auckland City Hospital,
Auckland, New Zealand

Foreword

Cardiovascular disease is destined to become an even more important cause of morbidity and mortality as the population of the first world ages and the prophesied epidemic of ischemic heart disease in the developing world sets in. To deal with this changing situation, it is fortunate that an extraordinary array of new cardiovascular therapies continues to become available. These drugs and devices are more efficacious and better tolerated than their predecessors not only in the management of established disease, but also increasingly in prevention. The result is that both students and practitioners of medicine have ever more difficulty in deciding how to choose the proper therapies for their patients. Professor Opie's book provides a rational approach to help with these important decisions. This marvelous book is a concise yet complete presentation of cardiac pharmacology and therapeutics. It presents, in a very readable and eminently understandable fashion, an extraordinary amount of important information on the effects of drugs on the heart and circulation. Professor Opie and his colleagues have the unique ability to explain in a straightforward manner the mechanism of action of drugs without oversimplifying these complex matters. Simultaneously, this book provides important practical information to the clinician.

The sixth edition of this now well-established book builds on the strengths of its predecessors. The excellent explanatory diagrams (an Opie trademark) are even better and more numerous than in previous editions, while the text and references in this rapidly moving field are as fresh as this morning's newspaper. For example, since the publication of the fifth edition the landscape of care of the patient with heart failure has changed considerably. The broadened role of beta-adrenoreceptor blockers, angiotensin receptor blockers, aldosterone blockers, cardiac resynchronization, and implantable cardioverter defibrillators have extended life and reduced morbidity and are presented in this edition. Important new information on the pharmacologic treatment of essential hypertension has also become available with the results of new clinical trials on both old drugs (diuretics) as well as newer drugs (angiotensin II receptor blockers). These are well described and placed in perspective. This concise volume should be of great value and interest to all—specialists, generalists, clinicians, students, teachers and scientists—who wish to gain a clear understanding of contemporary cardiovascular therapeutics and apply this information most effectively in the care of patients with cardiovascular disease.

EUGENE BRAUNWALD, MD
BOSTON, MASSACHUSETTS

ix

The Lancet
Editorial, 1980

(An Editorial from *The Lancet*, March 29, 1980, to introduce a series of articles on Drugs and the Heart)

Cardiovascular times are achanging. After a mere ten years' repose the medical Rip van Winkle would be thoroughly bewildered. For instance, there has been a big switch in attitudes to the failing heart. What would he make of those soft voices which now preach unloading or "afterload reduction"? Experience with beta-blockers has shown the fundamental importance of sympathetic activity in regulating cardiac contraction, and this activity can now be adjusted readily in either direction. Likewise, from calcium antagonists much has been discovered about the function of this ion at cellular level and its importance in the generation of necrosis and cardiac arrhythmia. Continuous ambulatory electrocardiography and special electrophysiological techniques have eased the assessment of arrhythmias, and, again, of drugs to stop or prevent them. Many new drugs have come on the scene, and increasingly they have been devised to act at specific points on pathways to cellular metabolism.

Dr van Winkle apart, there may be one or two other physicians who regard with alarm the new flood of cardioactive drugs. For such as these, Professor Lionel Opie has written the series of articles which begin on the next page. As Professor Opie remarks, drugs should be given not because they *ought* to work, but because they *do* work. We hope that this series will help stimulate the critical approach to cardiovascular pharmacology that will be much needed in the coming decade.

Preface

"What is the use of a book, thought Alice, without pictures?"
—ALICE'S ADVENTURES IN WONDERLAND, LEWIS CARROLL,
1832–1898

"Encouraged by the public reception of the former editions, the author has spared neither labour nor expense, to render this as perfect as his opportunities and abilities would permit. The progress of knowledge is so rapid, and the discoveries so numerous, both at home and abroad, that this may rather be regarded as a new work than as a re-publication of an old one. On this account, a short enumeration of the more important changes may possibly be expected by the reader."
—WILLIAM WITHERING, FROM BOTANY, 3RD EDITION, 1801

I think the advice of these two early authors is profound. Withering, the discoverer of digitalis, suggests that the changes should be enumerated, and Carroll suggests pictures. The changes for this new edition are:

1. By far the most important and major change is the introduction of an online version of the book that will be updated every six months. To access the book online, visit **www.opiedrugs.com** and register with the PIN code that comes with the print volume. Updates will appear immediately adjacent to the most relevant text of the book, and the website will feature a complete updates list for quick summary and review. The website will also feature an Image Library, home to all of the images featured in the book. All of these images will be downloadable into PowerPoint. A list of related websites will also be available on the website.

2. These steps promote our aim of providing a readily accessible guide to cardiovascular drugs in a unique style and format. This compact book, the hard copy again in the widely acclaimed Michelin size, gives crucial information in a readily accessible format for residents, cardiology fellows, and senior students (and, of course, consultants). We believe that the new sixth edition will be even more in demand and certainly better kept up to date than previous editions.

3. John DiMarco is the new lead author for the important arrhythmia chapter that considers the implications of the new trials on sudden cardiac death.

4. Illustrations. These are now in full color, almost all are either new or newly re-created with the aim of conveying maximum clarity, in keeping with the increasingly visual times in which we live. Sincerest gratitude to Jeanne Walker for her artistic genius, skills and patience.

5. References. A concerted effort has been made to provide the reader with all the major new references up to mid-2004 for each chapter. Almost all chapters have more new than old (2000 and before) references.

Acknowledgments

The rapid appearance of this newly revised sixth edition has once again been made possible by the willing and unstinting cooperation of many people. We thank our coauthors, Doctors Poole-Wilson, Kaplan, Pfeffer, White, and Gotto, for generously sharing their expertise and clinical skills on which this book is based and for undertaking their meticulous updating of the fifth edition. We extend a special welcome to Doctor DiMarco who has newly joined us.

We thank Anne Lenehan and the staff of Saunders-Elsevier for providing advice, skills and new ideas, and for so magnificently introducing color-illustrations.

LHO thanks the following. The figures (his copyright unless otherwise stated) are handdrawn by myself and recreated by Jeanne Walker, an illustrator without peer. LHO thanks Professor Patrick Commerford and his colleagues of the Department of Cardiology at Groote Schuur Hospital, Cape Town, for generous help, numerous discussions and for advice on Chapter 6. Victor Claasen provided an infallible reference-retrieval service. Last, but certainly not least, LHO's secretary Sylvia Dennis is thanked for prodigious patience and unfailing skills.

LIONEL H. OPIE
BERNARD J. GERSH

Contents

Foreword by Eugene Braunwald　ix
The Lancet Editorial, 1980　xi

1 **β-Blocking Agents**　1
Lionel H. Opie • Philip A. Poole-Wilson

2 **Nitrates**　33
Lionel H. Opie • Harvey D. White

3 **Calcium Channel Blockers (Calcium Antagonists)**　50
Lionel H. Opie

4 **Diuretics**　80
Lionel H. Opie • Norman M. Kaplan

5 **Angiotensin-Converting Enzyme (ACE) Inhibitors, Angiotensin-II Receptor Blockers (ARBs), and Aldosterone Antagonists**　104
Lionel H. Opie • Philip A. Poole-Wilson • Marc A. Pfeffer

6 **Digitalis, Acute Inotropes, and Inotropic Dilators. Acute and Chronic Heart Failure**　150
Philip A. Poole-Wilson • Lionel H. Opie

7 **Antihypertensive Drugs**　185
Norman M. Kaplan • Lionel H. Opie

8 **Antiarrhythmic Drugs and Strategies**　219
John P. DiMarco • Bernard J. Gersh • Lionel H. Opie

9 **Antithrombotic Agents: Platelet Inhibitors, Anticoagulants, and Fibrinolytics**　276
Harvey D. White • Bernard J. Gersh • Lionel H. Opie

10 **Lipid-Lowering and Antiatherosclerotic Drugs**　321
Antonio M. Gotto, Jr. • Lionel H. Opie

11 **Which Therapy for Which Condition?**　350
Bernard J. Gersh • Lionel H. Opie

Index　414

1

β-Blocking Agents

Lionel H. Opie • Philip A. Poole-Wilson

"Cardiac β-adrenergic signaling apparatus controls contractility."

DORN AND MOLKENTIN, 2004[1]

β-Adrenergic receptor antagonist agents remain a cornerstone in the therapy of all stages of ischemic heart disease, with the exception of Prinzmetal's vasospastic variant angina. β-Blockade is standard therapy for effort angina, mixed effort and rest angina, and unstable angina. β-Blockers decrease mortality in acute-phase myocardial infarction and in the postinfarct period. β-Blockers retain their position among basic therapies for numerous other conditions including hypertension, serious arrhythmias, and cardiomyopathy (Table 1-1). To this extensive list must be added the now firmly established role of β-blockers, cautiously titrated upward, in reducing mortality in heart failure.

MECHANISMS

The β₁-Adrenoceptor and Signal Transduction

Situated on the cardiac sarcolemma, the β_1-receptor is part of the adenylyl (adenyl) cyclase system (Fig. 1-1). The G-protein system links the receptor to adenylyl cyclase (AC), when the G-protein is in the stimulatory configuration (G_s or $G_{\alpha s}$). The link is interrupted by the inhibitory form (G_i or $G_{\alpha i}$), the formation of which results from muscarinic stimulation following vagal activation. When activated, adenylyl cyclase produces cyclic AMP from ATP. Cyclic AMP is the intracellular second messenger of β_1-stimulation; among its actions is the "opening" of calcium channels to increase the rate and force of myocardial contraction (the positive inotropic effect) and increased reuptake of cytosolic calcium into the sarcoplasmic reticulum (relaxing or lusitropic effect; Fig. 1-2). In the sinus node the pacemaker current is increased (positive chronotropic effect), while the rate of conduction is accelerated (positive dromotropic effect). The effect of a given β-blocking agent depends on the way it is absorbed, the binding to plasma proteins, the generation of metabolites, and the extent to which it inhibits the β-receptor (lock-and-key fit).

β₂-Receptors

Classically the β-receptors are divided into the β_1-receptors found in heart muscle and the β_2-receptors of bronchial and vascular smooth muscle. If the β-blocking drug selectively interacts better with the β_1- than with the β_2-receptors, then such a *β_1-selective blocker* is less likely to interact with the β_2-receptors in the bronchial tree, thereby giving a degree of protection from the tendency of nonselective β-blockers to cause pulmonary complications. There are sizable populations, about 20% to 25%, of β_2-receptors in the myocardium, with relative upregulation to about 50% in heart failure. Cardiac β_2-receptors, like the β_1-receptor, link to the stimulatory G_s protein. They also link to the inhibitory protein, G_i[1] with the possibility of protective G_i-mediated β_2-receptor effects. Hypothetically, this inhibitory path could help to limit the adverse effects of excess β_1-receptor catecholamine stimulation. *Inverse agonism* is a complex and still nascent concept

1

Table 1-1 Indications for β-Blockade and US FDA-Approved Drugs

Indications for β-Blockade	US FDA-Approved Drugs
1. Ischemic Heart Disease	
Angina pectoris	Propranolol, nadolol, atenolol, metoprolol
Silent ischemia	None
AMI, early phase	Atenolol, metoprolol
AMI, follow-up	Propranolol, timolol, metoprolol, carvedilol
Perioperative ischemia	(Bisoprolol, atenolol)
2. Hypertension	
Hypertension, systemic	Acebutolol, atenolol, bisoprolol, labetalol, metoprolol, nadolol, pindolol, propranolol, timolol
Hypertension, severe, urgent	Labetalol
Hypertension with LVH	Prefer angiotensin receptor blocker
Hypertension, isolated systolic	No outcome studies, prefer diuretic, CCB
Pheochromocytoma (already receiving α-blockade)	Propranolol
Hypertension, severe perioperative	Esmolol
3. Arrhythmias	
Excess urgent sinus tachycardia	Esmolol
Tachycardias (sinus, SVT and VT)	Propranolol
Supraventricular, perioperative	Esmolol
Recurrences of Afib, Afl	Sotalol
Control of ventricular rate in Afib, Afl	Propranolol
Digitalis-induced tachyarrhythmias	Propranolol
Anesthetic arrhythmias	Propranolol
PVC control	Acebutolol, propranolol
Serious ventricular tachycardia	Sotalol
4. Congestive Heart Failure	Carvedilol, metoprolol (bisoprolol)
5. Cardiomyopathy	
Hypertrophic obstructive cardiomyopathy	Propranolol
6. Other Cardiovascular Indications	
Neurocardiogenic syncope, aortic dissection, Marfan's syndrome, mitral valve prolapse, congenital QT prolongation, Tetralogy of Fallot, fetal tachycardia	(Propranolol; ? all)
7. Central Indications	
Anxiety	(Propranolol)
Essential tremor	Propranolol
Migraine prophylaxis	Propranolol, nadolol, timolol
Alcohol withdrawal	(Propranolol, atenolol)
8. Endocrine	
Thyrotoxicosis (arrhythmias)	Propranolol
9. Gastrointestinal	
Esophageal varices	(Propranolol)
10. Glaucoma (local use)	Timolol, betaxolol, carteolol, levobunolol, metipranolol

( ) = Well tested but not FDA approved; Afib = atrial fibrillation; Afl = atrial flutter; CCB = calcium channel blocker; PVC = premature ventricular contractions; SVT = supraventricular tachycardia; VT = ventricular tachycardia.

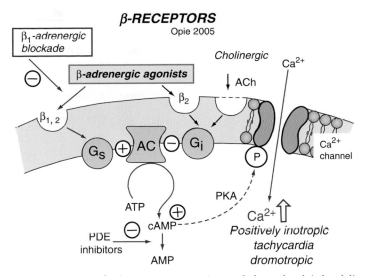

Figure 1-1 The β-adrenergic receptor is coupled to adenyl (adenylyl) cyclase (AC) via the activated stimulatory G-protein, G_s. Consequent formation of the second messenger, cyclic AMP (*cAMP*), activates protein kinase A (*PKA*) to phosphorylate (P) the calcium channel to increase calcium ion entry. Activity of adenyl cyclase can be decreased by the inhibitory subunits of the ACh-associated inhibitory G-protein, G_i. Cyclic AMP is broken down by phosphodiesterase (*PDE*) so that PDE-inhibitor drugs have a sympathomimetic effect. A current hypothesis is that the $β_2$-receptor stimulation additionally signals via the inhibitory G-protein, G_i, thereby modulating the harm of excess adrenergic activity. *ACh* = acetylcholine. (*Figure © LH Opie, 2005.*)

whereby, counterintuitively, a $β_2$-blocker could have stimulatory effects on the G_i-coupled form of the $β_2$-receptor in myocytes from failing human hearts.[2]

$β_3$-Receptors

Although the role of these receptors is well established in adipose tissue, their existence and function in the heart are not yet fully accepted. The proposal is that signals transmitted by these receptors exert a negative inotropic effect in heart failure by increasing the production of nitric oxide.[3]

Widespread Effects of β-Receptor Blockade

During physiologic β-adrenergic stimulation, the increased contractile activity, resulting from the greater and faster rise of cytosolic calcium, is coupled to increased breakdown of ATP by the myosin ATPase (Fig. 1-2). The increased rate of relaxation is linked to increased activity of the sarcoplasmic/endoplasmic reticulum calcium uptake pump, SERCA-2. Thus the uptake of calcium is enhanced with a more rapid rate of fall of cytosolic calcium, thereby accelerating relaxation. Increased cyclic AMP also increases the phosphorylation of troponin-I, so that the interaction between the myosin heads and actin ends more rapidly. Therefore, the β-blocked heart not only will beat more slowly because of inhibition of the depolarizing currents in the sino-atrial node but will also have a decreased force of contraction and a decreased rate of relaxation. Metabolically, β-blockade switches the heart from using oxygen-wasting fatty acids toward oxygen-conserving glucose.[4] All these *oxygen-conserving properties* are of special importance in the therapy of ischemic heart disease. Inhibition of lipolysis in adipose tissue explains why gain of body mass may be a side effect of chronic β-blocker therapy.

β-ADRENERGIC EFFECTS ON CONTRACTION

Opie 2005

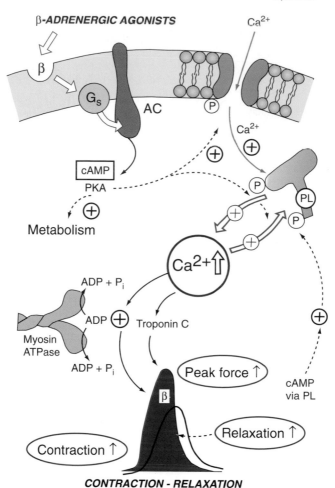

CONTRACTION - RELAXATION

Figure 1-2 β-Adrenergic signal systems involved in positive inotropic and lusitropic (enhanced relaxation) effects. These can be explained in terms of changes in the cardiac calcium cycle. When the β-adrenergic agonist interacts with the β-receptor, a series of G-protein–mediated changes lead to activation of adenylate cyclase and formation of the adrenergic second messenger, cyclic AMP (*cAMP*). The latter acts via protein kinase A to stimulate metabolism and to phosphorylate (*P*) the calcium channel protein, thus increasing the opening probability of this channel. More Ca^{2+} ions enter through the sarcolemmal (*SL*) channel, to release more Ca^{2+} ions from the sarcoplasmic reticulum (*SR*). Thus, the cytosolic Ca^{2+} ions also increase the rate of breakdown of adenosine triphosphate (*ATP*) and to adenosine diphosphate (*ADP*) and inorganic phosphate (*P_i*). Enhanced myosin ATPase activity explains the increased rate of contraction, with increased activation of troponin C explaining increased peak force development. An increased rate of relaxation (lusitropic effect) follows from phosphorylation of the protein phospholamban (*PL*), situated on the membrane of the SR, that controls the rate of calcium uptake into the SR. (*Figure © LH Opie, 2005.*)

Receptor Downregulation

In human heart failure, myocardial β-receptors respond to prolonged and excess β-adrenergic stimulation by internalization and downregulation, so that the β-adrenergic inotropic response is diminished.[5] This "endogenous antiadrenergic strategy" could be viewed as a self-protective mechanism in view of the known adverse effects of excess adrenergic stimulation.[5] The first step in internalization is the increased activity of *β₁-adrenergic receptor kinase* (β_1ARK) in response to excess β_1-agonist activity,[6] as occurs in advanced heart failure. β_1ARK then phosphorylates the β_1-receptor, which in the presence of β-arrestin becomes uncoupled from G_s and internalizes. If the β-stimulation is sustained, then the internalized receptors may undergo lysosomal destruction with a true loss of receptor density or downregulation. However, downregulation is a term also often loosely applied to any step leading to loss of receptor response.

Clinical β-receptor downregulation occurs during prolonged β-agonist therapy or in severe congestive heart failure (CHF). During continued infusion of dobutamine, a β-agonist, there may be a progressive loss or decrease of therapeutic efficacy, which is termed tachyphylaxis. The time taken and the extent of receptor downgrading depend on multiple factors including the dose and rate of infusion, the age of the patient, and the degree of preexisting downgrading of receptors as a result of CHF. For example, one third of the hemodynamic response may be lost after 72 hours (see Chapter 6). In CHF, the β_1-receptors are downregulated by the high circulating catecholamine levels, so that the response to β_1-stimulation is diminished.[5] Cardiac β_2-receptors, not being downregulated, are therefore increased in relative amounts, although there are some defects in the coupling mechanisms. Recent recognition of the dual signal path for the effects of β_2-receptor stimulation leads to the proposal that in CHF continued activity of the β_2-receptors may have beneficial effects such as protection from programmed cell death or apoptosis (see later in this chapter, Fig. 1-7).

Receptor Upregulation

Conversely, when β-receptors are chronically blocked, such as during sustained β-blocker therapy, then the number of β-receptors increases.[7] This change in the receptor density could explain the striking effect of long-term β-blockade in heart failure, namely, improved systolic function, in contrast to the short-term negative inotropic effect.[5] This effect is not shared by other agents such as the angiotensin-converting enzyme (ACE) inhibitors that reduce mortality in heart failure.

CARDIOVASCULAR EFFECTS OF β-BLOCKADE

β-Blockers were originally designed by the Nobel Prize winner Sir James Black to counteract the adverse cardiac effects of adrenergic stimulation. The latter, he reasoned, increased myocardial oxygen demand and worsened angina. His work led to the design of the prototype β-blocker *propranolol*. He showed that, by blocking the cardiac β-receptors, these agents could induce the now well-known inhibitory effects on the sinus node, atrioventricular node, and on myocardial contraction. These are respectively the negative chronotropic, dromotropic, and inotropic effects (Fig. 1-3). Of these, it is especially bradycardia and the negative inotropic effects that are relevant to the therapeutic effect in angina pectoris (Fig. 1-4). The inhibitory effect on the atrioventricular (AV) node is of special relevance in the therapy of supraventricular tachycardias (see Chapter 8), or when β-blockade is used to control the ventricular response rate in atrial fibrillation.

Effects on Coronary Flow and Myocardial Perfusion

Enhanced β-adrenergic stimulation, such as in exercise, leads to β-mediated coronary vasodilation. The signaling system in vascular smooth muscle again involves the formation of cyclic AMP, but

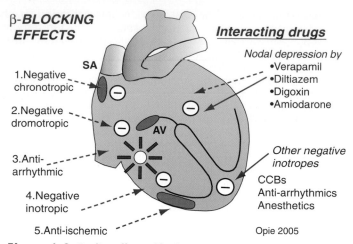

Figure 1-3 Cardiac effects of β-adrenergic blocking drugs at the levels of the SA node, AV node, conduction system, and myocardium. Major pharmacodynamic drug interactions are shown on the right. *AV* = atrioventricular; *SA* = sinoatrial. (*Figure* © *LH Opie, 2005.*)

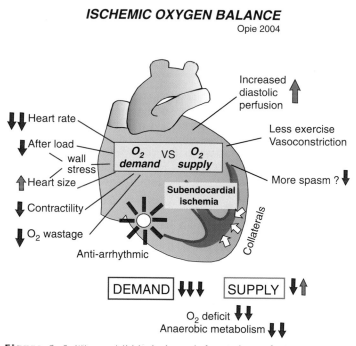

Figure 1-4 Effects of β-blockade on ischemic heart. β-Blockade has a beneficial effect on the ischemic myocardium, unless there is vasospastic angina in which case spasm may be promoted in some patients. Note proposal that β-blockade diminishes exercise-induced vasoconstriction. (*Figure* © *LH Opie, 2005.*)

whereas the latter agent increases cytosolic calcium in the heart, it paradoxically decreases calcium levels in vascular muscle cells (see Fig. 3-2). Thus, during exercise, the heart pumps faster and more forcefully, while the coronary flow is increased—a logical combination. Conversely, β-blockade should have a coronary vasoconstrictive effect with a rise in coronary vascular resistance. However, the longer diastolic filling time, resulting from the decreased heart rate in exercise, leads to better diastolic myocardial perfusion, to give an overall therapeutic benefit.

Effects on Systemic Circulation

The effects described in the preceding explain why β-blockers are antianginal, as predicted by their developers. Antihypertensive effects are less well understood. In the absence of the peripheral dilatory actions of some β-blockers (see section on vasodilatory β-blockers), β-blockers initially decrease the resting cardiac output by about 20% with a compensatory reflex rise in the peripheral vascular resistance. Thus, within the first 24 hours of therapy, the arterial pressure is unchanged. The peripheral resistance then starts to fall after 1 to 2 days, and the arterial pressure now starts to fall in response to decreased heart rate and cardiac output. Additional antihypertensive mechanisms may involve (1) inhibition of those β-receptors on the terminal neurons that facilitate the release of norepinephrine (prejunctional β-receptors), hence lessening adrenergic mediated vasoconstriction; (2) central nervous system effects with reduction of adrenergic outflow; and (3) decreased activity of the renin-angiotensin system, because β-receptors mediate renin release (the latter mechanism may explain part of the benefit in heart failure).

ANGINA PECTORIS

β-Blockade reduces the oxygen demand of the heart (Fig. 1-4) by reducing the double product (heart rate × blood pressure) and by limiting exercise-induced increases in contractility. Of these, the most important and easiest to measure is the reduction in heart rate. In addition, an aspect frequently neglected is the increased oxygen demand resulting from left ventricular (LV) dilation, so that any accompanying ventricular failure needs active therapy.

All β-blockers are potentially equally effective in angina pectoris (Table 1-1), and the choice of drug matters little in those who do not have concomitant diseases. But a minority of patients do not respond to any β-blocker, because of (1) underlying severe obstructive coronary artery disease, responsible for angina even at low levels of exertion and at heart rates of 100 beats per minute or lower; or (2) an abnormal increase in LV end-diastolic pressure resulting from an excess negative inotropic effect and a consequent decrease in subendocardial blood flow. Although it is conventional to adjust the dose of a β-blocker to secure a resting heart rate of 55 to 60 beats per minute, in individual patients heart rates below 50 beats per minute may be acceptable provided that heart block is avoided and there are no symptoms. The reduced heart rate at rest reflects the relative increase in vagal tone as adrenergic stimulation decreases. A major benefit is the restricted increase in the *heart rate during exercise*, which ideally should not exceed 100 beats per minute in patients with angina. In the case of β-blockers with added vasodilatory properties (see later), it may not be possible or desirable to achieve low resting heart rates, because reduction of the afterload plays an increasingly larger role in reducing the myocardial oxygen demand. Nonetheless, in general, vasodilatory β-blockers have not been well tested against angina. For example, carvedilol, which is now the most frequently used of the vasodilatory β-blockers, is licensed for treatment of angina in the United Kingdom but not in the United States.

Combination Anti-ischemic Therapy of Angina Pectoris

β-Blockers are often combined with nitrate vasodilators and calcium channel blockers (CCBs) in the therapy of angina. It is conventional to start drug therapy with two agents, nitrates plus β-blockers or CCBs, and then to go on to combined triple therapy while watching for adverse side effects, such as hypotension. The mechanism of action of the three types of agents is different and may be additive. Thus β-blockers act chiefly by decreasing the myocardial oxygen demand, whereas nitrates dilate coronary collaterals and reduce the preload (see Fig. 2-1), and CCBs prevent exercise-induced coronary constriction and reduce the afterload. β-Blockers may also improve myocardial blood flow by increased time for diastolic coronary blood flow.

Cotherapy in Angina

In the past, the emphasis was on triple–anti-ischemic therapy by nitrates, β-blockers, and CCBs. Although such combinations are still important, especially in those patients in whom intervention by angioplasty or bypass is not feasible, the emphasis has now shifted to the recognition that angina is basically a vascular disease that needs specific therapy designed to give long-term vascular protection. The following agents should be considered for every patient with angina: (1) aspirin and/or clopidogrel for antiplatelet protection; (2) statins and a lipid-lowering diet to decrease lipid-induced vascular damage; and (3) ACE inhibitors, choosing one that has proven protection from myocardial infarction and with the dose tested (see Chapter 5).

Prinzmetal's Variant Angina

β-Blockade is commonly held to be ineffective and even harmful, because of lack of efficacy. On the other hand, there is excellent evidence for the benefit of CCB therapy, which is the standard treatment. In the case of *exercise-induced anginal attacks in patients with variant angina*, a small prospective randomized study in 20 patients showed that nifedipine was considerably more effective than propranolol.[8]

Cold Intolerance and Angina

During exposure to severe cold, effort angina may occur more easily. Conventional β-blockade by propranolol is not as good as vasodilatory therapy using a CCB.[9]

Mixed Effort and Rest Angina

In the past, much was made of the possibility that coronary spasm contributes to the symptomatology of mixed or double-component angina in which, in addition to ordinary effort angina, there is angina at rest. However, two studies show that β-blockade remains the better therapy.

Silent Myocardial Ischemia

Increasing emphasis is now placed on the importance of silent myocardial ischemia in patients with angina. Attacks, monitored by continuous ECG recordings, may be precipitated by minor elevations of heart rate, probably explaining why β-blockers are very effective in reducing the frequency and number of episodes of silent ischemic attacks. In patients with silent ischemia and mild or no angina, atenolol given for 1 year lessened new events (angina aggravation, revascularization) and reduced combined end-points.[10]

β-Blockade Withdrawal

Chronic β-blockade increases β-receptor density. When β-blockers are suddenly withdrawn, angina may be exacerbated, sometimes resulting in myocardial infarction. Treatment of the withdrawal syndrome is by reintroduction of β-blockade.

ACUTE CORONARY SYNDROME

Acute coronary syndrome is an all-purpose term that includes unstable angina and other clinical entities, so that management is based on risk stratification (see Fig. 11-3). Plaque fissuring in the wall of the coronary artery with partial coronary thrombosis or platelet aggregation on an area of endothelial disruption is the basic pathology. Urgent antithrombotic therapy with heparin plus aspirin is the basic treatment. Currently, early platelet GPIIb/IIIa receptor blockade is standard in high-risk patients (see Fig. 9-5). In such patients early coronary angiography is increasingly performed and often leads to angioplasty with use of a drug-eluting stent, or to coronary artery bypass grafting.

β-Blockade is part of the ideal in-hospital quadruple therapy, the other three agents being statins, antiplatelet agents, and ACE inhibitors, a combination that reduces 6-month mortality by 90% compared with treatment using none of these.[11] β-Blockade is usually started early, especially in patients with elevated blood pressure and heart rate, to reduce the myocardial oxygen demand and to lessen ischemia (Fig. 1-5). The major argument for early β-blockade is that threatened infarction, into which unstable angina merges, may be prevented from becoming overt.[12] Logically the lower the heart rate, the less the risk of recurrent ischemia. The actual objective evidence favoring the use of β-blockers in unstable angina itself is limited to borderline results in one placebo-controlled trial,[13] with now the indirect evidence from the quadruple therapy observational study.[11]

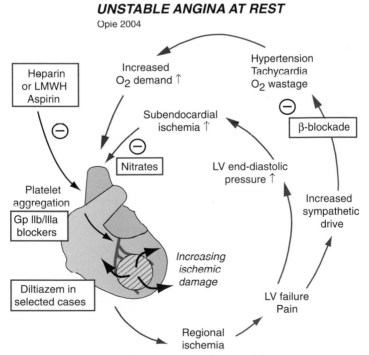

UNSTABLE ANGINA AT REST

Opie 2004

Figure 1-5 Hypothetical mechanisms for unstable angina at rest and proposed therapy. Increasing emphasis is being placed on the role of antithrombotics and antiplatelet agents, such as Gp IIb/IIIa blockers. β-Blockade may be particularly effective in the presence of sympathetic activation with increased heart rate and blood pressure. Calcium channel blockers need to be differentiated. Diltiazem, a heart rate–lowering calcium blocker, may be used intravenously or orally. Dihydropyridines such as nifedipine and amlodipine should be used with care and only in combination with β-blockade. *LMWH* = low molecular weight heparin. (*Figure* © *LH Opie, 2005.*)

ACUTE MYOCARDIAL INFARCTION (AMI)
Early AMI

According to a meta-analysis of 35 trials, in AMI without obvious clinical contraindications, early β-blockade has disappointingly little effect on mortality.[14] Furthermore, the strategy of urgent reperfusion (within the first hours of the onset of AMI) by angioplasty or by thrombolytic agents has overshadowed the possible benefits of early intravenous β-blockade given to inhibit adverse effects of catecholamines released in AMI. There are no good trial data on the early use of β-blockade in the reperfusion era. Logically, β-blockade should be of most use in the presence of ongoing pain,[15] inappropriate tachycardia, hypertension, or ventricular rhythm instability.[16] In others, early β-blockade has limited benefit,[14] especially because it is simpler to introduce it later when the hemodynamic situation has stabilized. Overall, intravenous β-blockade is now used in only about 10% of patients.[17] In the United States, metoprolol and atenolol are the only β-blockers licensed for intravenous use in AMI.

Benefits of Postinfarct β-Blockade

In the postinfarct phase, β-blockade reduced mortality by 23% according to trial data[14] and by 35% to 40% in an observational study on a spectrum of patients including diabetic individuals.[18] Timolol, propranolol, metoprolol, and atenolol are all effective and licensed for this purpose. Metoprolol has excellent long-term data.[19] Carvedilol is the only β-blocker studied in the reperfusion era and in a population also receiving ACE inhibitors.[17] As the LV dysfunction was an entry point, the carvedilol dose was gradually uptitrated, and all-cause mortality was reduced. The mechanisms concerned are multiple and include decreased ventricular arrhythmias[20] and decreased reinfarction.[17] β-Blockers with partial agonist activity are relatively ineffective, perhaps because of the higher heart rates.

The only outstanding questions are: (1) Do low-risk patients really benefit from β-blockade? However, those with non-Q infarcts, high ejection fractions, normal creatinine values, and normal systolic blood pressure values all benefit from postinfarct β-blockade.[18] (2) When should β-blockade start? This is flexible, and as data for early β-blockade are not strong,[14] oral β-blocker may be started when the patient's condition allows, say from 3 days onwards,[17] or even later at about 1 to 3 weeks. (3) For how long should β-blockade be continued? Bearing in mind the risk of β-blockade withdrawal in patients with angina, many clinicians continue β-blockade administration long term once a seemingly successful result has been obtained. The benefit in high-risk groups such as the elderly or those with low ejection fractions increased progressively over 24 months.[18]

The *high-risk patients* who should benefit most are those often thought to have contraindications to β-blockade.[18] Although congestive heart failure was previously regarded as a contraindication to β-blockade, postinfarct patients with heart failure benefited more than others from β-blockade.[18] Today this category of patient would be given a β-blocker cautiously, with gradually increasing doses of carvedilol, metoprolol, or bisoprolol. The SAVE trial[21] showed that ACE inhibitors and β-blockade are additive in reducing postinfarct mortality, at least in patients with reduced ejection fractions. The benefit of β-blockade when added to cotherapy with ACE inhibitors is a mortality reduction of 23% to 40%.[17,18] Concurrent therapy with calcium channel blockers or aspirin does not diminish the benefits of postinfarct β-blockade.

Despite all these strong arguments, and numerous recommendations, β-blockers are *still underused in postinfarct patients*, at the expense of many lives lost. Long-term, 42 patients have to be treated for

2 years to avoid one death, which compares favorably with other treatments.[14]

LACK OF OUTCOME STUDIES IN ANGINA

Solid evidence for a decrease in mortality in postinfarct follow-up achieved with β-blockade has led to the assumption that this type of treatment must also improve the outcome in effort angina and unstable angina. Regrettably, there are no convincing outcome studies to support this proposal. In unstable angina, the short-term benefits of metoprolol were borderline.[13] In effort angina, a meta-analysis of 90 studies showed that β-blockers and CCBs had equal efficacy and safety, but that β-blockers were better tolerated.[22] The possible benefit of β-blockade itself on clinical events in silent ischemia with mild or no angina seems settled by the ASIST study,[10] in which atenolol increased event-free survival at 1 year. In reality, major events, such as death, AMI, or unstable angina, were not reduced, perhaps because the study was underpowered.

β-BLOCKERS FOR HYPERTENSION

β-Blockers are no longer recommended as first-line treatment for hypertension by the Joint National Council of the United States but remain among second choices after diuretics (see Chapter 7). Currently JNC 7 lists the following as "compelling indications" for the use of β-blockers in hypertension: heart failure, post-MI hypertension, high coronary risk, and diabetes.[23] The European guidelines favor β-blocker use in angina, post-MI, heart failure, and tachyarrhythmias.[24] The exact mechanism of blood pressure lowering by β-blockers remains an open question. A sustained fall of cardiac output and a late decrease in peripheral vascular resistance (after an initial rise) are important. Inhibition of renin release may contribute, especially to the late vasodilation. Of the large number of β-blockers now available, all are antihypertensive agents but few have been the subject of outcome studies.[25]

Elderly Patients

In certain hypertension subgroups such as the elderly, especially those with LV hypertrophy, comparative studies show better outcome data with the other agents such as diuretics[26] and the angiotensin receptor blocker (ARB) losartan.[27] One possible reason is that at equivalent brachial artery pressures, β-blockade reduces the central aortic pressure less than do other agents.[28]

Black Patients

In elderly blacks, atenolol was only marginally more antihypertensive than placebo.[29] Unexpectedly, in younger blacks (age younger than 60 years), atenolol was the second most effective agent, following diltiazem, and more effective than the diuretic hydrochlorothiazide.[29] Thus, although β-blockade is generally held to be relatively ineffective as monotherapy in black patients, this reservation may be largely restricted to those older than 60 years.

Diabetic Hypertensive Patients

In the 9-year UK study, strict blood pressure reduction to a mean blood pressure of 144/82 mmHg substantially reduced macrovascular end-points.[30] Therapy based on atenolol versus captopril showed no major differences or even trends, although individuals in the β-blocker group had gained weight and more often needed additional glucose-lowering treatment to control blood sugar.[31] In reality, to achieve the new low blood pressure goals set in diabetic persons, such as 130/

80 mmHg,[23] will usually require multiple drug therapy, often with a diuretic and a CCB besides a β-blocker and an ACE inhibitor.

Combination Antihypertensive Therapy

To reduce blood pressure, β-blockers may be combined with CCBs, α-blockers, centrally active agents, and cautiously with diuretics. Because β-blockers reduce renin levels, combination with ACE inhibitors or an ARB is not so logical. Increased new diabetes is a risk during β-blocker–thiazide cotherapy.[32] For example, the combination of atenolol with a diuretic led to more new diabetes than the combination of an ARB with the same diuretic dose.[33] The major "antidiabetic" strategy is limiting the diuretic dose. Much less well tested is the use of carvedilol, which may increase insulin sensitivity.[34] *Ziac* is bisoprolol (2.5 to 10 mg) with a very low dose of hydrochlorothiazide (6.25 mg). The FDA approved as first-line therapy for systemic hypertension a drug combination starting with 2.5 mg of bisoprolol plus 6.25 mg of thiazide, an approval never before given to a combination product. To get this approval, there had to be a demonstration that both low-dose components (the diuretic and the β-blocker) were themselves only marginally effective with a response rate at 12 weeks of below 30%, and that when added together the agents were more efficacious with a response rate of 60% or more, and with a demonstration that each component contributed to the blood pressure lowering effect of the combination.[35] The side effects of each type of drug, β-blocker and diuretic, are dose dependent and different in nature. It makes sense that the combined low doses of each type gave fewer side effects than the higher doses of each agent alone that would be required to decrease the blood pressure by the same amount. Thus, key points are that the metabolic side effects of higher thiazide doses were minimized and that the side effect profile of the combination differed little from placebo, with only a small increase in fatigue and dizziness. In Europe, several combinations of β-blocker plus low-dose diuretic are available (Tenoret 50, Secadrex, Lopresoretic), yet none with a diuretic dose as low as in Ziac. In the United States, Tenoretic and Lopressor HCT are combinations widely used, yet they often contain diuretic doses that are higher than desirable (e.g., chlorthalidone 25 mg; see Chapter 7). Combinations of such prodiabetic doses of diuretics with β-blockade, in itself a risk for new diabetes,[36] is clearly undesirable.

β-BLOCKERS FOR ARRHYTHMIAS

Mechanisms

β-Blockers have multiple antiarrhythmic mechanisms (Fig. 1-6), being effective against many supraventricular and ventricular arrhythmias. Basic studies show that they counter the arrhythmogenic effects of excess catecholamine stimulation by countering the proarrhythmic effects of increased cyclic AMP and calcium-dependent triggered arrhythmias.[37,38] Logically, β-blockers should be particularly effective in arrhythmias caused by increased adrenergic drive (early phase AMI, heart failure, pheochromocytoma, anxiety, anesthesia, postoperative states, and some exercise-related arrhythmias, as well as mitral valve prolapse) or by increased cardiac sensitivity to catecholamines (thyrotoxicosis). β-Blockade may help in the prophylaxis of *supraventricular tachycardias* (SVTs) by inhibiting the initiating atrial ectopic beats and in the treatment of SVT by slowing the AV node and lessening the ventricular response rate.

Increasing Evidence

Although β-blockers have long been regarded as effective agents for supraventricular tachycardias, it was only recently that their remark-

ANTI-ARRHYTHMIC EFFECTS OF β-BLOCKERS
Opie 2004

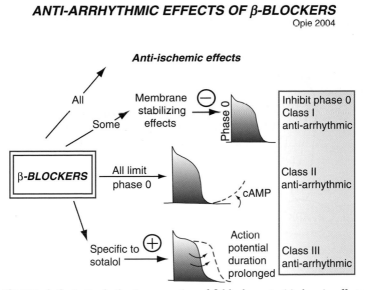

Figure 1-6 Antiarrhythmic properties of β-blockers. Anti-ischemic effects indirectly lessen arrhythmias. Note that only sotalol has added class III anti-arrhythmic effects. It is questionable whether the membrane stabilizing effects of propranolol confer additional antiarrhythmic properties. (*Figure © LH Opie, 2005.*)

able efficacy and safety as ventricular antiarrhythmics have come to be appreciated. Perhaps surprisingly, in sustained ventricular tachyarrhythmias the empirical use of metoprolol was as effective as electrophysiologically guided antiarrhythmic therapy.[39] Likewise, in ventricular tachyarrhythmias, the ESVEM study showed that sotalol, a β-blocker with added class III activity (Fig. 1-6), was more effective than a variety of class I antiarrhythmics.[40]

In *postinfarct patients*, β-blockers outperformed other antiarrhythmics[20] and decreased arrhythmic cardiac deaths.[41] In postinfarct patients with depressed LV function and ventricular arrhythmias, a retrospective analysis of data from the CAST study shows that β-blockade reduced all cause mortality and arrhythmia deaths.[42] Although the mechanism of benefit extends beyond antiarrhythmic protection,[43] it is very unlikely that β-blockers can match the striking results obtained with an implantable defibrillator (23% mortality reduction in class II and III heart failure).[43,44] As, however, amiodarone is ineffective[44] or only marginally effective (see Chapter 8, p. 239) in this patient group, β-blockade becomes the antiarrhythmic of choice.

In acute SVT, *the ultra-short–acting agent esmolol given intravenously* has challenged the previously standard use of verapamil or diltiazem in the perioperative period, although in the apparently healthy person with SVT, adenosine is still preferred (see Chapter 8). Intravenous esmolol may also be used acutely in atrial fibrillation or flutter to reduce the rapid ventricular response rate.

β-BLOCKERS IN CONGESTIVE HEART FAILURE

That β-blockers with their negative inotropic effects could increase cardiac contraction and decrease mortality in heart failure is certainly counterintuitive, especially bearing in mind that the β_1-receptor is downregulated (Fig. 1-7). Not only does the cardiac output increase, but in addition abnormal patterns of gene expression revert toward normal.[45] Several mechanisms are proposed.

EXCESS β-ADRENERGIC SIGNALS IN CHF
Opie 2004

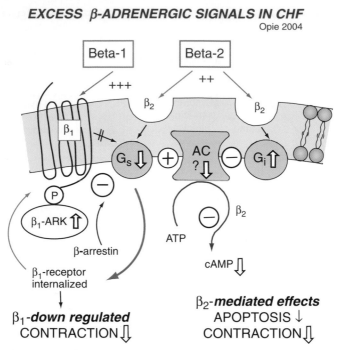

Figure 1-7 β-Adrenergic receptors in advanced heart failure. Down-regulation and uncoupling of β-adrenergic receptor signal systems result in depressed levels of cyclic AMP and decreased contractility, which may be viewed as an autoprotective from the adverse effects of cyclic AMP. Note: (1) $β_1$-receptor downregulation starts as a result of inhibitory $β_1$ARK-mediated phosphorylation; $β_1$ARK increases in response to excess $β_1$-adrenergic stimulation of the receptor; (2) β-receptor uncoupling from G_s due to β-arrestin activity; (3) $β_1$-receptor downregulation as a result of internalization; (4) increased G_i as a result of increased mRNA activity; (5) $β_2$-receptors are relatively upregulated and may hypothetically exert an inhibitory effect on apoptosis via enhanced G_i. (For details see LH Opie, Heart Physiology from Cell to Circulation. Lippincott Williams & Wilkins, Philadelphia, 2004:508.) (*Figure © LH Opie, 2005.*)

Mechanisms

1. *The hyperphosphorylation hypothesis.* The proposal is that continued excess adrenergic stimulation leads to overphosphorylation of the calcium-release channels (also known as the ryanodine receptor) on the sarcoplasmic reticulum (SR; Fig. 1-8). This causes defective functioning of these channels with excess calcium leak from the SR, with cytosolic calcium overload. Because the calcium pump that regulates calcium uptake into the SR is simultaneously down-regulated, the pattern of rise and fall of calcium ions in the cytosol is impaired, with poor contraction and delayed relaxation. These contractile and calcium abnormalities are reverted toward normal with β-blockade,[46,47] which also specifically normalizes the function of the calcium release channel.[48]

2. *Improved β-adrenergic signaling.* In advanced heart failure in humans, there is prominent downregulation of the $β_1$-adrenergic receptor and its signaling pathways with relative upregulation of the $β_2$- and $β_3$-receptors (Fig. 1-8). Prolonged excess stimulation of the $β_1$- leads to increased activity of βARK$_1$ (Fig. 1-7) that in turn phosphorylates and inhibits the $β_1$-receptors to decrease contractile activity.[49] Experimental $β_1$-blockade decreases the expression of βARK$_1$ and increases the activity of adenylyl cyclase, thereby improving contractile function. Relative upregulation of the $β_2$-receptor may have mixed effects (Fig. 1-7), including continued

HYPERPHOSPHORYLATION IN HF

Opie 2004

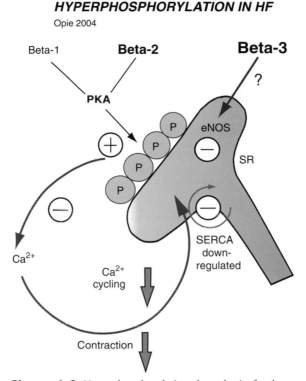

Figure 1-8 Hyperphosphorylation hypothesis for heart failure. Heart failure is a hyperadrenergic state. Excess β-stimulation acting via protein kinase A (*PKA*) hyperphosphorylates (*P*, example of phosphorylation site) the sarcoplasmic reticulum (*SR*), which causes a calcium leak and impaired cytosolic calcium cycling. β-Blockade, by lessening hyperphosphorylation, also lessens calcium leak from the SR, so that calcium stores in the SR improve and calcium release from the SR augments. Calcium uptake by the SERCA (sarcoendoplasmic reticulum calcium-ATPase) uptake pump may also improve. Note downregulated $β_1$-receptors, relative upregulation of $β_2$-receptors, and marked upregulation of inhibitory $β_3$-receptors. *eNOS* = endothelial nitric oxide synthase. (For details see LH Opie, Heart Physiology from Cell to Circulation. Lippincott Williams & Wilkins, Philadelphia, 2004:508.) (*Figure © LH Opie, 2005.*)

excess formation of hyperphosphorylated SR (Fig. 1-8). Upregulation of the $β_3$-receptor exerts a negative inotropic effect by increased formation of inhibitory nitric oxide in the SR.[3] It is speculated that a nonselective agent such as carvedilol restrains the excess activity of the $β_3$-receptor to exert an indirect inotropic effect.

3. *Protection from catecholamine myocyte toxicity.* The circulating concentrations of norepinephrine found in severe heart failure are high enough to be directly toxic to the myocardium,[5] experimentally damaging the membranes and promoting subcellular destruction, acting at least in part through cytosolic calcium overload.[50]

4. *Antiarrhythmic effects.* In experimental heart failure, ventricular arrhythmias are promoted via increased formation of cyclic AMP and calcium-mediated afterpotentials.[38]

5. *Bradycardia.* β-Blockade may act at least in part by reduction of the heart rate.[51,52] Metoprolol and carvedilol both reduce the heart rate by 8 to 10 beats per minute.[53,54] Bradycardia may improve coronary blood flow and decrease the myocardial oxygen demand. Experimentally, long-term heart rate reduction lessens extracellular matrix collagen, in addition to improving the LV ejection fraction.[55]

6. *Antiapoptosis.* Coupling of the β_2-receptor to the inhibitory G-protein, G_i, may be antiapoptotic.[56] Unexpectedly, even a combined β_1- and β_2-blocker can stimulate the β_2-receptor via inverse agonism.[2]

7. *Renin-angiotensin inhibition.* When added to prior ACE inhibitor or angiotensin receptor blocker therapy, β-blockade by metoprolol lessens circulating renin and angiotensin-II levels, thereby increasing the blockade of the renin-angiotensin system.[53]

How to Apply β-Blockers in Heart Failure

β-Blockers are now recognized as an integral part of therapy for heart failure; their mechanism of action is based on the principles of antagonism of the neurohumoral response.[57] They benefit a wide range of patients, including females, diabetic individuals, and (in several studies) black patients.[58] The following principles apply: (1) start slowly and uptitrate gradually (Table 1-2), watching for adverse effects and if necessary cutting back on the dose or titrating more slowly; (2) add β-blockade only to existing therapy including ACE inhibition and diuretics, and (in some studies) digoxin, when the patient is hemodynamically stable and ideally not in class IV or severe class III; (3) never stop the β-blocker abruptly (risk of ischemia and infarction); and (4) use only β-blockers whose doses are well understood and clearly delineated, and with proven benefit, notably carvedilol, metoprolol, and bisoprolol (Table 1-2). Of these, only carvedilol and long-acting metoprolol are approved in the United States. In large trials all three drugs have *reduced mortality* by about one third.[5] In the COMET trial,[54] carvedilol reduced mortality more than metoprolol (for assessment see Chapter 6, p. 178). The initiation of β-blockade is a slow process that requires careful supervision and may temporarily worsen the heart failure, so that we strongly advise that only the proven β-blockers should be used in the exact dose regimens that have been tested (Table 1-2). Propranolol, the original gold standard β-blocker, and atenolol, two commonly used agents, have not been well studied in heart failure.

OTHER CARDIAC INDICATIONS

In *hypertrophic obstructive cardiomyopathy*, high-dose propranolol is standard therapy, although verapamil and disopyramide are effective alternatives.

In *mitral stenosis with sinus rhythm*, β-blockade benefits by decreasing resting and exercise heart rates, thereby allowing longer diastolic filling and improved exercise tolerance. In mitral stenosis with chronic atrial fibrillation, β-blockade may have to be added to digoxin to

Table 1-2	Heart Failure: A New Indication for β-Blockade. Titration and Doses of Drugs			
β-Blocker	First Dose	Week 3	Week 5–6	Final Dose
Carvedilol	3.125	6.25×2	12.5×2	25×2
Metoprolol SR	25*	50	100	200
Bisoprolol	1.25	3.75	5.0	10.0

All daily doses are in milligrams. Data from placebo-controlled large trials, adapted from McMurray, Heart, 1999, 82 (Suppl IV), 14–22. Forced titration in all studies, assuming preceding dose tolerated. Dose once daily for metoprolol and bisoprolol and twice daily for carvedilol. Carvedilol doses from US package insert doses, taken with food to slow absorption; target dose may be increased to 50 mg bid for patients >85 kg. *Slow release metoprolol (CR/XL formulation); reduce initial dose to 12.5 mg in severe heart failure.

obtain sufficient ventricular slowing during exercise. Occasionally β-blockers, verapamil, and digoxin are all combined. Heart block is a risk during cotherapy of β-blockers with verapamil.

In mitral valve prolapse, β-blockade is the standard procedure for control of associated arrhythmias.

In dissecting aneurysms, in the hyperacute phase, intravenous propranolol has been standard, although it could be replaced by esmolol. Thereafter oral β-blockade is continued.

In Marfan's syndrome with aortic root involvement, β-blockade is likewise used against aortic dilation and possible dissection.

In neurocardiogenic syncope, β-blockade helps to control the episodic adrenergic reflex discharge believed to contribute to symptoms.

In Fallot's tetralogy, 2 mg/kg of propranolol twice daily is usually effective against the cyanotic spells, probably acting by inhibition of right ventricular contractility.

In congenital QT-prolongation, β-blockade is standard therapy,[59] perhaps acting to restore an imbalance between left and right stellate ganglia.

NONCARDIAC INDICATIONS FOR β-BLOCKADE

Vascular and Noncardiac Surgery

β-Blockade exerts an important protective effect in selected patients. Perioperative death from cardiac causes and myocardial infarction were reduced by bisoprolol in high-risk patients undergoing vascular surgery.[60] For noncardiac surgery, "we believe that beta-blockade should be given to all patients (unless contraindicated) at high risk for coronary events."[61]

Thyrotoxicosis

Together with antithyroid drugs or radioiodine, or as the sole agent before surgery, β-blockade is commonly used in thyrotoxicosis to control symptoms, although the hypermetabolic state is not decreased. β-Blockade controls tachycardia, palpitations, tremor, and nervousness and reduces the vascularity of the thyroid gland, thereby facilitating operation. In thyroid storm, intravenous propranolol can be given at a rate of 1 mg/minute (to a total of 5 mg at a time); circulatory collapse is a risk, so that β-blockade should be used in thyroid storm only if LV function is normal as shown by conventional noninvasive tests.

Anxiety States

Although propranolol is most widely used in anxiety (and is licensed for this purpose in several countries, including the United States), probably all β-blockers are effective, acting not centrally but by a reduction of peripheral manifestations of anxiety such as tremor and tachycardia.

Glaucoma

The use of local β-blocker eye solutions is now established for open-angle glaucoma; care needs to be exerted with occasional systemic side effects such as sexual dysfunction, bronchospasm, and cardiac depression. Among the agents approved for treatment of glaucoma in the United States are the nonselective agents timolol (Timoptic), carteolol, levobunolol, and metipranolol. The cardioselective betaxolol may be an advantage in avoiding side effects in patients with bronchospasm.

Migraine

Propranolol (80 to 240 mg daily, licensed in the United States) acts prophylactically to reduce the incidence of migraine attacks in 60% of patients. The mechanism presumably involves beneficial vaso-constriction. The antimigraine effect is prophylactic and not for attacks once they have occurred. If there is no benefit within 4 to 6 weeks, the drug should be discontinued.

PHARMACOLOGIC PROPERTIES OF VARIOUS β-BLOCKERS

β-Blocker Generations

First-generation agents, such as propranolol, nonselectively block all the β-receptors (both $β_1$ and $β_2$). Second-generation agents, such as atenolol, metoprolol, acebutolol, bisoprolol, and others, have relative selectivity when given in low doses for the $β_1$ (largely cardiac) receptors (Fig. 1-9). Third-generation agents have added vasodilatory properties (Fig. 1-10), acting chiefly through two mechanisms: (1) direct vasodilation, possibly mediated by release of nitric oxide as for nebivolol and for carvedilol[62]; and (2) added α-adrenergic blockade as in labetalol and carvedilol. A third vasodilatory mechanism, as in pindolol and acebutolol, acts via $β_2$-intrinsic sympathomimetic activity (ISA), which stimulates arterioles to relax; however, these agents are used less often at present and do not neatly fit into the division of the three generations. Acebutolol is a cardioselective agent with less ISA than pindolol that was very well tolerated in a 4-year antihypertensive study.[63]

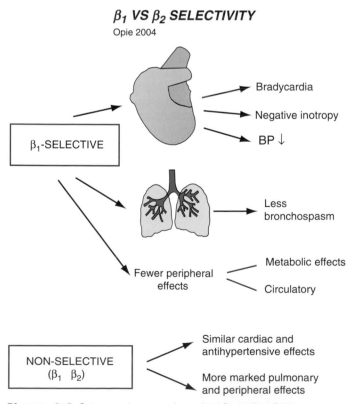

$β_1$ VS $β_2$ SELECTIVITY
Opie 2004

Bradycardia

Negative inotropy

BP ↓

$β_1$-SELECTIVE

Less bronchospasm

Metabolic effects

Fewer peripheral effects

Circulatory

NON-SELECTIVE ($β_1$ $β_2$)

Similar cardiac and antihypertensive effects

More marked pulmonary and peripheral effects

Figure 1-9 β-Antagonists may be either $β_1$-cardioselective or non-cardioselective ($β_1$-$β_2$ antagonism). In general, note several advantages of cardioselective β-blockers. Cardioselectivity is greatest at low drug doses. (*Figure © LH Opie, 2005.*)

VASODILATORY β-BLOCKERS

Opie 2004

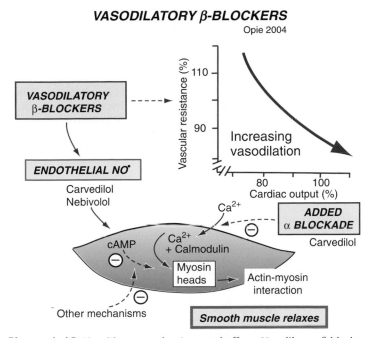

Figure 1-10 Vasodilatory mechanisms and effects. Vasodilatory β-blockers tend to decrease the cardiac output less as the systemic vascular resistance falls. Vasodilatory mechanisms include α-blockade (carvedilol), nonspecific mechanisms, and intrinsic sympathomimetic activity (*ISA*). ISA, as in pindolol, has a specific effect in increasing sympathetic tone when it is low, as at night, and increasing nocturnal heart rate, which might be disadvantageous in nocturnal angina or unstable angina   (*Figure © LH Opie, 2005.*)

Other marked differences between β-blockers lie in the pharmacokinetic properties, with half-lives varying from about 10 minutes (esmolol) to more than 30 hours, and in differing lipid or water solubility. Hence the side effects may vary from agent to agent. Nonetheless, there is no evidence that any of these ancillary properties has any compelling therapeutic advantage, although for the individual patient the art of minimizing β-blocker side effects may be of great importance. For example, a patient with chronic obstructive airways disease needs a cardioselective agent, whereas a patient with early morning angina may need an ultra-long–acting β-blocker. Likewise, a patient with cold extremities might benefit from a vasodilatory agent.

Nonselective Agents (Combined β₁-β₂-Blockers)

The prototype β-blocker is propranolol, which worldwide is still used more than any other agent and is a World Health Organization (WHO) essential drug. By blocking β₁-receptors it affects heart rate, conduction, and contractility, yet by blocking β₂-receptors it tends to cause smooth muscle contraction with risk of bronchospasm in predisposed individuals. This same quality might, however, explain the benefit in migraine when vasoconstriction could inhibit the attack. Among the nonselective blockers, nadolol and sotalol are much longer acting and are also lipid insoluble.

Cardioselective Agents (β₁-Selectivity)

Cardioselective agents (acebutolol, atenolol, betaxolol, bisoprolol, celiprolol, and metoprolol) are as antihypertensive as the nonselective ones (Fig. 1-9). Selective agents are preferable in patients with chronic lung disease or chronic smoking, and insulin-requiring diabetes mellitus. Cardioselectivity varies between agents, but is always greater at lower doses. Bisoprolol is among the most selective. Cardioselectivity declines or is lost at high doses. No β-blocker is completely safe in the presence of asthma; low-dose cardioselective agents can be used with care in patients with bronchospasm or chronic lung disease or chronic smoking. In angina and hypertension, cardioselective agents are just as effective as noncardioselective agents. In acute myocardial infarction (AMI) complicated by stress-induced hypokalemia, nonselective β-blockers theoretically should be better antiarrhythmics than β_1-selective blockers.

Antiarrhythmic β-Blockers

All β-blockers are potentially antiarrhythmic by virtue of class II activity (Fig. 1-6). Propranolol and some others have, in addition, a quinidine-like quality called membrane stabilizing activity (MSA), that is to say class I activity. Such experimental activity is not clinically relevant except in cases of overdose when MSA contributes to fatality. Sotalol is a unique β-blocker with prominent added class III antiarrhythmic activity (Fig. 1-6; see Chapter 8).

PHARMACOKINETIC PROPERTIES OF β-BLOCKERS
Plasma Half-Lives

Esmolol, given intravenously, has the shortest of all half-lives, at only 9 minutes. Esmolol may therefore be preferable in unstable angina and threatened infarction when hemodynamic changes may call for withdrawal of β-blockade. The half-life of propranolol (Table 1-3) is only 3 hours, but continued administration saturates the hepatic process that removes propranolol from the circulation; the active metabolite 4-hydroxypropranolol is formed, and the effective half-life then becomes longer. The biological half-life of propranolol and metoprolol (and that of all other β-blockers) exceeds the plasma half-life considerably, so that twice daily dosage of standard propranolol is effective even in angina pectoris. Clearly, the higher the dose of any β-blocker, the longer the biologic effects. Longer-acting compounds such as nadolol, sotalol, atenolol, and slow-release propranolol (Inderal-LA) or extended-release metoprolol (Toprol-XL) should be better for hypertension and effort angina.

Protein Binding

Propranolol is highly bound, as are pindolol, labetalol, and biso-prolol. Hypoproteinemia calls for lower doses of such compounds.

First-Pass Liver Metabolism

This is found especially with the highly lipid-soluble compounds, such as propranolol, labetalol, and oxprenolol. Acebutolol, metoprolol, and timolol have only modest lipid solubility, yet with hepatic clearance; first-pass metabolism varies greatly among patients and alters the dose required. In liver disease or low-output states the dose should be decreased. First-pass metabolism produces active metabolites with, in the case of propranolol, properties different from those of the parent compound. Acebutolol produces large amounts of diacetolol, also cardioselective with intrinsic sympathomimetic activity, but with a longer half-life and chiefly excreted by the kidneys (Fig. 1-11).

ROUTE OF ELIMINATION
Opie 2004

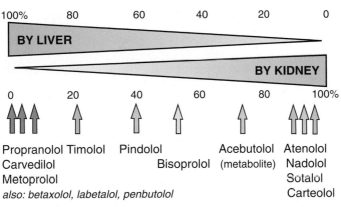

Figure 1-11 Comparative routes of elimination of β-blockers. Those most hydrophilic and least lipid-soluble are excreted unchanged by the kidneys. Those most lipophilic and least water-soluble are largely metabolized by the liver. Note that the metabolite of acebutolol, diacetolol, is largely excreted by the kidney, in contrast to the parent compound. (For derivation of data in figure, see the 3rd edition. Estimated data points for acebutolol and newer agents added). (Figure © LH Opie, 2005.)

Ideal Kinetics

Lipid-insoluble hydrophilic compounds (atenolol, sotalol, nadolol) are excreted only by the kidneys (Fig. 1-11) and have low brain penetration. In patients with renal or liver disease, the simpler pharmacokinetic patterns of lipid-insoluble agents make dosage easier. As a group, these agents have low protein binding (Table 1-3).

Drug Interactions with β-Blockers

Pharmacodynamic interactions can be predicted and occur in combinations of β-blockers with other drugs depressing the SA or AV nodes, or with other negative inotropic agents (Fig. 1-3). Pharmacokinetic interactions are chiefly at the level of the liver. Cimetidine reduces hepatic blood flow and increases blood levels of β-blockers highly metabolized by the liver, especially propranol. Verapamil inhibits the hepatic breakdown of metoprolol and propranolol, and possibly other β-blockers metabolized by the liver. To avoid such hepatic interactions, it is simpler to use those β-blockers not metabolized by the liver (Fig. 1-11). β-Blockers, in turn, depress hepatic blood flow so that the blood levels of lidocaine increase with greater risk of lidocaine toxicity.

CONCOMITANT DISEASES AND CHOICE OF β-BLOCKER

Respiratory Disease

Cardioselective $β_1$-blockers in low doses are best for patients with reversible bronchospasm. In patients with a history of asthma, no β-blocker can be considered safe.

Associated Cardiovascular Disease

In patients with *sick sinus syndrome*, pure β-blockade can be dangerous. Added ISA may be best. In patients with *Raynaud's phenomenon*, propranolol with its peripheral vasoconstrictive effects is best avoided. In active *peripheral vascular disease*, β-blockers are generally contraindicated, although the evidence is not firm.

Table 1-3 Properties of Various β-Adrenoceptor Antagonist Agents, Nonselective Versus Cardioselective and Vasodilatory Agents

Generic Name (Trade Name)	Extra Mechanism	Plasma Half-Life (h)	Lipid Solubility*	First-Pass Effect	Loss by Liver or Kidney	Plasma Protein Binding (%)	Usual Dose for Angina (Other Indications)	Usual Doses As Sole Therapy for Mild/Moderate Hypertension	Intravenous Dose (as Licensed in USA)
Noncardioselective									
Propranolol†‡ (Inderal)	—	1–6	+++	++	Liver	90	80 mg 2× daily usually adequate (may give 160 mg 2×)	Start with 10–40 mg 2× daily. Mean 160–320 mg/day, 1–2 doses	1–6 mg
(Inderal-LA)	—	8–11	+++	++	Liver	90	80–320 mg 1× daily (Not evaluated)	80–320 mg 1× daily	—
Carteolol† (Cartrol)	ISA +	5–6	0/+	0	Kidney	20–30	—	2.5–10 mg single dose	—
Nadolol†‡ (Corgard)	—	20–24	0	0	Kidney	30	40–80 mg 1× daily; up to 240 mg	40–80 mg/day 1× daily; up to 320 mg	—
Penbutolol (Levatol)	ISA +	20–25	+++	++	Liver	98	(Not studied)	10–20 mg daily	—
Sotalol§ (Betapace; Betapace AF)	—	7–18 (mean 12)	0	0	Kidney	5	(80–240 mg 2× daily in two doses for serious ventricular arrhythmias; up to 160 mg 2× daily for atrial fib, flutter)	80–320 mg/day; mean 190 mg	—
Timolol† (Blocadren)	—	4–5	+	+	L, K	60	(post-AMI 10 mg 2× daily)	10–20 mg 2× daily	—
Cardioselective									
Acebutolol* (Sectral)	ISA ++	8–13 (Diacetolol)	0 (Diacetolol)	++	L, K	15	(400–1200 mg/day in 2 doses for PVC)	400–1200 mg/day; can be given as a single dose	—

Drug		t½ (h)	*		Elimination	%	Dose in heart failure	Dose in hypertension	IV dose
Atenolol (Tenormin)†‡	—	6–7	0	0	Kidney	10	50–200 mg 1× daily	50–100 mg/day 1× daily	5 mg over 5 min; repeat 5 min later
Betaxolol (Kerlone)†	—	14–22	++	++	L, then K	50	—	10–20 mg 1× daily	—
Bisoprolol (Zebeta)†	—	9–12	+	0	L, K	30	10 mg 1× daily (not licensed in USA) (HF; see Table 1-2)	2.5–40 mg 1× daily (see also Ziac, p. 12)	—
Metoprolol (Lopressor)†‡	—	3–7	+	++	Liver	12	50–200 mg 2× daily (HF; see Table 1-2)	50–400 mg/day in 1 or 2 doses	5 mg 3× at 2 min intervals
Vasodilatory β-Blockers, Nonselective									
Labetalol (Trandate) (Normodyne)†	—	6–8	+++	++	L, some K	90	As for hypertension	300–600 mg/day in 3 doses; top dose 2400 mg/day	Up to 2 mg/min, up to 300 mg for severe HT
Pindolol (Visken)†	ISA +++	4	+	+	L, K	55	2.5–7.5 mg 3X daily (In UK, not USA)	5–30 mg/day 2× daily	—
Carvedilol (Coreg)†	β₁,β₂ α-block	6	+	++	Liver	95	(USA, UK license for heart failure, up to 25 mg 2× daily)	12.5–25 mg 2× daily	—
Vasodilatory β-Blockers, Selective									
Nebivolol (not licensed in USA; Nebilet in UK)	NO-vasodilation	10 (24 h, metabolites)	+++ (Genetic variation)	+++	L, K	98	Under investigation	5 mg once daily. 2.5 mg in renal disease or elderly	—

*Octanol-water distribution coefficient (pH 7.4, 37°C) where 0 = <0.5; + = 0.5–2 0; ++ = 2–10; ++ = >10.

†Approved by FDA for hypertension.

‡Approved by FDA for angina pectoris.

§Approved for life-threatening ventricular tachyarrhythmias.

fib = fibrillation; HT = hypertension; ISA = intrinsic sympathomimetic activity; K = kidney; L = liver; NO = nitric oxide; PVC = premature ventricular contractions.

Renal Disease

Ultimately β-blockers are usually excreted by the kidneys, so that in renal failure the dose may have to be altered, especially in the case of water-soluble agents excreted by the kidneys (atenolol, acebutolol, nadolol, sotalol) or agents partially excreted such as bisoprolol. In general, agents highly metabolized by the liver can be given in an unchanged dose.

Diabetes Mellitus

In diabetes mellitus, the risk of β-blockade in insulin-requiring diabetic individuals is that the symptoms of hypoglycemia might be masked. There is a lesser risk with the cardioselective agents. In persons with type 2 diabetes with hypertension, initial β-blocker therapy by atenolol was as effective as the ACE inhibitor captopril in reducing macrovascular end-points.[31] Whether *diabetic nephropathy* benefits as much from treatment with β-blockade is not clear. ARBs and ACE inhibitors have now been established as agents of first choice in diabetic nephropathy (see Chapter 5).

Those at Risk of New Diabetes

The β-blocker–diuretic combination poses a risk that should be lessened by using a truly low dose of the diuretic or by using another combination.

SIDE EFFECTS OF β-BLOCKERS

The *three major mechanisms for β-blocker side effects* are: (1) smooth muscle spasm (bronchospasm and cold extremities); (2) exaggeration of the cardiac therapeutic actions (bradycardia, heart block, excess negative inotropic effect); and (3) central nervous penetration (insomnia, depression). The *mechanism of fatigue* is not clear. When compared with propranolol, however, it is reduced by use of either a cardioselective β-blocker or a vasodilatory agent, so that both central and peripheral hemodynamic effects may be involved. When patients are appropriately selected, double-blind studies show few differences in side-effects between a cardioselective agent such as atenolol and placebo. This may be because atenolol is not lipid soluble and should have lesser effects on bronchial and vascular smooth muscle than propranolol. When *propranolol* is given for hypertension, the rate of serious side effects (bronchospasm, cold extremities, worsening of claudication) leading to withdrawal of therapy is about 10%.[64] The rate of withdrawal with atenolol is considerably lower (about 2%), but when it comes to dose-limiting side effects, both agents can cause cold extremities, fatigue, vivid dreams, worsening claudication, and bronchospasm. Increasing heart failure remains a potential hazard when β-blockade therapy is abruptly started at normal doses in a susceptible patient and not tailored in.

Central Nervous System (CNS) Side Effects

An attractive hypothesis is that the lipid-soluble β-blockers (epitomized by propranolol) with their high brain penetration are more likely to cause CNS side effects. An extremely detailed comparison of propranolol and atenolol showed that the latter, which is not lipid soluble, causes far fewer CNS side effects than does propranolol.[65] On the other hand, the lipid-solubility hypothesis does not explain why metoprolol, which is moderately lipid soluble, appears to interfere less with some complex psychological functions than does atenolol and may even enhance certain aspects of psychological performance.[66]

Quality of Life and Sex Life

In the first quality of life study reported in patients with hypertension, propranolol induced considerably more CNS effects than did the ACE inhibitor captopril.[67] Atenolol, with its far fewer CNS side effects, compares favorably with the ACE inhibitor enalapril.[68] It now appears that a variety of β-blockers, often with different fundamental properties, all leave the quality of life largely intact in hypertensive individuals. However, there are a number of negatives. First, *weight gain* is undesirable and contrary to the lifestyle pattern required to limit cardiovascular diseases including the metabolic syndrome and hypertension. Second, β-blockade may precipitate *diabetes*,[36] a disease that severely limits the quality of life. Third, during *exercise*, β-blockade reduces the total work possible by about 15% and increases the sense of fatigue. Vasodilatory β-blockers may be an exception. *Impotence* is a frequent complaint of aging men receiving β-blockade therapy. Problems with erection may take place in 11% of patients given a β-blocker, compared with 26% with a diuretic and 3% with placebo.[69] ACE inhibitors or ARBs give a better sex life.[70]

CONTRAINDICATIONS TO β-BLOCKADE

The absolute contraindications to β-blockade can be deduced from the profile of pharmacologic effects and side effects (Table 1-4). Cardiac absolute contraindications include severe bradycardia, preexisting high-degree heart block, sick sinus syndrome, and overt left ventricular failure unless already conventionally treated and stable (Fig. 1-12). Pulmonary contraindications are overt asthma or severe bronchospasm; depending on the severity of the disease and the cardioselectivity of the β-blocker used, these may be absolute or relative contraindications. The CNS contraindication is severe depression (especially for propranolol). Active peripheral vascular disease with rest ischemia is another contraindication.

OVERDOSE OF β-BLOCKERS

Bradycardia may be countered by 1 to 2 mg of intravenous atropine; if serious, temporary transvenous pacing may be required. When an

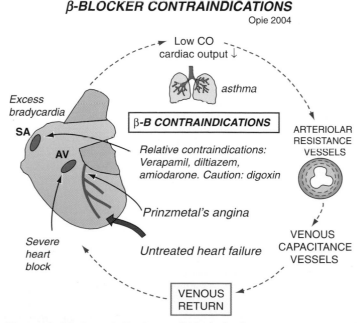

β-BLOCKER CONTRAINDICATIONS
Opie 2004

Figure 1-12 Contraindications to β-blockade. (*Figure © LH Opie, 2005.*)

Table 1-4 β-Blockade: Contraindications and Cautions

(NOTE: *Cautions may be overridden by the imperative to treat, as in postinfarct patients*)

Cardiac

Absolute: Severe bradycardia, high-degree heart block, cardiogenic shock, overt untreated left ventricular failure (versus major use in stabilized heart failure already conventionally treated)
Relative: Prinzmetal's angina (unopposed α-spasm), high doses of other agents depressing SA or AV nodes (verapamil, diltiazem, digoxin, antiarrhythmic agents); in angina, *avoid sudden withdrawal*, danger in unreliable patient.

Pulmonary

Absolute: Severe asthma or bronchospasm. *No patient* may be given a β-blocker without questions for past or present asthma. Fatalities have resulted when this rule was ignored.
Relative: Mild asthma or bronchospasm or chronic airways disease. Use agents with cardioselectivity plus $β_2$-stimulants (by inhalation).

Central Nervous System

Absolute: Severe depression (avoid propranolol).
Relative: Vivid dreams: avoid highly lipid-soluble agents (Fig. 1-11) and pindolol; avoid evening dose. Visual hallucinations: change from propranolol. Fatigue (all agents). If low cardiac output is cause of fatigue, try vasodilatory β-blockers. Impotence: may occur (check for diuretic use; consider change to ACE inhbitor/ARB). Psychotropic drugs (with adrenergic augmentation) may adversely interact with β-blockers.

Peripheral Vascular, Raynaud's Phenomenon

Absolute: Active disease: gangrene, skin necrosis, severe or worsening claudication, rest pain.
Relative: Cold extremities, absent pulses, Raynaud's phenomenon. Avoid nonselective agents (propranolol, sotalol, nadolol); prefer vasodilatory agents.

Diabetes Mellitus

Relative: Insulin-requiring diabetes: nonselective agents decrease reaction to hypoglycemia; use selective agents. Note successful use of atenolol in type 2 diabetes in prolonged UK trial.

Metabolic Syndrome

β-Blockers may increase blood sugar by 1.0–1.5 mmol/L and impair insulin sensitivity especially with diuretic cotherapy; adjust control accordingly or avoid combination.
Renal Failure
Relative: As renal blood flow falls, reduce doses of agents eliminated by kidney (Fig. 1-11).

Liver Disease

Relative: Avoid agents with high hepatic clearance (propranolol, carvedilol, timolol, acebutolol, metoprolol). Use agents with low clearance (atenolol, nadolol, sotalol). See Figure 1-11. If plasma proteins low, reduce dose of highly bound agents (propranolol, pindolol, bisoprolol).

Pregnancy Hypertension

β-Blockade increasingly used but may depress vital signs in neonate and cause uterine vasoconstriction. Labetalol and atenolol best tested. Preferred drug: methyldopa.

Surgical Operations

β-Blockade may be maintained throughout, provided indication is not trivial; otherwise stop 24 to 48 hours beforehand. May protect against anesthetic arrhythmias and perioperative ischemia. Preferred intravenous drug: esmolol. Use atropine for bradycardia, β-agonist for severe hypotension.

Table continued on opposite page

Table 1-4 β-Blockade: Contraindications and Cautions—*Continued*

Age

β-Blockade often helps to reduce blood pressure, but lacks positive outcome data and may harm versus comparator ARB as in LIFE study.* Watch pharmacokinetics and side effects in all elderly patients.

Smoking

In hypertension, β-blockade is less effective in reducing coronary events in smoking men.

Hyperlipidemia

β-Blockers may have unfavorable effects on the blood lipid profile, especially nonselective agents. Triglycerides increase and HDL-cholesterol falls. Clinical significance unknown, but may worsen metabolic syndrome. Vasodilatory agents, with intrinsic sympathomimetic activity or α-blocking activity, may have mildly favorable effects.

ARB = angiotensin receptor blocker; AV = atrioventricular; SA = sinoatrial.
*Kjeldsen SE, et al. For the LIFE Study Group. Effects of losartan on cardiovascular morbidity and mortality in patients with isolated systolic hypertension and left ventricular hypertrophy. *JAMA* 2002;288:1491–1498.

infusion is required, glucagon (2.5 to 7.5 mg/hour) is the drug of choice, because it stimulates formation of cyclic AMP by bypassing the occupied β-receptor. Logically an infusion of a phosphodiesterase (PDE) inhibitor, such as amrinone or milrinone, should help cyclic AMP to accumulate. Alternatively, dobutamine is given in doses high enough to overcome the competitive β-blockade (15 μg/kg/minute). In patients without ischemic heart disease, an infusion (up to 0.10 μg/kg/minute) of isoproterenol may be used.

SPECIFIC β-BLOCKERS

Of the large number of β-blockers, the ideal agent for hypertension or angina might have (1) advantageous pharmacokinetics (lipid insolubility); (2) a high degree of cardioselectivity; and (3) long duration of action. Vasodilatory properties should be of benefit in the treatment of hypertension in the elderly, but might be a disadvantage in the treatment of certain types of angina when the heart rate must be as slow as possible.

Propranolol (Inderal) is the historical gold standard because it is licensed for so many different indications, including angina, acute stage myocardial infarction, postinfarct follow-up, hypertension, arrhythmias, migraine prophylaxis, anxiety states, and essential tremor. However, propranolol is not $β_1$ selective. Being lipid-soluble, it has a high brain penetration and undergoes extensive hepatic first-pass metabolism. CNS side effects may explain its poor performance in quality-of-life studies. Propranolol also has a short half-life so that it must be given twice daily unless long-acting preparations are used. The chief of the other agents are dealt with alphabetically.

Acebutolol (Sectral) is the cardioselective agent with intrinsic sympathomimetic activity that gave a good quality of life in the 4-year TOMH study in mild hypertension. In particular, the incidence of impotence was not increased.[71]

Atenolol (Tenormin) was one of the first of the cardioselective agents and now in generic form is one of the most widely used drugs in angina, in postinfarct protection, and in hypertension. Its pharmacokinetic advantages include lipid-insolubility and a relatively long half-life. There are very few trials with outcome data for atenolol in these conditions with two exceptions, the ASIST study in silent ischemia[10] and when compared with verapamil in hypertensive individuals with coronary artery disease.[72] In the British Medical Research Council trial of hypertension in the elderly, atenolol did not reduce coronary events.[73] More recently, atenolol was inferior to the ARB losartan in the therapy of hypertensive patients with LVH.[74] Although atenolol is also widely used in postinfarct protection, there are in fact no randomized controlled trials to show that it works over a period longer than a few weeks.

Bisoprolol *(Zebeta in the United States, Cardicor or Emcor in the United Kingdom)* is a highly β₁-selective agent, more so than atenolol, licensed for hypertension and angina heart failure in the United Kingdom but only for hypertension in the United States. It was the drug used in the large and successful CIBIS-2 study in heart failure, in which there was a large reduction not only in total mortality but also in sudden death.[52] A combination of low-dose bisoprolol and low-dose hydrochlorothiazide (Ziac) is available in the Unites States (see Combination Therapy). The proposal is that antihypertensive efficacy can be reached at doses that cause few or no side effects.

Carvedilol *(Coreg in the United States, Eucardic in the United Kingdom)* is a nonselective β-blocker with antioxidant and α-mediated vasodilatory properties that has been extensively studied in CHF[54] and in postinfarct LV dysfunction.[17] In the United States, it is registered for hypertension, for CHF (mild to severe), and for post-MI LV dysfunction (ejection fraction ≤40%), but not for angina.

Celiprolol *(Celectol in the United Kingdom, not in the United States)* is a highly cardioselective β-blocker with low lipid solubility and a half-life similar to that of atenolol.

Labetalol *(Trandate, Normodyne)* is a combined α- and β-blocking antihypertensive agent that has now largely been supplanted by carvedilol.

Metoprolol *(Toprol-XL)* is cardioselective and particularly well studied in acute myocardial infarction and in postinfarct protection. Toprol-XL is approved in the United States for stable symptomatic class II or III heart failure.[75] It is also registered for hypertension and angina. *Lopressor, shorter acting,* is licensed for angina and myocardial infarction.

Nadolol *(Corgard)* is very long acting and water soluble, although nonselective. It is particularly useful when prolonged antianginal activity is required.

Nebivolol *(Nebilet in the United Kingdom, not licensed in the United States)* is a highly cardioselective agent with peripheral vasodilating properties mediated by nitric oxide. Hepatic metabolites probably account for the vasodilation[76] and the long biological half-life.[77] Nebivolol reverses endothelial dysfunction in hypertension.[78]

Penbutolol *(Levatol)*. This agent has modest ISA, similar to acebutolol, but is nonselective. It is highly lipid soluble and liver metabolized.

Sotalol *(Betapace, Betapace AF)* is a unique nonselective β-blocker that has class III antiarrhythmic activity. It is licensed for life-threatening ventricular arrhythmias as Betapace, and now also as Betapace AF for maintenance of sinus rhythm in patients with symptomatic atrial fibrillation or atrial flutter. Sotalol is a water-soluble drug, excreted only by the kidneys, so that Betapace AF is contraindicated in patients with a creatinine clearance of less than 40 ml/minute.

Timolol *(Blocarden)* was the first β-blocker shown to give postinfarct protection and it is one of the few licensed for this purpose in the United States. Other approved uses are for hypertension and in migraine prophylaxis.

ULTRA-SHORT–ACTING INTRAVENOUS β-BLOCKADE

Esmolol (Brevibloc) is an ultra-short–acting β₁-blocker with a half-life of 9 minutes, rapidly converting to inactive metabolites by blood esterases. Full recovery from β-blockade occurs within 30 minutes in patients with a normal cardiovascular system. *Indications* are situations in which on/off control of β-blockade is desired, as in supraventricular tachycardia in the peri-operative period, or sinus tachycardia (noncompensatory), or emergency hypertension in the perioperative period (all registered uses in the United States). Other logical indications are for emergency hypertension in other situations where pheochromocytoma is excluded, or in unstable angina.[79] *Doses* are as follows. For *supraventricular tachycardia*, a loading dose of 500 μg/kg/minute is given over 1 minute, followed by a 4-minute infusion of 50 μg/kg/minute (USA package insert). If this fails, repeat loading dose and increase infusion to 100 μg/kg/minute again over 4 minutes. If this fails, repeat loading dose and then infuse at rates up to 300 μg/kg/minute. Thereafter, to maintain control, infuse at adjusted rate for up to 24 hours. For *perioperative hypertension*, give 80 mg (about 1 mg/kg) over 30 seconds and infuse at 150 to 300 μg/kg/minute if needed. For more gradual control of blood pressure, follow the routine for supraventricular tachycardia. Higher doses are usually required for blood pressure control than for arrhythmias. Once the emergency is over, replace by conventional antiarrhythmic or antihypertensive drugs. *Cautions* include extravasation of the acid solution with risk of skin necrosis.

SUMMARY

1. *β-Blockers come closest among all cardiovascular agents to providing all-purpose therapy.* Licensed indications include angina, hypertension, AMI, postinfarct follow-up, arrhythmias, and now CHF. Data for postinfarct protection and for mortality reduction in CHF are particularly impressive.

2. *The major change in the clinical* use of β-blockers is the essential use of β-blockers in stabilized and treated patients with CHF, to counter the excessive adrenergic drive. Only three agents have been studied in detail, namely carvedilol, metoprolol, and biso-prolol, of which only the first two are approved for heart failure in the United States. It is essential to follow the recommended protocol, with slowly incremental doses of the chosen agent.

3. *Coronary heart disease.* β-Blockade is very effective treatment, alone or combined with other drugs, in 70% to 80% of patients with classic angina. β-Blockers are part of the essential postinfarct protection armamentarium. For acute coronary syndromes, indirect evidence suggests a quadruple follow-up regimen of aspirin, statin, ACE inhibitor, and β-blockade. However, there is no evidence that β-blockers slow the development of coronary artery disease.

4. *Hypertension.* β-Blockers reduce blood pressure effectively in 50% to 70% of those with mild to moderate hypertension. Elderly hypertensives, especially those of the black ethnic group, respond less well to β-blocker monotherapy. The previously recommended combination of β-blockers and diuretics may provoke diabetes, unless the diuretic dose is truly low.

5. *Arrhythmias.* There is renewed realization that β-blockers are among the more effective ventricular antiarrhythmics.

6. *Propranolol versus others.* Regarding choice of β-blocker, there is no particular advantage for this original "gold standard" drug, with its poor quality of life, unless hypertension or angina coexists with some other condition in which experience with propranolol is greater than with other β-blockers (e.g., hypertrophic cardiomyopathy, migraine prophylaxis, anxiety or essential tremor), or

unless cost is a major consideration when generic propranolol should be compared with other generics such as atenolol.

7. *Other β-blockers* are increasingly used because of specific attractive properties: cardio-selectivity (acebutolol, atenolol, bisoprolol, metoprolol); positive data in heart failure (carvedilol, metoprolol, bisoprolol) or postinfarct (metoprolol, carvedilol, timolol); lipid insolubility and no hepatic metabolism (atenolol, nadolol, sotalol); long action (nadolol) or long-acting formulations; intrinsic sympathomimetic activity (ISA) in selected patients to help avoid bradycardia (pindolol, acebutolol); added α-blockade to achieve more arterial dilation (carvedilol); and well-studied antiarrhythmic properties (sotalol). The antihypertensive combination bisoprolol-hydrochlorothiazide combines very low doses of two types of agents while maintaining efficacy and minimizing side effects. Esmolol is the best agent for intravenous use in the perioperative period because of its extremely short half-life.

8. *Evidence-based use.* Here the logic would be to use those agents established in large trials because of the known doses and clearly expected benefits. For example, for postinfarct protection propranolol, metoprolol, carvedilol, and timolol are the best studied, of which only carvedilol has been studied in the reperfusion era. For stabilized congestive heart failure, carvedilol, metoprolol, and bisoprolol have impressive data from large trials. Carvedilol especially merits attention, being licensed for a wide clinical range, from LV dysfunction to severe heart failure, and having best trial data. For arrhythmias, sotalol with its class III properties stands out.

R E F E R E N C E S

1. Dorn GW, 2nd, et al. Manipulating cardiac contractility in heart failure: data from mice and men. *Circulation* 2004;109:150–158.
2. Gong H, et al. Specific beta₂AR blocker ICI 118,551 actively decreases contraction through a Gᵢ-coupled form of the beta₂AR in myocytes from failing human heart. *Circulation* 2002;105:2497–2503.
3. Moniotte S, et al. Upregulation of beta₃-adrenoreceptors and altered contractile response to inotropic amines in human failing myocardium. *Circulation* 2001;103:1649–1655.
4. Wallhaus TR, et al. Myocardial free fatty acid and glucose use after carvedilol treatment in patients with congestive heart failure. *Circulation* 2001;103:2441–2446.
5. Bristow MR. β-Adrenergic receptor blockade in chronic heart failure. *Circulation* 2000;101:558–569.
6. Akhter S, et al. In vivo inhibition of elevated myocardial β-adrenergic receptor kinase activity in hybrid transgenic mice restores normal β-adrenergic signaling and function. *Circulation* 1999;100:648–653.
7. Heilbrunn SM, et al. Increased beta-receptor density and improved hemodynamic response to catecholamine stimulation during long-term metoprolol therapy in heart failure from dilated cardiomyopathy. *Circulation* 1989;79:483–490.
8. Kugiyama K, et al. Effects of propranolol and nifedipine on exercise-induced attack in patients variant angina: assessment by exercise thallium-201 myocardial scintigraphy with quantitative rotational tomography. *Circulation* 1986;74:374–380.
9. Peart I, et al. Cold intolerance in patients with angina pectoris: effect of nifedipine and propranolol. *Br Heart J* 1989;61:521–528.
10. ASIST Study. Effects of treatment on outcome in mildly symptomatic patients with ischemia during daily life. The Atenolol Silent Ischemia Study (ASIST). *Circulation* 1994;90:762–768.
11. Mukherjee D, et al. Impact of combination evidence-based medical therapy on mortality in patients with acute coronary syndromes. *Circulation* 2004;109:745–749.
12. Yusuf S, et al. Reduction in infarct size, arrhythmias and chest pain by early intravenous beta blockade in suspected acute myocardial infarction. *Circulation* 1983;67 (Suppl I):I-32–I-41.
13. HINT Study. Early treatment of unstable angina in the coronary care unit, a randomised, double-blind placebo controlled comparison of recurrent ischemia in patients treated with nifedipine or metoprolol or both. Holland Inter-university Nifedipine Trial. *Br Heart J* 1986;56:400–413.
14. Freemantle N, et al. β blockade after myocardial infarction: systemic review and meta regression analysis. *Br Med J* 1999;318:1730–1737.
15. Ryden L, et al. A double-blind trial of metoprolol in acute myocardial infarction. *N Engl J Med* 1983;308:614–618.
16. Norris RM, et al. Prevention of ventricular fibrillation during acute myocardial infarction by intravenous propranolol. *Lancet* 1984:883–886.

17. CAPRICORN Investigators. Effect of carvedilol on outcome after myocardial infarction in patients with left-ventricular dysfunction: the CAPRICORN randomised trial. *Lancet* 2001;357:1385–1390.
18. Gottlieb SS, et al. Effect of beta-blockade on mortality among high-risk and low-risk patients after myocardial infarction. *N Engl J Med* 1998;339:489–497.
19. Olsson G, et al. Long-term treatment with metoprolol after myocardial infarction: effect on 3-year mortality and morbidity. *J Am Coll Cardiol* 1985;5:1428–1437.
20. Teo KK, et al. Effects of prophylactic antiarrhythmic drug therapy in acute myocardial infarction. An overview of results from randomized controlled trials. *JAMA* 1993;270:1589–1595.
21. SAVE Study. Effect of captopril on mortality and morbidity in patients with left ventricular dysfunction after myocardial infarction. Results of the Survival and Ventricular Enlargement trial. *N Engl J Med* 1992;327:669–677.
22. Heidenreich PA, et al. Meta-analysis of trials comparing β-blockers, calcium antagonists, and nitrates for stable angina. *JAMA* 1999;281:1927–1936.
23. Chobanian AV, et al. The Seventh Report of the Joint National Committee on Prevention, Detection, Evaluation and Treatment of High Blood Pressure. *JAMA* 2003;289:2560–2572.
24. European Society of Hypertension Guidelines Committee. European Society of Cardiology guidelines for the management of arterial hypertension. *J Hypertens* 2003; 21:1011–1053.
25. Psaty BM, et al. Health outcomes associated with antihypertensive therapies uses as first-line agents. A systemic review and meta-analysis. *JAMA* 1997;277:739–745.
26. Messerli FH, et al. Are beta-blockers efficacious as first-line therapy for hypertension in the elderly? A systematic review. *JAMA* 1998;279:1903–1907.
27. Kjeldsen SE, et al. For the LIFE Study Group. Effects of losartan on cardiovascular morbidity and mortality in patients with isolated systolic hypertension and left ventricular hypertrophy. *JAMA* 2002;288:1491–1498.
28. Morgan T, et al. Effect of different antihypertensive drug classes on central aortic pressure. *Am J Hypertens* 2004;17:118–123.
29. Materson BJ, et al. Single-drug therapy for hypertension in men. A comparison of six antihypertensive agents with placebo. The Department of Veterans Affairs Cooperative Study Group on Antihypertensive Agents. *N Engl J Med* 1993;328:914–921.
30. UKPDS 38. UK Prospective Diabetes Study Group. Tight blood pressure control and risk of macrovascular and microvascular complications in type 2 diabetes: UKPDS 38. *Br Med J* 1998;317:703–713.
31. UKPDS 39. UK Prospective Diabetes Study Group. Efficacy of atenolol and captopril in reducing risk of macrovascular and microvascular complications in type 2 diabetes: UKPDS 39. *Br Med J* 1998;317:713–720.
32. Dunder K, et al. Increase in blood glucose concentration during antihypertensive treatment as a predictor of myocardial infarction: population based cohort study. *Br Med J* 2003;326:681–685.
33. Lindholm LH, et al. Risk of new-onset diabetes in the Losartan Intervention For Endpoint reduction in hypertension study. *J Hypertens* 2002;20:1879–1886.
34. Lithell H, et al. Metabolic effects of carvedilol in hypertensive patients. *Eur J Clin Pharmacol* 1997;52:13–17.
35. Frishman WH, et al. First-line therapy option with low-dose bisoprolol fumarate and low-dose hydrochlorothiazide in patients with stage I and stage II systemic hypertension. *J Clin Pharmacol* 1995;35:182–188.
36. Gress TW, et al. For the Atherosclerosis Risk in Communities Study. Hypertension and antihypertensives therapy as risk factors for type 2 diabetes mellitus. *N Engl J Med* 2000;342:905–912.
37. Lubbe WF, et al. Potential arrhythmogenic role of cyclic adenosine monophosphate (AMP) and cytosolic calcium overload: implications for prophylactic effects of beta-blockers in myocardial infarction and proarrhythmic effects of phosphodiesterase inhibitors. *J Am Coll Cardiol* 1992;19:1622–1633.
38. Pogwizd SM, et al. Arrhythmogenesis and contractile dysfunction in heart failure. *Circ Res* 2001;88:1159–1167.
39. Steinbeck G, et al. A comparison of electrophysiologically guided antiarrhythmic drug therapy with beta-blocker therapy in patients with symptomatic, sustained ventricular tachyarrhythmias. *N Engl J Med* 1992;327:987–992.
40. ESVEM Study. A comparison of seven antiarrhythmic drugs in patients with ventricular tachyarrhythmias. Electrophysiologic Study versus Electrocardiographic Monitoring Investigators. *N Engl J Med* 1993;329:452–458.
41. Boutitie F, et al. Amiodarone interactions with beta-blockers. Analysis of the merged EMIAT (European Myocardial Infarct Trial) and CAMIAT (Canadian Amiodarone Myocardial Infarct Trial) databases. *Circulation* 1999;99:2268–2275.
42. Kennedy HL, et al. β-Blocker therapy in the cardiac arrhythmia suppression trial. *Am J Cardiol* 1994;74:674–680.
43. Ellison KE, et al. Effect of beta-blocking therapy on outcome in the Multicenter UnSustained Tachycardia Trial (MUSTT). *Circulation* 2002;106:2694–2699.
44. Bardy G. SCD–HeFT: ICD cuts all-cause mortality by 23% in NYHA class 2–3 heart failure. *www.theheart.org* 2004;10 March.
45. Lowes BD, et al. Myocardial gene expression in dilated cardiomyopathy treated with beta-blocking agents. *N Engl J Med* 2002;346:1357–1365.
46. Kubo H, et al. Patients with end-stage congestive heart failure treated with β-adrenergic receptor antagonists have improved ventricular myocyte calcium regulatory protein abundance. *Circulation* 2001;104:1012–1018.
47. Doi M, et al. Propranolol prevents the development of heart failure by restoring FKBP 12.6-mediated stabilization of ryanodine receptor. *Circulation* 2002;105:1374–1379.

48. Reiken S, et al. β-Blockers restore calcium release channel function and improve cardiac muscle performance in human heart failure. *Circulation* 2003;107:2459–2466.
49. Koch WJ, et al. Exploring the role of the β-adrenergic receptor kinase in cardiac disease using gene-targeted mice. *Trends Cardiovasc Med* 1999;9:77–81.
50. Engelhardt S, et al. Altered calcium handling is critically involved in the cardiotoxic effects of chronic beta-adrenergic stimulation. *Circulation* 2004;109:1154–1160.
51. Nagatsu M, et al. Bradycardia and the role of β-blockade in the amelioration of left ventricular dysfunction. *Circulation* 2000;101:653–659.
52. Lechat P, et al. Heart rate and cardiac rhythm relationships with bisoprolol benefit in chronic heart failure in CIBIS II Trial. *Circulation* 2001;103:1428–1433.
53. RESOLVD Investigators. Effects of metoprolol CR in patients with ischemic and dilated cardiomyopathy. The Randomized Evaluation of Strategies for Left Ventricular Dysfunction Pilot Study. *Circulation* 2000;101:378–384.
54. Poole-Wilson PA, et al. Comparison of carvedilol and metoprolol on clinical outcomes in patients with chronic heart failure in the Carvedilol Or Metoprolol European Trial (COMET): randomised controlled trial. *Lancet* 2003;362:7–13.
55. Mulder P, et al. Long-term heart rate reduction induced by the selective I_f current inhibitor ivabradine improves left ventricular function and intrinsic myocardial structure in congestive heart failure. *Circulation* 2004;109:1674–1679.
56. Communal C, et al. Opposing effects of β_1- and β_2-adrenergic receptors on cardiac myocyte apoptosis. Role of a pertussis toxin–sensitive G protein. *Circulation* 1999; 100:2210–2212.
57. Packer M, et al. Consensus recommendations for the management of chronic heart failure. *Am J Cardiol* 1999;83 (2A):1A–38A.
58. Shekelle PG, et al. Efficacy of angiotensin-converting enzyme inhibitors and beta-blockers in the management of left ventricular systolic dysfunction according to race, gender, and diabetic status: a meta-analysis of major clinical trials. *J Am Coll Cardiol* 2003;41:1529–1538.
59. Moss AJ, et al. Effectiveness and limitations of β-blocker therapy in congenital long-QT syndrome. *Circulation* 2000;101:616–623.
60. Poldermans D, et al. The effect of bisoprolol on perioperative mortality and myocardial infarction in high-risk patients undergoing vascular surgery. *N Engl J Med* 1999;341:1789–1794.
61. Fleischer LA, et al. Lowering cardiac risk in non-cardiac surgery. *N Engl J Med* 2001;345:1677–1682.
62. Kalinowski L, et al. Third–generation beta-blockers stimulate nitric oxide release from endothelial cells through ATP efflux: a novel mechanism for antihypertensive action. *Circulation* 2003;107:2747–2752.
63. TOMH Study. Treatment of Mild Hypertension study (TOMH). Final results. *JAMA* 1993;270:713–724.
64. Simpson WT. Nature and incidence of unwanted effects with atenolol. *Postrgrad Med J* 1977;53:162–167.
65. Conant J, et al. Central nervous system side effects of beta-adrenergic blocking agents with high and low lipid solubility. *J Cardiovasc Pharmacol* 1989;13:656–661.
66. Streufert S, et al. Impact of β-adrenergic blockers on complex cognitive functioning. *Am Heart J* 1988;116:311–315.
67. Croog S, et al. The effects of antihypertensive therapy on the quality of life. *N Engl J Med* 1986;314:1657–1664.
68. Herrick AL, et al. Comparison of enalapril and atenolol in mild to moderate hypertension. *Am J Med* 1989;86:421–426.
69. TAIM Study, et al. The Trial of Antihypertensive Interventions and Management (TAIM) Study. Final results with regard to blood pressure, cardiovascular risk and quality of life. *Am J Hypertens* 1992;5:37–44.
70. Fogari R, et al. Sexual activity in hypertensive men treated with valsartan or carvedilol: A crossover study. *Am J Hypertens* 2001;14:27–31.
71. Grimm RH, et al. Long-term effects on sexual function of five antihypertensive drugs and nutritional hygienic treatment in hypertensive men and women. Treatment of Mild Hypertension Study (TOMHS). *Hypertension* 1997;29:8–14.
72. Pepine CJ, et al. A calcium antagonist vs a non–calcium antagonist hypertension treatment strategy for patients with coronary artery disease. The International Verapamil-Trandolapril Study (INVEST): a randomized controlled trial. *JAMA* 2003;290: 2805–2816.
73. MRC Working Party. Medical Research Council trial of treatment of hypertension in older adults: principal results. *Br Med J* 1992;304:405–412.
74. Dahlöf B. For the LIFE Study Group. Cardiovascular morbidity and mortality in the Losartan Intervention For Endpoint reduction in hypertension study (LIFE): a randomised trial against atenolol. *Lancet* 2002;359:995–1003.
75. MERIT-HF Study Group. Effect of metoprolol CR/XL in chronic heart failure: Metoprolol CR/XL Randomized Trial in Congestive Heart Failure (MERIT-HF). *Lancet* 1999;353:2001–2007.
76. Broeders MA, et al. Nebivolol: a third-generation beta-blocker that augments vascular nitric oxide release: endothelial beta(2)-adrenergic receptor-mediated nitric oxide production. *Circulation* 2000;102:677–684.
77. Van de Water A, et al. Pharmacological and hemodynamic profile of nebivolol, a chemically novel, potent, and selective beta 1-adrenergic antagonist. *J Cardiovasc Pharmacol* 1988;11:552–563.
78. Tzemos N, et al. Nebivolol reverses endothelial dysfunction in essential hypertension: a randomized, double-blind, crossover study. *Circulation* 2001;104:511–514.
79. Hohnloser SH, et al. For the European Esmolol Study Group. Usefulness of esmolol in unstable angina pectoris. *Am J Cardiol* 1991;67:1319–1323.

2

Nitrates

Lionel H. Opie • Harvey D. White

> *"When the remedy is used for a long time, the dose requires to be increased before the effect is produced."*
>
> BRUNTON, 1867[1]

MECHANISMS OF NITRATE ACTION IN ANGINA

Nitrates provide an exogenous source of vasodilator nitric oxide, a short-lived free radical (NO•, usually written as NO), thereby inducing coronary vasodilation even when endogenous production of nitric oxide is impaired by coronary artery disease. Thus nitrates act differently from the other classes of anti-anginals (see Fig. 11-1). Chronic use of nitrates produces tolerance, a significant clinical problem that is still not fully understood. The main focus of current clinical work remains on strategies to minimize or prevent the development of tolerance, with the major emphasis on the adverse role of excess nitric oxide that produces harmful peroxynitrite.[2] The major focus of basic work has shifted to the role of endogenously produced nitric oxide as a ubiquitous physiological messenger, as described by Furchgott, Iganarro, and Murad, the 1998 Nobel Prize winners in Medicine.[3] Although such endogenously produced nitric oxide has many functions, such as a role in vagal neurotransmission, that are quite different from the functions of nitric oxide derived from exogenous nitrates, they have important shared vasodilatory effects.

Vasodilatory Effects: Coronary and Peripheral

A distinction must be made between antianginal and coronary vasodilator properties. Nitrates dilate large coronary arteries and arterioles greater than 100 μm in diameter[4] to: (1) redistribute blood flow along collateral channels and from epicardial to endocardial regions and (2) relieve coronary spasm and dynamic stenosis, especially at epicardial sites, including the coronary arterial constriction induced by exercise. Exercise-induced myocardial ischemia is thereby relieved. Thus, nitrates are "effective" vasodilators for angina; dipyridamole and other vasodilators acting more distally in the arterial tree are not, rather having the risk of diverting blood from the ischemic area—a "coronary steal" effect.

The peripheral hemodynamic effects of nitrates, originally observed by Lauder Brunton,[1] cannot be ignored. Nitrates do reduce the afterload, in addition to the preload of the heart (Fig. 2-1). The arterial wave reflection from the periphery back to the aorta is altered in such a way that there is "true" afterload reduction, with the aortic systolic pressure falling even though the brachial artery pressure does not change.[5]

Reduced Oxygen Demand

Nitrates increase the venous capacitance, causing pooling of blood in the peripheral veins and thereby a reduction in venous return and in ventricular volume. There is less mechanical stress on the myocardial wall and the myocardial oxygen demand is reduced. Furthermore, a fall in the aortic systolic pressure also reduces the oxygen demand.

ACTION OF NITRATES ON CIRCULATION
Opie 2004

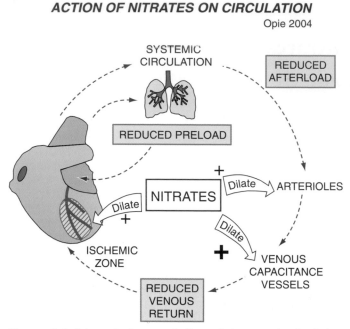

Figure 2-1 Schematic diagram of effects of nitrate on the circulation. The major effect is on the venous capacitance vessels, with additional coronary and peripheral arteriolar vasodilatory benefits. (*Figure © LH Opie, 2005.*)

Endothelium and Vascular Mechanisms

The chief vascular effect is the formation of NO$^\bullet$ (Fig. 2-2). An intact vascular endothelium is required for the vasodilatory effects of some vascular active agents (thus acetylcholine physiologically vasodilates but constricts when the endothelium is damaged). Nitrates vasodilate whether or not the endothelium is intact. Prolonged nitrate therapy does, however, inhibit endothelial nitric oxide synthase, which explains one of the mechanisms of nitrate tolerance.[2] Thus nitrate tolerance and endothelial dysfunction have shared pathogenetic mechanisms. Nitrates, after entering the vessel wall, are converted to nitric oxide (NO$^\bullet$), which stimulates guanylate cyclase to produce cyclic GMP (Fig. 2-2). Calcium in the vascular myocyte falls, and vasodilation results. Sulfhydryl (SH) groups are required for such formation of NO$^\bullet$ and the stimulation of guanylate cyclase. Nitroglycerin powerfully dilates when injected into an artery, an effect that is probably limited in humans by reflex adrenergic mediated vasoconstriction. Hence (1) nitrates are better venous than arteriolar dilators; and (2) there is an associated adrenergic reflex tachycardia[6] that can be attenuated by concurrent β-blockade.

Antiplatelet Effect

Increased platelet aggregation occurs in patients with angina.[7] The antiaggregating and cyclic GMP enhancing effects of nitrates are reduced in such patients, reflecting nitrate resistance at a platelet level.[7]

PHARMACOKINETICS OF NITRATES
Bioavailability and Half-Lives

The various preparations differ so much that each needs to be considered separately. As a group, nitrates are absorbed from the mucous membranes, the skin, and the gastrointestinal tract. The prototype

NITRATE MECHANISMS

Opie 2004

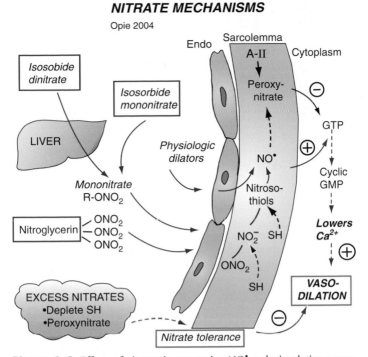

Figure 2-2 Effects of nitrates in generating NO• and stimulating guany-late cyclase to cause vasodilation. Note role of cysteine cascade in stimu-lating guanylate cyclase. Previously SH depletion was thought to explain nitrate tolerance. Current emphasis is on the generation of peroxynitrite, which in turn inhibits the conversion of GTP to cyclic GMP. Note that mononitrates bypass hepatic metabolism. *GMP* = guanosine monophos-phate; *GTP* = guanosine triphosphate; *SH* = sulfhydryl. (*Figure © LH Opie, 2005.*)

agent, nitroglycerin, has pharmacokinetics that are not well understood. It rapidly disappears from the blood with a half-life of only a few minutes, largely by extrahepatic mechanisms that convert the parent molecule to longer acting and active dinitrates.[8] Isosorbide, on the other hand, must first be converted in the liver to the active mononitrates (Fig. 2-3), which have half-lives of about 4 to 6 hours with ultimate renal excretion. The mononitrates are completely bioavailable without any hepatic metabolism, with half-lives of 4 to 6 hours. In reality, knowledge of pharmacokinetics is of limited inter-est, because of the highly variable relationship between the plasma concentrations of the nitrates, the levels of their active metabolites, and the onset and duration of pharmacologic action that matter most to the clinician.[8] Of the many nitrate preparations (Table 2-1), sub-lingual nitroglycerin remains the gold standard for acute anginal attacks.[9] In practice, patients are often also given long-acting nitrates. "No matter which long-acting preparation is used, physicians should prescribe the drug in a manner to decrease the likelihood of nitrate tolerance. This involves an on/off strategy of at least a 10-hour nitrate-free interval each day."[9] This policy does, however, entertain the risk of precipitation of angina during the nitrate-free interval, which is often at night.

NITRATE INTERACTIONS WITH OTHER DRUGS

Pharmacodynamics

The chief drug interactions of nitrates are pharmacodynamic. For example, during triple therapy of angina pectoris (nitrates, β-blockers,

Table 2-1 Nitrate Preparations; Doses, Preparations, and Duration of Effects

Compound	Route	Preparation and Dose	Duration of Effects and Comments
Amyl nitrite	Inhalation	2–5 mg	10 s to 10 min; for diagnosis of LV outflow obstruction in hypertrophic cardiomyopathy
Nitroglycerin (trinitrin, TNT, glyceryl trinitrate)	(a) Sublingual tablets	0.3–0.6 mg up to 1.5 mg	Peak blood levels at 2 min; $t^{1}/_{2}$ about 7 min; for acute therapy of effort or rest angina. Keep tightly capped. Use stabilized preparations.
	(b) Spray	0.4 mg/metered dose	Similar to tablets at same dose.
	(c) Ointment	2%; 6 × 6 ins or 15 × 15 cm or 7.5–40 mg	Apply 2× daily; 6-h intervals; effect up to 7 h after first dose. No efficacy data for chronic use.
	(d) Transdermal patches	0.2–0.8 mg/h patch on for 12 h, patch off for 12 h.	Effects start within minutes and last 3–5 h. No efficacy data for second or third doses during chronic therapy.
	(e) Oral: sustained release	2.5–13 mg 1–2 tablets 3× daily	4–8 h after first dose; no efficacy data for chronic therapy.
	(f) Buccal	1–3 mg tablets 3× daily	Effects start within minutes and last 3–5 h. No efficacy data for second or third doses during chronic therapy.
	(g) Intravenous infusion	5–200 µg/min (avoid PVC, absorbs nitrate; if used, start with 20 µg/min). Must dilute vials or ampules in dextrose or NaCl in glass containers. For severe hypertension, see Table 7-6	In unstable angina, increasing doses are often needed to overcome tolerance. High-concentration solutions contain propylene glycol; cross-reacts with heparin.

Isosorbide dinitrate (= sorbide nitrate)	(a) Sublingual	2.5–15 mg	Onset 5–10 min, effect up to 60 min or longer
	(b) Oral tablets	5–80 mg 2–3× daily	Up to 8 h (first dose; then tolerance) with 3× or 4× daily doses; 2× daily 7 h apart may be effective but data inadequate.
Isordil			
	(c) Spray	1.25 mg on tongue	Rapid action 2–3 min
	(d) Chewable	5 mg as single dose	Exercise time increased for 2 min–2½ h.
	(e) Oral; slow-release	40 mg once or 2× daily	Up to 8 h (first dose; 2× daily not superior to placebo)
	(f) Intravenous infusion	1.25–5.0 mg/h (care with PVC)	May need increasing doses for unstable angina at rest
	(g) Ointment	100 mg/24 h	Not effective during continuous therapy
Isosorbide 5-mononitrate	Oral tablets	20 mg 2× day (7 h apart)	12–14 h after chronic dosing for 2 wk
		120–240 mg 1× daily (slow release)	Efficacy up to 12 h after 6 wk
Pentaerythritol tetranitrate	Sublingual	10 mg as needed	No efficacy data

For references, see previous editions and text.
IV = intravenous; PVC = polyvinylchloride tubing.

SERIOUS NITRATE INTERACTION

Opie 2004

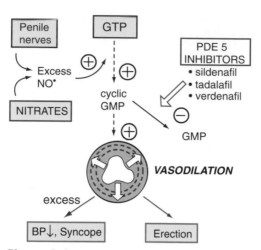

Figure 2-3 A serious nitrate drug interaction. The mechanism of normal erection involves penile vasodilation mediated by GTP and cyclic GMP. The phosphodiesterase-5 inhibitors *(PDE 5)* such as sildenafil (Viagra) act by inhibiting the enzymatic breakdown of penile cyclic GMP to GMP with increased vasodilation. This is not confined to the penis, and peripheral vasodilation added to that caused by nitrates gives rise to an excess fall of blood pressure *(BP)* and possible syncope. Hence the use of PDE 5 inhibitors in any patient taking nitrates *is contraindicated.* GMP = guanosine monophosphate; GTP = guanosine triphosphate. (*Figure © LH Opie, 2005.*)

calcium antagonists), the efficacy of the combination may be lessened, because each drug can predispose to excess *hypotension.* Individual patients vary greatly in their susceptibility to the hypotension of triple therapy. Even two components of triple therapy, such as diltiazem and nitrates, may interact adversely to cause moderate hypotension.[10] Another hypotensive interaction is between angiotensin-converting enzyme (ACE) inhibitors and nitrates in early phase acute myocardial infarction (AMI).

Interaction with Sildenafil, Tadalafil, and Vardenafil

Erectile dysfunction is commonly associated with endothelial dysfunction, and may be an early manifestation of systemic vascular disease.[11] Erectile dysfunction is often treated by one of these phosphodiesterase-5 (PDE-5) inhibitors, which are also systemic vasodilators, and can all cause serious hypotensive reactions when combined with nitrates (Fig. 2-3). Hence the package insert of all three agents forbids coadministration to patients taking nitrates in any form, either regularly or intermittently. For example, Viagra decreases the blood pressure by about 8.4/5.5 mmHg, and by much more in those taking nitrates. The exertion of intercourse also stresses the cardiovascular system further, which may explain why AMI has been found during the combined use with nitrates. As a group, these drugs should also not be given with α-adrenergic blockers. In case of *inadvertent phosphodiesterase-5 (PDE-5)–nitrate combinations*, administration of an α-adrenergic agonist or even of norepinephrine may be needed.

An Essential Question for Men with Acute Coronary Syndrome

Whenever a male patient presents with an anginal attack or acute coronary syndrome, whether or not precipitated by sexual intercourse, then one essential question is: Have you recently taken Viagra or Levitra or Cialis (the trade names for sildenafil, vardenafil, and tadalafil)? If so, how soon can a nitrate be given? The package insert for sildenafil, the prototype drug, indicates that plasma levels of sildenafil are much lower at 24 hours postdose, with the reservation that even then the safety of coadministration cannot be assured. Nonetheless, if the clinical situation requires the use of nitrates, then they may be cautiously started in low doses 24 hours or more after sildenafil.[9] Likewise for vardenafil a 24-hour interval can be inferred from data in the package insert. For the longer acting tadalafil the corresponding interval is 48 hours.[12]

High-Dose Intravenous Nitrate Interaction with Heparin

In patients receiving both drugs, as in unstable angina, the dose of heparin required is sometimes higher than anticipated, that is, there is *heparin resistance*. The dose of nitroglycerin required to produce heparin resistance is relatively high (>350 μg/minute). With lower doses (mean of 59 μg/minute), or with isosorbide dinitrate infusions (mean of 3.7 mg/hour), no tolerance was found.[13]

Beneficial Interaction with Hydralazine

There is a beneficial interaction between nitrates and hydralazine whereby the latter helps to lessen nitrate tolerance,[14] probably acting through inhibition of free radicals. This may explain why the combination of nitrates and hydralazine is effective in heart failure.

SHORT-ACTING NITRATES FOR ACUTE EFFORT ANGINA

Sublingual nitroglycerin is very well established in the initial therapy of angina of effort, yet may be ineffective, frequently because the patient has not received proper instruction or because of severe headaches. When angina starts, the patient should rest in the sitting position (standing promotes syncope; lying enhances venous return and heart work) and take sublingual nitroglycerin (0.3 to 0.6 mg) every 5 minutes until the pain stops or a maximum of four to five tablets have been taken. *Nitroglycerin spray* is an alternative mode of oral administration, which is more acceptable to some patients. It vasodilates sooner than does the tablet, which might be of special importance in those with dryness of the mouth.[15]

Isosorbide dinitrate may be given *sublingually* (5 mg) to abort an anginal attack and then exerts antianginal effects for about 1 hour. Because the dinitrate requires hepatic conversion to the mononitrate, the onset of antianginal action (mean time: 3.4 minutes) is slower than with nitroglycerin (mean time: 1.9 minutes), so that the manufacturers of the dinitrate recommend sublingual administration of this drug only if the patient is unresponsive to or intolerant of sublingual nitroglycerin. After oral ingestion, hemodynamic and antianginal effects persist for several hours. Single doses of isosorbide dinitrate confer longer protection against angina than can single doses of sublingual nitroglycerin (Table 2-1).

Table 2-2	Interval Therapy for Effort Angina by Eccentric Nitrate Dosage Schedules Designed to Avoid Tolerance	
Preparation	**Dose**	**Reference**
Isosorbide dinitrate	30 mg at 7 AM, 1 PM*	Thadani and Lipicky, 1994[†]
Isosorbide mononitrate (Robins-Boehringer-Wyeth-Ayerst; Pharma-Schwartz)	20 mg at 8 AM and 3 PM	Parker 1993[‡]
Isosorbide mononitrate, Extended-release (Key-Astra)	120–240 mg daily	Chrysant, 1993[§]
Transdermal nitrate patches	7.5–10 mg per 12 h patches removed after 12 h	DeMots, 1989[‖]
Phasic release nitroglycerin patch	15 mg, most released in first 12 h[¶]	Parker, 1989**

*Efficacy of second dose not established; no data for other doses.
[†]*Cardiovasc Drugs Ther* 1994;8:625–633.
[‡]*Am J Cardiol* 1993;72:871–876.
[§]*Am J Cardiol* 1993;72:1249–1256.
[‖]*J Am Coll Cardiol* 1989:13:786–793.
[¶]No data for other doses.
**Eur Heart J* 1989;10(Suppl A):43–49.

LONG-ACTING NITRATES FOR ANGINA PROPHYLAXIS

Long-acting nitrates are not continuously effective if regularly taken over a prolonged period, unless allowance is made for a nitrate-free or -low interval (Table 2-2).

Isosorbide dinitrate (oral preparation) is frequently given for the prophylaxis of angina. An important question is whether regular therapy with isosorbide dinitrate gives long-lasting protection (3 to 5 hours) against angina. In a crucial placebo-controlled study, exercise duration improved significantly for 6 to 8 hours after single oral doses of 15 to 120 mg isosorbide dinitrate, but for only 2 hours when the same doses were given repetitively four times daily.[16] Marked tolerance develops during sustained therapy, despite much higher plasma isosorbide dinitrate concentrations during sustained than during acute therapy.[16] With the extended-release formulation of isosorbide dinitrate *(Tembid)*, eccentric twice daily treatment with a 40-mg dose administered in the morning and 7 hours later was not superior to placebo in a large multicenter study.[17] Nonetheless eccentric dosing schedules of isosorbide dinitrate are still often used in an effort to avoid tolerance.

Mononitrates on the whole have dosage and effects similar to those of isosorbide dinitrate. Nitrate tolerance, likewise a potential problem, can be prevented or minimized when rapid-release preparations *(Monoket, Ismo)* are given twice daily in an eccentric pattern with doses spaced by 7 hours.[18] Using the slow-release preparation *(Imdur)*, the dose range 30 to 240 mg once daily was tested for antianginal activity. Only 120 and 240 mg daily improved exercise times at 4 and 12 hours after administration, even after 42 days of daily use.[19] These high doses were reached by titration over 7 days. A daily dose of 60 mg, still often used, was ineffective.

Transdermal nitroglycerin patches are designed to permit the timed release of nitroglycerin over a 24-hour period. Despite initial claims of 24-hour efficacy, major studies have failed to show prolonged improvement. The decisive study was a multicenter US Food and Drug Administration (FDA)-monitored trial evaluating chronic patch therapy in 562 patients, using patches that delivered up to 105 mg of nitroglycerin over a 24-hour period. There was no improvement in treadmill exercise duration measured at 4 and 24 hours after patch application when compared with placebo.[20] In patients with unstable anginal syndromes, a coronary event can rarely be precipitated in the nitrate-free period. However, eccentric dosage schedules of patches do work apparently without rebound at night in patients receiving concurrent β-blockade.[21]

LIMITATIONS: SIDE EFFECTS AND NITRATE FAILURE

Side Effects

The most common side effect is the development of headaches and the most serious side effect is hypotension (Table 2-3). Headaches characteristically occur with sublingual nitroglycerin, and at the start

Table 2-3	Precautions and Side Effects in Use of Nitrates

Precautions

Nitroglycerin tablets should be kept in *airtight containers.* Nitrate sprays are inflammable.

Common Side Effects

Headaches frequently limit dose. Arterial tolerance may exceed that on the veins. Therefore, headaches may cease while antianginal venous efficacy is sustained. Headaches often respond to aspirin. Facial flushing. Sublingual nitrates may cause halitosis.

Serious Side Effects

Syncope and *hypotension* from reduction of preload and afterload; alcohol or cotherapy with vasodilators may augment hypotension. Treat by recumbency.

Tachycardia frequent, but unexplained *bradycardia* occasionally occurs in AMI. Hypotension may cause cerebral ischemia. Prolonged high dosage can cause *methemoglobinemia* (nitrate ions can oxidize hemoglobin to methemoglobin); treat by intravenous methylene blue (1–2 mg/kg). High-dose intravenous nitrates can induce *heparin resistance.*

Contraindications

In angina caused by *hypertrophic obstructive cardiomyopathy,* nitrates may exaggerate outflow obstruction and are contraindicated except for diagnosis. *Acute inferior myocardial infarction* with right ventricular involvement: here a fall in the filling pressure may lead to hemodynamic and clinical deterioration. *Viagra* (or similar agents) may lead to excess hypotension or even AMI.

Relative Contraindications

In *cor pulmonale* and arterial hypoxemia, nitrates decrease arterial O_2 tension by venous admixture. Although *glaucoma* is usually held to be a contraindication, there is no objective evidence to show any increase in intraocular pressure (possible exception: amyl nitrite). *Cardiac tamponade* or constrictive pericarditis or tight mitral stenosis; the already compromised diastolic filling may be aggravated by reduced venous return.

Tolerance

Shown experimentally and clinically. Continuous therapy and high-dose frequent therapy leads to tolerance that eccentric dosage may avoid. Cross-tolerance occurs between the various formulations.

Withdrawal Symptoms

Established in munition workers, in whom withdrawal may precipitate symptoms and sudden death. Some evidence for a similar clinical syndrome. Therefore, long-term nitrate therapy should be gradually discontinued.

Recurrence of anginal pain in nitrate-free intervals during sustained therapy occurs in some patients, but is less common with β-blocker cotherapy.

of therapy with long-acting nitrates.[9] Often the headaches pass over while antianginal efficacy is maintained; yet often headaches lead to loss of compliance. Concomitant aspirin may protect from the headaches and from coronary events. In chronic lung disease, arterial hypoxemia may result from vasodilation and increased venous admixture. Occasionally, prolonged high-dose therapy can cause *methemoglobinemia* (Table 2-3), which reduces the oxygen carrying capacity of the blood and the rate of delivery of oxygen to the tissues. Treatment is by intravenous methylene blue (1 to 2 mg/kg over 5 minutes).

Failure of Nitrate Therapy

With short-acting preparations, the most common causes of failure are noncompliance (headaches), loss of potency of the tablets, and incorrect timing (nitrates are more effective if taken before the expected onset of anginal pain). Sometimes the diagnosis may be wrong, because nitrates also relieve the pain of esophageal spasm and, sometimes, renal or biliary colic. Nitrates may be less effective than expected owing to tachycardia, so that combination with β-blockade gives better results.

Nitrate Tolerance During therapy with long-acting preparations, the chief cause of failure is the development of tolerance, treated by decreasing the frequency of drug administration until there is a nitrate-free interval (see section on Tolerance). The other main cause of failure is worsening of the underlying disease process.

Management of Apparent Failure of Nitrate Therapy After exclusion of tolerance and poor compliance (headaches), therapy is stepped up (Table 2-4) while excluding aggravating factors such as hypertension, thyrotoxicosis, atrial fibrillation, or anemia.

NITRATES FOR UNSTABLE ANGINA AT REST

As Reichek stated, "The one setting in which intermittent nitrate therapy does not have a role is the treatment of the hospitalized patient with unstable ischemic symptoms with or without myocardial infarc-

---

Table 2-4 | Proposed Step-Care for Angina of Effort

1. **General**: History and physical examination to exclude valvular disease, anemia, hypertension, thromboembolic disease, thyrotoxicosis, and heart failure. Check risk factors for coronary artery disease (smoking, hypertension, blood lipids, diabetes). Must stop smoking.
2. **Prophylactic drugs.** Give aspirin if not contraindicated. Consider statins and ACE inhibitors. β-Blocker if prior infarct.
3. **Intermittent short acting nitrates**, as needed to control pain. Combination therapy with β-blockers (sometimes calcium blockers) often introduced here.
4. **Prophylactic long-acting nitrates** in eccentric doses known to avoid tolerance. Intermittent short-acting nitrates are still added as needed.
5. **Combination long-acting nitrate therapy.** May add (1) β-blocker (if not already used); or (2) calcium antagonist (preferably verapamil or diltiazem; second choice: long-acting dihydropyridine).
6. **Triple therapy**. Long-acting nitrates plus β-blockers plus calcium blockers. Care with combination of verapamil or diltiazem with β-blockers (Fig. 1-4). Use triple combination with caution when therapy with two agents ineffective; watch for hypotension.
7. **PCI with stenting** may be attempted at any stage in selected patients, especially for highly symptomatic single vessel disease.
8. **Consider bypass surgery** after failure to respond to medical therapy or for left main stem lesion or for triple vessel disease, especially if reduced LV function. Even response to medical therapy does not eliminate need for investigation.
9. **Nitrate failure.** Consider nitrate tolerance or worsening disease or poor compliance.

tion."[22] It is presumed that in the treatment of unstable angina, upward titration of the dose of intravenous nitrate can overcome tolerance.

Intravenous nitroglycerin is very effective in the management of pain in patients with unstable angina, although there is surprisingly little objective evidence of such efficacy in properly controlled trials. Furthermore, the manufacturers warn that continuous use of nitroglycerin leads to almost complete loss of hemodynamic effect (blood pressure reduction) within 48 hours. Intravenous therapy allows more rapid titration to an effective dose and the use of nitroglycerin rather than isosorbide dinitrate permits rapid reversal of hemodynamic effects if an adverse reaction occurs. The usual initial starting dose is 5 to 10 µg/minute, which can be titrated up to 200 µg/minute or occasionally higher up to 1000 µg/minute, depending on the clinical course and aiming at the relief of anginal pain. In patients who are already pain free, the aim is a fall of mean blood pressure by 10%, the infusion being maintained for up to 36 hours. A problem in dosing is that nitroglycerin is readily absorbed (40% to 80%) by polyvinyl chloride (PVC) tubing, but not onto polyethylene or glass.

Nitrostat infusion sets use nonabsorbent materials. The result is that the calculated dose will in reality be delivered to the patient, so that substantially lower doses than in many published series will be effective.

Intravenous isosorbide dinitrate (not licensed in the United States) is much more effective than the oral route. Oral isosorbide dinitrate has poor bioavailability owing to extensive presystemic metabolism.

Nitrate patches and *nitroglycerin ointment* should not be used. As there is no role for intermittent nitrate therapy in unstable angina, because eccentric dosage schedules cannot be used to avoid the development of tolerance. Intravenous therapy, which can be titrated upwards as needed, is far better for control of pain.

Percutaneous transluminal coronary angioplasty (PTCA): Intracoronary nitroglycerin is often used to avoid coronary spasm during PTCA. Some nitrate solutions contain high potassium that may precipitate ventricular fibrillation.

ACUTE MYOCARDIAL INFARCTION (AMI)
Selective Use of Nitrates

Nitrates have failed to give consistent benefit in large AMI trials, so that it would seem prudent to limit the use of intravenous nitrates in AMI to those complicated patients with ongoing anginal pain, when left ventricular (LV) end-diastolic pressure is thought to be elevated and suited for reduction of the preload, for those with LV failure when combined with ACE inhibition,[23] or severe hypertension, or when the differential diagnosis between early transmural AMI and Prinzmetal's angina is not clear. Initial low-dose therapy is required to avoid excess hypotension (blood pressure <90 mmHg). Nitroglycerin 5 µg/minute is increased by 5 to 20 µg/minute every 5 to 10 minutes to a ceiling of 200 µg/minute (using standard intravenous PVC sets with glass bottles) until the mean blood pressure is reduced by 10% in normotensive and by 30% in hypertensive patients.[24] The infusion should be maintained for 12 hours or longer. When the infusion is discontinued, the dose should be tapered over several hours. The *major danger is hypotension*, in which case the infusion must be stopped abruptly and restarted at 5 µg/minute. When doses of 200 µg/minute fail to reduce the blood pressure, there is *nitrate resistance* and the infusion should be abandoned.

AMI: Nitrate Contraindications

When there is right ventricular involvement in AMI, a nitrate-induced fall in filling pressure may cause hemodynamic and clinical deterioration. A systolic BP of less than 90 mmHg is also a contraindication. Recent ingestion of sildenafil or its equivalent means that nitrate therapy must be delayed or avoided (see section on Nitrate Interactions, this chapter, p. 39).

CONGESTIVE HEART FAILURE

Both short- and long-acting nitrates are used as unloading agents in the relief of symptoms in acute and chronic heart failure. Their dilating effects are more pronounced on veins than on arterioles, so they are best suited to patients with raised pulmonary wedge pressure and clinical features of pulmonary congestion. Combination of high-dose isosorbide dinitrate (60 mg four times daily) plus hydralazine was better than placebo in decreasing mortality, yet nonetheless inferior to an ACE inhibitor in severe congestive heart failure (CHF).[25] Dinitrate-hydralazine may, therefore, be chosen when a patient cannot tolerate an ACE inhibitor, while nitrates without hydralazine are selected for relief of pulmonary edema or to improve exercise time.[26]

Nitrate tolerance remains a problem. Intermittent dosing, designed to counter periods of expected dyspnea (at night, anticipated exercise), is one sensible policy.[26] Escalating doses of nitrates provide only a short-term solution. A third policy is cotherapy with ACE inhibitors or hydralazine or both, to blunt nitrate tolerance. *Nitrate patches* have given variable results in CHF. Tolerance is inevitable with sustained-release patches, unless these are given intermittently, for example, 12 hours on and 12 hours off.[26]

ACUTE PULMONARY EDEMA

In acute pulmonary edema from various causes, including AMI, nitroglycerin can be strikingly effective, with some risk of precipitous falls in blood pressure and of tachycardia or bradycardia. Sublingual nitroglycerin in repeated doses of 0.8 to 2.4 mg every 5 to 10 minutes can relieve dyspnea within 15 to 20 minutes, with a fall of LV filling pressure and a rise in cardiac output.[27] Intravenous nitroglycerin, however, is usually a better method to administer nitroglycerin, as the dose can be rapidly adjusted upward or downward depending on the clinical and hemodynamic response. Doses required may be higher than the maximal use for AMI (i.e., above 200 µg/minute).[24]

NITRATE TOLERANCE

Nitrate tolerance often limits nitrate efficacy. Thus, longer acting nitrates, although providing higher and better sustained blood nitrate levels, paradoxically often seem to lose their efficacy with time. This is the phenomenon of nitrate tolerance (Fig. 2-4). The major current hypotheses are as follows:

1. *Impaired bioconversion of nitrates to active form.* The donor nitrate compound undergoes intracellular transformation to the active NO* moiety that stimulates guanylate cyclase to produce vasodilatory cyclic GMP (Fig. 2-2). An early step in this process is the formation of 1,2-glyceryl dinitrate, under the influence of the mitochondrial enzyme aldehyde dehydrogenase.[28] This enzyme is hypothesized to function poorly in nitrate tolerance,[29] a defect that is associated with increased production of free radicals.[30]
2. *Free radical hypothesis.* Excess nitrate administration can lead to formation of superoxide by the endothelium, which in turn produces toxic superoxide and peroxynitrite,[29] the latter having multiple adverse effects, including inhibition of guanylyl cyclase with decreased formation of vasodilatory cyclic GMP (Fig. 2-3), impaired endothelial function,[29] and decreased activity of aldehyde dehydrogenase.[30] A further twist to the free radical hypothesis lies in the multiple sources of the free radicals, including increased

NITRATE TOLERANCE

Opie 2004

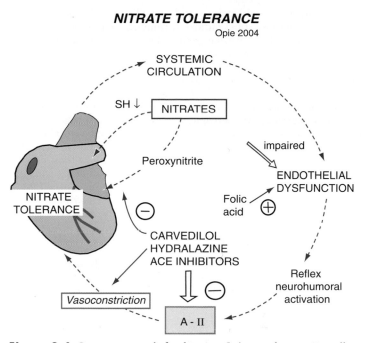

Figure 2-4 Current proposals for therapy of nitrate tolerance. For cellular mechanisms of peroxynitrite, see Fig. 2-3. Carvedilol, vitamin C, and hydralazine may all lessen free radical formation. ACE inhibitors oppose the neurohumoral activation that is thought to occur as a result of nitrate-induced vasodilation, possibly involving reflex arterial constriction and impaired renal blood flow. The SH depletion hypothesis (see Fig. 2-3), which gives a specific role for captopril, is relatively out of favor. (*Figure © LH Opie, 2005.*)

mitochondrial production of superoxide, an added pointer to a prominent role for mitochondrial dysfunction in nitrate tolerance.[30] The free radical hypothesis would explain why nitrate tolerance can be lessened by concurrent therapy by vitamin C[31,32] or hydralazine.[33]

3. *Vascular sulfhydryl depletion.* This classic hypothesis now seems outdated yet still merits consideration. The proposal is that the intracellular formation of NO• requires SH groups, derived from cysteine. Hypothetically, excess NO• formation depletes intracellular SH groups. Sulfhydryl donors, such as *acetylcysteine* or *methionine*, may counteract tolerance by providing SH groups. In unstable angina, *N*-acetylcysteine added to transdermal nitroglycerin reduced the probability of adverse outcome events over 4 months, but the severe headaches rendered the strategy impractical.[34]

4. *Neurohumoral hypothesis.* Marked venous dilation induced by nitrates could cause a reflex arterial vasoconstriction, with a reduction in renal perfusion and renin-angiotensin activation. Increased activity of angiotensin-II on the vascular wall may lead to increased formation of vasoconstrictive free radicals via the enzyme NAPDH.[30,35] Angiotensin-II blockade lessens tolerance and superoxide production[35] and in some clinical studies there is lessening of nitrate tolerance by simultaneous use of ACE inhibitors.

Prevention of Nitrate Tolerance

In effort angina, many studies now show that tolerance can be avoided by interval dosing. Eccentric twice daily doses of isosorbide mononitrate (Monoket, Ismo) or once daily treatment with 120 or 240 mg of the extended-release formulation of mononitrate (Imdur) prevents tolerance. Of the possible drug therapies, hydralazine is logical, especially in CHF, because (1) there are trial data favoring the nitrate-hydrazine combination; and (2) the hydralazine may over-come the impact of free radical formation. Addition of an ACE inhibitor is logical (see earlier section) but sometimes disappointing. Folic acid supplementation seems a simple procedure, and is thought to lead to improved function of nitric oxide synthase.[36] Likewise supplemental L-arginine is proposed as a "normalizer" of the activity of nitric oxide synthase.[37] Vitamin C should help,[31,32] is easy to obtain and without side effects. Rapidly increasing blood nitrate levels may overcome tolerance. For example, with established nitrate tolerance, sublingual nitrate can still have some therapeutic effect albeit diminished. Likewise, during treatment of unstable angina or CHF, dose escalation may be a short-term maneuver to minimize tolerance. Overall, present data do not give assurance that cotherapy with ACE inhibitors, carvedilol, hydralazine, folic acid, L-arginine, or vitamin C can prevent tolerance, although each may help the individual patient. Rather only the nitrate-free or -low interval works consistently.

Nitrate Cross-Tolerance

Short- and long-acting nitrates are frequently combined. In patients already receiving isosorbide dinitrate, addition of sublingual nitro-glycerin may give a further therapeutic effect, albeit diminished. Log-ically, as discussed in previous editions of this book, tolerance to long-acting nitrates should also cause cross-tolerance to short-acting nitrates, as shown for the capacitance vessels of the forearm, coronary artery diameter, and on exercise tolerance during intravenous nitro-glycerin therapy.

STEP-CARE FOR ANGINA OF EFFORT

A full history and physical examination is required to exclude a host of remediable factors (Table 2-4), not forgetting aortic stenosis that may be occult in the elderly. Risk factors must be managed and aspirin given. Nitrates remain the basis of symptomatic control of angina. Various combinations of short- and long-acting nitrates with β-blockers and/or calcium blockers are the successive choices. Percuta-neous intervention (PCI), now often with insertion of drug-eluting stents and bypass surgery, is increasingly taken as an escape route when coronary anatomy is appropriate. There are no long-term studies on the safety of nitrates alone in angina pectoris (see p. 47).

COMBINATION THERAPY FOR ANGINA

Existing data are inadequate to evaluate the overall efficacy of the com-bination of nitrates plus β-blockers or calcium blockers, when com-pared with optimal therapy using any one agent alone.

β-*Blockade and nitrates* are, nonetheless, usually combined in the therapy of angina (Table 2-4). Both β-blockers and nitrates decrease the oxygen demand, and nitrates increase the oxygen supply; β-blockers block the tachycardia caused by nitrates. β-Blockade tends to increase heart size, and nitrates tend to decrease it.

Calcium channel blockers (CCBs) and short-acting nitroglycerin are com-monly combined. In a double-blind trial of 47 patients with effort angina, 80 mg of verapamil three times daily decreased the use of nitroglycerin tablets by 25% and prolonged exercise time by 20%.[38]

CCBs and long-acting nitrates are also often given together. Yet there are no studies evaluating the objective benefits of current eccentric dosing schedules of long-acting nitrates plus CCBs. Long-acting nitrates are more readily combined with verapamil or diltiazem rather than with dihydropyridines (see Fig. 3-6), because of the powerful and sometimes excessive pre- and afterload reduction achieved by the latter combination. In contrast, dihydropyridines combine better with β-blockers.

Nitrates, β-blockers, and calcium antagonists may also be combined as triple therapy, frequently deemed to be "maximal." However, triple therapy may be no more effective or even less effective than any two of the components, possibly because of excess hypotension. Thus triple therapy should not be automatic when dual therapy fails because of individual variations among patients, as some will tolerate one type of combination therapy better than another. Thus various combinations of dual therapy should first be explored.

The ACTION study is a very large outcome study of the effects of addition of long-acting nifedipine (Adalat XL) to preexisting antianginal therapy, mostly β-blockers and nitrates. It is due at the European Society of Cardiology in September, 2004. It may revive interest in triple therapy and also prove that the CCB used is cardioprotective.

NEWER ANTIANGINAL AGENTS

Nicorandil (not licensed in the United States) is a nicotinamide nitrate, acting chiefly by dilation of the large coronary arteries, as well as by reduction of pre- and afterload. It has a double cellular mechanism of action, acting both as a potassium channel activator and having a nitrate-like effect, which may explain why experimentally it causes less tolerance than nitrates. It is widely used as an antianginal agent in Japan. In the IONA study, 5126 patients with stable angina were followed for a mean of 1.6 years. Major coronary events including acute coronary syndromes were reduced.[39]

Ranolazine (*under investigation in the United States and elsewhere*) is a metabolically active antianginal, thought to act by inhibition of oxygen-wasting fatty acid metabolism, thereby increasing the metabolism of protective glucose.[40]

Trimetazidine, available in some European countries but not in the United States and United Kingdom, has a similar mode of action. An interesting proposal is that, because it acts independently of any blood pressure reduction, it could be used as an antianginal in place of nitrates to allow free use of Viagra and similar agents.

Ivabradine, an inhibitor of the sinus node pacemaking current I_f, owes its antianginal properties to heart rate reduction. The proposal is that this specific effect is antianginal without the defects of β-blocker therapy such as depressed contractility and bronchoconstriction.

ARE NITRATES REALLY SAFE?

In contrast to the reasonable data for the safety of β-blockers and CCBs in effort angina,[41] logic would say that nitrate therapy that leads to excess production of free radicals, endothelial dysfunction, tachycardia, and renin-angiotensin activation may not be safe.[30] Analyses of two large databases showed that nitrate use was associated with increased mortality with hazard ratios of 1.6 and 3.8.[42] Such warnings do, however, have to be backed by prospective well-designed trials which are unlikely to be undertaken. Furthermore, there appear to be no data specifically on the mononitrates. At present the best policy may lie in combining mononitrate therapy with use of cardioprotective drugs such as aspirin, the ACE inhibitors and statins, as in the EUROPA study (see Chapter 5).

S U M M A R Y

1. *Mechanisms of action.* Nitrates act by venodilation and relief of coronary vasoconstriction (including that induced by exercise) to ameliorate anginal attacks. They are also arterial dilators, and reduce aortic systolic pressure. Their unloading effects also benefit patients with CHF with high LV filling pressures.

2. *Nitrates for effort angina.* Sublingual nitroglycerin remains the basic therapy, usually combined with a β-blocker or a CCB. As the duration of action lasts for minutes, nitrate tolerance is unusual because of the relatively long nitrate-free intervals between attacks. Isosorbide dinitrate has a delayed onset of action owing to the need for hepatic transformation to active metabolites, yet the duration of action is longer than with nitroglycerin. Some newer nitrate preparations are not substantial advances over the old, especially the nitrate patches, which clearly predispose to tolerance by sustained blood nitrate levels. By contrast, mononitrates are an advance over dinitrates because they eliminate variable hepatic metabolism on which the action of the dinitrates depends, and because the dose schedules required to avoid tolerance have been well studied. The longer the duration of nitrate action, the more tolerance is likely to develop, thus it effectively turns into a balancing act between duration of action and avoidance of tolerance.

3. *For unstable angina at rest,* a nitrate-free interval is not possible, and short-term treatment for 24 to 48 hours with intravenous nitroglycerin is frequently effective with, however, escalating doses often required to overcome tolerance.

4. *In early phase AMI,* the use of intravenous nitrates for selected and more ill patients must be differentiated from the failure of fixed dose nitrates in large trials. We suggest that intravenous nitrates be specifically reserved for more complicated patients.

5. *During the treatment of CHF,* tolerance also develops, so that nitrates are best reserved for specific problems such as acute LV failure, nocturnal dyspnea, or anticipated exercise.

6. *Acute pulmonary edema.* Nitrates are an important part of the overall therapy, acting chiefly by preload reduction.

7. *Nitrate tolerance.* The current understanding of the mechanism tolerance focuses on free radical formation (superoxide and peroxynitrite) with impaired bioconversion of nitrate to active nitric oxide. During the treatment of effort angina by isosorbide dinitrate or mononitrate, substantial evidence suggests that eccentric doses with a nitrate-free interval largely avoid tolerance. Other less well-tested measures include administration of folic acid.

8. *Serious interaction with Viagra-like agents.* Nitrates can interact very adversely with such agents, now often used to alleviate erectile dysfunction. The latter is common in those with cardiovascular disease, being a manifestation of endothelial dysfunction. The coadministration of these PDE-5 inhibitors with nitrates is therefore contraindicated. Every male presenting with acute coronary syndrome should be questioned about recent use of these agents (trade names: Viagra, Levitra, or Cialis). If so, there has to be an interval of 24 to 48 hours (the longer interval for Cialis) before nitrates can be given therapeutically if essential with reasonable safety but still with great care.

R E F E R E N C E S

1. Brunton TL. On the use of nitrite of amyl in angina pectoris. *Lancet* 1867;II:97–98.
2. Parker JD. Therapy with nitrates: increasing evidence of vascular toxicity. *J Am Coll Cardiol* 2003;42:1835–1837.
3. Ignarro LJ, et al. Nitric oxide donors and cardiovascular agents modulating the bioactivity of nitric oxide: an overview. *Circ Res* 2002;90:21–28.
4. Harrison DG, et al. The nitrovasodilators. New ideas about old drugs. *Circulation* 1993;87:1461–1467.
5. Kelly RP, et al. Nitroglycerin has more favourable effects on left ventricular afterload than apparent from measurement of pressure in a peripheral artery. *Eur Heart J* 1990;11:138–144.
6. Noll G, et al. Differential effects of captopril and nitrates on muscle sympathetic nerve activity in volunteers. *Circulation* 1997;95:2286–2292.
7. Chirkov YY, et al. Nitrate resistance in platelets from patients with stable angina pectoris. *Circulation* 1999;100:129–134.

8. Bogaert MG. Clinical pharmacokinetics of nitrates. *Cardiovasc Drugs Ther* 1994; 8:693–699.

9. Abrams J. How to use nitrates. *Cardiovasc Drugs Ther* 2002;16:511–514.

10. Bruce RA, et al. Excessive reduction in peripheral resistance during exercise and risk of orthostatic symptoms with sustained-release nitroglycerin and diltiazem treatment of angina. *Am Heart J* 1985;109:1020–1026.

11. Kaiser DR, et al. Impaired brachial artery endothelium-dependent and -independent vasodilation in men with erectile dysfunction and no other clinical cardiovascular disease. *J Am Coll Cardiol* 2004;43:179–184.

12. Kloner RA, et al. Time course of the interaction between tadalafil and nitrates. *J Am Coll Cardiol* 2003;42:1855–1860.

13. Koh KK, et al. Interaction of intravenous heparin and organic nitrates in acute ischemic syndromes. *Am J Cardiol* 1995;76:706–709.

14. Gogia H, et al. Prevention of tolerance to hemodynamic effects of nitrates with concomitant use of hydralazine in patients with chronic heart failure. *J Am Cardiol* 1995;26:1575–1580.

15. Ducharme A, et al. Comparison of nitroglycerin lingual spray and sublingual tablet on time of onset and duration of brachial artery vasodilation in normal subjects. *Am J Cardiol* 1999;84:952–954.

16. Thadani U, et al. Oral isosorbide dinitrate in angina pectoris: comparison of duration of action an dose-response relation during acute and sustained therapy. *Am J Cardiol* 1982;49:411–419.

17. Thadani U, et al. Short and long-acting oral nitrates for stable angina pectoris. *Cardiovasc Drugs Ther* 1994;8:611–623.

18. Parker JO. Eccentric dosing with isosorbide-5-mononitrate in angina pectoris. *Am J Cardiol* 1993;72:871–876.

19. Chrysant SG, et al. Efficacy and safety of extended-release isosorbide mononitrate for stable effort angina pectoris. *Am J Cardiol* 1993;72:1249–1256.

20. Transdermal Nitroglycerin Cooperative Study. Acute and chronic antianginal efficacy of continuous twenty-four-hour application of transdermal nitroglycerin. *Am J Cardiol* 1991;68:1263–1273.

21. Holdright DR, et al. Lack of rebound during intermittent transdermal treatment with glyceryl trinitrate in patients with stable angina on background beta blocker. *Br Heart J* 1993;69:223–227.

22. Reichek N. Intermittent nitrate therapy in angina pectoris. *Eur Heart J* 1989;10 (Suppl A):7–10.

23. GISSI-3 Study Group. GISSI-3: effects of lisinopril and transdermal glyceryl trinitrate singly and together on 6-week mortality and ventricular function after acute myocardial infarction. *Lancet* 1994;343:1115–1122.

24. Jugdutt BI. Nitrates in myocardial infarction. *Cardiovasc Drugs Ther* 1994;8:635–646.

25. V-HeFT II Study. A comparison of enalapril with hydralazine-isosorbide dinitrate in the treatment of chronic congestive cardiac failure. *N Engl J Med* 1991;325:303–310.

26. Elkayam U, et al. Double-blind, placebo-controlled study to evaluate the effect of organic nitrates in patients with chronic heart failure treated with angiotensin-converting enzyme inhibition. *Circulation* 1999;99:2652–2657.

27. Bussmann WD, et al. [Effect of sublingual nitroglycerin in emergency treatment of classic pulmonary edema]. *Minerva Cardioangiol* 1978;26:623–632.

28. Chen Z, et al. Identification of the enzymatic mechanism of nitroglycerin bioactivation. *Proc Natl Acad Sci USA* 2002;99:8306–8311.

29. Horowitz JD. Amelioration of nitrate tolerance: matching strategies with mechanisms. *J Am Coll Cardiol* 2003;41:2001–2003.

30. Parker JD. Nitrate tolerance, oxidative stress, and mitochondrial function: another worrisome chapter on the effects of organic nitrates. *J Clin Invest* 2004;113:352–354.

31. Fleming JW, et al. Muscarinic cholinergic-receptor stimulation of specific GTP hydrolysis related to adenylate cyclase activity in canine cardiac sarcolemma. *Circ Res* 1988;64:340–350.

32. Fink B, et al. Tolerance to nitrates with enhanced radical formation suppressed by carvedilol. *J Cardiovasc Pharmacol* 1999;34:800–805.

33. Münzel T, et al. Hydralazine prevents nitroglycerin tolerance by inhibiting activation of a membrane-bound NADH oxidase. *J Clin Invest* 1996;98:1465–1470.

34. Ardissino D, et al. Effect of transdermal nitroglycerin on N-acetylcysteine, or both, in the long-term treatment of unstable angina pectoris. *J Am Coll Cardiol* 1997;29:941–947.

35. Kurz S, et al. Evidence for a casual role of the renin-angiotensin system in nitrate tolerance. *Circulation* 1999;99:3181–3187.

36. Gori T, et al. Folic acid prevents nitroglycerin-induced nitric oxide synthase dysfunction and nitrate tolerance. *Circulation* 2001;104:1119–1123.

37. Parker JO, et al. The effect of supplemental L-arginine on tolerance development during continuous transdermal nitroglycerin therapy. *J Am Coll Cardiol* 2002;39:1199–1203.

38. Andreasen F, et al. Assessment of verapamil in the treatment of angina pectoris. *Eur J Cardiol* 1975;2:443–452.

39. IONA Study Group. Effect of nicorandil on coronary events in patients with stable angina: the Impact Of Nicorandil in Angina (IONA) Randomized Trial. *Lancet* 2002;359:1269–1275.

40. Chaitman BR, et al. Effects of ranolazine with atenolol, amlodipine, or diltiazem on exercise tolerance and angina frequency in patients with severe chronic angina: a randomized controlled trial. *JAMA* 2004;291:309–316.

41. Heidenreich PA, et al. Meta-analysis of trials comparing β-blockers, calcium antagonists, and nitrates for stable angina. *JAMA* 1999;281:1927–1936.

42. Nakamura Y, et al. Long-term nitrate use may be deleterious in ischemic heart disease: a study using the databases from two large-scale postinfarction studies. *Am Heart J* 1999;138:577–585.

3
Calcium Channel Blockers (Calcium Antagonists)

Lionel H. Opie

"Calcium antagonists have assumed a major role in the treatment of patients with hypertension or coronary heart disease."

ABERNETHY AND SCHWARTZ, 1999[1]

"There are none of the widely trumpeted dangers from dihydropyridine calcium channel blockers."

KAPLAN, 2003, COMMENTING ON THE RESULTS OF ALLHAT[2]

Calcium channel blockers (CCBs; calcium antagonists) act chiefly by vasodilation and reduction of the peripheral vascular resistance. They remain among the most commonly used agents for hypertension and angina. Their true place in these conditions is now well understood, based on the results of a series of large trials. CCBs are a heterogeneous group of drugs that can chemically be classified into the dihydropyridines (DHPs) and the non-DHPs (Table 3-1) their common pharmacologic property being selective inhibition of L-channel opening in vascular smooth muscle and in the myocardium (Fig. 3-1). Distinctions between the DHPs and non-DHPs are reflected in different binding sites on the calcium channel pores, and in the greater vascular selectivity of the DHP agents.[3] In addition, the non-DHPs by virtue of nodal inhibition are used in certain supraventricular arrhythmias, and tend to reduce the heart rate (heart rate-lowering agents, HRL). These agents, verapamil and diltiazem, more closely resemble the β-blockers in their therapeutic spectrum.

PHARMACOLOGIC PROPERTIES

Calcium Channels: L- and T-types

The most important property of all CCBs is selectively to inhibit the inward flow of charge-bearing calcium ions when the calcium channel becomes permeable or is "open." Previously, the term "slow channel" was used, but now it is realized that the calcium current travels much faster than previously believed, and that there are at least two types of calcium channels, the L and the T. The conventional long-lasting opening calcium channel is termed the L-channel, which is blocked by CCBs and increased in activity by catecholamines. The function of the L-type is to admit the substantial amount of calcium ions required for initiation of contraction via calcium-induced calcium release from the sarcoplasmic reticulum (Fig. 3-1). The T-type (T for transient) channel opens at more negative potentials than the L-type and probably plays an important role in the initial depolarization of sinus and atrioventricular (AV) nodal tissue. It is also relatively upregulated in the failing myocardium. A specific blocker for T-type calcium channels, mibefradil, was withdrawn when a large number of serious adverse hepatic interactions were discovered.

Cellular Mechanisms: β-Blockade versus CCBs

Both these categories of agents are used for angina and hypertension, yet there are important differences in their subcellular mode of action.

Table 3-1 Binding Sites for CCBs, Tissue Specificity, Clinical Uses, and Safety Concerns

Site	Tissue Specificity	Clinical Uses	Contraindications	Safety Concerns
DHP Binding				
Prototype: nifedipine site 1	Vessels > Myocardium > nodes *Vascular selectivity* 10× N, Nifedipine; A, amlodipine; 100× Nic, Nicardipine; 100× isradipine (I); 100× felodipine (F); 1000× Nis, Nisoldipine	Effort angina (N, A) Hypertension (N*, A, Nic, I, F, Nis) Vasospastic angina (N, A) Raynaud's phenomenon	Unstable angina, early phase AMI, systolic heart failure (possible exception: amlodipine)	*Nifedipine capsules*: excess BP fall especially in elderly; adrenergic activation in acute coronary syndromes (ACS) *Longer acting forms*: Safe in hypertension, no studies on ACS
Non-DHP Binding				
"Heart rate lowering" Site 1B, D, diltiazem Site 1C, V, verapamil	SA and AV nodes > myocardium = vessels	Angina: effort (V, D), unstable (V), vasospastic (V, D); Hypertension (D*, V); Arrhythmias; supra-ventricular (D†, V); Verapamil: postinfarct patients (no USA license).	Systolic heart failure; sinus bradycardia or SSS; AV nodal block; WPW syndrome. Acute myocardial infarction (early phase)	Systolic heart failure, especially diltiazem. Safety record of verapamil may equal that of β-blockade in elderly hypertensive patients[18]; also see ref. 25.

US FDA-approved drugs for listed indications in parentheses.
*Long-acting forms only.
†Intravenous forms only.
AV = atrioventricular; DHP = dihydropyridine; SA = sinoatrial; SSS = sick sinus syndrome; WPW = Wolff-Parkinson-White.

51

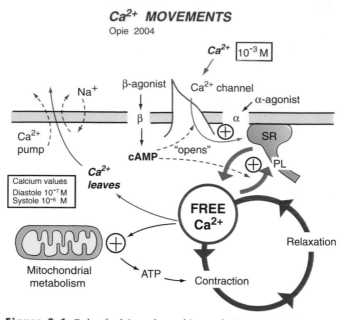

Figure 3-1 Role of calcium channel in regulating myocardial cytosolic calcium ion movements. α = α-adrenergic receptor; β = β-adrenergic receptor; *cAMP* = cyclic AMP; *PL* = phospholamban; *SR* = sarcoplasmic reticulum. (*Figure © LH Opie, 2005.*)

Both have a negative inotropic effect, whereas only CCBs relax vascular and (to a much lesser extent) other smooth muscle (Fig. 3-2). CCBs "block" the entry of calcium through the calcium channel in both smooth muscle and myocardium, so that less calcium is available to the contractile apparatus. The result is vasodilation and a negative inotropic effect, which in the case of the DHPs is usually modest due to the unloading effect of peripheral vasodilation.

β-blockade has contrasting effects on smooth muscle and on the myocardium. Whereas β-blockade tends to promote smooth muscle contraction, it impairs myocardial contraction. A fundamental difference lies in the regulation of the contractile mechanism by calcium ions in these two tissues. In the myocardium, calcium ions interact with troponin C to allow actin-myosin interaction; β-stimulation enhances the entry of calcium ions and the rate of their uptake into the sarcoplasmic reticulum, so that calcium ion levels rise and fall more rapidly. Hence both contraction and relaxation are speeded up as cyclic AMP forms under β-stimulation (see Fig. 1-2). Furthermore, a higher cytosolic calcium ion concentration at the time of systole means that the peak force of contraction is enhanced. β-Blockade opposes all these effects, and has a consistent and major inhibitory effect on the sinus and AV nodes (see Fig 1-4).

CCBs Inhibit Vascular Contraction In smooth muscle (Fig. 3-2), calcium ions regulate the contractile mechanism independently of troponin C. Interaction of calcium with calmodulin forms calcium-calmodulin, which then stimulates myosin light chain kinase (MLCK) to phosphorylate the myosin light chains to allow actin-myosin interaction and, hence, contraction. Cyclic AMP inhibits the MLCK. β-Blockade, by lessening the formation of cyclic AMP, removes the inhibition on MLCK activity and, therefore, promotes contraction in smooth muscle, which explains why asthma may be precipitated, and why the peripheral vascular resistance often rises at the start of β-blocker therapy (Fig. 3-3).

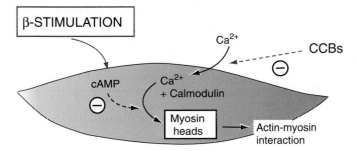

SMOOTH MUSCLE
beta-blockade promotes contraction

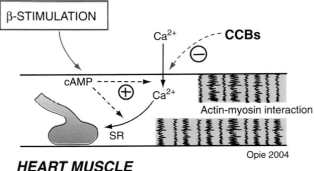

HEART MUSCLE
beta-blockade inhibits contraction

Figure 3-2 Proposed comparative effects of β-blockade and calcium channel blockers (CCBs) on smooth muscle and myocardium. The opposing effects on vascular smooth muscle are of critical therapeutic importance. *SR* = sarcoplasmic reticulum. (*Figure © LH Opie, 2005.*)

CCBs and Vascular Protection Experimentally, both nifedipine and amlodipine give endothelial protection and promote formation of nitric oxide. Furthermore, several CCBs including amlodipine, nifedipine, and lacidipine have inhibitory effects on carotid atheromatous disease.[4,5] Similar protective effects have not consistently been found with β-blockers. However, we don't yet know that such vascular protection leads to improved clinical outcomes.

CCBs versus β-Blockers: Hemodynamic and Neurohumoral Differences Hemodynamic differences are well defined (Fig. 3-3). Whereas β-blockers inhibit the renin-angiotensin system by decreasing renin release and oppose the hyperadrenergic state in heart failure, CCBs as a group have no such inhibitory effects.[6] This difference could explain why β-blockers but not CCBs are an important component of the therapy of heart failure. Of interest, new N-type CCBs that block neuronal channels with the aim of suppressing sympathetic activity are under test in Japan.

CLASSIFICATION OF CALCIUM CHANNEL BLOCKERS

Dihydropyridines

The dihydropyridines (DHPs) all bind to the same sites on the α_1-subunit (the N sites), thereby establishing their common property of calcium channel antagonism (Fig. 3-4). To a different degree, they exert a greater inhibitory effect on vascular smooth muscle than on the myocardium, conferring the property of vascular selectivity (Table

HEMODYNAMICS: β-BLOCKERS VS CCBs

Opie 2004

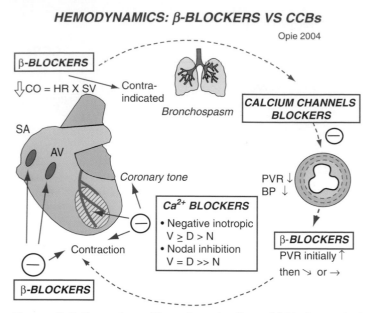

Figure 3-3 Comparison of hemodynamic effects of β-blockers and of CCBs, showing possibilities for combination therapy. *AV* = atrioventricular node; *BP* = blood pressure; *CO* = cardiac output; *D* = diltiazem; *HR* = heart rate; *N* = nifedipine as an example of dihydropyridines; *SA* = sinoatrial node; *SV* = stroke volume; *PVR* = peripheral vascular resistance; *V* = verapamil. (*Figure © LH Opie, 2005.*)

CALCIUM CHANNEL MODEL

Opie 2004

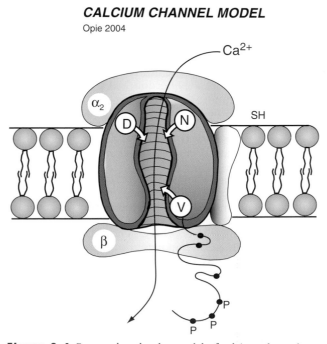

Figure 3-4 Proposed molecular model of calcium channel α_1-subunit with binding sites for nifedipine (*N*), diltiazem (*D*), and verapamil (*V*). It is thought that all DHPs bind to the same site as nifedipine. Amlodipine has additional subsidiary binding to the V and D sites. *P* indicates sites of phosphorylation in response to cAMP (Fig. 3-1), which acts to increase the opening probability of the calcium channel. (*Figure © LH Opie, 2005.*)

3-1, Fig. 3-5). There is nonetheless still the potential for myocardial depression, particularly in the case of agents with less selectivity and in the presence of prior myocardial disease and/or β-blockade. For practical purposes, effects on the sinoatrial (SA) and AV nodes can be ignored.

Nifedipine is the prototype of the DHPs. In the short-acting capsule form, originally available, it rapidly vasodilates to relieve severe hypertension and to terminate attacks of coronary spasm. The peripheral vasodilation and a rapid drop in blood pressure leads to rapid reflex adrenergic activation with tachycardia (Fig. 3-6). Such *proischemic effects* probably explain why the short-acting DHPs in high doses have precipitated serious adverse events in unstable angina. The inappropriate use of short-acting nifedipine can explain much of the adverse publicity that has surrounded the CCBs as a group,[7] so that the focus has now changed to the long-acting DHPs which are free of such dangers.[2]

Hence, the introduction of truly long-acting compounds, such as amlodipine or the extended-release formulations of nifedipine (GITS, XL, CC) and of others such as felodipine and isradipine, has led to substantially fewer symptomatic side effects. Two residual side effects of note are headache, as for all arteriolar dilators, and ankle edema, caused by precapillary dilation. There is now much greater attention to the appropriate use of the DHPs, with improved safety.[2]

Nondihydropyridines: Heart Rate–Lowering Agents

Verapamil and diltiazem bind to two different sites on the α_1-subunit of the calcium channel (Fig. 3-4), yet have many properties in common with each other. The first and most obvious distinction from the DHPs is that verapamil and diltiazem both act on nodal tissue, being therapeutically effective in supraventricular tachycardias. Both tend to decrease the sinus rate. Both inhibit myocardial contraction more than the DHPs or, put differently, are less vascular selective (Fig. 3-5). These properties, added to peripheral vasodilation, lead to substantial reduction in the myocardial oxygen demand. Such "oxygen conservation" makes the HRL agents much closer than the DHPs to the β-blockers, with whom they share a similar spectrum of

CARDIAC VS VASCULAR SELECTIVITY

Opie 2004

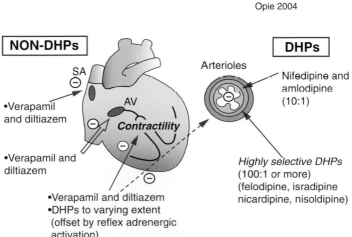

Figure 3-5 As a group, the DHPs (dihydropyridines) are more vascular selective, while the non-DHPs verapamil and diltiazem act equally on the heart and on the arterioles. (*Figure © LH Opie, 2005.*)

ISCHEMIC HEART: CCB EFFECT
Opie 2004

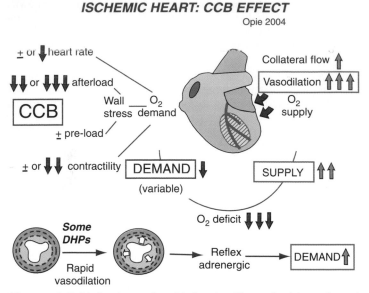

Figure 3-6 Mechanisms of anti-ischemic effects of calcium channel blockers. Note that the rapid arteriolar vasodilation resulting from the action of some short-acting dihydropyridines (*DHPs*) may increase myocardial oxygen demand by reflex adrenergic stimulation. (*Figure © LH Opie, 2005.*)

therapeutic activity. Two important exceptions are (1) the almost total lack of effect of verapamil and diltiazem on standard types of ventricular tachycardia, which rather is a contraindication to their use; and (2) the benefits of β-blockade in heart failure, in which the HRL agents are also clearly contraindicated. The salient features for the clinical use of these agents are shown in Table 3-2.

For *supraventricular tachycardias*, a frequency-dependent effect is important, so that there is better access to the binding sites of the AV node when the calcium channel pore is "open." During nodal reentry tachycardia, the channel of the AV node opens more frequently; the drug binds better and hence specifically inhibits the AV node to stop the reentry path.

Regarding side effects, the non-DHPs, being less active on vascular smooth muscle, also have less vasodilatory side effects than the DHPs, with less flushing or headaches or pedal edema (see later, Table 3-4). Reflex tachycardia is uncommon because of the inhibitory effects on the SA node. Left ventricular depression remains the major potential side effect, especially in patients with preexisting congestive heart failure (CHF). Why constipation occurs only with verapamil of all the CCBs is not known.

MAJOR INDICATIONS FOR CCBs

Effort Angina

Common to the effects of all types of CCBs is the inhibition of the L-calcium current in arterial smooth muscle, occurring at relatively low concentrations. Hence coronary vasodilation is a major common property (Fig. 3-3). Although the antianginal mechanisms are many and varied, the shared effects are (1) coronary vasodilation and relief of exercise-induced vasoconstriction, and (2) afterload reduction due to blood pressure reduction (Fig. 3-6). In addition, in the case of verapamil and diltiazem, slowing of the sinus node with a decrease in exercise heart rate and a negative inotropic effect also contribute (Fig. 3-7).

Table 3-2 Oral Heart Rate–Lowering CCBs; Salient Features for Cardiovascular Use

Agent	Dose	Pharmacokinetics and Metabolism	Side Effects and Contraindications	Kinetic and Dynamic Interactions
Verapamil				
Tablets (for IV use, see Table 8-2, p. 220)	180–480 mg daily in 2 or 3 doses (titrated)	Peak plasma levels within 1–3 h. Low bioavailability (10%–20%), high first-pass metabolism to long-acting norverapamil. Excretion: 75% renal, 25% GI. $t^{1}/_{2}$ 3–7 h	Constipation. C/I sick sinus syndrome, digoxin toxicity, excess β-blockade, IV failure. Obstructive cardiomyopathy. Levels ↑ in liver or renal disease.	Digoxin levels increase. Depression of SA, AV nodes and myocardium. SSS = care. Cardiodepressant drugs: β-blockers, disopyramide, flecainide. Liver metabolism, see text for interactions.
Slow release (SR) Verelan (Ver) Covera-HS (timed)	As above, 2 doses (SR) Single dose (Ver) Single bedtime dose	Peak effect 1–2 h (SR); 7–9 h (Ver). $t^{1}/_{2}$ 5–12 h; 12 h (Ver) Delayed 4–6 h release (Co)	As above	As above
Diltiazem				
Tablets (for IV use see Table 8-2, p. 221)	120–360 mg daily in 3 or 4 doses	Onset: 15–30 min. Peak: 1–2 h. $t^{1}/_{2}$ 5 h. Bioavailable: ≈45% (hepatic). Active metabolites. 65% GI loss	As for verapamil but no constipation	As for verapamil, except little/no effect on digoxin levels; liver interactions not so prominent. Cimetidine and liver disease increase blood levels. Propranolol levels ↑.
Prolonged SR, CD, XR Tiazac	As above, 1 (XR, CD, Tiazac) or 2 doses	Slower onset, longer $t^{1}/_{2}$, otherwise similar.	As above	As above

AV = atrioventricular; SA = sinoatrial; SSS = sick sinus syndrome; $t^{1}/_{2}$ = plasma elimination half-life.

VERAPAMIL or DILTIAZEM MULTIPLE EFFECTS
Opie 2004

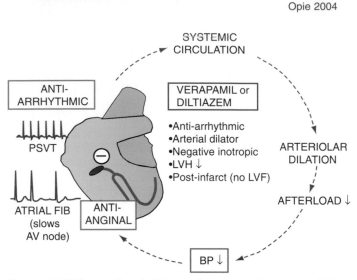

Figure 3-7 Verapamil and diltiazem have a broad spectrum of therapeutic effects. *Atrial fib* = atrial fibrillation; *LVF* = left ventricular failure; *LVH* = left ventricular hypertrophy; *PSVT* = paroxysmal supraventricular tachycardia. (*Figure © LH Opie, 2005.*)

Unstable Angina at Rest

Of the major CCBs, only verapamil has a license for unstable angina, although intravenous diltiazem has one good supporting study.[8] It must again be emphasized that the DHPs should not be used without concurrent β-blockade (risk of reflex adrenergic activation; see Fig. 3-6).

Coronary Spasm

The role of spasm as a major cause of the anginal syndromes has undergone revision. Once seen as a major contributor to transient ischemic pain at rest, coronary spasm is now relatively discounted because β-blockade was more effective than nifedipine in several studies.[9] The role of coronary spasm in unstable preinfarction angina has also been downplayed because nifedipine, in the absence of concurrent β-blockade, appeared to be harmful.[10] Coronary spasm remains important as a cause of angina precipitated by cold or hyperventilation, and in Prinzmetal's variant angina. All CCBs should be effective. Among those specifically licensed are verapamil and amlodipine.

Hypertension

CCBs are excellent antihypertensive agents, especially and among the best for elderly and black patients (see Chapter 7). Their effect is largely independent of sodium intake or of the concurrent use of anti-inflammatory agents such as nonsteroidal anti-inflammatory drugs (NSAIDs). The DHPs are recommended (among others) as favored agents by the European guidelines for the following groups of hypertensive cases: elderly patients, isolated systolic hypertension, angina pectoris, peripheral vascular disease, carotid atherosclerosis, and pregnancy.[11] The non-DHPs are favored for angina pectoris, carotid atherosclerosis, and supraventricular tachycardia. CHF is a contraindication only to the non-DHPs. The current American recommendations list only two "compelling indications" without separating DHPs and non-DHPs: high coronary risk patients and diabetes.[12] The most recent and largest meta-analysis finds as follows.[13] Compared with placebo, they reduce stroke, coronary heart disease, major cardiovascular events, and cardiovascular death. Compared with diuretics/β-blockade, there is the same total and cardiovascular-related mortality, and unchanged coronary heart disease. However, heart failure is increased, and stroke is borderline decreased.[13]

In hypertension with nephropathy, both DHPs and non-DHPs reduce the blood pressure, the primary aim, but non-DHPs reduce proteinuria better.[18]

Supraventricular Tachycardia

Verapamil and diltiazem inhibit the AV node, which explains their effect in supraventricular tachycardias. Nifedipine and other DHPs are clinically ineffective.

Postinfarct Protection

Although β-blockers remain the drugs of choice, both verapamil and diltiazem give some protection in the absence of prior left ventricular failure. Verapamil is better documented.[14,15] Data are lacking for DHPs.

Vascular Protection

Increased nitric oxide formation in cultured endothelial cells[16] and improved endothelial function in patients[17] may explain why CCBs slow down carotid atherosclerosis,[11] which in turn may be linked to decreased stroke found in several clinical studies. Whether coronary disease is limited, as suggested by early studies, is under investigation in the continuing arm of the ENCORE study[17] and in the forthcoming ACTION study (see p. 73).

SAFETY AND EFFICACY

The ideal cardiovascular drug is both efficacious in reducing hard endpoints, such as mortality, stroke, and myocardial infarction, and safe. Safety, not generally well defined, may be regarded as the absence of significant adverse effects when the drug is used with due regard for its known contraindications. In the case of CCBs, previous controversy regarding both efficacy and safety has been laid to rest by new studies that support the safety of long-acting CCBs, particularly in hypertension with coronary heart disease as end-point.[13] (Also see Table 3-6.)

A review of 100 reports leads to the following conclusions.[3] A distinction can be made between observational studies, including case control and cohort studies, and randomized controlled trials (RCTs). For example, observational data from a large British clinic suggest that angiotensin-converting enzyme (ACE) inhibitors are better able to reduce mortality in hypertensives than are CCBs.[19] But this hypothesis could not be confirmed in a large adequately powered RCT, the ALLHAT study, that found equal all-cause mortality when comparing amlodipine with lisinopril.[20] Here the RCT outweighs the observational study. The strongest evidence comes when experimental observations, observational studies, and RCTs all give concordant evidence, as when short-acting nifedipine is linked to poor outcomes in unstable angina. The proposed hypothesis for this adverse effect lies in abrupt vasodilation with reflex adrenergic activation[21] with increased risk of ischemia. By contrast, verapamil even in short-acting formulation gives much less adrenergic activation. This is important, because short-acting verapamil is widely available throughout the world as a relatively inexpensive generic drug that can now be classed as both safe and efficacious.

Safety in Ischemic Heart Disease and Hypertension

In stable effort angina, imperfect evidence based on RCTs and a meta-analysis suggests equivalent safety and efficacy of CCBs (other than short-acting nifedipine) to β-blockers. The largest trial, ACTION, due to be reported at the end of 2004, examines the effects of addition of long-acting nifedipine to existing therapy in effort angina. In unstable angina, a small trial supports the use of diltiazem.[8] There are no data to back the use of DHPs in unstable angina, and short-acting nifedipine remains totally contraindicated in the absence of β-blockade.[10] In postinfarct follow-up, β-blockers remain the agents of choice; with the non-DHP heart rate–lowering agents (especially verapamil) second choice if β-blockers are contraindicated or not tolerated. DHPs lack good evidence for safety and efficacy in post-MI patients.

In hypertension, four large outcome trials[4,22–24] show a reassuring efficacy and safety of longer acting DHPs (see later, Table 3-6). Amlodipine in ALLHAT exhibited the same outcomes regarding coronary heart disease and total mortality as did the diuretic, with, however, increased heart failure balanced by the decreased incidence of new diabetes.[20] A similar tit-for-tat balance was found in INSIGHT.[4] Verapamil-based therapy had effects on coronary disease similar to those of therapy based on atenolol in the INVEST trial, the primary end-points being all-cause deaths, nonfatal MI, or nonfatal stroke.[25] By the end of the study, to achieve the required blood pressure goals, combination therapy was required in most, so that the real comparison was between verapamil plus the ACE inhibitor trandolapril, and atenolol plus a thiazide. Verapamil and thiazide-based therapy were similar in the prematurely terminated and underpowered CONVINCE.[26] In *diabetic hypertensives* long-acting DHPs are also able to improve outcome.[24,27] In ALLHAT, amlodipine gave similar results in the diabetic and nondiabetic subgroups.[20] These findings make it difficult to agree with the view that CCBs have adverse effects in diabetic patients, in whom the major issue is adequate blood pressure reduction. In fact, diabetes may rather be a positive indication for preferential use of a CCB.[12] *Cancer, bleeding, and increased all-cause mortality, once proposed as serious and unexpected side effects of the CCBs, are now discounted.*[2,20]

VERAPAMIL

Verapamil (Isoptin, Calan, Verelan), the prototype non-DHP agent, remains the CCB that has the most licensed indications. Both verapamil and diltiazem have multiple cardiovascular effects (Fig. 3-7).

Electrophysiology Verapamil inhibits the action potential of the upper and middle regions of the AV node where depolarization is calcium mediated. Verapamil thus inhibits one limb of the reentry circuit, believed to underlie most paroxysmal supraventricular tachycardias (see Fig. 8-4). Increased AV block and the increase in effective refractory period of the AV node explain the reduction of the ventricular rate in atrial flutter and fibrillation. Verapamil is ineffective and harmful in the treatment of ventricular tachycardias except in certain uncommon forms. *Hemodynamically,* verapamil combines arteriolar dilation with a direct negative inotropic effect (Fig. 3-7). The cardiac output and left ventricular ejection fraction do not increase as expected following peripheral vasodilation, which may be an expression of the negative inotropic effect. At rest, the heart only drops modestly with a greater inhibition of exercise-induced tachycardia.

Pharmacokinetics and Interactions Oral verapamil tablets take 1–3 hours to act. Therapeutic blood levels (80 to 400 ng/ml) are seldom measured. The elimination half-life is usually 3 to 7 hours, but increases significantly during chronic administration and in patients with liver or advanced renal insufficiency. Despite nearly complete absorption of oral doses, bioavailability is only 10% to 20%. There is a high first-pass liver metabolism by multiple components of the P-450 system including CYP 3A4, the latter explaining why verapamil increases blood levels of several statins such as atorvastatin, simvastatin, and lovastatin, as well as ketoconazole. Ultimate excretion of the parent compound, as well as the active hepatic metabolite norverapamil, is 75% by the kidneys and 25% by the gastrointestinal (GI) tract. Verapamil is 87% to 93% protein bound, but no interaction with warfarin has been reported. When both verapamil and digoxin are given together, their interaction causes digoxin levels to rise, probably owing to a reduction in the renal clearance of digoxin (see p. 62). *Norverapamil* is the long-acting hepatic metabolite of verapamil, which appears rapidly in the plasma after oral administration of verapamil and in concentrations similar to those of the parent compound; like verapamil, norverapamil undergoes delayed clearance during chronic dosing.

Verapamil Doses The usual total oral daily dose is 180 to 360 mg daily, no more than 480 mg given once or twice daily (long-acting formulations) or three times daily for standard short-acting preparations (Table 3-2). Large differences of pharmacokinetics among individuals mean that dose titration is required, so that 120 mg daily may be adequate for those with hepatic impairment or for the elderly. During chronic oral dosing, the formation of norverapamil metabolites and altered rates of hepatic metabolism suggest that less frequent or smaller daily doses of short-acting verapamil may be used.[28] For example, if verapamil has been given at a dose of 80 mg three times daily, then 120 mg twice daily should be as good. Lower doses are required in elderly patients or in those with advanced renal or hepatic disease or when there is concurrent β-blockade. *Intravenous verapamil* is used much less often for supraventricular arrhythmias since the advent of adenosine and the ultra-short–acting β-blocker esmolol.

Slow-Release Preparations *Calan SR* or *Isoptin SR* releases the drug from a matrix at a rate that responds to food while *Verelan* releases the drug from a rate-controlling polymer at a rate not sensitive to food intake. The usual doses are 240 to 480 mg daily. The SR preparations are given once or twice daily and Verelan once daily. A controlled-onset extended-release formulation (*Covera-HS*; *COER-24*; 180 or 240 mg tablets) is taken once daily at bedtime, with the (unproven) aim of lessening adverse cardiovascular events early in the morning.

Side Effects Class side effects are those of vasodilation causing headaches, facial flushing, and dizziness. These may be lessened by the long-acting preparations, so that in practice they are often not troublesome. Tachycardia is not a side effect. Constipation is specific and causes the most trouble, especially in elderly patients. *Rare side effects* may include pain in the gums, facial pain, epigastric pain, hepatotoxicity, and transient mental confusion. In the elderly, verapamil may predispose to GI bleeding.[18]

Contraindications to Verapamil (Fig. 3-8, Table 3-3) Sick sinus syndrome; preexisting AV nodal disease; excess therapy with β-blockade, digitalis, quinidine, or disopyramide; or myocardial depression are all contraindications, especially in the intravenous therapy of supraventricular tachycardias. In the Wolff-Parkinson-White (WPW) syndrome complicated by atrial fibrillation, intravenous verapamil is contraindicated because of the risk of anterograde conduction through the bypass tract (see Fig. 8-2). Verapamil is also contraindicated in ventricular tachycardia (wide QRS-complex) because of excess myocardial depression, which may be lethal. An exception to this rule is exercise-induced ventricular tachycardia. Myocardial depression, if secondary to the supraventricular tachycardia, is not a contraindication, whereas preexisting left ventricular systolic failure is.

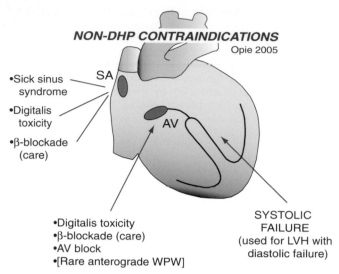

NON-DHP CONTRAINDICATIONS
Opie 2005

•Sick sinus syndrome
•Digitalis toxicity
•β-blockade (care)

SA

AV

•Digitalis toxicity
•β-blockade (care)
•AV block
•[Rare anterograde WPW]

SYSTOLIC FAILURE
(used for LVH with diastolic failure)

Figure 3-8 Contraindications to verapamil or diltiazem. For use of verapamil and diltiazem in patients already receiving β-blockers, see text. *AV* = atrioventricular node; *SA* = sinoatrial node; *WPW* = Wolff-Parkinson-White syndrome. (*Figure © LH Opie, 2005.*)

Dose reduction may be required in hepatic or renal disease (see Pharmacokinetics).

Drug Interactions with Verapamil

β-Blockers Verapamil by intravenous injection is now seldom given, so that the potentially serious interaction with preexisting β-adrenergic blockade is largely a matter of history. Depending on the dose and the state of the sinus node and the myocardium, the combination of oral verapamil with a β-blocker may be well tolerated or not. In practice, clinicians can often safely combine verapamil with β-blockade in the therapy of angina pectoris or hypertension, provided that due care is taken (monitoring for heart rate and heart block). In the elderly, prior nodal disease must be excluded. For hypertension, β-blocker plus verapamil works well, although heart rate, AV conduction, and LV function may sometimes be adversely affected. To avoid any hepatic pharmacokinetic interactions, verapamil is best combined with a hydrophilic β-blocker such as atenolol or nadolol, rather than one that is metabolized in the liver, such as metoprolol, propranolol, or carvedilol.

Digoxin Verapamil inhibits the digoxin transporter, P-glycoprotein, to increase blood digoxin levels, of special relevance when both are used chronically to inhibit AV nodal conduction. In digitalis toxicity, rapid intravenous verapamil is absolutely contraindicated because it can lethally exaggerate AV block. There is no reason why, in the absence of digitalis toxicity or AV block, oral verapamil and digitalis compounds should not be combined (checking the digoxin level). Whereas digoxin can be used for heart failure with atrial fibrillation, verapamil is negatively inotropic and should not be used.

Antiarrhythmics The combined negative inotropic potential of verapamil and *disopyramide* is considerable. Cotherapy with *flecainide* may also give added negative inotropic and dromotropic effects.

Statins Verapamil inhibits the hepatic CYP3A isoenzyme, and therefore potentially increases the blood levels of atorvastatin, simvastatin, and lovastatin, which are all metabolized by this isoenzyme.[29]

Table 3-3	Comparative Contraindications of Verapamil, Diltiazem, Dihydropyridines, and of β-Adrenergic Blocking Agents			
Contraindications	**Verapamil**	**Diltiazem**	**DHPs**	**β-Blockade**
Absolute:				
Severe sinus bradycardia	0/+	0/+	0	++
Sick sinus syndrome	++	++	0	++
AV conduction defects	++	++	0	++
WPW syndrome	++	++	0	++
Digoxin toxicity, AV block*	++	++	0	++
Asthma	0	0	0	+++
Bronchospasm	0	0	0	0/++
Heart failure	++	++	+	Indicated
Hypotension	+	+	++	+
Coronary artery spasm	0	0	0	+
Raynaud's and active peripheral vascular disease	0	0	0	+
Severe mental depression	0	0	0	+
Severe aortic stenosis	+	+	++	+
Obstructive cardiomyopathy	0/+	0/+	++	Indicated
Relative:				
Insulin resistance	0	0	0	Care
Adverse blood lipid profile	0	0	0	Care
Digoxin nodal effects	Care	Care	0	Care
β-Blockade	Care	Care	BP↓	N/A
(Quinidine therapy)[†]	(Care)	(Care)	(Care)	(Care)
Disopyramide therapy	Care	Care	0	Care
Unstable angina	Indicated	Indicated	++	Indicated
Postinfarct protection	Indicated	0 (+ if no LVF)	++	Indicated

Indicated means judged suitable for use by author (LH Opie), not necessarily FDA-approved.
*Contraindication to rapid intravenous administration.
[†]Not recommended for any purpose; see Chapter 8.
+++ = absolutely contraindicated; ++ = strongly contraindicated; + = relative contraindication; 0 = not contraindicated.
BP↓, hypotension; DHPs = dihydropyridines; LVF = left ventricular failure; N/A = not applicable.

Other Agents Phenobarbital, *phenytoin,* and *rifampin* induce the cytochrome systems metabolizing verapamil so that its blood levels fall. Conversely, verapamil inhibits hepatic CYP3A to increase blood levels of *cyclosporin, carbamazepine* (Tegretol), and *theophylline,* as mentioned in the package insert. This inhibition is also expected to increase blood levels of *ketoconazole* and *sildenafil.* Cimetidine has variable effects. Alcohol levels increase. Verapamil may sensitize to *neuromuscular blocking agents,* and to the effects of *lithium* (neurotoxicity).

Therapy of Verapamil Toxicity

There are few clinical reports on management of verapamil toxicity. Intravenous calcium gluconate (1 to 2 g) or half that dose of calcium chloride, given over 5 minutes, helps when heart failure or excess hypotension is present. If there is an inadequate response, positive inotropic or vasoconstrictory catecholamines (see Chapter 6) are given, or else glucagon. A novel alternative is hyperinsulinemic-euglycemic therapy.[30] Intravenous atropine (1 mg) or isoproterenol is used to shorten AV conduction. A pacemaker may be needed.

Clinical Indications of Verapamil

Angina In *chronic stable effort angina*, verapamil acts by a combination of afterload reduction and a mild negative inotropic effect, plus reduction of exercise-induced tachycardia and coronary vasoconstriction. The heart rate usually stays the same or falls modestly. In several studies, verapamil has been as effective as propranolol for effort angina. In *unstable angina* at rest with threat of infarction, verapamil has not been tested against placebo, although licensed for this purpose in the United States. In *Prinzmetal's variant angina* therapy is based on CCBs, including verapamil, and high doses may be needed.[31] Abrupt withdrawal of verapamil may precipitate rebound angina.

Hypertension Verapamil is approved for mild to moderate hypertension in the United States. There are now results from two major outcome studies. In CONVINCE, stopped early by the sponsors, verapamil-based therapy was similar to diuretic–β-blocker therapy with regard to all major outcomes.[26] In INVEST, verapamil-based therapy was compared with atenolol-based therapy, the former supplemented by an ACE inhibitor trandolapril, and the latter by a thiazide if required to reach the blood pressure goal.[25] Major outcomes were very similar without, however, reaching the strict criteria for noninferiority. Verapamil doses of 240 to 360 mg daily were the approximate equivalent of atenolol 50 to 100 mg daily. In another long-term double-blind comparative trial, mild to moderate hypertension was adequately controlled in 45% of patients given verapamil 240 mg daily,[32] versus 25% for hydrochlorothiazide 25 mg daily, versus 60% for the combination. Higher doses of verapamil might have had even better results.

Combinations can be with diuretics, β-blockers, ACE inhibitors, angiotensin receptor blockers, or centrally acting agents. During combination with α-blockers, a hepatic interaction may lead to excess hypotension.

Verapamil for Supraventricular Arrhythmias Verapamil is licensed for the prophylaxis of repetitive supraventricular tachycardias, and for rate control in chronic atrial fibrillation when given with digoxin (note interaction). For acute attacks of *supraventricular tachycardias*, when there is no myocardial depression, a bolus dose of 5 to 10 mg (0.1 to 0.15 mg/kg) given over 2 minutes restores sinus rhythm within 10 minutes in 60% of cases (see package insert). However, this use is now largely supplanted by intravenous adenosine (see Fig. 8-5). When used for uncontrolled *atrial fibrillation*, verapamil may safely be given (0.005 mg/kg/minute, increasing) or as an intravenous bolus of 5 mg (0.075 mg/kg) followed by double the dose if needed. If there is myocardial disease, and when cardioversion is not practical, verapamil can still be used with caution, if infused at a very low dose (0.0001 mg/kg/minute) and carefully titrated against the ventricular response. In *atrial flutter*, AV block is increased. In all supraventricular tachycardias, including atrial flutter and fibrillation, the presence of a bypass tract (WPW syndrome) contraindicates verapamil.

Other Uses for Verapamil In *hypertrophic cardiomyopathy*, verapamil has been the CCB best evaluated. It is licensed for this purpose in Canada. When given acutely, it lessens symptoms, reduces the outflow tract gradient, improves diastolic function, and enhances exercise performance by 20% to 25%. Verapamil should not be given to patients with resting outflow tract obstruction, when propranolol or disopyramide, which do not vasodilate, should be safer. No long-term placebo-controlled studies with verapamil are available. In retrospective comparisons with propranolol, verapamil appeared to decrease sudden death and gave better 10-year survival.[33] The best results were obtained by a combination of septal myectomy and verapamil. In current practice, propranolol and verapamil are often combined (see Chapter 11, p. 387). A significant number of patients on long-term verapamil develop severe side effects, including SA and AV nodal dysfunction, and occasionally overt heart failure.

Atypical ventricular tachycardia. Some patients with exercise-induced ventricular tachycardia due to triggered automaticity may respond well to verapamil, as may young patients with idiopathic right ventricular outflow tract ventricular tachycardia (right bundle branch block and left axis deviation). However, verapamil can be lethal for standard wide complex ventricular tachycardia, especially when given intravenously. Therefore, unless the diagnosis is sure, verapamil must be avoided in ventricular tachycardia.

For *postinfarct protection*, verapamil is approved in the United Kingdom and in Scandinavian countries when β-blockade is contraindicated. Verapamil 120 mg three times daily, started 7 to 15 days after the acute phase in patients without a history of heart failure and no signs of CHF (but with digoxin and diuretic therapy allowed), was protective and decreased reinfarction and mortality by about 25% over 18 months.[14]

For *diabetic nephropathy* in type 2 diabetics, verapamil was as good as an ACE inhibitor at slowing renal deterioration, but the numbers were low.[34]

In *intermittent claudication*, carefully titrated verapamil increased maximum walking ability.[35]

In *carotid atherosclerosis*, verapamil is among the CCBs tested. These agents as a group are now recommended by the European Society of Hypertension.[11]

Summary

Among CCBs, verapamil has the widest range of approved indications, including all varieties of angina (effort, vasospastic, unstable), supraventricular tachycardias, and hypertension. Indirect evidence suggests that is one of the safest of the CCBs with nonetheless risks of heart block and heart failure. Compared with propranolol in the therapy of effort angina, it is at least as effective, with, however, different side effects and contraindications. Verapamil is one of a number of early options in the therapy of hypertension, as confirmed by recent outcome studies. The combination with β-blockade can be more effective than either component in the therapy of angina or hypertension, but a number of cautions and contraindications such as increased risk of heart block and bradycardia must be observed.

DILTIAZEM

Although molecular studies show different channel binding sites for diltiazem and verapamil (Fig. 3-4), in clinical practice they have somewhat similar therapeutic spectra and contraindications, so that they are often classified as the non-DHPs or "heart rate lowering" agents (Fig. 3-5). Clinically, diltiazem is used for the same spectrum of diseases as is verapamil: angina pectoris, hypertension, supraventricular arrhythmias, and rate control in atrial fibrillation or flutter (Fig. 3-7). Of these, use of diltiazem for angina (effort and vasospastic) and hypertension is approved in the United States, with only the intravenous form approved for supraventricular tachycardias and for acute rate control. Diltiazem has a low side effect profile, similar to or possibly better than that of verapamil; specifically the incidence of constipation is much lower (Table 3-4). On the other hand, verapamil is registered for more indications. Is diltiazem less cardiodepressant than verapamil? There are no strictly comparable clinical studies to support this clinical impression.

Table 3-4 Reported Side Effects of the Three Prototypical CCBs and Long-Acting Dihydropyridines

	Verapamil Covera-HS (%)	Diltiazem Short-Acting (%)	Dittiazem XR or CD (%)	Nifedipine Capsules* (%)	Nifedipine XL, CC, GITS (%)	Amlodipine 10mg (%)	Felodipine ER 10mg (%)
Facial flushing	<1	0–3	0–1	6–25	0–4	3	5
Headaches	<Placebo	4–9	<Placebo	3–34	6	<Placebo	4
Palpitation	0	0	0	Low–25	0	4	1
Lightheadedness, dizziness	5	6–7	1–2	12	2–4	2	4
Constipation	12	4		0	1	0	0
Ankle edema, swelling	0	6–10	2–3	6	10–30	10	14
Provocation of angina	0	0	0	Low–14	0	0	0

Side effects are dose-related; no strict direct comparisons between the CCBs. Percentages are placebo-corrected.
*No longer used in the United States.
Data sources from Opie LH. Clinical Use of Calcium Antagonist Drugs, Kluwer, Boston, 1990, p. 197, and from package inserts.

Pharmacokinetics Following oral administration of diltiazem, more than 90% is absorbed, but bioavailability is about 45% (first-pass hepatic metabolism). The onset of action of short-acting diltiazem is within 15 to 30 minutes (oral), with a peak at 1 to 2 hours. The elimination half-life is 4 to 7 hours; hence, dosage every 6 to 8 hours of the short-acting preparation is required for sustained therapeutic effect. The therapeutic plasma concentration range is 50 to 300 ng/ml. Protein binding is 80% to 86%. Diltiazem is acetylated in the liver to deacyldiltiazem (40% of the activity of the parent compound), which accumulates with chronic therapy. Unlike verapamil and nifedipine, only 35% of diltiazem is excreted by the kidneys (65% by the GI tract).

Diltiazem Doses The dose of diltiazem is 120 to 360 mg, given as four daily doses of the short-acting formulation or once or twice a day with slow-release preparations. *Cardizem SR* permits twice daily doses. For once daily use, *Dilacor XR* is licensed in the United States for hypertension and *Cardizem CD* and *Tiazac* for hypertension and angina. *Intravenous diltiazem (Cardizem injectable)* is approved for arrhythmias but not for acute hypertension. For acute conversion of paroxysmal supraventricular tachycardia, after exclusion of WPW syndrome (see Fig. 8-2) or for slowing the ventricular response rate in atrial fibrillation or flutter, it is given as 0.25 mg/kg over 2 minutes with ECG and blood pressure monitoring. Then if the response is inadequate, the dose is repeated as 0.35 mg/kg over 2 minutes. Acute therapy is usually followed by an infusion of 5 to 15 mg/hour for up to 24 hours. *Diltiazem overdose* is treated as for verapamil (see p. 63).

Side Effects Normally side effects of the standard preparation are few and limited to headaches, dizziness, and ankle edema in about 6% to 10% of patients (Table 3-4). With high-dose diltiazem (360 mg daily), constipation may also occur. When the extended-release preparation (Dilacor XR) is used for hypertension, the side effect profile resembles that of placebo. Nonetheless, bradycardia and first degree AV block may occur with all diltiazem preparations. In the case of intravenous diltiazem, side effects resemble those of intravenous verapamil, including hypotension and the possible risk of asystole and high-degree AV block when there is preexisting nodal disease. In postinfarct patients with preexisting poor LV function, mortality is increased by diltiazem, not decreased. Occasionally, severe skin rashes such as exfoliative dermatitis are found.

Contraindications Contraindications resemble those of verapamil (Fig. 3-8, Table 3-3)—preexisting marked depression of the sinus or AV node, hypotension, myocardial failure, and the WPW syndrome. Use in nodal disease may require a pacemaker. Postinfarct, LV failure with an ejection fraction below 40% is a clear contraindication.[36]

Drug Interactions and Combinations Unlike verapamil, the effect of diltiazem on the blood digoxin level is often slight or negligible. As in the case of verapamil, there are the expected hemodynamic interactions with β-blockers. Nonetheless, diltiazem plus β-blocker may be used with care for angina, watching for excess bradycardia or AV block or hypotension. Diltiazem may increase the bioavailability of oral propranolol, perhaps by displacing it from its binding sites (see package insert). Occasionally diltiazem plus a DHP is used for refractory coronary artery spasm, the rationale being that two different binding sites on the calcium channel are involved (Fig. 3-4). Diltiazem plus long-acting nitrates may lead to excess hypotension. As in the case of verapamil, but probably less so, diltiazem may inhibit CYP3A cytochrome, which is expected to increase blood levels of cyclosporin, ketoconazole, carbamazepine (Tegretol), and sildenafil.[29] Conversely, cimetidine inhibits the hepatic cytochrome system, breaking down diltiazem to increase circulating levels.

Clinical Uses of Diltiazem

Ischemic Syndromes In chronic stable *effort angina*, the combination of vasodilation, reduced heart rate during exercise, and a modest negative inotropic effect is desirable (Figs. 3-5 and 3-6). The efficacy of diltiazem in chronic angina is at least as good as that of propranolol, and the dose is titrated from 120 to 360 mg daily (Table 3-2). In *unstable angina at rest*, there is a good albeit small study showing that intravenous diltiazem (not licensed for this purpose in the United States) gives better pain relief than does intravenous nitrate, with improved 1-year follow-up.[8] In *Prinzmetal's variant angina*, diltiazem 240 to 360 mg/day reduces the number of episodes of pain. In a pilot study on *early phase AMI*, intravenous diltiazem added to tissue plasminogen activator (t-PA) reduced postinfarct ischemia and reinfarction.[37] In the INTERCEPT study on thrombolysed patients with AMI, long-acting oral diltiazem plus aspirin, started within 36 to 96 hours of the onset of MI, was compared with aspirin alone, and given for 6 months.[18,38] Although there was a 24% reduction in the combined primary end-point of death, recurrent MI, or refractory ischemia, the confidence intervals just overlapped unity (CI, 0.59 to 1.02). Thus, a larger trial is required.

Diltiazem for Hypertension In the major long-term outcome study on more than 10,000 patients, the Nordic Diltiazem or NORDIL trial, diltiazem, followed by an ACE inhibitor if needed to reach blood pressure goals, was as effective in preventing the primary combined cardiovascular end-point as treatment based on a diuretic, a β-blocker, or both.[26] In the smaller multicenter VA study, diltiazem was the best among five agents (the others were atenolol, thiazide, doxazosin, and captopril) in reducing blood pressure, and was especially effective in elderly white patients and in black patients.[39] Nonetheless, reduction of LV hypertrophy was poor at 1-year of follow-up, possibly because a short-acting diltiazem formulation was used.[40]

Antiarrhythmic Properties of Diltiazem The electrophysiological properties of diltiazem closely resemble those of verapamil. The main effect is a depressant one on the AV node; the functional and effective refractory periods are prolonged by diltiazem, so that diltiazem is licensed for termination of an attack of supraventricular tachyarrhythmia and for rapid decrease of the ventricular response rate in atrial flutter or fibrillation. Only intravenous diltiazem is approved for this purpose in the United States (see p. 67). Oral diltiazem can be used for the elective as well as prophylactic control (90 mg three times daily) of most supraventricular tachyarrhythmias (oral diltiazem is not approved for this use in the United States or United Kingdom). Diltiazem is unlikely to be effective (and is contraindicated) in ventricular arrhythmias except in those complicating coronary artery spasm or in those few in whom verapamil works (see p. 65). In chronic atrial fibrillation, diltiazem may be added to digoxin to improve control of ventricular rate. As for verapamil, the presence of a bypass tract (WPW syndrome, Fig. 8-2) is a contraindication to diltiazem.

Cardiac Transplantation Diltiazem acts prophylactically to limit the development of post-transplant coronary atheroma, independently of any blood pressure reduction.[41]

Summary

Diltiazem, with its low side effect profile, is often regarded as having advantages in the therapy of angina pectoris. Like verapamil, it acts by peripheral vasodilation, relief of exercise-induced coronary constriction, a modest negative inotropic effect, and sinus node inhibition. In the therapy of hypertension, it is well tolerated, and has cardiovascular outcomes similar to those of conventional therapy by diuretics and/or β-blockers. The intravenous form is approved in the United States for acute supraventricular tachycardias and for acute decrease of the ventricular response rate in atrial fibrillation or flutter. The incidence of side effects (usually low) will depend on the dose and the underlying state of the sinus or AV nodes and the myocardium, as well as any possible cotherapy with β-blockers.

NIFEDIPINE: THE PROTOTYPICAL DHP

The major actions of the DHPs can be simplified to one: arteriolar dilation (Fig. 3-5). The direct negative inotropic effect is usually outweighed by arteriolar unloading effects and by reflex adrenergic stimulation (Fig. 3-6), except in patients with heart failure.

Short-Acting Capsular Nifedipine

Short-acting capsular nifedipine was first introduced in Europe and Japan as Adalat, and then became the best-selling Procardia in the United States. In angina, it was especially used for coronary spasm, at that time thought to be the basis of unstable angina. Unfortunately not enough attention was paid to three important negative studies,[10,42,43] which led to warnings against use in unstable angina in previous editions of this book. Nonetheless the widespread use of capsular nifedipine continued until an influential meta-analysis by Furberg stressed the increased mortality at high doses, 80 mg or more per day.[44] Although there were substantial arithmetical errors in the meta-analysis,[7] and although the excess of deaths amounted to only 16 in over 1000 patients, the message was clear: capsular nifedipine was potentially dangerous in acute ischemic situations (Fig. 3-6). The ensuing adverse reaction led to an examination of its overuse and off-license use in severe hypertension[45] with FDA warnings in the package inserts against any use in hypertension. Capsular nifedipine is now the treatment of choice only when taken intermittently for conditions such as attacks of vasospastic angina or Raynaud's phenomenon, or when in unstable angina it is desired to test the tolerability addition of a short-acting CCB to preexisting β-blockade.[10]

Long-Acting Nifedipine Formulations

The rest of this section largely focuses on long-acting nifedipine formulations (*Procardia XL in United States, Adalat LA elsewhere; Adalat CC*) that are now widely used in the treatment of hypertension, in effort angina, and in vasospastic angina.

Pharmacokinetics Almost all circulating nifedipine is broken down by hepatic metabolism by the cytochrome P-450 system to inactive metabolites (high first-pass metabolism) that are largely excreted in the urine. The long-acting osmotically sensitive tablet (nifedipine GITS, marketed as Procardia XL or Adalat LA) releases nifedipine from the inner core as water enters the tablet from the GI tract (Table 3-2). This process results in stable blood therapeutic levels of about 20 to 30 ng/ml over 24 hours. With a core-coat system (Adalat CC), the blood levels over 24 hours are more variable, with the trough/peak ratios of 41% to 91%.

Doses of Nifedipine In *effort angina*, the usual daily dose 30 to 90 mg of Procardia XL or Adalat LA (Adalat CC is not licensed in the United States for angina). Dose titration is important to avoid precipitation of ischemic pain in some patients. In cold-induced angina or in coronary spasm, the doses are similar and capsules (in similar total daily doses) allow the most rapid onset of action. In *hypertension*, standard doses are 30 to 90 mg once daily of Procardia XL or Adalat CC. In the *elderly or in severe liver disease*, doses should be reduced.

Contraindications and Cautions (Fig. 3-9, Table 3-5) These are tight aortic stenosis or obstructive hypertrophic cardiomyopathy (danger of exaggerated pressure gradient), clinically evident heart failure or LV dysfunction (added negative inotropic effect), unstable angina with threat of infarction (in the absence of concurrent β-blockade), and preexisting hypotension. Relative contraindications are subjective intolerance to nifedipine and previous adverse reactions. In pregnancy, nifedipine should be used only if the benefits are thought to outweigh the risk of embryopathy (experimental; pregnancy category C).

Minor Side Effects The bilateral ankle edema seen with nifedipine is distressing to patients but is not caused by cardiac failure; if required, it can be treated by dose reduction or conventional diuretics or an ACE inhibitor. Nifedipine itself has a mild diuretic effect. The incidence of subjective vasodilatory side effects is higher with nifedipine capsules than with verapamil or diltiazem. The manufacturers claim that with extended-release nifedipine preparations (Procardia XL), side effects are restricted to headache (nearly double that found in controls) and ankle edema (dose-dependent, 10% with 30 mg daily, 30% with 180 mg daily). The low incidence of acute vasodilatory side effects, such as flushing and tachycardia, is attributable to the slow rate of rise of blood DHP levels.

Severe or Rare Side Effects In patients with LV depression, the direct negative inotropic effect can be a serious problem. Occasionally, there are side effects compatible with the effects of excess hypotension and organ underperfusion, namely myocardial ischemia or even infarction, retinal and cerebral ischemia, and renal failure. Other unusual side effects include muscle cramps, myalgia, hypokalemia (via diuretic effect), and gingival swelling.

Drug Interactions *Cimetidine* and *grapefruit juice* (large amounts) inhibit the hepatic CYP3A4 P-450 enzyme system breaking down nifedipine, thereby substantially increasing its blood levels. *Phenobarbital, phenytoin,* and *rifampin* induce this system metabolizing so that nifedipine blood levels should fall (not mentioned in the package insert). In some reports, blood digoxin levels rise. Volatile anesthetics interfere

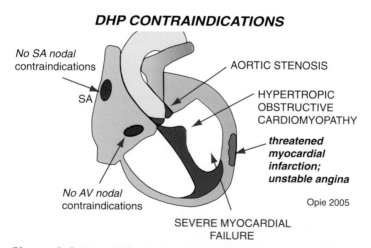

DHP CONTRAINDICATIONS

No SA nodal contraindications

SA

No AV nodal contraindications

AORTIC STENOSIS

HYPERTROPIC OBSTRUCTIVE CARDIOMYOPATHY

threatened myocardial infarction; unstable angina

Opie 2005

SEVERE MYOCARDIAL FAILURE

Figure 3-9 Contraindications to dihydropyridines are chiefly obstructive lesions such as aortic stenosis or hypertrophic obstructive cardiomyopathy, and heart failure. Unstable angina (threatened infarction) is a contraindication unless combined nifedipine plus β-blockade therapy is used or unless (rarely) coronary spasm is suspected. *SA* and *AV* as in Fig. 3-6. (*Figure © LH Opie, 2005.*)

Table 3-5 Long-Acting Dihydropyridines for Oral Use

Agent	Dose and Major Trial	Pharmacokinetics and Metabolism	Side Effects and Contraindications	Interactions and Precautions
Amlodipine (Norvasc, Istin)	5–10 mg once daily (ALLHAT, VALUE)	t max, 6–12h. Extensive but slow hepatic metabolism. 90% inactive metabolites. 60% renal. $t^1/_2$ 35–50h. Steady state in 7–8 days	Edema, dizziness, flushing, palpitation. C/I: severe aortic stenosis, obstructive cardiomyopathy, LV failure, unstable angina AMI. May use amlodipine in CHF class II or III, but best avoided	Prolonged $t^1/_2$ up to 56h in liver failure. Reduce dose, also in elderly and in heart failure. Grapefruit juice: caution, interaction not established.
Nifedipine Prolonged release XL, LA, GITS, Adalat CC Procardia XL	30–90 mg once daily (INSIGHT)	Stable 24-h blood levels. Slow onset, about 6h.	S/E headache, ankle edema. C/I: severe aortic stenosis, obstructive cardiomyopathy, LV failure. Unstable angina if no β-blockade	Added LV depression with β-blockade. Avoid in unstable angina without β-blockade. Cimetidine and liver disease increase blood levels
Felodipine ER (Plendil)	5–10 mg once daily (HOT)	t max, 3–5h. Complete hepatic metabolism (P-450) to inactive metabolites 75% renal loss, $t^1/_2$ 22–27h	Edema, headache, flushing. C/I as above except no evidence for benefit in CHF (mortality neutral).	Reduce dose with cimetidine, age, liver disease. Anticonvulsants enhance hepatic metabolism. Grapefruit juice markedly inhibits metabolism.

t max = time to peak blood level; $t^1/_2$ = plasma elimination half-life.

71

with the myocardial calcium regulation and have inhibitory effects additional to those of nifedipine.

Rebound After Cessation of Nifedipine Therapy In patients with vasospastic angina, abrupt cessation of nifedipine capsule therapy increased the frequency and duration of attacks. The evidence for rebound with the long-acting preparations is much less convincing, although the manufacturers recommend that the dose be tailed off.

Nifedipine Poisoning In one case there was hypotension, SA and AV nodal block, and hyperglycemia. Treatment was by infusions of calcium and dopamine (see also amlodipine).

Combination with β-Blockers and Other Drugs In patients with reasonable LV function, nifedipine may be freely combined with β-blockade (Fig. 3-10), provided that excess hypotension is guarded against. In LV depression, the added negative inotropic effects may precipitate overt heart failure. For unstable angina at rest, nifedipine can be used only if combined with a β-blocker.[10] In the therapy of effort or vasospastic angina, nifedipine is often combined with nitrates. In the therapy of hypertension, nifedipine may be combined with diuretics, β-blockers, methyldopa, ACE inhibitors, or angiotensin receptor blockers. Combination with prazosin or (by extrapolation) other α-blockers may lead to adverse hypotensive interactions.

Clinical Uses of Nifedipine

Ischemic Syndromes In the United States only Procardia XL and not Adalat CC is licensed for *effort angina*, when β-blockade and/or nitrates are ineffective or not tolerated. Whereas capsular nifedipine modestly increases the heart rate (that may aggravate angina), the extended-release preparations leave the heart rate unchanged.[46] Their

CCBs VERSUS β-BLOCKADE
Opie 2004

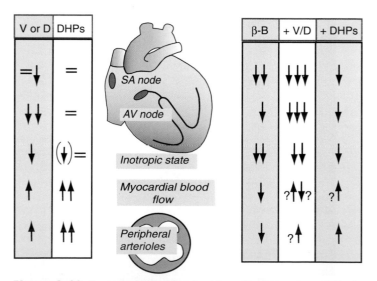

Figure 3-10 Proposed hemodynamic effects of calcium channel blockers, singly or in combination with β-blockade. Note that some of these effects are based on animal data, and extrapolation to humans needs to be made with caution. *βB* = β-blockade; *D* = diltiazem; *DHP* = dihydropyridines; *V* = verapamil. (*Figure © LH Opie, 2005.*)

antianginal activity and safety approximates that of the β-blockers, albeit at the cost of more subjective symptoms.[47] The ACTION study, to be announced in late 2004, will give more information on the long-term efficacy and safety of long-acting nifedipine in those with effort angina. The majority of patients will have had the nifedipine added to prior β-blockade, so that the expected result should be similar in direction to the much smaller PREVENT study with amlodipine, that is, decreased unstable angina and revascularization.[48] In addition, ACTION is powered to assess mortality and major cardiovascular events. In *Prinzmetal's angina* (vasospastic angina), nifedipine gives consistent relief. In *unstable angina*, nifedipine may be given only when combined with β-blockade.[10]

Systemic Hypertension Long-acting nifedipine and other DHPs are increasingly used. The major outcome study with nifedipine GITS, the INSIGHT study, showed equivalence in mortality and other major outcomes to the diuretic, with less new diabetes or gout or peripheral vascular disease and more heart failure.[4] Capsular forms are not licensed for hypertension in the United States because of the intermittent vasodilation and reflex adrenergic discharge, as well as the short duration of action. Procardia XL and Adalat CC are, however, approved and the dose is initially 30 mg once daily up to 90 mg daily.

Vascular Protection Intriguing basic and clinical work suggests that nifedipine and other CCBs have vascular protective qualities, especially in the carotid vessels.[49] Whether coronary disease is limited is still under investigation.

Off-License Uses of Nifedipine Capsules For severe hypertension (DBP > 120 mmHg), 5- to 10-mg nifedipine capsules, repeated once after 30 to 60 minutes, were widely used and abused.[45] Although nifedipine is quicker and less expensive than sodium nitroprusside infusion,[50] and when carefully used is safe,[51] it is no longer recommended for this purpose. In unstable angina, nifedipine in the absence of β-blockade by itself is contraindicated, as shown by the HINT study.[10]

Summary

Long-acting nifedipine is widely used as a powerful arterial vasodilator with few serious side effects and is now part of the accepted therapy of hypertension and of effort or Prinzmetal's vasospastic angina. In hypertension, it gives outcomes equivalent to those of a diuretic. Nifedipine is especially useful in angina patients with contraindications to β-blockade, such as bronchospasm, heart block, or active peripheral vascular disease. However, in unstable angina at rest, nifedipine in any formulation should not be used as monotherapy, although effective when added to preexisting β-blockade.

Contraindications to nifedipine are few (apart from severe aortic stenosis, obstructive cardiomyopathy, or LV failure), and careful combination with β-blockade is usually feasible. Vasodilatory side effects include headache and ankle edema.

AMLODIPINE: THE FIRST OF THE SECOND-GENERATION DHPs

The major specific advantage of amlodipine (*Norvasc; Istin* in the United Kingdom) compared with the original nifedipine capsules is the slower onset of action and the much longer duration of activity (Table 3-5). It was the first of the longer acting "second-generation" agents. It binds to the same site as do other DHPs (labeled "N" in Fig. 3-4). The charged nature of the molecule means that its binding is not entirely typical, with very slow association and dissociation, so that the channel block is slow in onset and offset. In addition, it also binds to the same sites as do verapamil and diltiazem, albeit to a lesser degree, so that with justification its binding properties are regarded as unique.[52] Because it is highly lipophilic, the membrane antioxidant effects[53] are of interest although not yet of proven clinical relevance.

Pharmacokinetics Peak blood levels are reached after 6 to 12 hours, followed by extensive hepatic metabolism to inactive metabolites. The plasma levels increase during chronic dosage, probably because of the very long half-life. The elimination half-life is 35 to 48 hours, increasing slightly with chronic dosage. In the elderly, the clearance is reduced and the dose may need reduction. Regarding *drug interactions*, no effect on digoxin levels has been found, nor is there any interaction with cimetidine (in contrast to verapamil and nifedipine). There is no known effect of grapefruit juice.

Clinical Uses of Amlodipine

Hypertension As initial monotherapy, a common starting dose is 5 mg daily going up to 10 mg. In a large 4-year trial on mild hypertension in a middle-aged group, amlodipine 5 mg daily was the best tolerated of the agents compared with an α-blocker, a β-blocker, a diuretic, and an ACE-inhibitor.[54] In the largest outcome study, ALLHAT, amlodipine had the same primary outcome (fatal and nonfatal coronary heart disease) as did the diuretic and ACE inhibitor groups, but with increased heart failure and decreased new diabetes.[20] Perhaps unexpectedly, amlodipine slowed renal deterioration better than other agents. In VALUE, amlodipine and valsartan gave equal benefit (see Table 3-6).

Effort Angina Amlodipine is well tested in *effort angina*, with an antianginal effect for 24 hours. In three relatively small comparative studies with β-blockers, amlodipine was well tolerated.[55-57] In PREVENT, amlodipine given to patients with coronary angiographic disease had reduced outcome measures after 3 years.[48] *Exercise-induced ischemia* was more effectively reduced by amlodipine than by the β-blocker atenolol, whereas ambulatory ischemia was better reduced by atenolol, and for both settings the combination was the best.[56] Exercise-induced ischemia is at the basis of effort angina. After the anginal pain is relieved by nitrates, the ejection fraction takes about 30 minutes to recover, a manifestation of *postischemic stunning*. Amlodipine markedly attenuates such stunning,[58] hypothetically because cellular calcium overload underlies stunning. In *Prinzmetal's vasospastic angina*, another licensed indication, amlodipine 5 mg daily lessens symptoms and ST changes.

Contraindications, Cautions, and Side Effects Amlodipine has the same contraindications as other DHPs (Fig. 3-9). It is untested in *unstable angina, AMI, and follow-up*. First principles strongly suggest that it should not be used in the absence of concurrent β-blockade. In *heart failure* patients otherwise fully treated, amlodipine could be added without overall adverse effects.[59] In ALLHAT, amlodipine increased heart failure compared with the diuretic.[20] CCBs as a group are best avoided in CHF but amlodipine may be added, for example, for better control of angina. In established hypertension with nephrosclerosis in black patients, amlodipine gave poorer outcomes than ramipril.[60] By contrast, in ALLHAT the glomerular filtration rate was better preserved in the amlodipine than in the diuretic or ACE inhibitor arms. In *liver disease* the dose should be reduced. Of the *side effects*, peripheral edema is most troublesome, occurring in about 10% of patients at 10 mg daily (Table 3-4). In women there is more edema (15%) than in men (6%). Next in significance are dizziness (3% to 4%) and flushing (2% to 3%). Compared with verapamil, edema is more common but headache and constipation are less common. Compared with placebo, headache is not increased (package insert). Amlodipine gave an excellent quality of life compared with other agents in the TOMH study.[54]

Summary

The very long half-life of amlodipine, good tolerability, excellent trial data, and virtual absence of drug interactions makes it an effective once-a-day antihypertensive and antianginal agent, setting it apart from agents that are used either twice or thrice daily. Nonetheless, the introduction of extended-release preparations of all other DHPs has narrowed these differences.

FELODIPINE

Felodipine (*Plendil ER*) shares the standard properties of other long-acting DHPs. In the United States it is licensed only for hypertension, in a starting dose of 5 mg once daily, then increasing to 10 mg or decreasing to 2.5 mg as needed. As monotherapy, it is approximately as effective as nifedipine. Initial felodipine monotherapy was the basis of a very large outcome study in Scandinavia in which the aim was to compare blood pressure reduction to different diastolic levels: 90, 85, or 80 mmHg.[24] Combination with other agents such as ACE inhibitors and β-blockers was often required to attain the goals. The best results were found with the lowest blood pressure group in diabetic individuals, in whom hard end-points such as cardiovascular mortality were reduced. Felodipine, like other DHPs, combines well with β-blockers.[61] Regarding *drug interactions*, there are two of note: cimetidine, which increases blood felodipine levels, and anticonvulsants, which markedly decrease levels, both probably acting at the level of the hepatic enzymes. *Grapefruit juice* markedly inhibits the metabolism. The high vascular selectivity of felodipine led to extensive testing in *heart failure*, yet achieving no sustained benefit in the large Ve-HeFT-III trial in which it was added to conventional therapy.[62]

OTHER DIHYDROPYRIDINES

These include, in alphabetical order, isradipine, lacipidine, lercanidipine, nicardipine, and nisoldipine. There appears to be no particular reason for choosing any of these above the much better studied agents such as amlodipine, nifedipine, and felodipine. *Lacidipine* (only in Europe and the United Kingdom), however, deserves a comment in that it is highly lipophilic and may therefore exert more marked vascular protection than other agents. In the ELSA trial (European Lacidipine Study of Atherosclerosis) the progression of carotid atherosclerosis was slowed when compared with atenolol, even though the ambulatory blood pressure reduction of −7/−5 mmHg was less than with the β-blocker (−10/−9 mmHg).[5] Lacidipine is also claimed to cause less ankle edema than amlodipine.

LARGE OUTCOME TRIALS AND CCB SAFETY

In hypertension, there are a large number of outcome studies, which taken together attest to the safety of CCBs in treating this condition (Table 3-6). The only outstanding trial, ASCOT, compares "new therapy," amlodipine ± perindopril, versus "old" therapy by atenolol ± diuretic. In angina, the major study is ACTION with long-acting nifedipine added to existing therapy, due for report at the European Congress of Cardiology in August 2004. For both studies, recruitment has been excellent and the safety committees have seen no reason to stop either study.

Table 3-6 CCBs: Major Outcome Trials in Hypertension

Acronym and Drug	Numbers and Duration	Comparison	End-points
ALLHAT, amlodipine[20]	33,357 patients. 9048 in amlodipine arm	A vs others (diuretic, ACE inhibitor, α-blocker)	Equal CHD, stroke, all cause mortality, at same BP target. More HF; less new diabetes
ASCOT, amlodipine	18,000 patients, 5 years, BP > 160/100 or 140/90 on drug: age 40–80. 3+ risk factors for CHD	Amlodipine vs atenolol; 2nd: A + perindopril vs atenolol + thiazide	Amlodipine ± perindopril delivered superior risk reductions in hypertension patients compared with the atenolol ± bendroflumethuczide combination. Endpoints included: fatal CHD and nonfatal MI, total mortality fatal and nonfatal stroke, new onset diabetes.
CONVINCE verapamil[63]	16,602 patients, aim for 4–6 years, but stopped after 3 years by sponsor	Verapamil Covera-HS vs thiazide or atenolol	Similar combined end-point, but no strict equivalence.
ELSA, lacidipine[5]	2334 patients. BP 150–210/95–115 mmHg	Lacidipine vs atenolol ± diuretic if needed	Caroid wall thickness ultrasound; lacidipine better
INSIGHT, nifedipine GITS[4]	6321 patients; BP↑ plus one other risk factor (smoking, diabetes, angina, hyperlipidemia); 3 years	Nifedipine vs thiazide; then add atenolol or enalapril to control BP	Equal CV events, ↑heart failure, ↓ new diabetes and gout
INVEST verapamil[25]	22,576 for 2 years; hypertension + coronary disease	Verapamil ± ACE inhibitor vs atenolol ± diuretic	Similar in all major end-points: CAD, all-cause mortality.
NORDIL, diltiazem[26]	10,881 patients, up to 5 years, mild to moderate BP↑, ages 50–74	Diltiazem vs β-blocker/diuretic	Equal CV mortality, ↓ stroke
SHELL, lacidipine[64]	1882 patients, age 60+, isolated systolic hypertension	Lacidipine vs diuretic ± ACE inhibitor if needed	CV morbidity and mortality similar
VALUE, amlodipine[65]	15,245 patients, age 50+, initial BP 155/87 mmHg	Amlodipine vs valsartan; both ± thiazide	Equal cardiac and mortality outcomes.

ALLHAT = Antihypertensive and Lipid-Lowering treatment to prevent Heart Attack Trial; ASCOT = Anglo Scandinavian Cardiac Outcomes Trial; CONVINCE = Controlled Onset Verapamil Investigation for Cardiovascular Endpoints; ELSA = European Lacidipine Study on Atherosclerosis; HF = heart failure; NORDIL = Nordic Diltiazem study. INSIGHT = International Nifedipine-GITS Study Intervention as a Goal in Hypertension Treatment; INVEST = International Verapamil SR/Trandolapril study; SHELL = Systolic Hypertension in the Elderly Long-term Lacidipine; VALUE = Valsartan Antihypertensive Long-term Use Evaluation trial.

SUMMARY

1. *Spectrum of use.* Calcium channel blockers (CCBs; calcium antagonists) are widely used in the therapy of hypertension and effort angina. The major mechanism of action is by calcium channel blockade in the arterioles, with peripheral or coronary vasodilation thereby explaining the major effects in hypertension and in effort angina. The heart rate–lowering (HRL) CCBs also have more β-blocking with a more prominent negative inotropic effect and inhibit the sinus and the atrioventricular nodes. These inhibitory cardiac effects are absent or muted in the dihydropyridines (DHPs), of which nifedipine is the prototype, now joined by amlodipine and felodipine, and others. As a group, the DHPs are more vascular selective and more often used in hypertension than the HRL agents, which are also called the non-DHPs. Only the non-DHPs, verapamil and diltiazem, have antiarrhythmic properties by inhibiting the AV node. Both DHPs and non-DHPs are used against effort angina, albeit acting through different mechanisms.

2. *Safety and efficacy.* Previous serious concerns about the long-term safety of the CCBs as a group have been annulled by a series of large-outcome studies in hypertension, with one still to come in angina pectoris. Nonetheless, cautions and contraindication need to be honored for correct use.

3. *Ischemic heart disease.* All the CCBs work against effort angina, with efficacy and safety rather similar to those of β-blockers. In unstable angina the DHPs are specifically contra-indicated in the absence of β-blockade, because of their tendency to vasodilation-induced reflex adrenergic activation. By contrast, the use of the heart rate–lowering agents, the non-DHPs, in unstable angina is relatively well supported. In postinfarct patients, data also favor verapamil, although the number of trials is not nearly as impressive as the many favoring β-blockade. Thus, when there is no heart failure postinfarct verapamil can be used when β-blockade is not tolerated or contraindicated, although not licensed for this purpose in the United States. DHPs do not have good postinfarct data.

4. *Hypertension.* Overall evidence from a series of large-outcome studies, including ALLHAT, favors the safety and efficacy on hard end-points, including coronary heart disease, of longer acting DHPs. One large-outcome study on coronary heart disease shows that the non-DHP verapamil gives results overall as good as atenolol.

5. *In diabetic hypertensive patients,* ALLHAT showed that amlodipine was as effective as the diuretic or the ACE inhibitor in reducing coronary heart disease. Other data suggest that initial antihypertensive therapy in diabetic patients should be based on an ACE inhibitor, especially in those with nephropathy. To achieve current blood pressure goals in diabetic patients, it is almost always necessary to use combination therapy, which would include an ACE inhibitor and often a CCB besides a diuretic and/or β-blocker.

6. *Heart failure* remains a class contraindication to the use of all CCBs, with two exceptions: diastolic dysfunction based on left ventricular hypertrophy, and otherwise well-treated systolic heart failure, when amlodipine may be cautiously added if essential, for example, for control of angina.

REFERENCES

1. Abernethy DR, et al. Calcium-antagonist drugs. *N Engl J Med* 1999;341:1447–1455.
2. Kaplan NM. The meaning of ALLHAT. *J Hypertens* 2003;21:233–234.

3. Opie LH, et al. Calcium channel antagonists in the treatment of coronary artery disease: fundamental pharmacological properties relevant to clinical use. *Prog Cardiovasc Dis* 1996;38:273–290.

4. Brown MJ, et al. Morbidity and mortality in patients randomised to double-blind treatment with a long-acting calcium-channel blocker or diuretic in the International Nifedipine GITS study: intervention as a Goal in Hypertension Treatment. *Lancet* 2000;356:366–372.

5. Zanchetti A, et al. On behalf of the ELSA Investigators. Calcium antagonist lacidipine slows down progression of asymptomatic carotid atherosclerosis. Principal results of the European Lacidipine Study on Atherosclerosis (ELSA), a randomized, double-blind, long-term trial. *Circulation* 2002;106:2422–2427.

6. Binggeli C, et al. Effects of chronic calcium channel blockade on sympathetic nerve activity in hypertension. *Hypertension* 2002;39:892–896.

7. Opie LH, et al. Nifedipine and mortality. Grave defects in the dossier. *Circulation* 1995;92:1068–1073.

8. Göbel EJ, et al. Long-term follow-up after early intervention with intravenous diltiazem or intravenous nitroglycerin for unstable angina pectoris. *Eur Heart J* 1998;19:1208–1213.

9. Ardissino D, et al. Transient myocardial ischemia during daily life in rest and exertional angina pectoris and comparison of effectiveness of metoprolol versus nifedipine. *Am J Cardiol* 1991;6:946–952.

10. HINT Study. Early treatment of unstable angina in the coronary care unit, a randomised, double-blind placebo controlled comparison of recurrent ischemia in patients treated with nifedipine or metoprolol or both. Holland Inter–university Nifedipine Trial. *Br Heart J* 1986;56:400–413.

11. European Society of Hypertension Guidelines Committee. European Society of Cardiology guidelines for the management of arterial hypertension. *J Hypertens* 2003; 21:1011–1053.

12. JNC VII. The Seventh Report of the Joint National Committee on Prevention, Detection, Evaluation and Treatment of High Blood Pressure. *JAMA* 2003;289: 2560–2572.

13. BP Trialists. Effects of different blood-pressure lowering regimens on major cardiovascular events: results of prospectively-designed overviews of randomised trials. *Lancet* 2003;362:1527–1535.

14. Fischer Hansen J, et al. Treatment with verapamil during and after an acute myocardial infarction: a review based on the Danish verapamil infarction trials I and II. *J Cardiovasc Pharmacol* 1991;18 (Suppl.6):S20–S25.

15. Pepine CJ, et al. Verapamil use in patients with cardiovascular disease: an overview of randomized trials. *Clin Cardiol* 1998;21:633–641.

16. Brovkovych V, et al. Synergistic antihypertensive effects of nifedipine on endothelium. *Hypertension* 2001;37:34–39.

17. ENCORE Investigators. Effect of nifedipine and cerivastatin on coronary endothelial function in patients with coronary artery disease: the ENCORE I Study (Evaluation of Nifedipine and Cerivastatin On Recovery of coronary Endothelial function). *Circulation* 2003;107:422–428.

18. Bakris GL, et al. Differential effects of calcium antagonist subclasses on markers of nephropathy progression. *Kidney Int* 2004;65:1991–2002.

19. McInnes GT, et al. Mortality differences between ACE inhibitor and calcium channel blocker treated hypertensive patients (Abstract). *JACC* 2000;35:333A.

20. ALLHAT Collaborative Research Group. Major outcomes in high–risk hypertensive patients randomized to angiotensin-converting enzyme inhibitor or calcium channel blocker vs diuretic. The Antihypertensive and Lipid–Lowering Treatment to Prevent Heart Attack Trial (ALLHAT). *JAMA* 2002;288:2981–2997.

21. Grossman EH, et al. Effect of calcium antagonists on plasma norepinephrine levels, heart rate and blood pressure. *Am J Cardiol* 1997;80:1453–1458.

22. STOP-2 Study. Randomised trial of old and new antihypertensive drugs in elderly patients: cardiovascular mortality and morbidity in the Swedish Trial in Old Patients with Hypertension-2 study. *Lancet* 1999;354:1751–1756.

23. Syst-Eur Trial. Randomised double-blind comparison of placebo and active treatment for older patients with isolated systolic hypertension (Syst-Eur Trial). *Lancet* 1997;350:757–764.

24. HOT Study. Effects of intensive blood-pressure lowering and low-dose aspirin in patients with hypertension: principal results of the Hypertension Optimal Treatment (HOT) randomised trial. *Lancet* 1998;351:1755–1762.

25. Pepine CJ, et al. A calcium antagonist vs a non-calcium antagonist hypertension treatment strategy for patients with coronary artery disease. The International Verapamil-Trandolapril Study (INVEST): a randomized controlled trial. *JAMA* 2003;290: 2805–2816.

26. Black HR, et al. Principal results of the Controlled Onset Verapamil Investigation of Cardiovascular End Points (CONVINCE) trial. *JAMA* 2003;289:2073–2082.

27. Tuomilehto J, et al. Effects of calcium-channel blockade in older patients with diabetes and systolic hypertension. *N Engl J Med* 1999;340:677–684.

28. Schwartz JB, et al. Prolongation of verapamil elimination kinetics during chronic oral administration. *Am Heart J* 1982;104:198–203.

29. Opie LH. Adverse cardiovascular drug reactions. *Curr Probl Cardiol* 2000;25:621–676.

30. Boyer EW, et al. Treatment of calcium-channel-blocker intoxication with insulin infusion. *N Engl J Med* 2001;344:1721–1722.

31. Freedman SB, et al. Long-term follow-up of verapamil and nitrate treatment for coronary artery spasm. *Am J Cardiol* 1982;50:711–715.

32. Holzgreve H, et al. Verapamil versus hydrochlorothiazide in the treatment of hypertension: results of long term double blind comparative trial. Verapamil versus Diuretic (VERDI) Trial Research Group. *Br Med J* 1989;299:881–886.

33. Seiler C, et al. Long-term follow-up of medical versus surgical therapy for hypertrophic cardiomyopathy: a retrospective study. *J Am Coll Cardiol* 1991;17:634–642.
34. Bakris GL, et al. Calcium channel blockers versus other antihypertensive therapies on progression of NIDDM associated nephropathy. *Kidney Int* 1996;50:1641–1650.
35. Bagger JP, et al. Effect of verapamil in intermittent claudication. A randomized, double-blind, placebo-controlled, cross-over study after individual dose-response assessment. *Circulation* 1997;95:411–414.
36. Multicenter Diltiazem Postinfarction Trial Research Group. The effect of diltiazem on mortality and reinfarction after myocardial infarction. *N Engl J Med* 1988;319: 385–392.
37. Théroux P, et al. Intravenous diltiazem in acute myocardial infarction. Diltiazem as Adjunctive Therapy to Activase (DATA) trial. *J Am Coll Cardiol* 1998;32:620–628.
38. Boden WE, et al. Incomplete Infarction Trial of European Research Collaborators Evaluating Prognosis Post-Thrombolysis (INTERCEPT Trial). Diltiazem in acute myocardial infarction treated by thrombolytic agents. *Lancet* 2000;355:1751–1756.
39. Materson BJ, et al. Single-drug therapy for hypertension in men. A comparison of six antihypertensive agents with placebo. The Department of Veterans Affairs Co-operative Study Group on Antihypertensive Agents. *N Engl J Med* 1993;328:914–921.
40. Gottdiener JS, et al. For the VA Cooperative Study Group on Antihypertensive Agents. Effect of single-drug therapy on reduction of left ventricular size in mild to moderate hypertension. Comparison of six antihypertensive agents. *Circulation* 1998;98:140–148.
41 Schroeder J, et al. A preliminary study of diltiazem in the prevention of coronary artery disease in heart transplant recipients. *N Engl J Med* 1993;328:164–170.
42. Muller J, et al. Nifedipine therapy for patients with threatened and acute myocardial infarction: a randomized, double-blind, placebo-controlled comparison. *Circulation* 1984;69:740–747.
43. Muller J, et al. Nifedipine and conventional therapy for unstable angina pectoris: a randomized, double-blind comparison. *Circulation* 1984;69:728–733.
44. Furberg CD, et al. Nifedipine dose-related increase in mortality in patients with coronary heart disease. *Circulation* 1995;92:1326–1331.
45. Grossman E, et al. Should a moratorium be placed on sublingual nifedipine capsules given for hypertensive emergencies and pseudoemergencies. *JAMA* 1996;276:1328–1331.
46. de Champlain J, et al. Different effects of nifedipine and amlodipine on circulating catecholamine levels in essential hypertensive patients. *J Hypertens* 1998;16: 1357–1369.
47. Heidenreich PA, et al. Meta-analysis of trials comparing β-blockers, calcium antagonists, and nitrates for stable angina. *JAMA* 1999;281:1927–1936.
48. Pitt B, et al. Effect of amlodipine on the progression of atherosclerosis and the occurrence of clinical events. *Circulation* 2000;102:1503–1510.
49 Simon A, et al. Differential effects of nifedipine and co-amilozide on the progression of early carotid wall changes. *Circulation* 2001;103:2949–2954.
50. Franklin C, et al. A randomized comparison of nifedipine and sodium nitroprusside in severe hypertension. *Chest* 1986;90:500–503.
51. Schneider E, et al. Captopril, nifedipine and their combination for therapy of hypertensive urgencies. *S Afr Med J* 1991;80:265–270.
52. Nayler WG, et al. The unique binding properties of amlodipine: a long-acting calcium antagonist. *J Hum Hypertens* 1991;5 (Suppl 1):55–59.
53. Mason RP. Calcium channel blockers, apoptosis and cancer: Is there a biologic relationship? *JACC* 1999;34:1857–1866.
54. TOMH Study. Treatment of Mild Hypertension study (TOMH). Final results. *JAMA* 1993;270:713–724.
55. Singh S. Long-term double-blind evaluation of amlodipine and nadolol in patients with stable exertional angina pectoris. The Investigators Study 152. *Clin Cardiol* 1993;16:54–58.
56. Davies RF, et al. Effect of amlodipine, atenolol and their combination on myocardial ischemia during treadmill exercise and ambulatory monitoring. *J Am Coll Cardiol* 1995;25:619–625.
57. Midtbo K, et al. Amlodipine versus slow release metoprolol in the treatment of stable exertional angina pectoris (AMSA). *Scand Cardiovasc J* 2000;34:475–479.
58. Rinaldi CA, et al. Randomized, double-blind crossover study to investigate the effects of amlodipine and isosorbide mononitrate on the time course and severity of exercise-induced myocardial stunning. *Circulation* 1998;98:749–756.
59. Udelson JE, et al. Effects of amlodipine on exercise tolerance, quality of life, and left ventricular function in patients with heart failure from left ventricular systolic dysfunction. *Am Heart J* 2000;139:503–510.
60. Agodoa LY, et al. Effect of ramipril vs amlodipine on renal outcomes in hypertensive nephrosclerosis: a randomized controlled trial. *JAMA* 2001;285:2719–2728.
61. Emanuelsson H, et al. For the TRAFFIC Study Group. Antianginal efficacy of the combination of felodipine-metoprolol 10/100 mg compared with each drug alone in patients with stable effort-induced angina pectoris: a multicenter parallel group study. *Am Heart J* 1999;137:854–862.
62. Cohn JN, et al. Effect of the calcium antagonist felodipine as supplementary vasodilator therapy in patients with chronic heart failure treated with enalapril (V-HeFT III Study). *Circulation* 1997;96:856–863.
63. Izzo JJ, et al. Clinical advisory statement: importance of systolic blood pressure in older Americans. *Hypertension* 2000;35:1021–1024.
64. Malacco E, et al. Treatment of isolated systolic hypertension: the SHELL study results. *Blood Press* 2003;12:160–167.
65. Julius S, et al. Outcomes in hypertensive patients at high cardiovascular risk treated with regimens based on valsartan or amlodipine: the VALUE randomised trial. *Lancet* 2004;363:2022–2031.

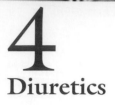

4
Diuretics

Lionel H. Opie • Norman M. Kaplan

"Little benefit is to be derived from using large doses of oral diuretics to reduce blood pressure."

CRANSTON ET AL., 1963[1]

"Low dose diuretics are the most effective first-line treatment for preventing cardiovascular morbidity and mortality (in hypertension).

PSATY ET AL., 2003[2]

Diuretics are agents that alter the physiological renal mechanisms that form urine in such a way that there is increased flow of urine with greater excretion of sodium (natriuresis; Fig. 4-1). Diuretic therapy has traditionally been the first choice in the treatment of symptomatic congestive heart failure, now usually in conjunction with angiotensin-converting enzyme (ACE) inhibitors. In hypertension, diuretics continue to be used as first-line therapy, albeit in much lower doses—a position supported by recent meta-analyses.[2,3]

Differing Effects of Diuretics in Heart Failure and Hypertension

In *heart failure,* diuretics are given to control pulmonary and peripheral symptoms and signs of congestion. Diuretics should rarely be used as monotherapy, rather being combined with ACE inhibitors and generally a β-blocker.[4] Often the loop diuretics (Fig. 4-2) are used preferentially, for three reasons: (1) the superior fluid clearance for the same degree of natriuresis (Table 4-1); (2) loop diuretics work even in the presence of renal impairment that often accompanies severe heart failure; and (3) there is an increasing diuretic response to increasing doses, so that they are "high ceiling" diuretics. Yet in mild heart failure thiazides may initially be preferred, especially when there is a background of hypertension. In general, diuretic doses are higher than those used in hypertension. Besides the induction of renal sodium and water loss, furosemide given to previously untreated patients with severe congestive heart failure (CHF) calls forth two opposing stimuli. The vasoconstrictory renin-angiotensin system is stimulated, and there are also increased levels of vasodilatory prostaglandins. Hence, the addition of ACE inhibitors to offset the renin rise should be beneficial.

In *hypertension,* to exert an effect, the diuretic must provide enough natriuresis to shrink fluid volume at least to some extent. Diuretics may also work as vasodilators and in other ways. Some persistent volume depletion is required to lower the blood pressure. Therefore, once daily furosemide is usually inadequate because the initial sodium loss is quickly reconstituted throughout the remainder of the day. Thus, a longer acting thiazide-type diuretic is usually chosen for hypertension.[5,6]

Benefit/Risk Ratio

The benefit/risk ratio of diuretics is high in CHF. In hypertension, their use has been questioned because of certain "wrong way" blood

NEPHRON FUNCTION
Opie 2004

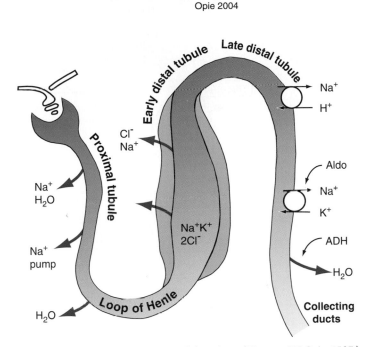

Figure 4-1 Nephron anatomy and function. (*Figure © LH Opie, 2005.*)

Table 4-1 | Urinary Electrolyte Composition During Diuresis

	Volume (ml/min)	pH	Na$^+$ (mmol/L)	K$^+$ (mmol/L)	Cl$^-$	HCO$_3^-$	Ca^{2+}
Control	1	6.0	50	15	60	1	Variable
Thiazides	3	7.4	150	25	150	25	0
Furosemide	8	6.0	140	10	155	1	+
Triamterene	3	7.2	130	5	120	15	0
Amiloride	2	7.2	130	5	110	15	0

0 = decreased; + = increased.
Modified from Mudge[62] with permission.

biochemical changes. Nonetheless, they retain their primacy as first-line agents when used in low daily doses, such as 12.5 to 25 mg of hydrochlorothiazide, that reduce total and cardiovascular mortality, stroke, coronary heart disease, and congestive heart failure.[2] Higher doses, 50 to 200 mg, as used in the past, did not reduce coronary heart disease nor total mortality. The value of diuretics is particularly well established in certain groups of hypertensive patients—the elderly, the obese, and blacks—and those already receiving ACE inhibitors or angiotensin receptor blockers (ARBs). Furthermore, low doses of diuretics can be given over prolonged periods with minimal changes in blood lipids, glucose, and potassium. Thus the American Joint National Committee[7] and the WHO/ISH Committee[6] recommend that diuretics should be considered for first choice in the treatment of hypertension not complicated by other conditions (see Chapter 7).

For practical purposes, the three major groups of diuretics are the loop diuretics, the thiazides, and the potassium-sparing agents. Each type of diuretic acts at a different site of the nephron (Fig. 4-2), leading to

DIURETIC SITES OF ACTION

Opie 2004

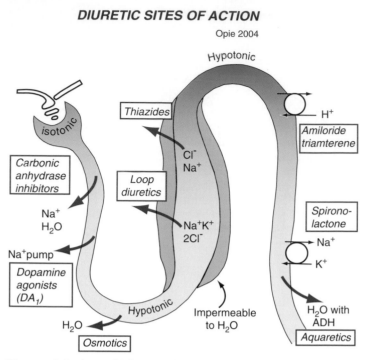

Figure 4-2 The multiple sites of action of diuretic agents from which follows the principle of sequential nephron block. A common maximal combination, using this principle, is a loop diuretic plus a thiazide plus a K⁺-sparing agent. (*Figure © LH Opie, 2005.*)

the concept of *sequential nephron blockade*. All but the potassium sparers must be transported to the luminal side; this process is blocked by the buildup of organic acids in renal insufficiency so that progressively larger doses are needed. Especially thiazides lose their potency as renal function falls.

LOOP DIURETICS

Furosemide

Furosemide (frusemide in the United Kingdom; *Lasix, Dryptal, Frusetic, Frusid*) is one of the standard loop diuretics for severe CHF. It is a sulfonamide derivative. Furosemide is initial therapy in acute pulmonary edema and in the pulmonary congestion of left-sided failure of acute myocardial infarction (AMI). Relief of dyspnea even before diuresis results from venodilation and preload reduction.[8]

Pharmacologic Effects and Pharmacokinetics Loop diuretics including furosemide inhibit the $Na^+/K^+/2Cl^-$ cotransporter concerned with the transport of chloride across the lining cells of the ascending limb of the loop of Henle (Fig. 4-2). This site of action is reached intraluminally, after the drug has been excreted by the proximal tubule. The effect of the cotransport inhibition is that chloride, sodium, potassium, and hydrogen ions all remain intraluminally and are lost in the urine with the possible side effects of hyponatremia, hypochloremia, hypokalemia, and alkalosis. However, in comparison with thiazides there is a relatively greater urine volume and relatively less loss of sodium (Table 4-1). For equinatriuretic doses, loop diuretics actually lose less potassium than do thiazides, despite their image of provoking hypokalemia. The plasma half-life of furosemide is 1.5 hours; the duration of action is 4 to 6 hours. Diuresis starts within 10 to 20 minutes of an intravenous dose and peaks 1 to 1.5 hours after an oral dose. Venodilation reduces the preload in acute LV failure within 5 to 15 minutes; the mechanism is not well understood. Conversely, there may follow a reactive vasoconstriction.

Dose

Intravenous furosemide is usually started as a slow 40-mg injection (no more than 4 mg/minute to reduce ototoxicity; give 80 mg over 20 minutes IV 1 hour later if needed). When renal function is impaired, as in elderly patients, higher doses are required, with much higher doses for renal failure and severe CHF. *Oral furosemide* also has a wide dose range (20 to 240 mg/day or even more; 20-, 40-, and 80-mg tablets in the United States; in Europe, also scored 500-mg tablets). A short duration of action (4 to 5 hours) means that frequent doses are needed when sustained diuresis is required. When two daily doses are required, they should be given in the early morning and mid-afternoon to obviate nocturia and to protect against volume depletion. Because of variable responses, such as a brisk initial diuresis with a residual resistant component, the dose regimen must be individualized. For *hypertension*, furosemide 20 mg twice daily is the approximate equivalent of hydrochlorothiazide 25 mg. In healthy subjects, furosemide causes a greater earlier (0 to 6 hours) absolute loss of sodium than does hydrochlorothiazide but, because of its short duration of action, the total 24-hour sodium loss may be insufficient to maintain the slight volume contraction that is needed for a sustained antihypertensive action.[9] This observation supports the practice of giving furosemide twice daily in hypertension. In the presence of *oliguria* (not induced by volume depletion), as the glomerular filtration rate (GFR) drops below 20 ml/minute, from 240 mg up to 2000 mg of furosemide may be required because of decreasing luminal excretion. Similar arguments lead to increasing doses of furosemide in *severe refractory heart failure*.

Indications Furosemide is frequently the diuretic of choice for *severe heart failure* for reasons already discussed. Similarly, it is the initial drug of choice in *acute pulmonary edema*. After initial intravenous use, oral furosemide is usually continued as standard diuretic therapy, sometimes to be replaced by thiazides as the heart failure ameliorates. In *AMI* with clinical failure, intravenous furosemide has rapid beneficial hemodynamic effects and is often combined with ACE inhibition.[10] In *hypertension*, twice daily low-dose furosemide can be effective even as monotherapy or combined with other agents and is increasingly needed as renal function deteriorates.[11] In *hypertensive crisis*, intravenous furosemide is used if fluid overload is present. It is widely believed that in *severe renal failure* high dose furosemide increases the GFR, yet the subject is poorly understood.

Contraindications Anuria, although listed as a contraindication to the use of furosemide, is sometimes treated (as is oliguria) by furosemide in the hope of evoking a diuresis; first exclude dehydration and a history of hypersensitivity to furosemide or sulfonamides. Furosemide (like other sulfonamides) may precipitate photosensitive skin eruptions or may cause blood dyscrasias. Furosemide should not be used intravenously when electrolytes cannot be monitored.

Hypokalemia with Furosemide Clearly, much depends on the doses chosen and the degree of diuresis achieved. A lesser degree of hypokalemia than expected occurs because (1) the actual potassium concentration lost per unit volume during the diuresis is low (Table 4-1), and (2) the short action of furosemide allows for post-diuresis correction of potassium and magnesium balance. The risk of hypokalemia is greatest with high-dose furosemide, especially when given intravenously, and at the start of myocardial infarction when hypokalemia with risk of arrhythmias is common even in the absence of diuretic therapy. Carefully regulated intravenous potassium supplements may be required in these circumstances. In heart failure, digitalis toxicity may be precipitated by overdiuresis and hypokalemia.

Other Side Effects The chief side effects, in addition to *hypokalemia*, are *hypovolemia* and *hyperuricemia*. Hypovolemia can be lessened by a low starting initial dose (20 to 40 mg); if hypovolemia occurs, prerenal azotemia may develop (monitor blood urea). A few patients on high-dose furosemide have developed severe hyperosmolar nonketotic *hyperglycemic states*. *Atherogenic blood lipid changes*, similar to those found with thiazides, may also be found with loop diuretics, although this is not so well documented. Occasionally, gout or diabetes may be precipitated. It is not clear whether furosemide causes fewer metabolic side effects than conventional thiazides. First principles suggest that minimizing hypokalemia should lessen the risk of glucose intolerance. Reversible dose-related *ototoxicity* (electrolyte disturbances of the endolymphatic system) can be avoided by infusing furosemide at rates not greater than 4 mg/minute and keeping the oral dose below 1000 mg daily. *Urinary retention* may result from vigorous diuresis in the elderly. In *nursing mothers*, furosemide is excreted in the milk.

Loss of Diuretic Potency Braking is the phenomenon whereby after the first dose, there is a decrease in the diuretic response caused by renin-angiotensin activation and prevented by restoring the diuretic-induced loss of blood volume.[12] *Long-term tolerance* refers to increased reabsorption of sodium associated with hypertrophy of the distal nephron segments (see section on Diuretic Resistance). The mechanism may be increased growth of the nephron cells induced by increased aldosterone.[9]

Drug Interactions with Furosemide Cotherapy with certain *aminoglycosides* can precipitate ototoxicity. *Probenecid* may interfere with the effects of thiazides or loop diuretics by blocking their secretion into the urine of the proximal tubule. *Indomethacin* and other nonsteroidal anti-inflammatory drugs (*NSAIDs*) lessen the renal response to loop diuretics, presumably by interfering with formation of vasodilatory prostaglandins.[13] High doses of furosemide may competitively inhibit the excretion of *salicylates* to predispose to salicylate poisoning with tinnitus. *Steroid* or adrenocorticotropic hormone (ACTH) therapy may predispose to hypokalemia. Furosemide, unlike thiazides, does not decrease renal excretion of *lithium*, so that lithium toxicity is not a risk. Loop diuretics do not alter blood digoxin levels, nor do they interact with warfarin.

Bumetanide

The site of action of bumetanide (*Bumex, Burinex*) and its effects (and side effects) are very similar to those of furosemide (Table 4-2). The onset of diuresis is within 30 minutes, with a peak at 75 to 90 minutes, and a total duration of action of 270 minutes. In practice, as with furosemide, low-dose therapy need not occasion undue concern regarding hypokalemia as a possible side effect, while higher doses can cause considerable electrolyte disturbances, including hypokalemia. Again, as in the case of furosemide, a combined diuretic effect is obtained by addition of a thiazide diuretic.

Dosage and Clinical Uses In CHF, the usual oral dose is 0.5 to 2 mg, with 1 mg bumetanide being equal to 40 mg of furosemide. In acute pulmonary edema, a single dose of 1 to 3 mg can be effective; usually it is given intravenously over 1 to 2 minutes, and the dose can be repeated at 2- to 3-hour intervals to a maximum of 10 mg daily. In *renal edema*, the effects of bumetanide are similar to those of furosemide. In the United States, bumetanide is not approved for hypertension.

Table 4-2 Loop Diuretics; Doses and Kinetics

Drug	Dose	Pharmacokinetics
1. Furosemide (USA) Frusemide (UK) = Lasix	10–40 mg oral, 2× for BP; 20–80 mg 2–3× for CHF; Up to 250–2000 mg oral or IV	Diuresis within 10–20 min Peak diuresis at 1.5 h Total duration of action 4–5 h Renal excretion
2. Bumetanide = Bumex (USA) = Burinex (UK)	0.5–2 mg oral 1–2× daily for CHF; 5 mg oral or IV for oliguria (not licensed for BP)	Peak diuresis at 75–90 min Total duration of action 4–5 h Renal excretion
3. Torsemide = Demadex (USA)	5–10 mg oral 1× daily for BP; 10–20 mg oral 1× daily or IV for CHF (up to 200 mg daily)	Diuresis within 10 min of IV dose Peak diuresis at 60 min Oral peak effect at 1–2 h Oral duration of diuresis 6–8 h

BP = blood pressure control; CHF = congestive heart failure.

Side Effects and Cautions Side effects associated with bumetanide are similar to those of furosemide; ototoxicity may be lower and renal toxicity greater. The combination with other potentially nephrotoxic drugs, such as aminoglycosides, must be avoided. In patients with renal failure, high doses have caused myalgia, so that the dose should not exceed 4 mg/day when the GFR is below 5 ml/minute. Patients allergic to sulfonamides may also be hypersensitive to bumetanide. In pregnancy, the risk is similar to that of furosemide (category C).

Summary Most clinicians will continue to use the agent they know best (i.e., furosemide). Because furosemide is widely available in generic form, its cost is likely to be less than that of bumetanide.

Torsemide

This loop diuretic (*Demadex*) has a longer duration of action than furosemide (Table 4-2). Although initial studies suggested that a subdiuretic daily dose of 2.5 mg was antihypertensive and free of changes in plasma potassium or glucose, in the United States the only doses registered for antihypertensive efficacy are 5 to 10 mg daily. These natriuretic doses decrease plasma potassium, increase uric acid, and transiently increase serum cholesterol, while the 10-mg dose mildly increases plasma glucose (package insert). The information available is not enough to state whether torsemide or other loop diuretics cause less metabolic disturbances than do thiazides in equihypotensive doses.

In *heart failure*, an intravenous dose of torsemide 10 to 20 mg initiates a diuresis within 10 minutes that peaks within the first hour. Similar oral doses (high availability) give an onset of diuresis within 1 hour and a peak effect within 1 to 2 hours, and a total duration of action of 6 to 8 hours. Torsemide 10 mg gives about the same degree of natriuresis as does furosemide 40 mg.[13a] In these doses and in a 12-month open-label cohort study, torsemide was associated with a better functional class, less evident potassium loss and a lower mortality than furosemide.[13a] Properly designed long-term outcome studies are required to confirm this proposed superiority of torsemide.

In *renal failure*, as in the case of other loop diuretics, the renal excretion of the drug falls, as does the renal function. Yet the plasma half-life torsemide is unaltered, probably because hepatic clearance increases. In *hepatic cirrhosis*, the dose is 5 to 10 mg daily, titrated upwards to a maximum of 200 mg daily. Torsemide is given with an aldosterone antagonist. In *pregnancy*, torsemide may be relatively safe (category B versus category C for furosemide).

Regarding *metabolic side effects*, the FDA-approved package insert for torsemide claims that antihypertensive doses (5 to 10 mg) reduce plasma potassium only by 0.1 mEq/L after 6 weeks, yet the higher dose increases plasma glucose by 5.5 mg/dl (0.3 mmol/L) after 6 weeks with a further increase of 1.8 mg/dl during the subsequent year. Other side effects, cautions, and contraindications are similar to those of furosemide.

Class Side Effects of Loop Diuretics

Sulfonamide Sensitivity Ethacrynic acid (*Edecrin*) is the only non-sulfonamide diuretic and is used only in patients allergic to other diuretics. It closely resembles furosemide in dose (25- and 50-mg tablet), duration of diuresis, and side effects (except for more ototoxicity). If ethacrynic acid is not available for a sulfonamide-sensitive patient, a gradual challenge with furosemide or, even better, torsemide may overcome sensitivity.[14]

Metabolic Changes Loop diuretics all produce a powerful and rapid natriuresis and can be used in the therapy of acute and chronic heart failure. They are also used for hepatic cirrhosis and hypertension. The important question is whether or not the loop diuretics, like the thiazides, can induce adverse metabolic changes, such as an increased plasma cholesterol, glucose, and uric acid. The answer is yes.

Hypokalemia This may cause vague symptoms such as fatigue and listlessness, besides electrocardiographic and rhythm abnormalities. In the doses used for mild hypertension (furosemide 20 mg twice daily, torsemide 5 to 10 mg), hypokalemia is limited and possibly less than with hydrochlorothiazide 25 to 50 mg daily. Nonetheless, it does make sense to combine a loop diuretic with a potassium-retaining agent or with an ACE inhibitor or ARBs unless these are contraindicated. In heart failure, hypokalemia is more likely; similar cautions apply.

Hyperglycemia Diuretic-induced glucose intolerance is likely related to hypokalemia, and/or to total body potassium depletion.[15] An interesting proposal is that the transient postprandial fall of potassium impairs the effect of insulin at that time and hence leads to intermittent hyperglycemia.[16] Although there are no large prospective studies on the effects of loop diuretics on insulin insensitivity or glucose tolerance in hypertensive patients, it is clearly prudent to avoid hypokalemia and to monitor both serum potassium and blood glucose values.

Blood Lipid Profile Loop diuretics may cause blood lipid changes similar to thiazides. For torsemide, the package insert indicates that short-term treatment with doses of 5 to 20 mg daily increased plasma cholesterol by only 4 to 8 mg/dL (0.1 to 0.2 mmol/L) and that the changes subsided during chronic therapy over 1 year. Likewise, triglycerides rose and then reverted to normal. These transient changes are rather similar to the situation described with low-dose thiazides.

Metabolic Changes with Loop Diuretics—Recommendations The overall evidence suggests that loop diuretics, like the thiazides, can cause dose-related metabolic disturbances. High doses used for heart failure might therefore pose problems. It makes sense to take special precautions against the hypokalemia of high-dose loop diuretics because of the link between intermittent falls in plasma potassium and hyperglycemia. A sensible start is addition of an ACE inhibitor or ARB.

THIAZIDE DIURETICS

Thiazide diuretics (Table 4-3) remain the most widely recommended first-line therapy for hypertension,[5,6] although challenged by other agents such as ACE inhibitors, angiotensin receptor blockers, β-blockers, and calcium channel blockers. Thiazides are also standard therapy for chronic CHF, when edema is modest, either alone or in combination with loop diuretics.

Pharmacologic Action and Pharmacokinetics Thiazide diuretics act to inhibit the reabsorption of sodium and chloride in the more distal part of the nephron (Fig. 4-2). This cotransporter is insensitive to the loop diuretics. More sodium reaches the distal tubules to stimulate the exchange with potassium, particularly in the presence of an activated renin-angiotensin-aldosterone system. Thiazides may also increase the active excretion of potassium in the distal renal tubule. Thiazides are rapidly absorbed from the gastrointestinal (GI) tract to produce a diuresis within 1 to 2 hours, which lasts for 16 to 24 hours in the case of the prototype thiazide, hydrochlorothiazide.[17] Some major differences from the loop diuretics are (1) the longer duration of action; (2) the different site of action (Fig. 4-2); (3) the fact that thiazides are *low ceiling diuretics* because the maximal response is reached at a relatively low dosage (Fig. 4-3); and (4) the much decreased capacity of thiazides to work in the presence of renal failure (serum creatinine >2.0 mg/dL or about 180 μmol/L; GFR below 15 to 20 ml/min).[12] The fact that thiazides, loop diuretics, and potassium-sparing agents all act at different tubular sites explains their additive effects *(sequential nephron block)*.

Thiazide Doses and Indications In *hypertension*, diuretics are regaining their primacy as the initial agent of choice, especially in the elderly

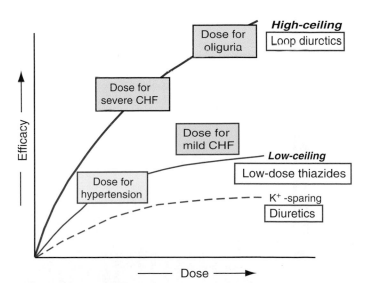

LOW VS HIGH CEILING DIURETICS
Opie 2004

Figure 4-3 The differences between high- and low-ceiling diuretics, and the doses of each group used for various indications. The lowest doses are used for hypertension. (*Figure © LH Opie, 2005.*)

Table 4-3 Thiazide Diuretics: Doses and Duration of Action

	Trade Name (UK-Europe)	Trade Name (USA)	Dose	Duration of Action (h)
Hydrochlorothiazide	Esidrex HydroSaluric	HydroDiuril; Esidrix	12.5–25 mg; 12.5 mg preferred (BP); 25–100 mg (CHF)	16–24
Hydroflumethazide	Hydrenox	Saluron; Diucardin	12.5–25 mg; 12.5 mg preferred (BP); 25–200 mg (CHF)	12–24
Chlorthalidone	Hygroton	Hygroton	12.5–50 mg; 12.5–15 preferred (BP)	48–72
Metolazone	Metenix; Diulo	Zaroxolyn; Diulo	2.5–5 mg (BP) 5–20 mg (CHF)	24
Bendrofluazide = bendroflumethiazide	Aprinox; Centyl; Urizide	Naturetin	1.25–2.5 mg; 1.25 preferred (BP); 10 mg (CHF)	12–18
Polythiazide	—	Renese	1*–2 mg (BP)	24–48
Benthiazide	—	Aquatag; Exna	50*–200 mg	12–18
Chlorothiazide	Saluric	Diuril	250*–1000 mg	6–12
Cyclothiazide	—	Anhydron	1*–2 mg	18–24
Trichlormethiazide	Fluitran (not in UK)	Metahydrin; Naqua	1*–4 mg	24
Cyclopenthiazide	Navidrex	—	0.125–0.25 mg (0.125 mg preferred, BP)	6–12
Indapamide	Natrilix	Lozol	1.25–2.5 mg; 1.25 mg preferred (BP); 2.5–5 mg (CHF)†	24
Xipamide	Diurexan	—	10–20 mg (5 mg preferred for BP)	6–12

Note: The doses given here for antihypertensive therapy are generally *lower* than those recommended by the manufacturers (exception: Lozol 1.25 mg is recommended).
*Lowest effective antihypertensive dose not known; may prefer to use other agents for BP control.
†Not licensed for CHF in the UK.
BP = use for blood-pressure-lowering; CHF = use for congestive heart failure.

and in black patients. By contrast, in younger whites (mean age 51 years) only one third responded to escalating doses of hydrochloro-thiazide over 1 year.[18] The thiazide doses generally used have been too high. Lower doses with fewer biochemical alterations provide full antihypertensive as shown in several large trials. In the SHEP study, chlorthalidone 12.5 mg was initially used, and after 5 years 30% of the subjects were still on this lower dose; in 16% the dose was doubled.[19] Overall, documented biochemical changes were small, including a 0.3 mmol/L fall in potassium, a rise in serum uric acid, and small increases in serum cholesterol and in glucose (1.7% more new diabetes than in placebo). These changes found after 1 year of treatment do not necessarily predict changes over a longer period. Regarding hydrochlorothiazide, exceeding 25 mg daily clearly creates metabolic problems,[20,21] whereas increasing the dose from 12.5 to 25 mg may give only a borderline better reduction of blood pressure.[22] In the case of cyclopenthiazide, widely used in the United Kingdom, only 0.125 mg (the approximate equivalent of hydrochloro-thiazide 8 mg) gives as much antihypertensive effect as 0.5 mg daily with fewer metabolic side effects. Higher doses of all these agents are marginally more effective, with greater risks of undesirable side effects (Table 4-4). In the case of bendrofluazide, a lower dose (1.25 mg daily) causes less metabolic side effects and no effects on blood glucose or insulin when compared with the conventional 5-mg dose.[23]

The *response rate in hypertension* to thiazide monotherapy is variable and may be disappointing, being only about 45% in one trial with 12.5 to 25 mg chlorthalidone daily.[24] The response depends in part on the age and race of the patient and probably also on the sodium intake. A common error in diuretic therapy is *"premature step therapy"* (i.e., going on to the next step too soon). With hydrochlorothiazide, the full antihypertensive effect of low-dose 12.5 mg daily may take up to 6 weeks. Increasing the dose of hydrochlorothiazide up to a maximum of 100 mg daily may improve the response, but the risk of metabolic side effects is unacceptably high, so that combination therapy, for example, with an ACE inhibitor or ARB becomes prefer-able rather than increasing the dose beyond 25 mg daily[17] or even beyond 12.5 mg daily.[22] In *CHF,* higher doses are justified (50 to 100 mg hydrochlorothiazide daily are probably ceiling doses), while watching the serum potassium. Considerable advantage can result from combining a loop diuretic with a thiazide.[12] Specifically, the thia-zides block the nephron sites at which hypertrophy occurs during long-term loop diuretic therapy (see section on Diuretic Resistance).

In the United States, hydrochlorothiazide is the most popular thiazide but chlorthalidone was chosen for the two most important

---

Table 4-4 Side Effects of Diuretic Therapy for Hypertension

Causing Withdrawal of Therapy

Impaired glucose tolerance
Gout
Impotence
Nausea, dizziness, or headache

Blood Biochemical Changes

Potassium: hypokalemia
Glucose: hyperglycemia
Uric acid: hyperuricemia
Urea, creatinine: prerenal fall in GFR
Lipid profile: rise in serum cholesterol, triglyceride and ratio
  apolipoprotein B to A; fall in HDL-cholesterol

All effects are minimized by appropriately lower doses such as hydrochlorothiazide 12.5 mg daily. See also references in previous edition.

trials—SHEP and ALLHAT.[24] Chlorthalidone lasts longer,[17] and no more than 15 mg should be used. Hydrochlorthiazide 12.5 mg is a good alternative (see Chapter 7, p. 194).

Contraindications These include severe renal insufficiency, hypokalemia, ventricular arrhythmias, and cotherapy with proarrhythmic drugs. In hypokalemia (including early AMI), thiazide diuretics may precipitate arrhythmias. Relative contraindications include pregnancy hypertension, because of the risk of a decreased blood volume; moreover, thiazides can cross the placental barrier with risk of neonatal jaundice. In mild renal impairment, the GFR may fall further as thiazides decrease the blood volume.

Side Effects Besides the "wrong way" metabolic side effects seen with higher doses (Table 4-4) such as hypokalemia, hyponatremia, increased insulin resistance, and increased blood triglyceride and cholesterol levels, thiazide diuretics rarely cause sulfonamide-type immune side effects including intrahepatic jaundice, pancreatitis, blood dyscrasias, angiitis, pneumonitis, and interstitial nephritis. Impotence is newly emphasized, seen more commonly than with any other class of drugs in the TOMH study.[25]

Thiazide Drug Interactions *Steroids* may cause salt retention to antagonize the action of thiazide diuretics. *Indomethacin* and other NSAIDs blunt the response to thiazide diuretics.[13] *Antiarrhythmics* that prolong the QT-interval, such as class IA or III agents including sotalol, may precipitate torsades de pointes in the presence of diuretic-induced hypokalemia. The *nephrotoxic effects of certain antibiotics*, such as the aminoglycosides, may be potentiated by diuretics. *Probenecid* (for the therapy of gout) and *lithium* (for mania) may block thiazide effects by interfering with thiazide excretion into the urine. Thiazide diuretics also interact with lithium by impairing renal clearance with risk of lithium toxicity.

OTHER THIAZIDE-LIKE AGENTS

Metolazone (*Zaroloxyn, Diulo, Metenix*) is a powerful diuretic with a quinazoline structure yet falling within the overall thiazide family. There may be an additional site of action beyond that of the standard thia-zides. An important advantage of metolazone is efficacy even *despite reduced renal function.* There are, however, no strict studies comparing metolazone with standard thiazides in renal impairment. The duration of action is up to 24 hours. The standard dose is 5 to 20 mg once daily for CHF or renal edema and 2.5 to 5 mg for hypertension. In combination with furosemide, metolazone may provoke a profound diuresis, with the risk of excessive volume and potassium depletion. Nonetheless, metolazone may be added to furosemide with care, especially in patients with renal as well as cardiac failure. The side effect profile of metolazone closely resembles that of the ordinary thiazides. Metolazone 1.25 to 10 mg once daily was given in titrated doses to 17 patients with severe CHF, almost all of whom were already on furosemide, captopril, and digoxin; most responded by a brisk diuresis within 48 to 72 hours.[26] Consequently, metolazone is often used in addition to a prior combination of a loop diuretic, a thiazide, and aldosterone inhibitor in patients with chronic heart failure and resistant peripheral edema.

Mykrox is a rapidly acting formulation of metolazone with high bioavailability, registered for use in hypertension only in a dose of 0.5 to 1 mg once daily. The maximum antihypertensive effect is reached within 2 weeks.

Indapamide (*Lozol, Natrilix*) is a thiazide-like diuretic albeit with a different indoline structure. It has two properties beyond diuresis. First, there is added vasodilation.[27] A second unusual property is a high concentration class I and III antiarrhythmic effect.[28] If this were also clinically relevant, it could protect from ventricular arrhythmias, while also carrying a theoretical risk of torsades de pointes in the presence of hypokalemia or cotherapy with certain other antiarrhythmics (see Fig. 8-8). Indapamide has a terminal half-life of 14 to 16 hours, and effectively lowers the blood pressure over 24 hours. The initial dose is 1.25 mg once daily for 4 weeks, then if needed 2.5 mg daily. Indapamide appears to be more lipid neutral than other thiazides[29] but seems equally likely to cause other metabolic problems such as hypokalemia, hyperglycemia, or hyperuricemia. With a reduced but still antihypertensive dose of only 0.625 to 1.25 mg combined with the ACE inhibitor perindopril 2–4 mg, the serum potassium fell by only 0.11 mmol/L over 1 year, while the blood glucose was unchanged from placebo.[30] Regarding *regression of LV hypertrophy*, indapamide was better than enalapril in the LIVE study (LVH with Indapamide Versus Enalapril).[31] In *cardiac edema*, higher doses such as 2.5 to 5 mg give a diuresis. However, the drug has little advantage over other well-tried diuretics, although approved for this purpose. There are no strict comparisons with low-dose thiazides concerning effects on glucose tolerance. In general, its side effect profile resembles that of the thiazides, including the low risk of sulfonamide sensitivity reactions. In Europe, a sustained-release preparation (1.5 mg) gives blood pressure reduction equal to that of 2.5 mg indapamide, yet the incidence of hypokalemia <3.4 mmol/L is more than 50% lower.[32]

METABOLIC AND OTHER SIDE EFFECTS OF THIAZIDES

Many side effects of thiazides are similar to those of the loop diuretics: electrolyte disturbances, including hypokalemia, hyponatremia, and hyperuricemia; the precipitation of gout and diabetes; a decreased blood volume; and alkalosis. *Atherogenic blood lipid changes* and especially impotence have recently been emphasized. *Hyponatremia* may sometimes occur in the elderly, even with low diuretic doses. Most side effects are dose dependent. Doses as low as 6.25 mg of hydrochlorothiazide potentiate the efficacy of other drugs such as β-blockers[33] or ACE inhibitors with no obvious adverse effects.

Hypokalemia As in the case of loop diuretics, hypokalemia is probably an over-feared complication, especially when low doses of thiazides are used.[34] Many physicians remain impressed by the risk of fall in plasma potassium that may become covert only when dietary potassium decreases or intercurrent diarrhea develops, hence the frequent choice of combination of thiazides with the potassium-retaining agents including the ACE inhibitors and ARBs. This choice in turn brings about the alternative but lesser risk that some patients will develop *hyperkalemia*, especially in the presence of renal impairment and the concomitant use of ACE inhibitors.

Ventricular Arrhythmias Diuretic-induced hypokalemia can contribute to torsades de pointes and hence to sudden death, especially when there is cotherapy with agents prolonging the QT-interval (see Fig. 8-4). The proarrhythmic risk seems much more serious in patients with pre-existing clinical coronary disease or heart failure. Of importance, in the SOLVD study on heart failure, the baseline use of a non–potassium-retaining diuretic was associated with an increased risk of arrhythmic death compared with a potassium-retaining diuretic.[35] In mild to moderate hypertension, the degree of hypokalemia evoked by low-dose thia-zides seldom matters.

Therapeutic Strategies to Avoid Hypokalemia Common sense says that in patients with a higher risk of arrhythmias, as in ischemic heart disease, heart failure on digoxin, or hypertension with LV hypertrophy, a potassium- and magnesium-sparing diuretic should be part of the therapy unless contraindicated by renal failure or by cotherapy with an ACE inhibitor or ARB. A potassium sparer may be better than potassium supplementation, especially because the supplements do not avoid hypomagnesemia; yet these issues are not completely resolved. Of note, several antihypertensive combination diuretic tablets contain too much thiazide (see Table 7-5).

Hypomagnesemia Conventional doses of diuretics rarely cause magnesium deficiency,[36] but hypomagnesemia, like hypokalemia, is blamed for arrhythmias of QT prolongation during diuretic therapy. Animal data suggest that hypomagnesemia can be prevented by the addition of a potassium-retaining component such as amiloride to the thiazide diuretic.

Diabetogenic Effects The thiazides are more likely to provoke diabetes if combined with a β-blocker.[37–41] This risk presumably depends on the thiazide dose and possibly on the type of β-blocker, in that vasodilators such as carvedilol may be exceptions. Patients with a familial tendency to diabetes or those with the metabolic syndrome are probably more prone to the diabetogenic side effects, so that thiazides should be avoided or be given only in low doses, such as hydrochlorothiazide 12.5 mg daily or chlorthalidone 15 mg daily. In addition, plasma potassium and glucose should be monitored. The "transition" dose of hydrochlorothiazide from low-dose benefit to high-dose precipitation of hyperglycemia and diabetes is not clearly defined, but lower than previously thought. Hydrochlorothiazide doses exceeding 25 mg daily may precipitate glucose intolerance[20] or frank diabetes.[21] Common sense but no good trial data suggest that the lowest effective dose of hydrochlorothiazide (12.5 mg) should be used with the expectation that a significant proportion of the antihypertensive effect should be maintained without impairing glucose tolerance as found in the case of low-dose bendrofluazide.[23] There is no evidence that changing from a thiazide to a loop diuretic improves glucose tolerance.

Urate Excretion and Gout Most diuretics decrease urate excretion with the risk of increasing blood uric acid, causing gout in those predisposed; thus a personal or family history of gout further requires that only low-dose diuretics should be used. Cotherapy with *losartan* lessens the rise in uric acid.[42] When *allopurinol* is given for gout, or when the blood urate is high with a family history of gout, it must be remembered that the standard dose of 300 mg daily is for a normal creatinine clearance. With a clearance of only 40 ml/minute, the allopurinol dose drops to 150 mg daily and for 10 ml/minute down to 100 mg every 2 days. *Dose reduction is essential* to avoid serious dose-related reactions, which can be fatal.

Atherogenic Changes in Blood Lipids Thiazides may increase the total blood cholesterol in a dose-related fashion.[43] Low-density lipoprotein (LDL)-cholesterol and triglycerides increase after 4 months with hydrochlorothiazide (40 mg daily mean dose).[20] In the TOMH study, low-dose chlorthalidone (15 mg daily) increased cholesterol levels at 1 year but not at 4 years.[44] By contrast, high diuretic doses clearly have an adverse effect. Thus a high dose of hydrochlorothiazide, above 25 mg daily, unequivocally increases hyperlipidemia compared with a calcium channel blocker (CCB), both given for several years.[21] But even if total cholesterol does not change, triglycerides and the ratio of apolipoprotein B to A may rise, while high-density lipoprotein (HDL)-cholesterol may fall.[40] During prolonged thiazide therapy occasional checks on blood lipid profile are ideal and a lipid-lowering diet is advisable.

Hypercalcemia Thiazide diuretics tend to retain calcium by increasing proximal tubular reabsorption (along with sodium). The benefit is a decreased risk of hip fractures in the elderly.[45] Conversely, especially in hyperparathyroid patients, hypercalcemia can be precipitated.

Impotence Impotence was unexpectedly found in the large British anti-hypertension trial that used a high-dose diuretic (Table 4-4). The hope was that decreasing diuretic doses would avoid this unexplained problem. Yet in the TOMH study, low-dose chlorthalidone (15 mg daily given over 4 years) was the only one of several antihypertensive agents that doubled impotence.[25] Pragmatically, sildenafil or similar drugs should help, provided the patient is not also receiving nitrates. However, in hypertension when diuretic therapy may not be essential, a change of agent may be preferred.

Do Diuretics Cause Renal Cancer?

Overall, regarding cancer, the answer is no, as suggested by the large West of Scotland observational study that lasted up to 15 years; or at least they caused no more cancer than did β-blockers or calcium antagonists.[46] According to an observational study, the incidence of renal cell carcinoma is increased.[47] Although the risk ratio was 1.55, the absolute incidence of renal cell carcinoma was only 0.065%, not of great absolute statistical significance. It should be considered that observational studies such as these usually extend over years, going back to the era when high- rather than low-dose diuretics were the rule.

Prevention of Metabolic Side Effects

Reduction in the dose of diuretic is the basic step. In addition, restriction of dietary sodium and additional dietary potassium will reduce the frequency of hypokalemia. Combination of a thiazide with a potassium sparer lessens hypokalemia, as does the addition of an ACE inhibitor or ARB. In the treatment of hypertension, standard doses of diuretics should not be combined, if possible, with other drugs with unfavorable effects on blood lipids, such as the β-blockers, but rather with ACE inhibitors, ARBs, or CCBs which are lipid neutral (see Table 10-2).

POTASSIUM-SPARING AGENTS

Potassium-retaining agents lessen the incidence of serious ventricular arrhythmias in heart failure[35] and in hypertension.[48]

Amiloride and Triamterene

Amiloride and triamterene inhibit the sodium-proton exchanger, which is concerned with sodium reabsorption in the distal tubules and collecting tubules. Potassium loss is thereby indirectly decreased (Table 4-5). Relatively weak diuretics on their own, they are almost always used in combination with thiazides (Table 4-6). Advantages are that (1) the loss of sodium is achieved without a major loss of potassium or magnesium, and (2) there is an action independent of the activity of aldosterone. Side effects are few: hyperkalemia (a contraindication) and acidosis may seldom occur, and then mostly in those with renal disease. In particular, the thiazide-related risks of diabetes mellitus and gout have not been reported with these agents. There are suggestions that amiloride may be preferable to triamterene (the latter is excreted by the kidneys with risks of renal casts on standard doses and occasional renal dysfunction); amiloride helps to retain magnesium and may be of special benefit to the small percentage of blacks with a genetic defect in the epithelial sodium channel.[49] In practice, compounds with triamterene have been widely and extensively used without detectable risks.

Table 4-5 Potassium-Sparing Agents (Generally Also Spare Magnesium)

	Trade Names	Dose	Duration of Action
Spironolactone	Aldactone	25–200 mg	3–5 days
Amiloride	Midamor	2.5–20 mg	6–24 h
Triamterene	Dytac, Dyrenium	25–200 mg	8–12 h
Eplerenone	Inspra	50–100 mg	24 h

Table 4-6 Some Combination K+-Retaining Diuretics

	Trade Name	Combination (mg)	Preferred Daily Dose
Hydrochlorothiazide	Dyazide	25	$\frac{1}{2}$ (up to 4 in
+ triamterene		50	CHF)
Hydrochlorothiazide	Moduretic	50	$\frac{1}{4}$ (up to 2 in
+ amiloride		5	CHF)
Hydrochlorothiazide	Maxzide	50	$\frac{1}{4}$
+ triamterene		75	
Hydrochlorothiazide	Maxzide-25	25	$\frac{1}{2}$
+ triamterene		37.5	
Spironolactone	Aldactazide	25	1–4/day
+ hydrochlorothiazide		25	
Furosemide	Frumil*	40	1–2/day
+ amiloride		5	

For hypertension, see text; low doses are generally preferred and high doses are **contraindicated.**
*Not licensed in the United States.
CHF = congestive heart failure.

Spironolactone and Eplerenone

Spironolactone and eplerenone are both aldosterone antagonists and potassium sparers. In patients with severe CHF,[50] spironolactone has increasingly been chosen for its blocking effects on aldosterone-mediated damage in the heart, kidneys, and vasculature.[51] More recently, eplerenone, a more specific blocker of the aldosterone receptor (thereby preventing the gynecomastia and sexual dysfunctions seen in up to 10% of those given spironolactone) has been marketed. Eplerenone provided additional benefit in the large EPHESUS trial of post-MI patients by further reducing mortality.[52] Eplerenone was also as effective as enalapril, 40 mg daily, in regressing left ventricular hypertrophy and lowering blood pressure,[53] so that it could become a primary drug for treatment of hypertension, as well as a mortality reducer in CHF and in postinfarct patients, except for its exceedingly high cost. These aldosterone receptor blockers also have an obvious place in the treatment of primary aldosteronism and perhaps in the larger population of patients with resistant hypertension.[54]

ACE Inhibitors and ARBs

Because these agents ultimately exert an antialdosterone effect, they too act as mild potassium-retaining diuretics. Combination therapy with other potassium retainers should be avoided in the presence of renal impairment, but can successfully be undertaken with care and monitoring of serum potassium, as in the RALES study.[50]

Hyperkalemia—A Specific Risk Amiloride, triamterene, spironolactone, and eplerenone may all cause hyperkalemia (serum potassium equal to or exceeding 5.5 mEq/L), especially in the presence of preexisting renal disease, diabetes, in elderly patients during cotherapy with ACE inhibitors or ARBs, or in patients receiving possible nephrotoxic agents. Hyperkalemia is treated by drug withdrawal, infusions of glucose-insulin, and cation-exchange resins such as sodium, polystyrene, sulfonate, and sometimes dialysis. Intravenous calcium chloride may be required to avoid ventricular fibrillation.

COMBINATION DIURETICS

Besides the added diuresis achieved by addition of one class of diuretic to another, the fear of hypokalemia has increased the use of potassium-retaining agents and diuretic combinations (Table 4-6), such as *Dyazide, Maxzide, Moduretic,* and *Aldactazide.* For *heart failure,* a standard combination daily therapy might be one to two tablets of Moduretic (hydrochlorothiazide 50 mg, amiloride 5 mg), or two to four tablets of Dyazide (hydrochlorothiazide 25 mg, triamterene 50 mg), or one to two tablets of Maxzide (hydrochlorothiazide 50 mg, triamterene 75 mg). When used for *hypertension,* special attention must be given to the thiazide dose (25 mg hydrochlorothiazide in Dyazide; 50 mg in Moduretic; while Maxzide has both 25 mg and 50 mg), where the initial aim is only 12.5 mg hydrochlorothiazide. A potassium-retaining furosemide combination is available and much used in Europe (*Frumil,* furosemide 40 mg, amiloride 5 mg). A logical combination is that of an ACE inhibitor or ARB with low-dose thiazide, for example, low-dose perindopril with low-dose indapamide.[30] Thiazide diuretics increase renin levels and ACE inhibitors or ARBs decrease the metabolic side effects of thiazides (see Chapter 5).

MINOR DIURETICS

Carbonic anhydrase inhibitors such as acetazolamide (*Diamox*) are weak diuretics. They decrease the secretion of hydrogen ions by the proximal renal tubule, with increased loss of bicarbonate and hence of sodium. These agents, seldom used as primary diuretics, have found a place in the therapy of *glaucoma* because carbonic anhydrase plays a role in the secretion of aqueous humor in the ciliary processes of the eye. In *salicylate poisoning,* the alkalinizing effect of carbonic anhydrase inhibitors increases the renal excretion of lipid-soluble weak organic acids.

Calcium channel blockers of the dihydropyridine group have a direct diuretic effect that contributes to the long-term antihypertensive effect. For example, nifedipine increases urine volume and sodium excretion and may inhibit aldosterone release by angiotensin.

Dopamine has a diuretic action apart from the improvement in cardiac function and indirect diuresis that it induces. The mechanism of the diuresis, found only in conditions of fluid retention, appears to involve DA_1-receptors on the renal tubular cells where dopamine stimulation opposes the effects of antidiuretic hormone.

A_1-Adenosine receptor antagonists, another new approach to diuresis, increase urine flow and natriuresis. They may act by afferent arteriolar dilation, thereby increasing glomerular filtration.[55]

POTASSIUM SUPPLEMENTS

In the treatment of heart failure, the routine practice in many centers of giving potassium supplements with loop diuretics is usually unnecessary and does not appear to protect from the adverse effects of non–K-sparing diuretics. Supplements lead to extra cost and loss of compliance. Rather, addition of low-dose potassium-retaining agents is usually better (Table 4-5) and can often be accompanied by a lower dose of the loop diuretic. Even high doses of furosemide may not automatically require potassium replacement because such doses are usually given in the presence of renal impairment or severe CHF when renal potassium handling may be abnormal. Clearly potassium levels need periodic checking during therapy with all diuretics. A high-potassium, low-salt diet is advised and can be simply and inexpensively achieved by choosing fresh rather than processed foods and by the use of salt substitutes. Sometimes, despite all reasonable care, problematic hypokalemia develops, especially after prolonged diuretic therapy or in the presence of diarrhea or alkalosis. Then a potassium supplement may become necessary. Persistent hypokalemia in hypertension merits investigation for primary aldosteronism.

Potassium chloride in liquid form is theoretically best because (1) coadministration of chloride is required to correct fully potassium deficiency in hypokalemic hypochloremic alkalosis[56]; (2) slow-release tablets may cause gastrointestinal (GI) ulceration, which liquid KCl does not.[57] The dose is variable. At least 20 mEq daily are required to avoid potassium depletion and 60 to 100 mEq are required to treat potassium depletion. Absorption is rapid and bioavailability good. To help avoid the frequent GI irritation, liquid KCl needs dilution in water or another liquid and titration against the patient's acceptability. KCl may also be given in some effervescent preparations. *Slow-release potassium chloride wax-matrix tablets* (Slow-K, each with 8 mEq or 600 mg KCl; Klotrix, K-Tab, and Ten-K each contain 10 mEq KCl; Kaon-CL, 6.7 or 10 mEq KCl) are widely used and well tolerated. Nonetheless, the United States package insert cautions against the use unless liquid or effervescent potassium preparations are not tolerated. To avoid esophageal ulceration, tablets should be taken upright or sitting, with a meal or beverage, and anticholinergic therapy should be avoided. *Microencapsulated KCl* (Micro-K, Extencaps, 8 mEq KCl or 10 mEq KCl) may reduce GI ulceration to only 1 per 100,000 patient years. Nonetheless, high doses of Micro-K may cause GI ulcers, especially during anticholinergic therapy.

Effervescent preparations lessen the risk of GI ulceration and those with KCl include Klor-Con EF (25 mEq of K per tablet). *Extended release preparations* (e.g., K-Tab, 10 mEq K per tablet) may be used if effervescent tablets are not tolerated, but there is a bold package insert warning against GI ulcerations. GI intolerance frequently limits the use of these agents, which are best given with liquid meals and in relatively small doses. *Potassium gluconate* (with citrate), Bi-K 20 mEq, or Twin-K tends to minimize the GI irritative effects of the effervescent preparations.

Recommendations Diet is the simplest, with high-potassium low-sodium intake achieved by consuming fresh foods and using salt substitutes. When K^+ supplements become essential, KCl is preferred. The best preparation will be one well tolerated by the patient and that is inexpensive. No comprehensive adequately controlled studies of the relative efficacy of the various KCl preparations in clinical settings are available.

SPECIAL DIURETIC PROBLEMS
Overdiuresis

During therapy of edematous states, overvigorous diuresis is common and may reduce intravascular volume and ventricular filling so that the cardiac output drops and tissues become underperfused. The renin-angiotensin axis is further activated. Probably many patients are protected against the extremely effective potent diuretics by poor compliance. Overdiuresis is most frequently seen during hospital admissions when a rigid policy of regular administration of diuretics is carried out. Symptoms include fatigue and listlessness. Sometimes the addition of ACE inhibitors or ARBs to diuretics enhances the risk of overdiuresis.

Fixed diuretic regimens are largely unsatisfactory in edematous patients. Often intelligent patients can manage their therapy well by tailoring a flexible diuretic schedule to their own needs, using a simple bathroom scale. Knowing how to recognize pedal edema and the time course of maximal effect of their diuretic often allows a patient to adjust his or her own diuretic dose and administration schedule to fit in with daily activities. A *practical approach* is to stabilize the patient on a combination of drugs, and then to allow self-modification of the furosemide dose, within specified limits, and according to body weight.

Adverse effects due to overdiuresis include (1) those with mild chronic heart failure overtreated with potent diuretics; (2) patients requiring a high filling pressure particularly those with a "restrictive" pathophysiology as in restrictive cardiomyopathy, hypertrophic cardiomyopathy, or constrictive pericarditis; and (3) patients in early phase AMI, when excess diuresis by potent intravenous diuretics can cause a pressor response that attenuated by ACE inhibition.[10] It may be necessary to administer cautiously a *"fluid challenge"* with saline solution or a colloid preparation while checking the patient's cardiovascular status. If the resting heart rate falls, renal function improves, and blood pressure stabilizes, the ventricular filling pressure has been reduced too much by overdiuresis.

Diuretic Resistance

Diuretic tolerance includes late resistance and early "braking," the latter occurring even after one dose of a diuretic and resulting from intravascular fluid contraction.[12] Repetitive diuretic administration leads to a leveling off of the diuretic effect, because (in the face of a shrunken intravascular volume) the part of the tubular system not affected reacts by reabsorbing more sodium (Fig. 4-4). Such decreased sodium diuresis is associated with hypertrophy of distal nephron cells,[12] thought to be the result of aldosterone-induced growth.[9] Of therapeutic interest, the thiazides block the nephron sites at which the hypertrophy occurs,[12] thereby providing another argument for combined thiazide-loop therapy.[58] Additional mechanisms for diuretic resistance are an abnormally low cardiac output in patients with heart failure; prominent activation of the renin-angiotensin axis; or an electrolyte-induced resistance. Apparent resistance can also develop during incorrect use of diuretics (Table 4-7), or when there is concomitant therapy with indomethacin or with other NSAIDs or with probenecid. The thiazide diuretics will not work well if the GFR is below 20 to 30 ml/minute; metolazone is an exception (Table 4-7). When potassium depletion is severe, all diuretics work poorly for complex reasons.

Is there compliance with dietary salt restriction? Is complete bed rest required? Is the optimal agent being used, avoiding thiazide diuretics (except metolazone), when the GFR is low? Is the optimal dose being used? Are there interfering drugs or severe electrolyte or volume imbalances that can be remedied? Has the general cardiovascular status been made optimal by judicious use of unloading or inotropic drugs? *To achieve diuresis*, an ACE inhibitor or ARB may have to be added cautiously to thiazide and/or loop diuretics, or metolazone may have to be combined with loop diuretics, all following the principle of sequential nephron blockade. Sometimes spironolactone is also required. Furthermore, intravenous *dopamine* may through its action on DA_1-receptors help induce a diuresis acting in part by increasing renal blood flow. In outpatients, compliance and dietary salt restriction must be carefully checked, while all unnecessary drugs are eliminated. Sometimes fewer drugs work better than more (here the prime sinners are potassium supplements, sometimes requiring many daily tablets frequently not taken).

DIURETIC RESISTANCE IN CHF

Opie 2004

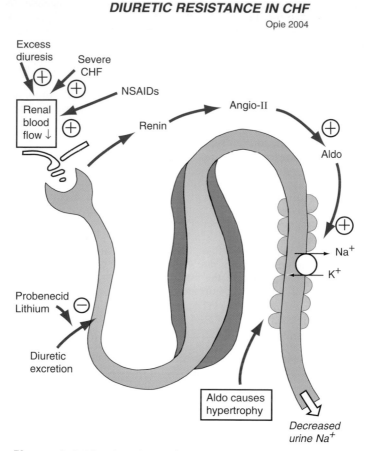

Figure 4-4 Diuretic resistance has several causes including reduced renal blood flow and the stimulation of the renin-angiotensin-aldosterone system. Hypothetically, increased aldosterone *(aldo)* may promote distal tubular hypertrophy to reabsorb greater amounts of sodium. For early "braking," not shown here, see text. *Angio-II* = angiotensin-II. *(Figure © LH Opie, 2005.)*

Hyponatremia

In heart failure, hyponatremia may occur in patients severely ill with CHF and in some elderly patients who consume large amounts of water despite an increased total body sodium in heart failure. Predominant water retention is caused by (1) the inappropriate release of arginine vasopressin-antidiuretic hormone (see ADH in Fig. 4-1); and (2) increased activity of angiotensin-II.[59] The best treatment seems to be the combination of furosemide and an ACE inhibitor (see Chapter 5, p. 124); restriction of water intake is also critical. *In hypertension*, hyponatremia may occur, especially in elderly women receiving a thiazide dose of 25 mg daily or more.[60]

LESS COMMON USES OF DIURETICS

Less common indications are:

1. Intravenous furosemide in *malignant hypertension*, especially if there is associated CHF and fluid retention.
2. High-dose furosemide for *acute or chronic renal failure* when it is hoped that the drug may initiate diuresis.
3. In *hypercalcemia*, high-dose loop diuretics increase urinary excretion of calcium; intravenous furosemide plus saline is used in the emergency treatment of severe hypercalcemia.

Table 4-7 Some Causes of Apparent Resistance to Diuretics in Therapy of Cardiac Failure

Incorrect Use of Diuretic Agent

Combination of two thiazides or two loop diuretics instead of one of each type
Use of thiazides when GFR is low* (exception: metolazone)
Excessive diuretic dose
Poor compliance, especially caused by multiple tablets of oral K⁺ supplements

Electrolyte and/or Volume Imbalance

Hyponatremia, hypokalemia, hypovolemia
Hypomagnesemia may need correction to remedy hypokalemia

Poor Renal Perfusion Diuretic-Induced Hypovolemia

Cardiac output too low
Excess hypotension (ACE inhibitors)

Excess Circulating Catecholamines

Frequent in severe CHF
Correct by additional therapy for CHF

Interfering Drugs

Nonsteroidal anti-inflammatory agents inhibit diuresis
Probenecid and lithium inhibit tubular excretion of thiazides and loop diuretics

*GFR = glomerular filtration rate below 15 to 20 ml/minute.

4. Thiazides for the *nephrogenic form of diabetes insipidus*—the mechanism of action is not clear, but there is a diminution in "free water" clearance.
5. Thiazide diuretics decrease the urinary calcium output by promoting proximal reabsorption, so that they are used in *idiopathic hypercalciuria* to decrease the formation of renal stones (in contrast, loop diuretics increase urinary excretion of calcium).

The inhibitory effect of thiazides on urinary calcium loss may explain why these agents may increase bone mineralization and decrease the incidence of hip fractures.[61] The latter benefit is another argument for first-line low-dose diuretic therapy in elderly hypertensive patients.

DIURETICS IN STEP-CARE THERAPY OF CHF

In *mild to moderate CHF*, diuretics are standard first-line therapy. The choice of diuretic lies between standard thiazide, a K-retainer plus thiazide, furosemide, spironolactone and eplerenone. The latter two are known to save lives in severe CHF when added to otherwise standard therapy.[50,51] Furthermore, a retrospective analysis showed that use of non–K-retaining diuretics in the SOLVD study was associated with increased arrhythmic death.[35] By contrast, a K-retainer alone or in combination with a non-K retainer, gave no such increase in risk of arrhythmic death. ACE inhibition plus a non–K-retaining diuretic also did not protect from arrhythmic death. These studies, although retrospective and observational, are bound to influence clinicians toward the preferential use of spironolactone, eplerenone, or combination diuretics containing K-retainers (Tables 4-5 and 4-6).

Step-care diuretic therapy in symptomatic heart failure (see Fig. 6-2) with fluid retention is not clearly delineated by adequate trials, but could be: (1) thiazide diuretics with ACE inhibitors; (2) low-dose furosemide with ACE inhibitors; (3) thiazides together with low-dose furosemide with ACE inhibitors; and (4) spironolactone or eplerenone added to the others, that is, four agents. High-dose furosemide is now less used, chiefly for acute heart failure. The current practice is to add ACE inhibitors or an ARB whenever the patient is given a diuretic, unless there is a contraindication. ACE inhibition should offset the deleterious renin-angiotensin activation induced by diuretics. Modest *sodium restriction* is advisable throughout, starting with no added salt, then cutting out obvious sources of salt as in processed or fast foods, and then going onto salt-free bread. Down-regulation of the salt-sensitive taste buds means that after about 6 weeks of modest sodium restriction, a low-salt diet becomes the preferred norm.

For *severe congestive heart failure*, when congestion and edema are prominent symptoms, initial therapy is usually with furosemide, especially when renal perfusion may be impaired. In severely ill patients complete bed rest, although old-fashioned, may promote an early diuresis. The dose of furosemide required in resistant CHF may be very high (500 to 1500 mg daily). Alternatively, the principle of sequential nephron blockade may be used with a lower dose of furosemide, and consideration should be given to intermittent dopamine.

Sequential nephron blockade is the principle whereby addition of a diuretic acting at a different site, such as a thiazide to a loop diuretic, is logical. Thus, the addition of amiloride to hydrochlorothiazide and digoxin improved hemodynamics in patients with CHF.

ACE inhibitors or ARBs are now standard agents for all stages of heart failure. In CHF, the action of diuretics may be inhibited by poor renal perfusion and vasoconstrictive formation of renin, with a low GFR lessening sodium excretion. Hence ACE inhibitors are logical additions to diuretics. They have an indirect diuretic effect ultimately by inhibiting aldosterone release. They also help to maintain normal cell potassium and magnesium concentrations.

Acknowledgment

We thank Professor Ariel Reyes, Institute of Cardiovascular Theory, Montevideo, Uruguay, for advice on diuretic doses.

S U M M A R Y

1. *In hypertension*, diuretics remain the best tested of the potential first-line antihypertensive agents, achieving better results when used in low doses (below 25 mg hydrochlorothiazide or chlorthalidone). Nonetheless, being powerful therapeutic agents, they have the potential for major and serious side effects at higher doses. The benefit/risk ratio of diuretics in the therapy of mild hypertension has been particularly well documented in three groups of patients: the elderly, black patients, and the obese. Patients with renal impairment also require a diuretic (loop or metolazone). For most hypertensive patients, a low-dose thiazide diuretic, probably with a potassium-retaining component (amiloride, triamterene, spironolactone, or eplerenone) is appropriate. Most combination diuretic tablets contain too much hydrochlorothiazide, so that the tablet must be divided with only 12.5 mg hydrochlorothiazide as the initial and ideal dose. Thiazide diuretics combine well with ACE inhibitors, in which case a potassium-sparing component is not advisable.

2. *In heart failure*, the benefit/risk ratio of diuretics is high and their use for fluid retention remains standard. Yet not all patients require vigorous diuresis; rather, each patient needs careful clinical evaluation with a specific cardiological diagnosis so that surgically correctable defects are appropriately handled. First choice of therapy

is a thiazide (for mild heart failure) or a loop diuretic (for severe heart failure). A logical practice in mild heart failure is to start low doses of diuretic and ACE inhibitor therapy together. With intermediate severities of failure, increasing doses of thiazide may be used before switching to or combining with a loop diuretic such as furosemide.

3. *Sequential nephron block* is an important principle. Basically, this calls for the addition of thiazide to loop diuretics, and then aldosterone antagonists, as the severity of heart failure increases. When spironolactone is added to ACE inhibition, there is a possible danger of hyperkalemia, which was limited in the RALES study by the low dose of spironolactone used. Nonetheless, mortality was reduced by aldosterone antagonism.

4. *Hypokalemia* remains one of the frequent complications of diuretic therapy. In hypertension this is avoided by the use of a low-dose potassium-retaining agent, amiloride, triamterene, spironolactone, or eplerenone. We stress that in heart failure, automatic addition of oral potassium supplements is far from ideal practice. Rather, the combination with ACE inhibitors or ARBs counters hypokalemia by an antialdosterone effect. Today, some combination of diuretics plus ACE inhibitors, often with β-blockade, is standard therapy in mild to moderate heart failure. In more severe heart failure or in postinfarct patients, the addition of the aldosterone antagonists spironolactone or eplerenone, respectively, improves prognosis.

REFERENCES

1. Cranston W, et al. Effects of oral diuretics on raised arterial pressure. *Lancet* 1963;2:966–969.
2. Psaty BM, et al. Health outcomes associated with various antihypertensive therapies used as first-line agents. *JAMA* 2003;289:2534–2544.
3. BP Trialists. Effects of different blood-pressure lowering regimens on major cardiovascular events: results of prospectively-designed overviews of randomised trials. *Lancet* 2003;362:1527–1535.
4. Hunt SA, et al. ACC/AHA Guidelines for the Evaluation and Management of Chronic Heart Failure in the Adult: Executive Summary: A Report of the American College of Cardiology/American Heart Association Task Force on Practice Guidelines (Committee to Revise the 1995 Guidelines for the Evaluation and Management of Heart Failure); developed in Collaboration with the International Society for Heart and Lung Transplantation; endorsed by the Heart Failure Society of America. *Circulation* 2001;104:2996–3007.
5. JNC VII. The Seventh Report of the Joint National Committee on Prevention, Detection, Evaluation and Treatment of High Blood Pressure. *JAMA* 2003;289:2560–2572.
6. WHO/ISH Writing Group. 2003 World Health Organisation (WHO)/ International Society of Hypertension (ISH) statement on management of hypertension. *J Hypertens* 2003;21:1983–1992.
7. JNC VI. Joint National Committee on Prevention, Detection, Evaluation and Treatment of High Blood Pressure. The Sixth Report of the Joint National Committee on Prevention, Detection, Evaluation and Treatment of High Blood Pressure. *Arch Intern Med* 1997;157:2413–2446.
8. Gammage M. Treatment of acute pulmonary oedema: diuresis or vasodilation? (Commentary). *Lancet* 1998;351:382–383.
9. Reyes AJ, et al. Diuretics in cardiovascular therapy: the new clinicopharmacological bases that matter. *Cardiovasc Drugs Ther* 1999;13:371–398.
10. Goldsmith SR, et al. Attenuation of the pressor response to intravenous furosemide by angiotensin converting enzyme inhibition in congestive heart failure. *Am J Cardiol* 1989;64:1382–1385.
11. Vlase HL, et al. Effectiveness of furosemide in uncontrolled hypertension in the elderly: role of renin profiling. *Am J Hypertens* 2003;16:187–193.
12. Brater DC. Diuretic therapy. *N Engl J Med* 1998;339:387–395.
13. Johnson AG. NSAIDs and blood pressure. Clinical importance for older patients. *Drugs Aging* 1998;12:17–27.
13a. Cosin J, et al. Torasemide in chronic heart failure: results of the TORIC study. *Eur J Heart Fail* 2002;4:507–513. Erratum in: *Eur J Heart Fail* 2002;4:667.
14. Wall GC, et al. Ethacrynic acid and the sulfa-sensitive patient. *Arch Intern Med* 2003;163:116–117.
15. Helderman JR, et al. Prevention of the glucose intolerance of thiazide diuretics by maintenance of body potassium. *Diabetes* 1983;32:106–111.

16. Santoro D, et al. Effects of chronic angiotensin-converting enzyme inhibition on glucose tolerance and insulin sensitivity in essential hypertension. *Hypertension* 1992;20:181–191.

17. Carter BL, et al. Hydrochlorothiazide versus chlorthalidone: evidence supporting their interchangeability. *Hypertension* 2004;43:4–9.

18. Materson BJ, et al. Single-drug therapy for hypertension in men. A comparison of six antihypertensive agents with placebo. The Department of Veterans Affairs Cooperative Study Group on Antihypertensive Agents. *N Engl J Med* 1993;328:914–921.

19. SHEP Cooperative Research Group. Prevention of stroke by antihypertensive drug treatment in older persons with isolated systolic hypertension Final results of the Systolic Hypertension in the Elderly Program (SHEP). *JAMA* 1991;265:3255–3264.

20. Pollare T, et al. A comparison of the effects of hydrochlorothiazide and captopril on glucose and lipid metabolism in patients with hypertension. *N Engl J Med* 1989;321:868–873.

21. Brown MJ, et al. Morbidity and mortality in patients randomised to double-blind treatment with a long-acting calcium-channel blocker or diuretic in the International Nifedipine GITS study: Intervention as a Goal in Hypertension Treatment. *Lancet* 2000;356:366–372.

22. Lacourciere Y, et al. Antihypertensive effects of two fixed-dose combinations of losartan and hydrochlorothiazide versus hydrochlorothiazide monotherapy in subjects with ambulatory systolic hypertension. *Am J Hypertens* 2003;16:1036–1042.

23. Harper R, et al. Effects of low dose versus conventional dose thiazide diuretic on insulin action in essential hypertension. *Br Med J* 1994;309:226–230.

24. ALLHAT Collaborative Research Group. Major outcomes in high-risk hypertensive patients randomized to angiotensin-converting enzyme inhibitor or calcium channel blocker vs diuretic. The Antihypertensive and Lipid-Lowering Treatment to Prevent Heart Attack Trial (ALLHAT). *JAMA* 2002;288:2981–2997.

25. Grimm RH, et al. Long-term effects on sexual function of five antihypertensive drugs and nutritional hygienic treatment in hypertensive men and women. Treatment of Mild Hypertension Study (TOMHS). *Hypertension* 1997;29:8–14.

26. Sica DA, et al. Diuretic combinations in refractory oedema states: pharmacokinetic-pharmacodynamic relationships. *Clin Pharmacokinet* 1996;30:229–249.

27. Kreeft JH, et al. Comparative trial of indapamide and hydrochlorothiazide in essential hypertension with forearm plethysmography. *J Cardiovasc Pharmacol* 1984;6: 622–626.

28. Lu Y, et al. Effects of the diuretic agent indapamide on Na+, transient outward and delayed rectifier currents in canine atrial myocytes. *Circ Res* 1998;83:158–166.

29. Ames RP. A comparison of blood lipid and blood pressure responses during the treatment of systemic hypertension with indapamide and with thiazides. *Am J Cardiol* 1996;77:12B–16B.

30. Chalmers J, et al. Long-term efficacy of a new, fixed, very-low-dose angiotensin-converting enzyme inhibitor/diuretic combination as first-line therapy in elderly hypertensive patients. *J Hypertens* 2000;18:327–337.

31. Gosse P, et al. On behalf of the LIVE investigators. Regression of left ventricular hypertrophy in hypertensive patients treated with indapamide SR 1.5 mg versus enalapril 20 mg: the LIVE study. *J Hypertens* 2000;18:1465–1475.

32. Ambrosioni E, et al. Low-dose antihypertensive therapy with 1.5 mg sustained-release indapamide: results of randomised double-blind controlled studies. *J Hypertens* 1998;16:1677–1684.

33. Frishman WH, et al. A multifactorial trial design to assess combination therapy in hypertension. *Arch Intern Med* 1994;154:1461–1468.

34. Franse LV, et al. Hypokalemia associated with diuretic use and cardiovascular events in the Systolic Hypertension in the Elderly Program. *Hypertension* 2000;35:1025–1030.

35. Domanski M, et al. Diuretic use, progressive heart failure, and death in patients in the Studies Of Left Ventricular Dysfunction (SOLVD). *J Am Coll Cardiol* 2003;42: 705–708.

36. Wilcox CS. Metabolic and adverse effects of diuretics. *Semin Nephrol* 1999;19: 557–568.

37. Gress TW, et al. For the Atherosclerosis Risk in Communities Study. Hypertension and antihypertensives therapy as risk factors for type 2 diabetes mellitus. *N Engl J Med* 2000;342:905–912.

38. Swislocki ALM, et al. Insulin resistance, glucose intolerance and hyperinsulinemia in patients with hypertension. *Am J Hypertens* 1989;2:419–423.

39. Dahlöf B, et al. For the LIFE study group. Cardiovascular morbidity and mortality in the Losartan Intervention For Endpoint reduction in hypertension study (LIFE): a randomised trial against atenolol. *Lancet* 2002;359:995–1003.

40. Lindholm LH, et al. Metabolic outcome during 1 year in newly detected hypertensives: results of the Antihypertensive Treatment and Lipid Profile in a North of Sweden Efficacy Evaluation (ALPINE study). *J Hypertens* 2003;21:1563–1574.

41. Holzgreve H, et al. Antihypertensive therapy with verapamil SR plus trandolapril versus atenolol plus chlorthalidone on glycemic control. *Am J Hypertens* 2003;16: 381–386.

42. Owens P, et al. Comparison of antihypertensive and metabolic effects of losartan and losartan in combination with hydrochlorothiazide—a randomized controlled trial. *J Hypertens* 2000;18:339–345.

43. Kasiske BL, et al. Effects of antihypertensive therapy on serum lipids. *Ann Intern Med* 1995;122:133–141.

44. TOMH Study. Treatment of Mild Hypertension study (TOMH). Final results. *JAMA* 1993;270:713–724.

45. LaCroix AZ, et al. Thiazide diuretic agents and the incidence of hip fracture. *N Engl J Med* 1990;322:286–290.
46. Lever AF, et al. Do inhibitors of angiotensin-I-converting enzyme protect against risk of cancer? *Lancet* 1998;352:179–184.
47. Grossman E, et al. Does diuretic therapy increase the risk of renal cell carcinoma in women? *Am J Cardiol* 1999;88:1090–1093.
48. Siscovick DS, et al. Diuretic therapy for hypertension and the risk of primary cardiac arrest. *N Engl J Med* 1994;330:1852–1857.
49. Baker EH, et al. Amiloride, a specific drug for hypertension in black people with T594M variant? *Hypertension* 2002;40:13–17.
50. RALES Study. For the Randomized Aldactone Evaluation Study Investigators. The effect of spironolactone on morbidity and mortality in patients with severe heart failure. *N Engl J Med* 1999;341:709–717.
51. Pitt B. Aldosterone blockade in patients with systolic left ventricular dysfunction. *Circulation* 2003;108:1790–1794.
52. Pitt B, et al. Eplerenone, a selective aldosterone blocker in patients with left ventricular dysfunction after myocardial infarction. *N Engl J Med* 2003;348:1309–1321.
53. Pitt B, et al. Effects of eplerenone, enalapril, and eplerenone/enalapril in patients with essential hypertension and left ventricular hypertrophy: the 4E-left ventricular hypertrophy study. *Circulation* 2003;108:1831–1838.
54. Ouzan J, et al. The role of spironolactone in the treatment of patients with refractory hypertension. *Am J Hypertens* 2002;15:333–339.
55. Gottlieb SS, et al. Effects of BG9719 (CVT-124), an A_1-adenosine receptor antagonist, and furosemide on glomerular filtration rate and natriuresis in patients with congestive heart failure. *J Am Coll Cardiol* 2000;35:56–59.
56. Stanaszek WF, et al. Current approaches to management of potassium deficiency. *Drug Intell Clin Pharm* 1985;19:176–184.
57. Patterson DJ, et al. Endoscopic comparison of solid and liquid potassium chloride supplements. *Lancet* 1983;2:1077–1078.
58. Dormans TPJ, et al. Combination of high-dose furosemide and hydrochlorothiazide in the treatment of refractory congestive heart failure. *Eur Heart J* 1996;17:1867–1874.
59. Ray WA, et al. Long-term use of thiazide diuretics and risk of hip fractures. *Lancet* 1989;1:687–690.
60. Sharabi Y, et al. Diuretic induced hyponatraemia in elderly hypertensive women. *J Hum Hypertens* 2002;16:631–635.
61. LaCroix AZ, et al. Low-dose hydrochlorothiazide and preservation of bone mineral density in older adults. A randomized, double-blind, placebo-controlled trial. *Ann Intern Med* 2000;133:516–526.
62. Mudge GH. Diuretics and other agents employed in the mobilization of edema fluid. In: The Pharmacological Basis of Therapeutics. Gilman AG, et al., editors. New York: Macmillan, 1980; pp. 892–915.

5

Angiotensin-Converting Enzyme (ACE) Inhibitors, Angiotensin-II Receptor Blockers (ARBs), and Aldosterone Antagonists

Lionel H. Opie • Philip A. Poole-Wilson • Marc A. Pfeffer

> "Angiotensin-converting enzyme inhibitors have been shown to have the broadest impact of any drug in cardiovascular medicine."
>
> HARVEY WHITE, 2003[1]

> "The ultimate question raised is whether high-risk patients should receive ACE inhibitors or angiotensin-receptor blockers after myocardial infarction."
>
> MANN, 2003[2]

Since the description in 1977 of the first angiotensin-converting enzyme (ACE) inhibitor, captopril, by the Squibb Group led by Ondetti and Cushman, ACE inhibitors have not only become the cornerstone of the treatment of heart failure, but increasingly also play a major role in hypertension therapy and in cardiovascular protection.[3,4] The purpose of this chapter is to survey the pharmacology, the use, and the limitations of these agents and their new relatives, the angiotensin receptor blockers (ARBs). Frequent reference will be made to the role of the renin-angiotensin-aldosterone system (RAAS) in cardiovascular pathology, with excess activities of angiotensin-II and of aldosterone playing major adverse maladaptive roles. ACE inhibitors act on the crucial enzyme that generates angiotensin-II, whereas the ARBs act directly on the major angiotensin-II receptor subtype-1 (AT_1 subtype) that responds to angiotensin-II stimulation. In addition, spironolactone and eplerenone antagonize the effects of aldosterone. As the result of many careful long and large trials, it is now clear that ACE inhibitors give both primary and secondary protection from cardiovascular disease, thereby interrupting the vicious circle from risk factors to left ventricular failure at many sites (Fig. 5-1). The ARBs are very well tolerated, and in several but not all outcome trials give benefits equal to those of the ACE inhibitors. The final step in the RAAS, aldosterone, is increased in heart failure. Aldosterone inhibitors have protective effects additive to those of ACE inhibitors in heart failure and in high-risk post–myocardial infarction (post-MI) patients.

MECHANISMS OF ACTION OF ACE INHIBITORS

Logically, ACE inhibition should work by lessening the complex and widespread effects of angiotensin-II (Table 5-1). This octapeptide is formed from its precursor, a decapeptide *angiotensin-I*, by the activity of the ACE. ACE activity is found chiefly in the vascular endothelium of the lungs, but occurs in all vascular beds including the coronary arteries. Angiotensin-I originates in the liver from *angiotensinogen* under the influence of the enzyme *renin*, a protease that is formed in the renal juxtaglomerular cells. Classic stimuli to the release of renin

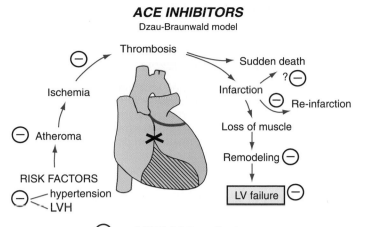

ACE INHIBITORS
Dzau-Braunwald model

Figure 5-1 Dual role of ACE inhibitors, both preventing and treating cardiovascular disease. Note multiple sites of action in both primary and secondary prevention. ACE inhibitors have an indirect effect in primary prevention by lessening hypertension and by decreasing left ventricular hypertrophy. They protect the blood vessels indirectly by an antihypertensive effect, and directly inhibit carotid atherogenesis and thrombogenesis. Given at the start of myocardial infarction, they improve mortality in high-risk patients. By an antiarrhythmic effect, they may act to prevent postinfarct sudden death. By lessening wall stress, they beneficially improve postinfarct remodeling and decrease the incidence of left ventricular failure. The concept of sequential changes leading to a chain of events from risk factors to left ventricular failure is based on Dzau and Braunwald.[126] *LVH* = left ventricular hypertrophy. (*Figure © LH Opie, 2005.*)

Table 5-1	Potential Pathogenic Properties of Angiotensin II

Heart

Myocardial hypertrophy
Interstitial fibrosis

Coronary Arteries

Endothelial dysfunction with deceased release of nitric oxide
Coronary constriction via release of norepinephrine
Increased oxidative stress; oxygen-derived free radicals formed via NADH
  oxidase
Promotion of inflammatory response and atheroma
Promotion of LDL-cholesterol uptake

Kidneys

Increased intraglomerular pressure
Increased protein leak
Glomerular growth and fibrosis
Increased sodium reabsorption

Adrenals

Increased formation of aldosterone

Coagulation System

Increased fibrinogen
Increased PAI-1 relative to tissue plasminogen factor

include (1) impaired renal blood flow as in ischemia or hypotension; (2) salt depletion or sodium diuresis; and (3) β-adrenergic stimulation.

The Angiotensin-Converting Enzyme

This protease has two zinc groups, of which only one participates in the high-affinity binding site that interacts with angiotensin-I or with the ACE inhibitors. This converting enzyme not only converts angiotensin-I to angiotensin-II but also inactivates the breakdown of bradykinin, hence the alternate name of *kininase*. ACE inhibition is vasodilatory by decreased formation of angiotensin-II and potentially by decreased degradation of bradykinin (Fig. 5-2).

Alternate Modes of Angiotensin-II Generation

Not all angiotensin-II is generated as a result of the activity of ACE. Non-ACE pathways, involving chymase-like serine proteases, can do the same job and also form angiotensin-II. The exact role of such non-ACE pathways is still the subject of controversy. One view is that more than 75% of the cardiac angiotensin-II formed in severe human heart failure is formed by chymase activity, and that inhibition of chymase prevents cardiac fibrosis and limits the progression of experimental heart failure.[5] However, if this path were really so important in human heart failure, why does therapy by an ARB that would block all the angiotensin-II formed both by chymase and by ACE not give results clinically superior to those of ACE-inhibitor therapy?

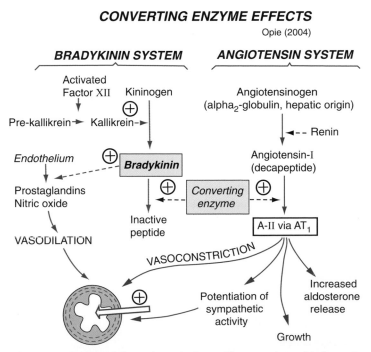

CONVERTING ENZYME EFFECTS

Opie (2004)

Figure 5-2 ACE inhibitors have dual vasodilatory actions, chiefly on the renin-angiotensin system with ancillary effects on the breakdown of bradykinin. The result of the former action is the inhibition of the vasoconstrictory systems and the result of the latter is the formation of vasodilatory nitric oxide and prostacyclin. These effects of bradykinin may protect the endothelium. (*Figure © LH Opie, 2005.*)

Angiotensin-II and Intracellular Messenger Systems

Just as there are many intermediate steps between occupation of the β-adrenoceptor and increased contractile activity of the myocardium, so there are many complex steps between occupation of the angiotensin-II receptor and ultimate mobilization of calcium with a vasoconstrictor effect in vascular smooth muscle. Activity of the signaling system starts when occupation of the angiotensin-II receptor stimulates the phosphodiesterase (called phospholipase C) that leads to a series of signals that activate a specialized enzyme, *protein kinase C*, which in turn evokes the activity of mitogen-activated protein (MAP)-kinase pathway to stimulate ventricular hypertrophy.[6] In blood vessels, phospholipase C activates the *inositol trisphosphate (IP₃) signaling pathway* to liberate calcium from the intracellular sarcoplasmic reticulum to promote vasoconstriction.

Angiotensin-II Receptor Subtypes: The AT_1 and AT_2 Receptors

There are two angiotensin-II receptor subtypes, the AT_1 and AT_2 receptors (Fig. 5-3). Note the potentially confusing nomenclature: both receptors respond to angiotensin-II, but are subtypes 1 and 2. These link to separate internal signaling paths.[7] Clinically used ARBs should be considered as AT_1-blockers. The effects of angiotensin-II acting via

ANGIOTENSION-II RECEPTOR SUBTYPES

Opie 2004

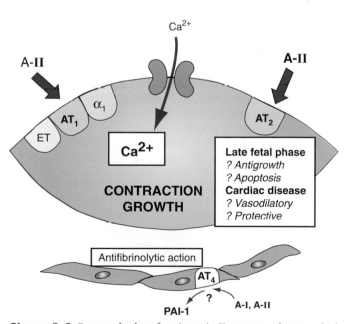

Figure 5-3 Proposed roles of angiotensin II receptor subtypes, which are called AT-1, AT-2 and (putative) AT-4 subtypes. Most of the physiological effects in adult vascular smooth muscle cells are conveyed by the AT-1 receptor subtype. The AT-2 receptor is of substantial importance in late fetal vascular growth, exerting an antigrowth effect. Hypothetically, these receptors may also play a beneficial role in various myocardial pathophysiological conditions (see text). AT-4 receptors are postulated to have an antifibrinolytic effect. (*Figure © LH Opie, 2005.*)

AT_1-receptors on the diseased heart and failing circulation are often regarded as adverse, such as stimulation of contraction, vasoconstriction, myocyte hypertrophy,[6] and antinatriuresis. In fetal life, these AT_1-receptors act as growth stimulators, which explains why ACE inhibitors and ARBs are prohibited therapy in pregnancy. The physiological role of the AT_2 receptor includes the inhibition of growth in the late fetal phase (growth can't keep on forever). In adult life, the role of the AT_2 receptors is much less well understood, but could become more relevant in pathophysiological conditions, the receptors being upregulated in hypertrophy and in heart failure. It is postulated by Dzau and others that the AT_2 receptors may reduce some of the adverse effects of AT_1 receptor stimulation by a Yin-Yang effect. Controversially, other workers suggest that there could be mixed or even adverse consequences of long-term AT_2 stimulation as occurs during therapy with an ARB when only the AT_1 receptor is blocked.[8] By contrast, during ACE inhibitor administration the activity of both receptors is restricted because the formation of angiotensin-II is inhibited.

Renin-Angiotensin-Aldosterone System

The major factors stimulating *renin release* from the juxtaglomerular cells of the kidney are (Fig. 5-4): (1) increased β_1-sympathetic activity; (2) a low arterial blood pressure; (3) decreased sodium reabsorption in the distal tubule, as when dietary sodium is low or during diuretic therapy; and (4) decreased blood volume. Local formation of angiotensin-II following renin release seems to explain efferent arteriolar vasoconstriction in the renal glomerulus. Thus, for example, during a state of arterial hypotension, the increased efferent arteriolar vasoconstriction resulting from increased angiotensin-II will help to preserve renal function by maintaining the intraglomerular pressure.

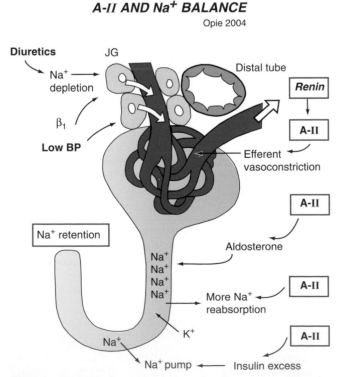

Figure 5-4 Renal mechanisms whereby renin-angiotensin-aldosterone system promotes sodium retention. *Jg* = juxtaglomerular cells. (*Figure © LH Opie, 2005.*)

Feedback inhibition of renin by angiotensin-II means that renin release is suppressed both directly by angiotensin-II and indirectly by the sodium retention associated with the increased aldosterone levels. *Stimulation of aldosterone by angiotensin-II* means that the latter stimulus releases the sodium-retaining hormone aldosterone from the adrenal cortex. Hence, ACE inhibition is associated with aldosterone reduction and has potential indirect natriuretic and potassium-retaining effects. Aldosterone formation does not, however, stay fully blocked during prolonged ACE inhibitor therapy. This late "escape" does not appear to compromise the antihypertensive effects achieved by ACE inhibitors; nonetheless it might detract from the prolonged benefit of these agents in heart failure. In the RALES study, added low-dose spironolactone (mean: 25 mg daily) on top of diuretics and ACE inhibition reduced mortality (see p. 141 of this chapter).

Adverse Effects of Excess Aldosterone

Aldosterone, released either in response to angiotensin-II or to stimulation by adrenocorticotropic hormone (ACTH), has major effects on electrolyte balance. It retains sodium and helps to excrete potassium by inhibition of sodium-potassium exchange in the distal renal tubule (Fig. 5-4). Water is retained with sodium. In heart failure, plasma aldosterone rises up to 20 times normal, in response to increased angiotensin-II, coupled with decreased hepatic clearance.[9] Aldosterone, some of it locally produced, may adversely alter the structure of the myocardium by promotion of cardiac fibrosis.[9] Aldosterone also promotes endothelial dysfunction.[10]

Sodium Status, Renin, and ACE Inhibitor Efficacy

Renin secretion from the juxtaglomerular cells is enhanced by sodium depletion, which in turn increases the hypotensive effect of ACE inhibition. Therefore, in the therapy of hypertension, ACE inhibitors are often combined with either a diuretic or a low-sodium diet or both. *Salt sensitivity* means that certain individuals, especially the elderly, react adversely to a high salt intake by increasing the arterial blood pressure. In normal subjects, a high-sodium diet leads to increased tubular reabsorption of sodium, which inhibits renin release, which decreases efferent arteriolar vasoconstriction, so that renal blood flow increases with increased sodium excretion. Furthermore, less formation of angiotensin-II leads to a lower level of aldosterone to promote sodium diuresis. In some hypertensive patients, the above sequence does not happen in response to sodium so that there is sodium retention with increased sodium-calcium exchange and vasoconstriction. In the elderly, minor but significant degrees of sodium retention may result from impaired renal function. The result is a low renin status, common in the elderly and in ethnic groups of African origin.

Autonomic Interactions of Angiotensin-II

ACE inhibitors have indirect permissive antiadrenergic effects. Angiotensin-II promotes the release of norepinephrine from adrenergic terminal neurons, and also enhances adrenergic tone by central activation and by facilitation of ganglionic transmission. Furthermore, angiotensin-II amplifies the vasoconstriction achieved by α_1-receptor stimulation. Thus, angiotensin-II has facilitatory adrenergic actions leading to increased activity of vasoconstrictory norepinephrine. ACE inhibitors have vagomimetic effects that could explain why tachycardia is absent despite peripheral vasodilation. The combined antiadrenergic and vago-mimetic mechanisms could contribute to the *antiarrhythmic effects* of ACE inhibitors and the reduction of sudden death in several trials in congestive heart failure (CHF), especially post-MI.[11] An additional factor is probably better potassium retention (as a result of aldosterone inhibition).

Kallikrein-Kinin System and Bradykinin

Besides decreased formation of angiotensin-II, increased bradykinin is another possible alternate site of action of ACE inhibitors (see Fig. 5-2; Table 5-2). This nonapeptide, originally described as causing slow contractions in the gut (hence the *brady* in the name) is of potential cardiovascular importance. Bradykinin is inactivated by two kininases, kininase I and II. The latter is identical to ACE. ACE inhibition, therefore, leads to increased local formation of bradykinin, which has major vasodilatory properties. Bradykinin acts on bradykinin receptors in the vascular endothelium to promote the release of two vasodilators (Table 5-2). First, there is increased formation of nitric oxide. Second, there is increased conversion of arachidonic acid to vasodilatory prostaglandins, such as prostacyclin and prostaglandin E_2 (PGE_2). Indomethacin, which inhibits prostaglandin synthesis, partially reduces the hypotensive effect of ACE inhibitors. The current concept is that bradykinin formation, occurring locally and thus not easily measured, can participate in the hypotensive effect of ACE inhibitors and may act via nitric oxide to protect the endothelium. This is one of the several mechanisms whereby bradykinin can lessen the adverse myocardial effects of pacing-induced heart failure in dogs.[12] Conversely, in a bradykinin B2 receptor knockout mouse, spontaneous heart failure develops.[13] Bradykinin formed during ACE inhibition may also contribute to the protective effect of preconditioning on the heart,[14] and to the vasodilator effects of ACE inhibition in heart failure.[15] *Renal prostaglandins* may respond to bradykinin. During ACE inhibition there is increased local synthesis of the active bradykinin in the kidney. Such bradykinin stimulates the formation of vasodilatory prostaglandins. These potentially favorable actions of an ACE inhibitor would not occur with an ARB (but there would also be fewer adverse effects of bradykinin such as cough and angioedema).

Tissue Renin-Angiotensin Systems

Although the acute hypotensive effects of ACE inhibition can clearly be linked to decreased circulating levels of angiotensin-II, during chronic ACE inhibition there is a reactive hyperreninemia linked to reemergence of circulating angiotensin-II and aldosterone. Hence, the present proposal is that ACE inhibitors exert their sustained antihypertensive and anti-heart failure effects at least in part by lessening formation of angiotensin-II within the target organ, acting on the tissue renin-angiotensin systems. Likewise, this is the proposed site of

Table 5-2	Actions of Bradykinin	
Organ(elle)	Cellular Effect	Consequence
Gut	Ca^{2+} mobilization	Slow contraction (*brady*, slow; *kinin*, movement)
Vascular endothelium	Formation of nitric oxide (NO), prostacyclin	Vasodilation; antiplatelet aggregation; endothelial protection
Respiratory tract	Formation of prostaglandins	Cough, angioedema
Heart, vessels	Endothelial protection	Participates in experimental coronary dilation induced by ACE-inhibition.[123]
Heart, myocardium	Preconditioning[14]	Protects against repeat ischemia

STRETCH AND CARDIAC GROWTH

Opie 2004

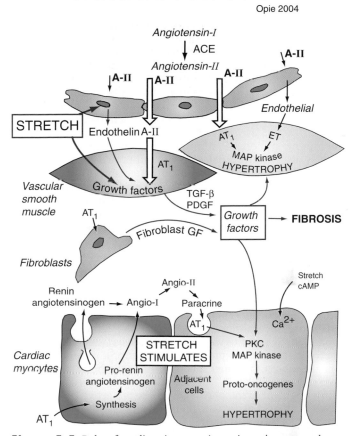

Figure 5-5 Role of cardiac tissue renin-angiotensin system, hypothetically as in left ventricular hypertrophy (*LVH*), involving myocytes, fibroblasts, vascular smooth muscle, and endothelium. AT_1 = angiotensin-II receptor subtype-1; *ET* = endothelin; *GF*, growth factor; *MAP kinase* = mitogen activated protein kinase; *PDGF* = platelet-derived growth factor; *PKC* = protein kinase C; *TGF* = transforming growth factor; other abbreviations as in Fig. 5-2. (*Figure © LH Opie, 2005.*)

action, in addition to blood pressure reduction, in the regression of LV hypertrophy and vascular remodeling (Fig. 5-5).

Genotypes and Response to ACE Inhibitors

ACE gene polymorphism is often considered as a possible genetic factor that could predispose to cardiovascular disease, although the evidence remains controversial. A different issue is whether the ACE genotype could regulate the response, for example, to exercise training, and whether the response to ACE inhibitors could likewise be sensitive to the genotype. The DD genotype (where D = deletion) is associated with greater myocardial ACE levels than its presence,[16] the latter being the ACE II (I = insertion) genotype. In a series of normotensive British army recruits subjected to intense exercise training, the DD genotype was associated with a greater degree of exercise-induced left ventricular hypertrophy.[17] Controversially, DD may be associated with increased myocardial infarction. Thus variable clinical responses in different individuals to the same dose of an ACE inhibitor could potentially be explained on a genetic base. However, much more data would be needed formally to link DD to structural heart disease.

Angiotensin-II Receptor Type AT₁ Blockers (ARBs)

Angiotensin-II has been called a "molecular murderer" with serious adverse effects on the heart, the coronary arteries, the renal glomeruli, and on thrombosis (Table 5-1). Because ACE inhibitors have their major effects by inhibiting the formation of angiotensin-II, it follows that direct antagonism of these receptors should duplicate many or most of the effects of ACE inhibition. One advantage of ARBs over ACE inhibitors is the much lower incidence of cough and angioedema, the latter hypothetically being induced by bradykinin and prostaglandins. ARBs might, again theoretically, be able to avoid the hormonal "escape" (hyperreninemia and increase in angiotensin-II) found during prolonged administration of ACE inhibitors. This concept is also controversial, and not supported by data from one trial.[18] Furthermore, ARBs should be better able to act against the non–ACE-dependent chymase paths,[5] because of more complete inhibition of the synthesis of angiotensin-II. But it is proposed that the lesser formation of bradykinin with the ARBs than with the ACE inhibitors may lead to correspondingly less endothelial protection.

PHARMACOLOGY OF ACE INHIBITORS

Major Indications and Classes

These are heart failure, hypertension, acute myocardial infarction, and postinfarct follow-up; renoprotection, diabetic nephropathy, and hypertension; and cardiovascular protection (Table 5-3). From the pharmacokinetic point of view, there are *three classes of ACE inhibitors* (Table 5-4). The first is represented by captopril, a compound active as it is, yet subject to further metabolism in the body to metabolites that are also active (class I). The next category consists of the prodrugs of which enalapril is the prototype. These are active only once converted to the diacid by hepatic metabolism (class II, Fig. 5-6). Third, in a class of its own, lisinopril is water-soluble and not metabolized, and excreted unchanged by the kidneys (class III). Probably the major site of ACE inhibition is in the vascular endothelium, accessible to all ACE inhibitors, whether lipid-soluble or not. Yet it must be admitted that ramipril and perindopril, the agents linked to major cardiovascular protection in the HOPE and EUROPA studies, are both lipid-soluble so that penetration of myocardial cells to reach the tissue ACE is theoretically more feasible.[19,20] The major outcome trials with ACE inhibitors and other inhibitors of the RAAS system are listed in Table 5-5.

Side Effects of ACE Inhibitors

Cough has emerged as one of the most troublesome and common of the various side effects (Table 5-6; Fig. 5-7), some serious and some not. This side effect took a long time to be discovered. Patients with heart failure often cough as a result of pulmonary congestion (which may need more rather than less ACE inhibitor), and in patients with

---

Table 5-3 | Indications for ACE Inhibitors, Based on Trial Data

1. Heart failure, all stages
2. Hypertension especially in high-risk and in diabetic patients
3. AMI, acute phase for high-risk patients, postinfarct LV dysfunction
4. Nephropathy, nondiabetic and diabetic type 1
5. Cardiovascular protection in specified doses (ramipril, perindopril; trandolapril pending)

Caution: Not all the above are licensed indications and the license for a specific ACE inhibitor will vary from the above. Check the package insert.
AMI = acute myocardial infarction.

Table 5-4 Summary of Pharmacologic Properties, Clinical Indications, and Doses of ACE Inhibitors

Drug	Zinc Ligand	Active Drug	Elim $t\frac{1}{2}$ (hours)	T/P ratio % (FDA)	Hypertension (usual daily dose)	Heart failure or postinfarct, target doses used in large trials
Class I: Captopril-Like						
Captopril	SH	Captopril	4–6 (total captopril)	—	25–50 mg 2× or 3×	50 mg 3×
Class II: Prodrugs						
Alacepril	Carboxyl	Captopril	8 (total captopril)	—	12.5–25 mg 2×	Not established
Benazepril	Carboxyl	Benazeprilat	11	—	10–40 mg in 1–2 doses	Not established
Cilazepril	Carboxyl	Cilazeprilat	9	—	2.5–5 mg 1×	Not established
Delapril	Carboxyl	Delaprilat 5-OH-delaprilat	1.21.4	—	7.5–30 mg in 1–2 doses	Not established
Enalapril	Carboxyl	Enalaprilat	6; 11 (accum)	—	5–20 mg in 1–2 doses	10 mg 2×
Fosinopril	Phosphoryl	Fosinoprilat	12	50–80	10–80 mg 1× (or 2×)	Not established
Perindopril	Carboxyl	Perindoprilat	3–10	75–100	4–8 mg 1×	Not established
Quinapril	Carboxyl	Quinaprilat	1.8	50	10–80 mg in 1–2 doses	Not established
Ramipril	Carboxyl	Ramiprilat	13–17	50–60	2.5–10 mg in 1–2 doses	5 mg 2×
Spirapril	Carboxyl	Spiraprilat	<2	—	3–6 mg 1 dose*	Not established
Trandolapril	Carboxyl	Trandoprilat	10	50–90	0.5–4 mg 1×, then 4 mg 2×†	4 mg 1×
Class III: Water-Soluble						
Lisinopril	Carboxyl	Lisinopril	7; 12 (accum)	—	10–40 mg 1× (may need high dose if given 1×)	10–35 mg 1×

Data based on FDA-approved information where available.

accum = accumulation half-life; Elim $t\frac{1}{2}$ = elimination half-life; T/P ratio = trough/peak ratios, FDA-approved values.

*Thurmann, *Hypertension*, 1996;28:450.

†Initial dose 1 mg, 2 mg in black patients.

113

Table 5-5 Major Outcome Trials with Renin-Angiotensin-Aldosterone Inhibitors

Renin-angiotensin-aldosterone blocker	Risk prevention	HPT	Chronic Heart Failure	Heart Failure, Post-MI	AMI, Early Phase	Diabetic Nephropathy	Chronic Renal Disease
ACE Inhibitor							
Captopril		✓ CAPP		✓✓ SAVE		✓✓ type 1	✓
Enalapril		✓✓ ANBP2	✓✓ SOLVD, V-HeFT, CONSENSUS				✓
Lisinopril		✓ ALLHAT	✓ ATLAS		✓✓ GISSI		
Perindopril	✓✓ EUROPA						
Ramipril	✓✓ HOPE			✓✓ AIRE		✓ MICROHOPE	✓✓ REIN, AASK
Trandolapril	✓✓? PEACE pending	✓ INVEST		✓✓ TRACE			
ARBs							
Candesartan			✓✓ CHARM				
Irbesartan						✓✓ IDNT, IRMA	
Losartan		✓✓ with LVH, LIFE	?✗ ?✓ ELITE 1 & 2 (?dose too low)	✗, OPTIMAAL (?dose too low)		✓✓ RENAAL	
Valsartan	? VALUE		✓✓ VALHeFT	✓✓ VALIANT			
Aldosterone Antagonist							
Spironolactone			✓✓ RALES				
Eplerenone				✓✓ EPHESUS			

✓✓ = strongly indicated; ✓ = indicated; ✗ = not indicated.

CLASS II: PRO-DRUGS
Opie 2004

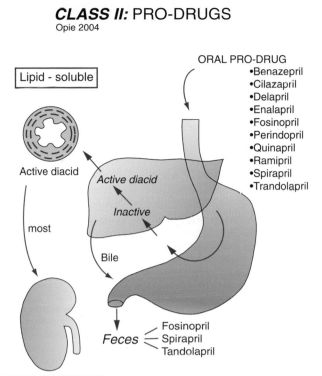

Figure 5-6 Pharmacokinetic patterns of prodrugs that are converted to active diacids and then excreted (class II). The predominant pattern for most is renal excretion but with some drugs, especially fosinopril, biliary and fecal excretion may be as important. (*Figure © LH Opie, 2005.*)

Table 5-6 | **ACE Inhibitors and ARBs: Side Effects and Contraindications**

1. ACEi, Side Effects, Class

Cough: common
Hypotension: variable (care with renal artery stenosis; severe heart failure)
Deterioration of renal function (related in part to hypotension)
Angioedema (rare; but potentially fatal)
Renal failure (rare, risk with bilateral renal artery stenosis)
Hyperkalemia (in renal failure, especially with K-retaining diuretics)
Skin reactions (especially with captopril)

2. ACEi, Side Effects First Described for High-Dose Captopril

Loss of taste
Neutropenia especially with collagen vascular renal disease
Proteinuria
Oral lesions; scalded-mouth syndrome (rare)

3. ACEi and ARBs, Shared Contraindications and Cautions

Pregnancy (NB: prominent FDA warning)
Severe renal failure (caution if creatinine >2.5–3.0 mg/dL, 220–265 μmol/L)
Hyperkalemia requires caution
Bilateral renal artery stenosis or equivalent lesions
Preexisting hypotension
Severe aortic stenosis or obstructive cardiomyopathy
Often less effective in black persons without added diuretic

ACE INHIBITORS: POTENTIAL SIDE EFFECTS
Opie 2004

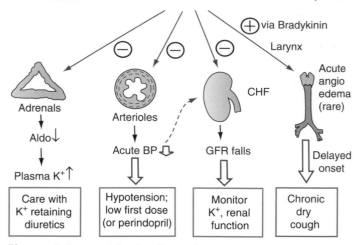

Figure 5-7 Potential side effects of ACE inhibitors include cough, hypotension, and renal impairment. Angioedema is rare. To avoid hypotension in heart failure patients, a low first test dose is usually given. *aldo* = aldosterone; *CHF* = congestive heart failure; *GFR* = glomerular filtration rate. (*Figure © LH Opie, 2005.*)

hypertension such side effects are generally discovered only if volunteered. In some centers, the incidence of cough is thought to be as high as 10% to 15%, whereas others report a much lower incidence, such as 5.5% in HOPE.[21] The cough is due to an increased sensitivity of the cough reflex resulting in a dry irritating nonproductive cough, quite different from bronchospasm. Increased formation of bradykinin and prostaglandins may play a role (Table 5-2). Several studies suggest relief of the cough by added nonsteroidal anti-inflammatory drugs,[22] with the downside of diminished antihypertensive effects. As an alternative, the combination of low-dose ACE inhibitor and the calcium channel blocker (CCB) nifedipine lessens the cough through unknown mechanisms. Logically, and most often tried with success, a change to an angiotensin-II receptor blocker consistently lessens the cough.[23]

Hypotension Particularly in CHF, orthostatic symptoms attributable to excess hypotension are common and may necessitate dose reduction or even cessation of ACE inhibitor therapy. In general, so long as orthostatic symptoms do not occur, the absolute blood pressure is not crucial and many patients do well with systolic pressures of 80 to 90 mmHg. *Hyponatremia* can be an indicator of heightened renin-angiotensin-aldosterone activity, and when present, there is an increased risk of inducing hypotension.

Hyperkalemia Hyperkalemia is a risk when ACE inhibitors are given with potassium-sparing diuretics or in the presence of renal failure. Thus potassium supplements or retainers should be used with care in the presence of ACE inhibition, especially when there is renal failure. The RALES study did, however, show the safety and efficacy of low doses of spironolactone when carefully added to ACE inhibitors and diuretics in the therapy of severe systolic heart failure.[24] Careful monitoring of the serum potassium level is essential because of the potentially serious harm caused by hyperkalemia.

Renal Side Effects Renal side effects with reversible renal failure can be precipitated by hypotension. Predisposing are a fixed low renal blood flow as in severe congestive heart failure (CHF) or severe sodium and volume depletion, or underlying renal disease including renal artery stenosis. In these conditions, efferent glomerular arterial constriction resulting from angiotensin-II may be crucial in retaining the GFR (glomerular filtration rate). Rarely, irreversible renal failure has occurred in patients with bilateral renal artery stenosis, which is therefore a contraindication to ACE inhibitors. In unilateral renal artery disease, with high circulating renin values, ACE inhibitors may also cause excessive hypotensive responses with oliguria and/or azotemia. To obviate such problems, and especially when there is unilateral renal artery stenosis or a low sodium state, a low first test dose is required with blood pressure checks. An arbitrary high value of serum creatinine is often taken as a contraindication (Table 5-6). A slight stable increase in serum creatinine after the introduction of an ACE inhibitor should not limit use.

Serious but Rare: Angioedema Although rare (about 0.3% in ALLHAT, rising to 0.6% to 1.6% in black individuals), angioedema can be life threatening.[25,26] This condition can very rarely be fatal, the incidence of death increasing from zero in a large study on 12,634 patients given enalapril for 24 weeks,[26] to about one in 5000 to 10,000 patients.[25,27] The mechanism depends on bradykinin.[28] Prompt subcutaneous epinephrine and rarely even intubation may be needed.[29] The ACE inhibitor must be stopped and an ARB can be considered. Although with a switch to an ARB, more than 90% may become free of ACE-inhibitor–induced angioedema,[23] there are isolated instances of an ARB also being associated with angioedema.

Pregnancy Risks All ACE inhibitors (and ARBs) are embryopathic and contraindicated in pregnancy, with the greatest risk in the second and third trimesters. The FDA requires a boxed warning in the package insert.

Neutropenia Whether the SH-groups in the captopril molecule really are the specific cause of neutropenia and/or agranulocytosis is still not clear. The association with high-dose captopril, usually occurring in patients with renal failure and especially those with a collagen vascular disorder, is undoubted. In the case of all other ACE inhibitors, the American package inserts all warn that available data for noncaptopril ACE inhibitors (i.e., all the rest) are not sufficient to exclude agranulocytosis at rates similar to those found with captopril. In reality, neutropenia seems to have disappeared with high-dose captopril.

Contraindications These include bilateral renal artery stenosis, pregnancy, known allergy, or hypersensitivity and hyperkalemia. Often a high serum creatinine above 2.5 to 3.0 mg/dL (220 to 265 µmol/L) is taken as an arbitrary cutoff point for the use of ACE inhibitors and for ARBs, especially in heart failure. However, overall benefits can be attained with lesser degrees of renal insufficiency.[30]

ACE INHIBITORS FOR HEART FAILURE
Neurohumoral Effects of Overt Heart Failure

A crucial problem in CHF is the inability of the left ventricle in severe failure to maintain a normal blood pressure and organ perfusion. *Enhanced activity of the renin-angiotensin system* (Fig. 5-8) follows from: (1) hypotension, which evokes baroreflexes to increase sympathetic adrenergic discharge, thereby stimulating the β_1 renal receptors involved in renin release; (2) activation of chemoreflexes and ergoreflexes; and (3) decreased renal perfusion, resulting in renal ischemia which enhances renin release. However, even in severe CHF, plasma renin may not be elevated.[31] Rather, to achieve consistent stimulation of the renin-angiotensin system requires simultaneous diuretic

NEUROHUMORAL EFFECTS OF HEART FAILURE

Opie 2004

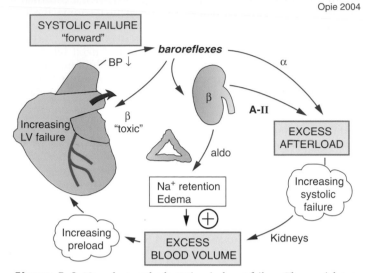

Figure 5-8 Neurohumoral adaptation in heart failure. The crucial consequence of LV failure is the inability to maintain a normal blood pressure and normal organ perfusion. As a result of reflex baroreflex activation and excess adrenergic stimulation, there is alpha (α) mediated peripheral vasoconstriction that increases the afterload and leads to increased LV failure. Excess alpha (α) adrenergic stimulation leads to peripheral vasoconstriction. Furthermore, excess β-adrenergic stimulation promotes renin release with increased vasoconstrictive angiotensin-II (*A-II*) and release of aldosterone. Increasing preload and afterload leads to increasing LV failure. (*Figure © LH Opie, 2005.*)

therapy. Angiotensin-II promotes secretion of aldosterone, and also the release of vasopressin, to contribute to abnormal fluid retention and volume regulation in severe CHF. Generally, such changes are thought to be adverse because of increased vasoconstriction following enhanced levels of angiotensin-II and norepinephrine, because of fluid and sodium retention associated with increased aldosterone levels, and the dilutional hyponatremia associated with increased vasopressin levels.

Great Increase in Peripheral Vascular Resistance Thus the greater afterload against which the failing heart must work is explained by (1) increased formation of angiotensin-II, (2) reflex release of norepinephrine, (3) release of vasoconstrictor *endothelin* from the dysfunctional vascular endothelium, (4) reduced muscle mass, (5) thickened capillary membranes, and (6) altered endothelial cell response to muscle metabolites. Systemic vasoconstriction reduces renal plasma flow, which detrimentally affects salt excretion and further promotes renin formation. Vasodilator hormones of cardiac origin, such as atrial and brain natriuretic peptides, and prostaglandins of vascular origin, are also activated, but fail to achieve compensatory vasodilation for complex reasons including receptor downgrading.

Increase in LV Wall Stress Especially during exertion, both systolic and diastolic wall stresses become too high for the depressed contractility of the failing myocardium. The inability of the left ventricle to empty itself during systole increases the preload. The combination of increased pre- and afterload, so common in CHF, leads to progressive ventricular dilation with wall remodeling (myocyte hypertrophy and slippage with matrix changes), so that the ejection fraction progressively declines with time. Load reduction and in particular angiotensin-II inhibition may retard this detrimental process. According to the *Laplace law*, the stress on the wall of a thin-walled sphere is proportional to the product of the intraluminal pressure and the radius, and inversely related to the wall thickness:

$$\text{Wall stress} = \frac{\text{Pressure} \times \text{Radius}}{2 \times \text{Wall thickness}}$$

Wall stress is one of the major determinants of myocardial oxygen uptake. Afterload and preload reduction, by decreasing the radius of the left ventricle, decreases the myocardial oxygen demand. ACE inhibition, by reducing the preload and the afterload, lessens excessive LV wall stress, limits remodeling, and enhances ventricular emptying.[32] All these factors improve the myocardial oxygen balance. Long term, further LV chamber enlargement is attenuated.

Beneficial Neurohumoral Effects of ACE Inhibitors Administration of ACE inhibitors has a consistent effect in increasing plasma renin, decreasing angiotensin-II and aldosterone, with a fall in norepinephrine and/or epinephrine, and in vasopressin. Angiotensin-II production falls. Parasympathetic activity, reduced in heart failure, is improved by ACE inhibition. Although there are some exceptions to the patterns noted, most of the results are reasonably consistent. From these data it can be concluded that chronic ACE inhibition ameliorates the neurohumoral changes found in congestive heart failure.

Possible Use of ACE Inhibitors as First-Line Therapy in Early Heart Failure

In the SOLVD prevention study[33] on more than 4000 patients, only 17% were taking diuretics and 67% were in NYHA class I, so that the question was whether enalapril could prevent the development of overt heart failure (Table 5-7). Not surprisingly, the most striking benefits were found in patients with the lowest initial ejection fractions, below 28%, with only borderline results in those with values of 33% to 35%. Enalapril in a mean daily dose of 17 mg was associated with less hospitalization and less development of symptomatic heart failure. Data from this arm of SOLVD influence the meta-analysis of Flather and Yusuf to show that the mortality benefit of ACE inhibitors can be found even in the absence of initial diuretic therapy.[34]

How Do Diuretics Compare with ACE Inhibitors? In postinfarct patients without clinical heart failure but with modestly depressed left ventricular function, the ACE inhibitor captopril was better able to maintain left ventricular function and size than the diuretic furosemide.[35] There could be many adverse effects of diuretics including activation of the renin-angiotensin axis. Yet in overt left ventricular failure and in congestive heart failure, diuretic therapy is still universally accepted as first-step and first-line therapy. This is because of symptomatic benefit, and because diuretics are superior to ACE inhibitors in diminishing sodium and water retention. There is only limited evidence that life is prolonged by diuretics, although it is clinically evident that an intravenous loop diuretic is life-saving when given to a patient with severe left ventricular failure and pulmonary edema. Long term, it is now clear that ACE inhibitors prolong life (Tables 5-7 to 5-9) whereas digoxin does not, so that the automatic choice current choice of agent to combine with a diuretic in CHF would be an ACE inhibitor.

ACE Inhibitors Plus β-Blockers (and Diuretics) for Heart Failure

As ACE inhibitors are so effective in suppressing the neurohumoral response, it is no surprise that β-blockers, which also inhibit renin and

Table 5-7	Major Outcome Trials of ACE Inhibitors in Heart Failure				
Acronym and Drug	Condition	No. of Patients	Mean Duration of Trial	Major Result	
CONSENSUS Enalapril	Severe heart failure	253	6 mo	40% mortality reduction at 6 months, 31% at 1 yr	
SOLVD (treatment) enalapril	Mild to moderate heart failure	2369	41 mo	18% mortality reduction	
SOLVD (prevention) enalapril	Asymptomatic LV dysfunction	4228	37 mo	37% reduction in risk of CHF; mortality unchanged	
X-SOLVD	Follow-up of both SOLVD arms	5165	12 yr	10% death risk fall in both SOLVD arms	
V-HeFT-II enalapril	Chronic heart failure	804	24 mo	18% reduction in death vs. nitrate-hydralazine	
SAVE Captopril	Postinfarct LV dysfunction	2231	42 mo	37% reduction in risk of CHF; 19% mortality reduction	
TRACE Trandolapril	Postinfarct LV dysfunction	1749	4 yr	22% decrease in mortality	
AIRE Ramipril	Postinfarct clinical heart failure	1986	15 mo	27% mortality reduction	

AIRE = Acute Infarction Ramipril Efficacy[61]; CHF = congestive heart failure; CONSENSUS = Cooperative North Scandinavian Enalapril Survival Study[45]; LV dysfunction = low ventricular ejection fraction; SAVE = Survival and Ventricular Enlargement[69]; SOLVD = Studies of Left Ventricular Dysfunction[33,85]; TRACE = Trandolapril Cardiac Evaluation[62]; V-HeFT-II = VA Cooperative Vasodilator Heart Failure Trial[124]; X-SOLVD, Extended Studies Of Left Ventricular Dysfunction.[84]

the effects of norepinephrine, also benefit heart failure. The consistently positive results of the CIBIS II study with bisoprolol,[36] the MERIT study with metoprolol,[37] and several carvedilol studies,[38] were such that β-blockers are now viewed as an integral part of the standard therapy for heart failure. The chosen drug should be introduced carefully at a very low dose which is then increased over several months (see Table 1-2). The β-blocker should be introduced when the patient is stable, not when there is hemodynamic deterioration. *Should the β-blocker be combined with an ACE inhibitor?* The answer is certainly yes, as almost all the patients in these trials were already receiving an ACE inhibitor. Furthermore, in the Flather meta-analysis, mortality reduction with the combination of an ACE inhibitor and a β-blocker (relative risk of 0.68) was better than with an ACE inhibitor alone (relative risk of 0.83).[34]

Aldosterone Inhibition by Spironolactone or Eplerenone: A New Imperative?

In RALES, a low dose of *spironolactone*, often only 25 mg daily, was given to patients in NYHA class III-IV.[24] Prior therapy was an ACE inhibitor, a loop diuretic and digoxin (in 75%). There was only a small rise in serum potassium, but it should be stressed that these patients did not have renal impairment, a risk factor for serious hyperkalemia. Risk of all cause mortality fell by 30% ($P < 0.001$), owing

Table 5-8	Comparison of Some Properties of Angiotensin-Receptor Blockers (ARBs) versus ACE Inhibitors Relevant to Use in Hypertension	
Property	**ARB**	**ACE Inhibitor**
Major site of block	AT-1 receptor	Converting enzyme
Major claims, basic science	More complete AT-1 block, AT-2 activity increased; latter may increase bradykinin	Block of two receptors: AT-1, AT-2. Inhibition of bradykinin breakdown
Side effects	Generally similar to placebo; angioedema rare but found (CHARM)[23]	Dry cough; angioedema higher in black (1.6%) than non-black patients (0.6%), enalapril data from OCTAVE[26]
Licensed for hypertension?	Yes	Yes
First line therapy, JNC VII[125]	No	No
Compelling indications, JNC VII[125]	Heart failure, diabetes, chronic renal disease; post-MI likely in future	As for ARB plus post-MI, high coronary risk, recurrent stroke prevention
Favored therapy in hypertension, European Guidelines[76]	LVH; ACE inhibitor-cough; diabetic type 2 nephropathy or microalbuminuria; proteinuria	CHF; LV dysfunction; post-MI; nondiabetic renal disease; diabetic type 1 nephropathy; proteinuria
Major clinical claims in hypertension	Equal BP reduction to ACE inhibitors, little/no cough, excellent tolerability, well tested in LVH and in diabetic nephropathy	Well tolerated, years of experience especially in CHF; good quality of life. Used in coronary prevention trials (HOPE, EUROPA, PEACE)
Effect on LVH, vs. β-blockers	Better (losartan, valsartan); Major outcome trial, LIFE[91]	Better (lisinopril, ramipril)
Effect on sex life, vs. β-blockers	Better	Better
Less new diabetes	Losartan; valsartan; candesartan	CAPPP,[58] STOP-2[59]
Outcome trials (death, stroke, coronary events, etc.)	LIFE (losartan better than atenolol, stroke less, deaths less in diabetics).[91] VALUE[91a] (valsartan similar to amlodipine)	Enalapril > diuretic,[56] Diuretic > lisinopril in ALLHAT[25]

>, better than; AT-1 = angiotensin-II receptor, subtype one; CHF = congestive heart failure; LVH = left ventricular hypertrophy.

to decreases in both progressive heart failure and sudden death. The benefit was found irrespective of β-blocker use. The surprise is that the standard advice to doctors prescribing ACE inhibitors has been to avoid the addition of potassium retainers because of the implicit danger of hyperkalemia. A similar picture unfolded in the case of EPHESUS, in which addition of the more specific aldosterone blocker eplerenone to prior therapy of those with postinfarct heart failure reduced mortality.[39] Yet in RALES and in EPHESUS, the rise in serum potassium was limited and the results positive. However, serum potassium *must be* carefully monitored, with reduction of the dose of the ACE inhibitor or the aldosterone blocker in case of hyperkalemia. Note that an initial serum potassium value exceeding 5.0 mmol/L was an exclusion criterion in both RALES and EPHESUS.

Table 5-9	Comparison of Angiotensin Receptor Blockers (ARBs) vs ACE Inhibitors in Heart Failure, in CV Prevention, and in Stroke	
Property	**ARB**	**ACE Inhibitor**
Heart failure: Licensed in USA?	Valsartan for ACEi-intolerant patients; candesartan under evaluation	Yes, several but not all
Major clinical claims in heart failure	Use in ACEi-intolerant patients; noninferiority to ACEi not yet established	Many studies with large data base, at least 12,000 patients, definite mortality reduction of 20%, prevents reinfarction
Post-MI: Major studies	VALIANT, valsartan noninferior to captopril in postinfarct heart failure.[83]	Several large studies, definite protection including LV dysfunction
Diabetic nephropathy: Major claims	Renoprotective in type 2 diabetes independently of hypertension[109,114]; slows progress of microalbuminuria[113]	Renoprotective in type 1 diabetes independently of hypertension
Nondiabetic renal disease	No outcome data	Better outcome, REIN, AASK
Prevention of CV complications (MI, heart failure, stroke, or CV death)	No data, ON TARGET evaluating telmisartan vs. ramipril in HOPE-like study	HOPE reduction of this primary end-point by 22%; EUROPA, reduction of MI and combined end-points; PEACE underway
Prevention of stroke	LIFE, less stroke in LVH treated by losartan usually with diuretic versus atenolol	PROGRESS, less repeat stroke with perindopril only if with diuretic
Major warnings	Pregnancy, all trimesters	Pregnancy, all trimesters
Additional warnings	Hypotension; hyperkalemia; renal function	Angioedema; hypotension; hyperkalemia; renal function

CV = cardiovascular; MI = myocardial infarction.

Quadruple Therapy as the Ideal?

Increasingly the optimal therapy of heart failure is seen as a combination of the three drugs known to reduce mortality (ACE inhibitors, β-blockers, aldosterone blockers) and one type that improves symptoms (diuretics), with digoxin for selected patients (atrial fibrillation or persistent symptoms). Such combined therapy receives support from the EHPESUS study,[39] in which eplerenone was added to prior medication with ACE inhibition or an ARB (86%), β-blockers (75%), and diuretics (60%) but no digoxin. An alternate multiple therapy with an added high dose ARB replacing the aldosterone blocker, receives some support from the CHARM-Added study.[40]

Potential Problems with Drug Combinations in CHF

Diuretics plus ACE Inhibitors Additive effects on the preload may lead to syncope or hypotension so that the diuretic dose is usually halved before starting ACE inhibitors. The result may be a true diuretic-sparing effect in about half of patients with mild CHF on addition of the ACE inhibitor, while in others the full diuretic dose must be reinstituted.

ACE Inhibitors plus Spironolactone or Eplerenone Here the major danger is hyperkalemia and the lesser is an increasing serum creatinine,[24,39] so that frequent checks are needed. Exclusion criteria are the prior use of potassium-retaining diuretics, a serum creatinine exceeding 2.5 mg/dL (220 μmol/L), and a serum potassium exceeding 5.0 mm/L. Sometimes the dose of the ACE inhibitor must be adjusted downwards.

ACE Inhibitors and Aspirin or Nonsteroidal Anti-inflammatories (NSAIDs) Formation of bradykinin and thereby prostaglandins may play an important role in peripheral and renal vasodilation. Hence, nonsteroidal anti-inflammatories, especially indomethacin, lessen the effectiveness of ACE inhibitors in hypertension.[41] Sulindac may have less effect and ARBs seem to interact less.[41] These strictures probably also apply to the newer COX-2 inhibitors. In CHF the interaction with NSAIDs is less studied. Restrictions on renal blood flow invoked by NSAIDs are most likely to be serious in those with major renin-angiotensin inhibition receiving high-dose diuretics and with hyponatremia.[42] If an NSAID has to be used in heart failure, frequent checks of renal function are required. Regarding aspirin, despite the persuasive meta-analysis on 22,000 patients showing similar beneficial effects in heart failure irrespective of baseline aspirin use,[43] the issue of an aspirin-ACE inhibitor interaction is not dead (Ch 9, p. 282). In practice, low-dose (about 80 mg daily) aspirin is often combined with an ACE inhibitor in the therapy of ischemic heart failure. Alternatively, replacement of aspirin by clopidogrel may be considered.

How to Start an ACE Inhibitor in CHF

First the patient must be fully assessed clinically, including measurements of serum creatinine and urea, and electrolytes. It is important to avoid first-dose hypotension and thereby to lessen the risk of temporary renal failure. Patients at high *risk of hypotension* include those with serum sodium <130 mmol/L, and increased serum creatinine in the range of 1.5 to 3.0 mg/dL or 135 to 265 μmol/L. Patients with creatinine values exceeding 3.0 mg/dL should be considered separately (see later). Other groups at high risk include those on multiple diuretics or high-dose furosemide (exceeding 80 mg daily), those with pre-existing hypotension and a systolic blood pressure <90 mmHg, and those 70 years of age or older (UK package insert, enalapril). All these patients need to have diuretic therapy stopped for 1 to 2 days and are then ideally given a test dose under close supervision, often in hospital. Alternatively, a low initial dose of a very low dose of enalapril (1.25 mg) or 2 mg of perindopril (with its slow onset of action) is given.[44] If there is no symptomatic hypotension, the chosen drug is continued, renal function monitored, and the dose gradually increased.[45] Absence of first-dose hypotension suggests but does not securely establish that the subsequent course will be smooth. If the patient is fluid overloaded with an elevated jugular venous pressure, then the test dose of the ACE inhibitor can be given without first having to stop diuretic therapy. The addition of the ACE inhibitor may call forth a diuresis, in which case the diuretic dose is decreased to avoid hypotension. Although these procedures are often undertaken in hospital, it is becoming more common in selected patients to undertake outpatient monitoring.

Preexisting Renal Failure In general, the serum creatinine can be expected to rise modestly and then to stabilize. In severe CHF, in which renal function is already limited by hypotension and by poor renal blood flow, it may be a difficult decision to know whether or not to introduce ACE inhibitor therapy. For example, the serum creatinine may exceed 2.5 to 3.0 mg/dL or 220 to 265 μmol/L. The danger of exaggeration of renal failure must be balanced against the possible benefit from an improved cardiac output and decreased renal afferent arteriolar vasoconstriction resulting from ACE inhibitor therapy. Problems can be expected especially when the glomerular filtration rate (GFR) is low and the renin-angiotensin axis highly stimulated. The best policy may be to improve the hemodynamic status as far as possible by the combined use of optimal doses of diuretics and other agents. Then the diuretic dose could be briefly reduced or stopped, and a very low dose of an ACE inhibitor introduced.

Hypotensive Response to ACE Inhibition Temporary renal failure is most likely to develop in patients with excess diuretic therapy and volume depletion, in whom there is a greater hypotensive response to ACE inhibitor therapy. Thus it is logical to start ACE inhibitors with low initial doses, such as captopril 6.25 mg or enalapril 2.5 mg or even 1.25 mg. In elderly patients, a low initial dose of perindopril (2 mg) is less likely to cause initial hypotension than a low first dose of either enalapril (2.5 mg) or captopril (6.25 mg) for reasons that are unknown.[44] Special caution is required in diabetic individuals in whom renal failure is a particular hazard.

Hyponatremia: Salt and Water Limitation Patients with severe hyponatremia are 30 times more likely to develop hypotension in response to ACE inhibitor therapy and require special care. The cause of the hyponatremia is at least in part release of vasopressin (antidiuretic hormone) as can result from renin-angiotensin activation following intense diuretic therapy.[42] Although the combination of furosemide and ACE inhibitor may work safely, it is essential to avoid excess diuresis and volume depletion. Modest, tolerable *salt restriction* is standard practice. Patients already on strict low sodium diets are at increased risk of first dose hypotension. In patients who are not volume-depleted, restriction of water intake is advisable because delayed water diuresis may contribute to hyponatremia in severe CHF.

Outstanding Clinical Problems in the Therapy of Heart Failure

Drug Dose Whereas in hypertension the dose-response curve is flat and can be monitored from the blood pressure response, in CHF the problem of the optimal dose does arise. Is the dose large enough to give as complete renin-angiotensin inhibition as possible? In the ATLAS study a high dose of lisinopril (about 35 mg daily) gave fewer hospitalizations but no lower mortality than low-dose (2.5 or 5 mg daily).[46] Standard medium doses were not tested. In the case of enalapril, the standard target dose is 10 mg twice daily. Increasing this to 60 mg/day did not alter death rate or hemodynamic parameters.[47] In clinical practice lower doses than in the trials are commonly used, below those found to work in trials. Although the optimal doses of ACE inhibitors in CHF have not been established by clinical studies, our opinion is that the dose should be titrated upwards to the effective trial doses without going higher.

Diastolic Dysfunction Most heart failure studies have concentrated on the role of ACE inhibition in systolic heart failure and the indices of improvement in systolic function. Diastolic heart failure is thought to be an early event particularly in left ventricular hypertrophy (LVH) in response to hypertension or aortic stenosis, as well as in the elderly. Intracoronary enalaprilat improves diastolic function in patients with LVH due to either aortic stenosis[48] or hypertension.[49]

Skeletal Muscle Metabolism in Heart Failure The skeletal muscle myopathy found in heart failure is associated with increased proton production that stimulates the ergoreflexes that worsen the symptoms of exertional intolerance.[50] The causes of the myopathy are not clear. Increased circulating angiotensin-II may play a role.[51] Clinical studies with ACE inhibitors or ARBs geared to this problem are needed.

Anemia A low hemoglobin is a poorly understood risk factor for cardiovascular disease.[52] A small decrease in hemoglobin, to the order of 0.3 g/dL, may occur with enalapril therapy (package insert), and ACE inhibitors may be used therapeutically to treat the erythrocytosis that follows renal transplantation. Perhaps more attention should be paid to the possible development of anemia during ACE inhibitor therapy.

Ethnic and Gender Differences Most large heart failure trials have studied Caucasian males. Are black patients less likely to respond to ACE inhibitors than others, as in the case of hypertension? However, in a large meta-analysis, there were similar clinical outcomes in black as in white subjects,[53] the probable explanation being that diuretic cotherapy sensitizes black patients to ACE inhibitors. Women respond in a similar way to men, without, however, evidence of mortality benefit in those with asymptomatic LV systolic dysfunction.[53]

Established Adverse Role of Aldosterone The RALES and EPHESUS studies have shown that aldosterone excess may have serious adverse effects in heart failure of various etiologies.[24,54]

ACE INHIBITORS FOR HYPERTENSION

The renin-angiotensin-aldosterone system (RAAS) is one of several major mechanisms that help to maintain the blood pressure both in normal persons and in those with essential hypertension, especially when sodium is restricted or diuretics are in use. In malignant hypertension or in renal artery stenosis, renal ischemia stimulates the release of renin from the juxtaglomerular apparatus and drives the blood pressure up. Although ACE inhibition leads to the most dramatic falls of blood pressure in the presence of such an underlying renal mechanism, ACE inhibition is also an effective antihypertensive therapy in mild to moderate hypertension even when plasma renin is not high. ACE inhibitors appear to lower blood pressure by multiple mechanisms as discussed in Chapter 7 (see Fig. 7-9). In general, ACE inhibitors are more effective in white patients who would also respond to β-blockers.[55] Lesser efficacy in black patients, especially in the elderly, can be overcome by addition of low-dose diuretics. The somewhat lesser efficacy of an ACE inhibitor in the ALLHAT trial than the diuretic[25] may be ascribed to (1) the trial design, which did not allow addition of a diuretic or CCB to the ACE inhibitor so that blood pressure control was not good enough in the ACE inhibitor group; and (2) to the relatively high proportion of black patients, about one third, in whom the lack of diuretic would be more serious. In the Australian study on elderly Caucasian subjects, enalapril gave overall better results than did the diuretic at exactly equal blood pressure control.[56] As ACE inhibitors do not alter glucose tolerance, blood uric acid, or cholesterol levels, and as these agents seldom cause subjective side effects apart from cough, their use in hypertension has rapidly increased. ACE inhibitors generally give a good quality of life, and are among the best tolerated of the antihypertensive drugs,[57] apart from the development of cough as an irritating side effect. For further details of the use of ACE inhibitors in hypertension, see Chapter 7.

Less New Diabetes

Rather than precipitating diabetes as may occur with diuretic or β-blocker therapy, ACE inhibitors may lessen the development of new diabetes in hypertensive individuals,[58,59] in heart failure,[60] and in those at risk of cardiovascular disease.[21] Because similar protection is found with ARBs, the mechanism is likely to involve AT-1 receptor blockade rather than bradykinin.

ACE INHIBITORS FOR EARLY PHASE AMI OR POSTINFARCT LV DYSFUNCTION OR FAILURE

ACE Inhibition Within 24 Hours of Onset of AMI

ACE inhibitors are now virtually mandatory for overt left ventricular failure or LV dysfunction after the early acute phase of myocardial infarction is over.[61-63] The only possible controversy surrounds their use within 24 hours of onset of AMI. The selective policy, favored by the present authors, is to give ACE inhibitors to all high-risk patients: diabetic individuals, and those with anterior infarcts[64] or tachycardia or overt LV failure. Logically, the sicker the patient, the greater the activation of the renin-angiotensin-system, and the better the expected result with the use of an ACE inhibitor. The selective policy receives a class 1 (highest) recommendation from the American Heart Association and American College of Cardiology, and is based on results from several major trials. For example, in nearly 19,000 patients in GISSI-3,[65] lisinopril reduced mortality at 6 weeks from the already low value of 7.1% in controls to 6.3%. Later subgroup analysis showed that the mortality reduction was largely confined to the diabetic patients.[66] Nonetheless, nondiabetic individuals can also benefit, as found in an overview of nearly 100,000 high-risk patients with AMI.[67] Of note, the benefit of early ACE inhibition is not annulled by early administration of aspirin.[63] Nor is the benefit explained by reduction of infarct size, which is better accomplished by β-blockade.[68]

ACE Inhibitors in Postinfarct LV Dysfunction or Clinical Failure

ACE inhibitors attenuate LV remodeling and reduce the risk of subsequent MI. If ACE inhibitors have not been started within 24 hours of the onset of AMI, then the next opportunity is a few days later. Three major trials used rather different entry criteria, one being clinical[61] and two based on LV functional measurements.[62,69] All three showed major mortality reduction. Long term follow-up of the AIRE patients, over 42 to 59 months, gave "robust evidence" that all-cause mortality was reduced by 36% (relative risk reduction) with an absolute reduction of 11.4%.[70] In a 6-year follow-up to the TRACE study,[71] the mean prolongation of life was 15.3 months. These are impressive data, and very strongly argue for the compulsory prolonged use of ACE inhibitors in postinfarct patients with clinical or echocardiographic LV failure. The mechanism of these beneficial effects is likely to be a combination of load reduction (Fig. 5-9) and removal of the local cardiac effects of angiotensin-II in promoting myocyte growth and fibroblastic proliferation (see Fig. 5-5).

ACE INHIBITORS: LONG-TERM CARDIOVASCULAR PROTECTION

Whether ACE inhibitors can give protection against myocardial infarction, as unexpectedly suggested by studies such as SOLVD[33] and SAVE,[69] has now received prospective confirmation by two adequately powered studies, namely HOPE with ramipril[21] and EUROPA with perindopril.[20] The PEACE study with trandolapril is still to be disclosed. As proposed mechanisms, ACE inhibitors could (1) enhance fibrinolysis, acting to reduce plasminogen activator inhibitor-1[72]; (2) act via bradykinin to increase nitric oxide formation to reverse endothelial dysfunction; (3) confer a preconditioning-like protection, acting via bradykinin BK$_2$-receptor activation, as suggested by short-term observations on human

POST-INFARCT REMODELING

Opie 2004

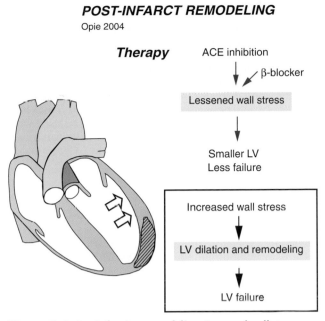

Figure 5-9 Postinfarction remodeling. Increased wall stress promotes adverse remodeling and left ventricular (*LV*) failure by the Laplace Law (see equation). The proposal, based on substantial animal data and human studies, is that ACE inhibition will attenuate postinfarct left ventricular enlargement and promote beneficial remodeling with better LV mechanical function. (*Figure © LH Opie, 2005.*)

atrial tissue[14]; or (4) reduce the blood pressure. In HOPE, the patients were at high risk, and there was reduction of multiple end-points besides myocardial infarction such as stroke and all-cause mortality. In EUROPA the risk was lower in that the patients selected had stable coronary artery disease, and the major effect was reduction of nonfatal myocardial infarction. In both HOPE and in EUROPA, the addition of the ACE inhibitor decreased the blood pressure, and some blood pressure experts argue that simple blood pressure reduction could have achieved the widespread cardiovascular protection. However, no other antihypertensive agents have shown this degree of reduction in major cardiovascular events starting at an initial blood pressure of only about 139/79 mmHg as in HOPE.

ACE inhibitors are not direct antianginal agents. It must be emphasized that these agents have only an indirect anti-ischemic effect by lessening the afterload on the myocardial oxygen demand,[73] by decreasing adrenergic activation, and by improving endothelial function. They are not antianginals.[74] Long term, they reduce the need for coronary revascularization procedures,[21,69] perhaps because of their antithrombotic properties.

DIABETES: PREVENTION OF COMPLICATIONS AND RENOPROTECTION

In diabetic individuals, the blood pressure aims are lower than in nondiabetic persons. JNC VII recommends a goal blood pressure of 130/80 mmHg. Both diabetes (type 2; maturity onset; non–insulin-dependent) and hypertension are associated with insulin resistance. Both high-dose thiazides and β-blockers can impair insulin sensitivity in nondiabetic hypertensive individuals. Therefore, there are arguments for the preferential use of ACE inhibition or an ARB.[75]

Diabetics with Nephropathy

In type 1 diabetic nephropathy, ACE inhibitors have repeatedly been shown to reduce proteinuria and protect against progressive glomerular sclerosis and loss of renal function.[75] In type 2 diabetic nephropathy, four trials with ARBs have shown similar renal protection.[75] Evidence-based guidelines therefore suggest ACE inhibitors for type I and ARBs for type 2 diabetic renal disease.[76] The strong likelihood that ACE inhibitors would be as effective in type 2 patients if they had been tested means that in practice ACE inhibitors will be used whenever ARBs cannot be afforded. They will often have to be combined with other drugs including diuretics, β-blockers, and CCBs to reduce the blood pressure to below 130/80 mmHg.

Diabetic Microalbuminuria

Renoprotective therapy, it is proposed, may be adjusted by the decline in proteinuria, just as antihypertensive therapy is adjusted by blood pressure levels.[77] Therefore the therapeutic attack should start whenever there is microalbuminuria. In MICRO-HOPE, one of the entry criteria was diabetes with microalbuminuria, but not macroalbuminuria.[78] In the overall diabetic population, the marked benefits of prolonged prophylactic ACE inhibition by ramipril supported the concept of renoprotection by ACE inhibition in diabetes.

ACE INHIBITION FOR NONDIABETIC RENAL FAILURE

In progressive renal failure, from whatever cause, there is a steady rise in serum creatinine, fall in glomerular function, and increasing proteinuria. Angiotensin-II may play a crucial role in the progression of glomerular injury and the growth and destruction of the glomeruli (Fig. 5-10). Besides dietary protein restriction, a variety of drugs have been used with a blood pressure goal of 125/75 mmHg.[79] There is good evidence from a meta-analysis on 1594 patients showing that ACE inhibitors beneficially alter the course of end-stage renal failure (ESRF), although better blood pressure reduction could also contribute to the results.[80]

Ramipril Nephropathy Study (REIN)

To this must be added the very impressive REIN study (Ramipril Efficacy In Nephropathy) and its long-term follow-up.[81] In the initial core study, patients with proteinuria of more than 3 g per 24 hours were selected. Ramipril reduced the rate of GFR decline more than expected from the blood pressure drop. In the follow-up study, those originally allocated to non-ramipril therapy and then switched to ramipril at the end of the initial core study never "caught" up with those kept on ramipril from the start. This occurred even though the blood pressure reduction in the "switched" group was greater than in those who stayed on ramipril throughout. In those with lesser degrees of proteinuria (1 to 3 g per day), there was slower progression to overt proteinuria.[30] Thus: (1) the earlier ACE inhibitor therapy is started, the better; (2) the sickest patients benefit most; (3) all degrees of proteinuria (1 g and more per day) benefit; and (4) the benefit cannot fully be explained by reduction of the blood pressure. Of importance, a relatively high serum creatinine was not a contraindication to ramipril. Nonetheless, clinicians often stop ACE inhibitor therapy after only a modest rise in serum creatinine.

African American Study of Kidney Disease and Hypertension (AASK)

Here the entry point was established hypertension with a low glomerular filtration rate (GFR). The primary outcome was the rate of

GLOMULAR INJURY AND GROWTH
Opie 2004

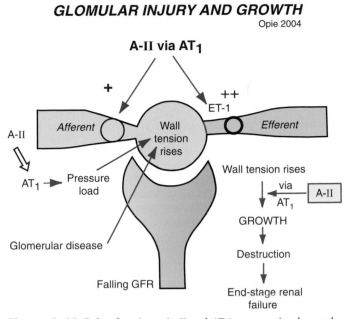

Figure 5-10 Role of angiotensin-II and AT-1 receptor in glomerular injury and progressive renal failure. An increased intraglomerular pressure as from a pressure load in hypertension or primary renal disease or diabetes can evoke mesangial growth with threat of complete glomerular closure. Angiotensin-II may be an important growth signal accelerating the disease process. (*Figure © LH Opie, 2005.*)

change of GFR, while the secondary end-points included end-stage renal disease and death.[82] Ramipril-based therapy was more effective than amlodipine at equal blood pressure levels in reducing the clinical end-points and proteinuria, while the GFR fell less but only in those with more severe renal failure in whom the mean initial serum creatinine was high at 2.76 mg/dL. Thus there was greater renoprotection with the ACE inhibitor, independent of the blood pressure reduction and despite the high serum creatinine.

PROPERTIES OF SPECIFIC ACE INHIBITORS
Captopril (Kinetic Class I)

Captopril (Capoten; Lopril in France; Lopirin in Germany; Captopril in Japan), the first widely available ACE inhibitor and now generically available, was originally seen to be an agent with significant and serious side effects such as loss of taste, renal impairment, and neutropenia. Now it is recognized that these are rather rare side effects that can be avoided largely by reducing the daily dose and by appropriate monitoring. Captopril is licensed in the United States for hypertension, heart failure, postinfarct LV dysfunction, and type 1 diabetic nephropathy. It is the best studied ACE inhibitor and has the widest range of approved indications. In the United Kingdom, it is also licensed for prevention of reinfarction and for diabetic microproteinuria. Pharmacokinetically, it belongs to class 1. After absorption from the stomach, captopril is largely excreted by the kidneys, about half as is and half as active metabolites formed in liver and kidney. The elimination half-life is approximately 4 to 6 hours (Table 5-4). In hypertension, its biological half-life is long enough to allow twice daily dosage.

Dose and Indications In *hypertension*, captopril has an average daily dose of 25 to 50 mg orally given twice or three times daily (instead of much higher previous doses). For maximum bioavailability, captopril should be taken on an empty stomach, yet food has little influence on antihypertensive effects. The risk of excess hypotension is highest in patients with high renin states (renal artery stenosis, preexisting vigorous diuretic therapy, severe sodium restriction, or hyponatremia) when the initial dose should be low (6.25 to 12.5 mg). Whether captopril can improve hard end-points in hypertension is not clear. In the CAPP study, the stroke rate was higher with captopril than in the conventional group (β-blocker, diuretic), but captopril was given only once or twice daily and the blood presure control was inferior to that in conventional therapy.[58] In *CHF*, captopril may cause excessive hypotension especially in vigorously diuresed patients so that a *test dose* of 6.25 mg may be required followed by 12.5 mg three times daily, and working up to 50 mg three times daily if tolerated. The diuretic may have to be stopped for 24 to 48 hours prior to captopril to avoid an excess renin state. In *postinfarct patients with LV dysfunction* (ejection fraction 40% or lower), captopril is licensed to prevent overt heart failure and, in the United Kingdom, to reduce recurrent myocardial infarction and coronary revascularization procedures. In VALIANT, captopril was noninferior to valsartan.[83] In *diabetic nephropathy*, captopril improves proteinuria and decreases hard end-points, such as death, transplantation, or dialysis. However, captopril is largely renal-excreted, so that doses should be reduced. In *renal disease*, when captopril is not contraindicated (next section), the dose is reduced.

Contraindications to Captopril These include bilateral renal artery stenosis; renal artery stenosis in a single kidney; immune-based renal disease, especially collagen vascular disease; severe renal failure (serum creatinine >3 mg/dL or >265 μmol/L; this chapter, p. 123); preexisting neutropenia; and systemic hypotension. Pregnancy is an absolute contraindication for all ACE inhibitors.

Side Effects In general, the side effects are seldom serious provided that the total daily dose is 150 mg daily or less. Cough is the most common and frequently troublesome side effect. Other class side effects include transient renal failure, angioedema, and hyperkalemia. Immune-based side effects are probably specific to captopril, such as taste disturbances, certain immune-based skin rashes, and (in a subgroup of patients) neutropenia. *Neutropenia* ($<1000/mm^3$) may occur with captopril, extremely rarely in hypertensive patients with normal renal function (1/8600 according to the package insert), more commonly (1/500) with preexisting impaired renal function with a serum creatinine of 1.6 mg/dL or more, and as a grave risk (1/25) in patients with both collagen vascular disease and renal impairment. When captopril is discontinued, recovery from neutropenia is usual except when there is associated serious disease, such as severe renal or heart failure or collagen vascular disease. *Proteinuria* occurs in about 1% of patients receiving captopril, especially in the presence of preexisting renal disease or with high doses of captopril (>150 mg/day). There is a double mechanism for renal damage induced by captopril: first, an altered immune response, and second, excess hypotension. Paradoxically, captopril is used in the therapy of diabetic type 1 nephropathy with proteinuria. *Other side effects* include hypotension (frequent in the treatment of CHF), impaired taste (2% to 7%), skin rashes (4% to 10%) sometimes with eosinophilia, and rarely serious angioedema (1/100 to 1/1000). Hepatic damage is also very rare.

Pretreatment Precautions Bilateral renal artery stenosis and pregnancy must be excluded as far as possible. Patients with renal impairment caused by collagen disease, or patients receiving immunosuppressives or immune system modifiers such as steroids and hydralazine, should probably be excluded, as should patients with a history of hematological disease or pretreatment depression of neutrophils or platelets. Pretreatment hypotension excludes therapy.

Precautions During Treatment Regular monitoring of neutrophil counts is required in patients with preexisting serious renal impairment, especially on the basis of collagen vascular disease (pretreatment count, then two weekly counts for 3 months). The risk of renal damage from captopril is reduced by limiting total daily doses to 150 mg/day, as is now standard practice.

Enalapril

Enalapril (Vasotec in the United States; Innovace in the United Kingdom; Xanef, Renitec, or Pres elsewhere in Europe; Renivace in Japan) is the standard prodrug, and is also generically available. The major trials have been in heart failure where it saved lives over a 12-year period of follow-up,[84] and in hypertension where it was at least as good and in some ways better than a diuretic.[56] The chief differences from captopril are: (1) a longer half-life, (2) a slower onset of effect because of the requirement of hydrolysis in the liver of the prodrug to the active form, enalaprilat, so that the therapeutic effect depends on hepatic metabolism (class II pattern of pharmacokinetics, Table 5-4), and (3) the absence of the SH-group from the structure, thus theoretically lessening or removing the risk of immune-based side effects. Enalapril is approved for hypertension, heart failure, and to decrease the development of overt heart failure in symptomatic patients with LV dysfunction (ejection fraction equal to or less than 35%). In the latter group of patients, enalapril is also licensed in the United Kingdom to prevent coronary ischemic events.

Pharmacokinetics About 60% of the oral dose is absorbed with no influence of meals. Enalapril is deesterified in the liver and kidney to the active form, enalaprilat. Time to peak serum concentration is about 2 hours for enalapril, and about 5 hours for enalaprilat, with some delay in CHF. Excretion is 95% renal as enalapril or enalaprilat (hence the lower doses in renal failure). The elimination half-life of enalaprilat is about 4 to 5 hours in hypertension and 7 to 8 hours in CHF. Following multiple doses, the effective elimination half-life of enalaprilat is 11 hours (package insert). One oral 10-mg dose of enalapril yields sufficient enalaprilat to cause significant ACE inhibition for 19 hours. In hypertension and in CHF, the peak hypotensive response to enalapril occurs about 4 to 6 hours after the oral dose, and may account for the marked depression of renal function that may occur at that time.

Dose and Indications In *hypertension*, the dose is 2.5 to 20 mg as one or two daily doses. In some patients the effect wanes over 24 hours so that twice daily dosing may be better. Doses higher than 10 to 20 mg daily give little added benefit. A low initial dose (2.5 mg) is a wise precaution, especially when enalapril is added to a diuretic or the patient is salt-depleted, in the elderly, or when high-renin hypertension is suspected. In *asymptomatic LV dysfunction and in CHF*, in the SOLVD trials,[33,85] enalapril was started with an initial dose of 2.5 mg twice daily and worked up to 10 mg twice daily (mean daily dose 17 mg). In renal failure (glomerular filtration rate below 30 ml/minute), the dose of enalapril must be reduced. In severe liver disease, the dose may have to be increased (impaired conversion of enalapril to enalaprilat). In early phase AMI, within 24 hours of symptoms, an initial dose of only 1.25 mg at 2-hour intervals for three doses was followed by 5 mg three times daily with long-term benefits.

Contraindications, Precautions, and Side Effects Pregnancy is a clear contraindication (see Captopril). In hypertensive persons, bilateral renal artery stenosis or stenosis in a single kidney must be excluded. *Precautions:* to avoid the major risks of excess hypotension, use a low initial dose and evaluate pretreatment renal function and drug cotherapy including diuretic dose. It is presumed that enalapril, without the

SH-group found in captopril, does not produce the same immune-based toxic effects. Thus monitoring of the neutrophil count is not essential, although it is advisable according to the package insert. *Side effects:* Cough is most common, as for all ACE inhibitors. Enalapril may be safer when captopril has induced a skin rash. As for all ACE inhibitors, angioedema is a rare but serious risk[26] as highlighted in the package insert.

OTHER PRODRUGS (KINETIC CLASS II)

Perindopril (Coversyl in the United Kingdom, Aceon in the United States)

The recommended dosage of 4 to 8 mg once daily for hypertension is long-acting with a good peak-to-trough ratio. Experimentally it is well studied in relation to beneficial effects on the vascular structure in hypertension. A low dose diuretic combination is perindopril 2 mg plus indapamide 0.625 mg. In CHF, the effect of a first dose of 2 mg is well documented and appears to cause little or no hypotension, in contrast to low-dose enalapril or captopril.[44] This interesting property warrants further study. Perindopril was used in PROGRESS, a large trial aimed at prevention of repeat stroke. The combination of perindropil with indapamide reduced stroke. In EUROPA, a large prophylactic trial in those with stable coronary artery disease, perindopril 8 mg daily markedly reduced myocardial infarction.[20] Of note, the relative risk reduction of 20% (p = 0.0003) in the primary endpoint of cardiovascular death, myocardial infarction or cardiac arrest was achieved on top of existing prophylactic therapy, usually platelet inhibitors, lipid-lowering therapy, and beta-blockers. The prescribed dose of 8 mg was well tolerated. An important landmark trial, ASCOT-BPLA (Anglo-Scandinavian Cardiac Outcomes Trial-Blood Pressure Lowering Arm), compared the effects on major outcomes of antihypertensive therapy by amlodipine ± perindopril versus atenolol ± a thiazide.[87] Thus 'modern' therapy was pitted against the "old" or conventional therapy. This was the largest large trial thus far undertaken, on 19,257 high risk hypertensive patients. The trial had to be stopped prematurely because all-cause mortality (a secondary end-point) was reduced by 11%. However, the primary end-point, fatal coronary heart disease and non-fatal myocardial infarction, was not significantly reduced. The benefits among secondary and tertiary end-points included reductions in cardiovascular mortality (24%), stroke (23%), unstable angina (32%) and new diabetes (30%). 'Modern' therapy was also associated with a higher HDL- cholesterol, a lower body weight, lower creatinine, and better BP lowering by a mean of 2.7/1.9 mmHg.

Quinapril (Accupril in the United States; Accupro in the United Kingdom)

In *hypertension*, the dose recommended in the package insert is initially 10 mg/day given once or twice daily up to a maximum of 80 mg/day. Dosage should be adjusted by measuring both the peak response (2 to 6 hours after the dose) and the trough (before the next dose). When quinapril is combined with a diuretic, the initial dose may be reduced to 5 mg/day (package insert) In *congestive heart failure*, the initial dose of 5 mg twice daily is titrated upwards to the usual maintenance dose of 10 to 20 mg twice daily (package insert). Mortality data are not available. *Impaired endothelial function* in normotensive patients with coronary artery disease could be reversed by 6 months of therapy with quinapril, 40 mg once daily.[87]

Ramipril (Altace in the United States; Ramace, Tritace Elsewhere)

This very well studied agent is a long-acting antihypertensive in a dose of 2.5 to 20 mg in one or two daily doses. It is also licensed for post-MI heart failure (dose 12.5 to 5 mg twice daily) and for cardiovascular protection (see later). It is proposed as a relatively tissue-specific ACE inhibitor. In early postinfarct heart failure in the AIRE study,[61] ramipril 2.5 mg twice daily and then 5 mg twice daily, as tolerated, was used to show a major fall (27%) in mortality of patients with heart failure diagnosed clinically. The mortality benefit was maintained over a 5-year follow-up.[70] It is also the drug used in the REIN nephropathy study to show an excellent long-term benefit (see earlier section on Renal Failure). In the landmark prophylactic HOPE trial,[21] ramipril given to high-risk patients, starting with 2.5 mg daily and working up to 10 mg once daily at night, gave markedly positive results including reduction in all-cause mortality. As a result of this study, the specific cardioprotective license given to ramipril in the United States is to reduce the risk of myocardial infarction, stroke, and death from cardiovascular causes in those at high risk, defined as patients 55 years or older with a history of coronary artery disease, stroke, peripheral vascular disease, or diabetes that is accompanied by one other risk factor (hypertension, high total cholesterol or low HDL-cholesterol, cigarette smoking or microalbuminuria). The dose is 2.5 mg, 5.0 mg, and then 10 mg once daily (the latter for prophylaxis, given at night).

Trandolapril

Trandolapril has one of the longest durations of action. It has been studied in one positive postinfarct trial[62] (TRACE) and is under study in a large prophylactic trial in those with coronary artery disease (PEACE). *In hypertension*, the initial dose is 1 mg daily in non-black patients and 2 mg daily in black patients (packet insert). Most patients will require 2 to 4 mg once daily. If once daily dosing at 4 mg is inadequate, twice daily divided dosing may be tried, or the agent combined with a diuretic. *In postinfarct heart failure or LV dysfunction* (United States license) the package insert recommends an initial dose of 1 mg going up to 4 mg. *In the elderly* with normal renal function, dose adjustment is not needed. *In chronic renal failure*, despite the predominant biliary excretion, there is some accumulation of trandolaprilat. The initial dose should be reduced to 0.5 mg daily when the creatinine clearance falls below 30 ml/minute or in hepatic cirrhosis (USA package insert).

Some Others

Benazepril (*Lotensin* in the United States) has an optimal dose of 10 mg twice daily in hypertension. *Cilazapril* (*Vasace* in the United Kingdom) has kinetics similar to those of enalapril. The half-life of the active form appears to be 8 to 24 hours. *Zofenopril* contains a sulfhydryl group. It is especially able to inhibit cardiac ACE.[88] The dose in the SMILE study on severe AMI was 7.5 mg initially, then repeated after 12 hours, then doubled to a target of 30 mg twice daily.[64] Over 48 weeks of follow-up there was a 29% reduction in the risk of mortality.

LISINOPRIL: KINETIC CLASS III

This ACE inhibitor (*Zestril, Prinivil*) is approved for hypertension, CHF, and AMI in the United States, and in the United Kingdom also for diabetic nephropathy. It differs from all the others in its unusual pharmacokinetic properties (Table 5-4). It is not a prodrug, it is not metabolized by the liver, it is water-soluble, and it is excreted unchanged by the kidneys (reminiscent of the kinetic patterns of water-soluble β-blockers). Therefore, it can be given a class of its own, class III. The half-life is sufficiently long to give a duration of action exceeding 24 hours. Once daily dosing for *CHF* is licensed in the United States. The initial dose is 2.5 to 5 mg in heart failure, and the maintenance dose is 5 to 20 mg per day. In *hypertension*, the initial dose is 10 mg once daily and the usual dose range is 20 to 40 mg per day. In *renal impairment* and in the *elderly*, the dose should be reduced. *Regarding large trials*, lisinopril was the drug used in the GISSI-3 mega-study in acute phase AMI[65] and in the ATLAS study (Assessment of Treatment with Lisinopril and Survival). The latter study in CHF showed modest benefits for even higher doses of lisinopril (35 mg daily or more) than those usually used.[46] In the ALLHAT antihypertensive study, lisinopril was compared with a diuretic and a CCB and, unexpectedly, failed to reduce the development of heart failure when compared with the diuretic,[25] possibly because of the high percentage of black patients.

CHOICE OF ACE INHIBITOR

In general, we see little advantage for any one agent compared with others. But when a specific ACE inhibitor is very well tested in a major outcome trial, we are more sure of the dosage of that drug for that indication. All those tested work in hypertension and heart failure. However, some drugs are much better tested for specific situations than others. *Captopril*, the first agent available, is now much less used than before despite its wide range of approved indications, probably in part because it requires 2–3 daily doses. In postinfarct heart failure or LV dysfunction, it gave protection from death equal to that of the ARB valsartan,[83] and is much less expensive. Not being a prodrug, it has a rapid onset of action, thus creating the risk of hypotension especially in heart failure. Note that captopril in high doses may incur the risk of certain side effects specific to the SH-group, including ageusia and neutropenia. *Enalapril* is very well tested for all stages of heart failure in several landmark studies including the CONSENSUS study, V-HeFT II, and the SOLVD studies (prevention and treatment arms) including the remarkable 12-year follow-up.[84] It is the drug with the best data on reduction of mortality in CHF. Yet (and this point is often forgotten) it is not clearly a once-a-day drug and was used twice daily (total dose 20 mg) in all these studies. *Ramipril* is especially well tested in (1) early postinfarct clinical heart failure, where it reduced mortality substantially; (2) renoprotection; and in (3) cardiovascular prophylaxis, where in the HOPE trial it gave such striking results at a dose of 10 mg daily. *Perindopril* was the agent used in another landmark prophylactic study, EUROPA, on stable coronary artery disease, at a dose of 8 mg, higher than usual. *Lisinopril* has simple pharmacokinetics, being water-soluble, with no liver transformation and renal excretion, making it an easy drug to use and understand. Thus there is no risk of hepatic pharmacokinetic interactions, and it has been studied in several major postinfarct and heart failure trials.

ANGIOTENSIN II RECEPTOR BLOCKERS (ARBs)

Because ACE inhibitors exert most of their major effects by inhibiting the formation of angiotensin-II, it follows that direct antagonism of the receptors for angiotensin-II should duplicate many or most of the effects of ACE inhibition. They should largely avoid the bradykinin-related side effects of ACE inhibitors such as cough and angioedema so that they are virtually free of subjective side effects. Hence these new ARBs, of which the prototype is losartan, are being used more and more, both in hypertension and in heart failure (Tables 5-8 and 5-9).

Use in Hypertension

ARBs have the capacity to reduce blood pressure with "an astonishing lack" of side effects,[89] and, in particular, the absence or much lower incidence of cough. In recent trials with hard end-points such as end-stage renal failure in diabetic nephropathy and stroke in left ventricular hypertrophy, they have been better than comparators,[90,91] with greater reduction of stroke and heart failure (Table 5-8). They are already regarded as possible first-line therapy by the European Guidelines, but not by the American JNC VII committee which nonetheless recognizes the following compelling indications for ARBs: heart failure, diabetes, and chronic kidney disease (see Chapter 7). All of these are also recognized as compelling indications for ACE inhibitors, so that patient tolerability and price (higher for the ARBs than generic ACE inhibitors) are likely to be the deciding factors. Note that the established contraindications to ACE inhibitor therapy such as pregnancy and bilateral renal artery stenosis are the same for the ARBs. The vast VALUE trial on 15,245 high risk patients compared the ARB valsartan with CCB amlodipine and found no difference in the composite primary endpoint (time to first cardiac endpoint) nor in total mortality.[91a] The hypothesis had been that the ARB would reduce cardiac events beyond BP reduction.

Use in Diabetic Nephropathy

In the European guidelines, ARBs have better supporting documentation for type 2 diabetes, a point of view supported by at least one of the present authors.[92] On the other hand, in type I diabetes, the ACE inhibitors have better evidence.[93] In neither situation are there direct comparisons between ARBs and ACE inhibitors.

Less New Diabetes

In hypertension, losartan was associated with less new diabetes than atenolol,[94] candesartan with less than hydrochlorothiazide,[95] and valsartan less than amlodipine.[91a] In heart failure, there was less new diabetes with candesartan than with placebo.[96]

Use in Heart Failure

Both ACE inhibitors and ARBs inhibit the RAAS and are now well tested in heart failure (Table 5-9). Major arguments for using ARBs are: (1) The adverse effects of major renin-angiotensin activation in heart failure are mediated by the stimulation by angiotensin-II of the receptor subtype, AT-1, which the ARBs specifically block (Fig. 5-11). This is potentially a more efficient and sure mechanism than inhibition of ACE in reducing the effects of angiotensin-II, especially bearing in mind the potential synthesis of angiotensin-II by non-ACE dependent paths catalyzed by chymase. For example, the malignant properties of angiotensin-II in causing apoptosis in cardiomyocytes are mediated solely by the AT-1 receptor.[97] (2) The AT-2 receptor is not blocked and can still respond to the increased concentrations of angiotensin-II as result of the AT-1 receptor block. Unopposed AT-2 receptor activity unexpectedly and through an unknown mechanism leads to formation of protective bradykinin and vasodilation.[98,99] Dzau and others regard AT-2 stimulation by angiotensin-II as potentially cardioprotective. (3) Non-ACE paths may be of substantial importance in the generation of angiotensin-II,[5] also in vascular tissues.[100] (4) Angiotensin-II may play a direct pathogenic role in vascular disease. The vascular AT-1 receptors can be upregulated by insulin[101] or by low-density lipoprotein (LDL),[102] thereby increasing the sensitivity to circulating or locally generated angiotensin-II.

Hence in severe heart failure when there is strong activation of the RAAS, as complete a block of cardiac and vascular AT-1 receptors as possible should be of special benefit. These proposed benefits are bought almost without the cost of any side effects and, in particular a consistently lower incidence of cough. Thus ARBs are even better tolerated than ACE inhibitors and of all drug classes, patients are most likely to stay on the ARBs, at least in hypertension.[57] Yet despite these cogent arguments, "in large-scale randomized clinical trials, ARBs have

ACE, A-II EFFECTS and ARBs

Opie 2004

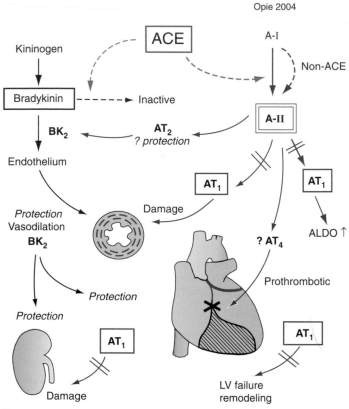

Figure 5-11 Mechanisms whereby angiotensin-II (*A-II*) exerts adverse effects on cardiovascular system. Most of the damaging effects are via the AT-1 receptor, with possible protection via the unopposed AT-2 receptor (see Fig. 5-3) that may unexpectedly lead to relatively small amounts of bradykinin formation. The putative AT-4 receptor may mediate prothrombotic effects. Bradykinin (*BK*), formed especially during inhibition of ACE (angiotensin-converting enzyme), mediates protection by activation of the BK-2 receptor.

failed to live up to the high expectations that they would prove superior to ACE inhibitors in the context of chronic heart failure."[8] One possible reason is that the role of the AT-2 receptor is still not fully understood[7] and that unopposed AT-2 receptor stimulation may not be as desirable as previously thought.[8] Another possibility is that although protective bradykinin might still be formed by AT-2 activity during ARB therapy, the amounts formed may not be clinically relevant as shown by the much lower incidence of cough and angioedema.

The overall data from two major trials, Val-HeFT[103] and VALIANT,[83] show that ARBs give outcome results as good as those of ACE inhibitors (Table 5-9). However, only one of these trials, VALIANT, was designed to show non-inferiority (for mortality, $P = 0.004$). Therefore ARBs become a reasonable alternative for use in heart failure, not only in ACE inhibitor intolerant patients where the case for their use is very strong.[23] Although ACE inhibitors remain the logical first-line therapy[2] because of the vast experience with these agents in heart failure, including postinfarction LV dysfunction, this prime position is gradually being eroded by the better tolerated ARBs.

Combination of ARBs with ACE Inhibitors

In heart failure, an ARB added to an ACE inhibitor achieves better neurohumoral and hemodynamic control, including reduction of circulating aldosterone levels.[18] If there are progressive symptoms despite high dose of an ACE inhibitor, then losartan 50 mg improves exercise capacity.[104] Regarding data from large trials, in the CHARM-added study[96] and in Val-HeFT[103] the ARB-ACE-inhibitor combination was beneficial, while in VALIANT it was not.[83] The difference may lie in intensity of the heart failure, the majority in CHARM and Val-HeFT having ejection fractions much lower than in VALIANT. The more severe the heart failure, the more the activation of RAAS, so that added inhibition by the ARB-ACE inhibitor combination may give greater benefit. Note, however, that it remains controversial whether this combination should be used in the presence of prior β-blockade.[40,96,103] *In nondiabetic renal disease,* combination of losartan (100 mg) and trandolapril (3 mg) strikingly decreased proteinuria and lessened the risk of reaching the primary end-point which was doubling the serum creatinine or reaching end-stage renal disease.[105]

SPECIFIC ANGIOTENSIN RECEPTOR BLOCKERS (ARBs)

Losartan (Cozaar)

This is the prototype ARB, historically the first, with numerous clinical studies to support its efficacy in blood pressure reduction, and now in diabetic nephropathy, left ventricular hypertrophy, and possibly in heart failure (Table 5-10). For hypertension, the standard start-up dose is 50 mg once daily, with an increase to 100 mg if needed. The package insert allows for twice daily dosing, the half-life being 6 to 9 hours. As with all the ARBs, a dose increase is usually less effective than the addition of a low-dose diuretic in achieving greater blood pressure control.[106] When there is volume depletion or liver disease (risk of decreased plasma clearance), the starting dose should be only 25 mg. The combination with hydrochlorothiazide is Hyzaar (losartan 50, thiazide 12.5 mg; or losartan 100, thiazide 25 mg). As for all the ARBs, the major antihypertensive effect is present within 1 week. The full effect may take up to 3 to 6 weeks, and is potentiated by diuretic action or low salt diet more than by dose increase. Losartan 50 mg daily has been thoroughly compared with captopril in heart failure (ELITE I and II studies),[107] and in high-risk postinfarct patients, the majority with heart failure.[108] In none of these studies was losartan superior to captopril, and in some aspects inferior, possibly owing to underdosing,[2] thus allowing the investigator's claim that losartan in that dose can be used only in case of ACE inhibitor intolerance. Higher doses are now under study. In diabetic nephropathy, in the RENAAL study, losartan in a higher dose (50 to 100 mg daily) reduced end-stage renal disease and proteinuria.[109] In hypertensives with LV hypertrophy, losartan (mean dose 82 mg daily) protected from stroke when compared with equivalent blood pressure reduction by atenolol, both agents mostly with a diuretic.[91] In addition, mortality was reduced in diabetic persons[110] and in the elderly with isolated systolic hypertension.[111] In the United States losartan is registered for hypertension, including the subgroup with LV hypertrophy, in the latter only for stroke reduction, and for diabetic nephropathy with a history of hypertension.

Candesartan (Atacand)

Pharmacologically, it differs from the others in that active candesartan is formed during the process of GI absorption, with a somewhat longer half-life than losartan (Table 5-10). In hypertension, the usual starting dose is 16 mg once daily (lower in volume depletion), with a top dose of 32 mg daily, given in one or two doses according to the package insert. However, when given once daily (dose 16 mg) there is still at 48 hours about two thirds of the effect seen at 24 hours.[112] Note that full hypotensive effect may take several weeks. This drug was chosen in

Table 5-10 Specific Angiotensin Receptor Blockers (ARBs). Key Pharmacologic and Clinical Properties

Compound and Indications	Major Trials	Pharmacokinetics	Doses (FDA-Approved)	Side Effects and Contraindications
Losartan potassium (Cozaar) Hypertension	ELITE II and OPTIMAAL in HF; LIFE (LVH, end-points vs. atenolol); RENAAL (diabetic nephropathy)	Converted in liver to active metabolite with $t^{1}/_{2}$ 6–9 h; dominant fecal excretion; minimal food effect	25–100 mg total in one or two doses; usual start with 50 mg, half if volume depletion or liver disease	S/E in hypertension = placebo; C/I = pregnancy, bilateral renal artery stenosis; Care: liver disease
Candesartan cilexetil (Atacand) Hypertension	CHARM (three studies in HF: ACEi-intolerant; diastolic dysfunction; *vs.* ACEi);	Converted to active candesartan by ester hydrolysis during GI absorption, then excreted unchanged in bile and feces; $t^{1}/_{2}$ 9 h; no food effect	8–32 mg total in one or two doses; usual start with 16 mg; less if volume depletion	As above
Irbesartan (Avapro) Hypertension Diabetic type 2 nephropathy	Diabetic nephropathy, diabetic microalbuminuria (type 2 for both)	No metabolite. Rapid oral absorption, high bioavailability; $t^{1}/_{2}$ 11–15 h; 80% excreted unchanged in bile and feces. High tissue distribution.	150 mg once daily; half if volume depletion; up to 300 mg daily; no changes for moderate hepatic or severe renal disease	As above
Valsartan (Diovan) Hypertension; HF; ACEi-intolerant	ValHeFT, HF; VALIANT (post-MI, LVF): VALUE (high risk hypertensives vs. amlodipine)	Rapid absorption. Food effect (AUC↓40%, C_{max}↓50%). No metabolite, $t^{1}/_{2}$ 6 h, 83% biliary and fecal excretion. Low tissue distribution.	80 mg up to max 320 mg once daily; less in severe hepatic or renal failure (*caution*: volume depletion)	As above but in VALUE similar withdrawal rate to amlodipine Care: severe renal disease
Telmisartan (Micardis) Hypertension	ON TARGET (HOPE-like trial vs. ramipril)	No active metabolite, $t^{1}/_{2}$ 24 h, food effect (6–20%), almost all excreted unchanged (bile, feces). Nonlinear kinetics, ↑ AUC and C_{max} with higher dose	40–80 mg daily, can't go below 40 mg for volume depletion or liver failure	As above

ACEi = angiotensin-converting enzyme inhibitors; HF = heart failure; LVH = left ventricular hypertrophy.

three large heart failure trials, the CHARM studies, at a target dose of 32 mg. In the CHARM-alternative trial, in patients with ACE intolerance, candesartan significantly reduced the combined end-point of cardiovascular death or hospitalization for CHF by 23%, with much less cough and angioedema.[23] In CHARM-added,[40] candesartan added to prior ACE-inhibitor therapy reduced cardiovascular death at the cost of an increase in creatinine (3.7% above placebo) and hyperkalemia (2.7% above placebo). Of note, the effects of candesartan were more marked in those receiving both an ACE inhibitor and a β-blocker. Thus the triple neurohumoral inhibitor therapy (ARB plus ACE inhibitor plus β-blocker) was successful. In the United States it is registered for hypertension, with the CHARM results in heart failure under review.

Irbesartan (Avapro)

This drug has no active metabolite, a terminal half-life of 11 to 15 hours, and for hypertension there is a single daily dose of 150 to 300 mg (Table 5-10). There are the usual caveats: lower dose for volume depletion, initial rapid hypotensive effect, then a full effect in weeks, and a better response to added diuretic than to an increased dose. The diuretic combination, Avalide, contains irbesartan 150 or 300 mg combined with 12.5 mg of hydrochlorothiazide. In an important study on type 2 diabetic nephropathy, irbesartan reduced the rate of progression of microalbuminuria to overt proteinuria.[113] In established diabetic nephropathy, it lessened the primary renal end-point which included the rate of rise of serum creatinine and end-stage renal disease.[114] These benefits were found both in comparison to placebo and to amlodipine therapy, and were not explained by blood pressure changes. Irbesartan is licensed in the United States for hypertension and for nephropathy in type 2 diabetic patients.

Valsartan (Diovan)

This drug also has no active metabolite (Table 5-10). Despite the food effect of up to 50%, the package insert indicates that the drug may be given with or without food. The $t\frac{1}{2}$ is shorter than that of irbesartan, yet the dose is also only once daily (80 to 320 mg). Like the others, added diuretic is more effective than a dose increase. Diovan HCT has a fixed dose of 12.5 mg hydrochlorothiazide with valsartan 80 or 160 mg. There are the usual caveats about volume depletion and the length of time for a full response. Two heart failure trials have been completed, Val-HeFT[103] and VALIANT.[83] In the former, there was a better prognosis (versus placebo) when valsartan was combined with prior ACE inhibitor therapy. However, in contrast to CHARM-added, the triple combination of ARB, ACE inhibitor, and β-blocker was detrimental. However, this was a post-hoc analysis, whereas CHARM was prospective and a larger series. In the United States Val-Heft is recognized as the basis of a license, besides the standard one for hypertension, for use in ACE-intolerant patients with heart failure, with the caveat that there is no evidence that valsartan confers benefits if used with an adequate dose of the ACE inhibitor. Also, note it is not approved as an add-on to ACE inhibition. VALUE is the largest ARB trial on 15,425 high risk hypertensives,[91a,115] in which valsartan challenged the CCB, amlodipine, but with almost identical outcomes except for less new diabetes with valsartan (Table 5-10).

Telmisartan (Micardis)

With no active metabolite, and a very long half-life of 24 hours, this drug is attractive at 40 to 80 mg once daily (Table 5-10). However, the formulation is such that the dose cannot be reduced below 40 mg even when there is hypovolemia. There is a small increase in hypotensive effect going from 40 to 80 mg daily, with the expected response to added thiazide (Micardis HCT tablets 40/12.5 mg, 80/12.5 mg). Other caveats are much the same as for all the ARBs. The USA license is for hypertension, with the proviso that the fixed dose combination is not indicated for initial therapy. This is the ARB used in the ongoing ON TARGET trial which is comparing the preventative effects of ramipril with those of an ARB with a giant HOPE-like design.

Other ARBs

Eprosartan (Teveten) is registered for hypertension, the usual dose being 600 mg once daily, but varying from 400 to 800 mg and given once or twice daily. *Olmesartan (Benicar)* is likewise licensed for hypertension, with a half-life of 13 hours, and the dose being 20 to 40 mg once daily. These newer agents in general have little support from large trial data but may offer a price advantage.[116]

Caveats for Use of ARBs in Hypertension

There are a number of caveats common to ACE inhibitors and ARBs: reduce the dose in volume depletion, watch out for renal complications, check for hyperkalemia, and don't use in pregnancy or bilateral renal artery stenosis. In general, care is required in liver or renal disease (most ARBs are either metabolized by the liver or directly excreted by the bile or the kidneys). A good antihypertensive effect can be expected in 1 week with a full effect over 3 to 6 weeks, and if needed a diuretic is added rather than increasing the ARB dose. As in the case of ACE inhibitors, and in the absence of diuretic cotherapy, there is relative resistance to the antihypertensive effects of ARBs in black patients.[117]

ARBs: The Future

In view of the large number of careful trials now completed with various ARBs (Table 5-10), the true place of these more specific inhibitors of the RAAS has emerged as follows. In hypertension, there is no question of the excellent tolerability of the ARBs, which makes them an especially attractive early option for hypertension therapy. ARBs have outcome benefit versus several other different modes of blood pressure reduction in specialized situations such as diabetic type 2 nephropathy or LV hypertrophy. However, there have been no direct comparisons with ACE inhibitors on outcome in hypertension, nor are any planned. In general they are more expensive than ACE inhibitors. In heart failure, they are excellent in ACE-intolerant patients, yet also increasingly used instead of ACE inhibitors on the grounds of better tolerance and extrapolation of the benefit of candersartan in ACE-intolerant patients to the overall population of those with heart failure. Furthermore, there is a case for combining an ARB with an ACE inhibitor in severe heart failure (see CHARM-Added study).[40] In high-risk postinfarct patients, valsartan met the criteria for noninferiority versus captopril.[83] Whether the ARBs will be as good as or better than the ACE inhibitors in improving outcome in high-risk patients, as in HOPE or in coronary patients as in EUROPA, is a tough challenge. This hypothesis is under study in the ON TARGET trial.

ALDOSTERONE, SPIRONOLACTONE, AND EPLERENONE

The RALES and EPHESUS studies have focused on the fact that aldosterone is the final link in the overactive renin-angiotensin-aldosterone system that underlies the lethality of heart failure.[24,39] Aldosterone production increases in response to increased stimulation by angiotensin-II, and hepatic clearance decreases.[9] Initially increased aldosterone values fall with ACE inhibitor therapy, but later may "escape" during prolonged therapy. Because there is a correlation between aldosterone

ALDOSTERONE IN CHF

Opie 2004

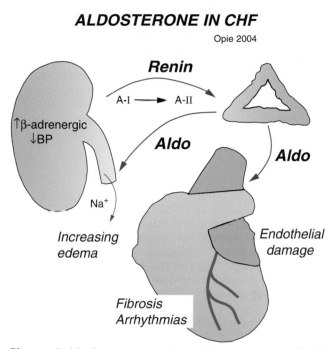

Figure 5-12 The renin-angiotensin-aldosterone system (*RAAS*), showing the adverse effects of excess aldosterone as an end-effector of this system. Angiotensin-II (*A-II*) again exerts harm via AT-1 induced release of aldosterone and also increased local synthesis in the heart. Cardiac fibrosis and arrhythmias are based on experimental data, not yet established in humans. (*Figure © LH Opie, 2005.*)

production and mortality in heart failure, the addition of the aldosterone antagonists spironolactone or eplerenone is logical (Table 5-5).

Mechanism of Benefit: Diuresis or Tissue Effects?

Aldosterone, by sodium and water retention will tend to worsen edema (Fig. 5-12). Nonetheless, the benefit of spironolactone in the RALES trial was due not only to a diuretic effect. Rather, there are several other beneficial mechanisms. Thus locally produced aldosterone may be linked to myocardial fibrosis by autocrine/paracrine effects.[9] In addition, aldosterone also has adverse vascular effects including inhibition of release of nitric oxide, and possibly an increased response to vasoconstrictor doses of angiotensin-I in human heart failure.[10] Myocardial fibrosis associated with experimental myocardial infarction is lessened both by spironolactone and by the AT$_1$ blocker, losartan, showing that locally produced aldosterone is fibrogenic.[118] This sequence may also occur in patients.[119] In addition, spironolactone decreases the release of cardiac norepinephrine, which should reduce ventricular arrhythmias and sudden death. The small rise of plasma potassium may also be antiarrhythmic. Furthermore, spironolactone also has vasodilator properties.[10]

All these effects together may explain the therapeutic benefit of even the low dose of spironolactone used in the treatment of severe heart failure in RALES and why sudden cardiac death was less. It should be stressed that the patients selected did not have renal impairment, a risk factor for serious hyperkalemia. Serum potassium was carefully monitored, and there was provision for reduction of the dose of the ACE inhibitor or the aldosterone blocker in case of hyperkalemia. These precautions are *essential*.

Eplerenone (Inspra)

Because antiandrogenic (gynecomastia, impotence) and antiprogesta-
tional (oligomenorrhea) side effects are found with spironolactone,
the derivative compound eplerenone with fewer of these side effects
is better tolerated. *In postinfarct heart failure*, in EPHESUS,[39] eplerenone
was added to optimal medical treatment including usually an ACE
inhibitor, a diuretic, and a β-blocker. Morbidity and mortality were
reduced. The USA license is for (1) hypertension and (2) to improve
survival of stable patients with left ventricular (LV) systolic dysfunction (ejection fraction ≤ 40%) and clinical evidence of congestive
heart failure after an acute myocardial infarction. The *major danger is
hyperkalemia*, so that in heart failure the dose is based on the serum
potassium level. The starting dose of 25 mg daily is increased to 50 mg
if the potassium is below 5.0 mEq/L, aiming for 5.0 to 5.4 mEq/L. If
the serum potassium is higher at 5.5 to 5.9 mEq/L, the dose must be
decreased, and the dose withheld if the potassium exceeds 6 mEq/L
(package insert). The dose for hypertension is 50 to 100 mg once daily,
and it is equally effective in Caucasian and black patients.[120] As
expected, LV hypertrophy was reduced and better achieved by combination with an ACE inhibitor (enalapril) in the 4E-study.[121] LV hypertrophy is also regressed and diastolic dysfunction improved by the
related compound, canrenone (available in Europe).[122] In hypertension as in heart failure, the major risk is hyperkalemia. Thus there is
a specific warning in the package insert against the use of eplerenone
in type 2 diabetes with hypertension and microalbuminuria, because
of the risk of hyperkalemia.

SUMMARY

1. *Inhibition of the renin-angiotensin-aldosterone system* is established
   for the treatment and now possible prevention of a wide range
   of cardiovascular diseases. The basic concept hinges on the
   adverse effects of excess angiotensin-II and aldosterone. ACE
   inhibitors have a twofold action, to decrease the formation of
   angiotensin-II and to increase the formation of protective
   bradykinin. Angiotensin-receptor blockers (ARBs) directly block
   the angiotensin-II subtype one receptor, thereby largely avoiding the side effects of excess bradykinin such as cough and
   angioedema. Aldosterone blockers oppose the cellular effects of
   aldosterone including sodium retention and myocardial fibrosis.

2. *In congestive heart failure* (CHF), thousands of patients have been
   studied in many large trials that have focused attention on the
   important therapeutic and potential prophylactic role of the ACE
   inhibitors. These trials have shown that reduction of "hard" end-
   points, such as mortality, hospitalization, and prevention of
   disease progression, can be achieved in certain patient populations. In a minority of patients, ACE inhibitors fail to benefit.
   Careful use is needed to avoid potentially harmful hypotension.
   The benefits of ACE inhibitors can best be explained by inhibition of the activated renin-angiotensin-aldosterone system. The
   strong argument is to start therapy with ACE inhibition as early
   as possible in the course of heart failure, even when only mild to
   moderate, and whether symptomatic or asymptomatic. ACE
   inhibitors are increasingly used with other life-conserving (death
   delaying) drugs such as β-blockers and now spironolactone or
   eplerenone.

3. *In hypertension*, ACE inhibitors are effective as monotherapy in
   blood pressure reduction in most patient groups except blacks.
   There are few side effects and contraindications. A particularly
   attractive combination is that with diuretics, because diuretics
   increase circulating renin activity and angiotensin-II levels, which

ACE inhibitors counterregulate by inhibiting the conversion of angiotensin-I to angiotensin-II. Adding a low-dose diuretic to a standard dose of ACE inhibitor seems more effective than increasing the ACE inhibitor dose and also sensitizes black patients to the antihypertensive effects.

4. In *early phase acute myocardial infarction*, ACE inhibitors achieve a modest but statistically significant reduction in mortality (6% to 11%). Best results are obtained in high-risk patients such as those with a large anterior infarct or with diabetes. *In postinfarct heart failure*, ACE inhibitors give a striking reduction of 26% in mortality.[83]

5. In *asymptomatic left ventricular (LV) dysfunction*, whether postinfarct or otherwise, ACE inhibitors can prevent the development of overt CHF, as shown by two large trials, SAVE and SOLVD. The latter now has a 12-year follow-up.

6. In *diabetic nephropathy, type 1*, ACE inhibition added to other antihypertensives has achieved reduction of hard end-points, such as death, dialysis, and renal transplantation. Indirect evidence suggests similar protection in type 2 nephropathy, but direct evidence for a blood pressure-independent protection is still missing.

7. *In nondiabetic nephropathy*, renoprotection occurred independently of any blood pressure reduction with ramipril in the REIN and AASK studies.

8. *Cardiovascular prophylaxis in high- and moderate-risk patients.* A large-scale preventative trial on patients at high risk of cardiovascular events, the HOPE study with ramipril found definitive benefits on hard end-points such as myocardial infarction, stroke, and all-cause mortality. In the EUROPA study with perindopril, the entry point was existing but stable coronary artery disease. Even in the presence of frequent cotherapy with statins and β-blockers, perindopril reduced myocardial infarction and the combined primary end-point. The third study, PEACE, with trandolapril, is still awaited.

9. *Angiotensin Receptor Blockers* (ARBs) act at a different site from ACE inhibitors to block the effects of angiotensin-II, namely the AT-1 receptor. Substantial experimental evidence shows that angiotensin-II promotes vascular and myocardial hypertrophy. Theoretically AT-1 receptor blockade gives all the benefits of ACE inhibition, except for formation of protective bradykinin. Hence ARBs are virtually without bradykinin-related adverse side effects such as cough and angioedema, the latter rare but potentially fatal. Although ACE inhibitors remain the gold standard in heart failure and hypertension, the ARBs are increasingly seen as having similar efficacy with fewer side effects. Therefore ARBs are increasingly used not only for ACE-intolerant patients, but also when avoidance of symptomatic side effects is crucial and when these drugs can be afforded. They have the same contraindications as the ACE inhibitors, and there is also relative resistance to their blood pressure lowering effects in blacks.

10. *ARBs and heart failure.* ARBs have been tested in an era when ACE inhibitors were already the established therapy of choice for heart failure. Had the ARBs come earlier, they would probably have been first choice. At present, the only licensed indication for an ARB in heart failure is valsartan for intolerance to ACE inhibition. Yet, taking together the results of several large trials such as Val-HeFT, CHARM, and VALIANT, the ARBs in the specific doses used are not inferior to ACE inhibitors, whether the basic problem is heart failure or postinfarct protection. In practice, there is increasing use of ARBs in heart failure, and not only in ACE inhibitor–intolerant patients.

11. *ARBs and post-MI heart failure.* Valsartan was equivalent to captopril in reducing death and adverse cardiovascular outcomes as captopril, with decreased cough, rash, and taste disturbances (VALIANT trial). The downside was increased hypotension and renal problems.

12. *Combination therapy with an ACE inhibitor and ARB.* Adding the ARB to the ACE-inhibitor gave better results in more severe heart failure with the mean ejection fraction about 25% (Val-HeFT and CHARM trials), but not in postinfarct LV dysfunction when the ejection fraction was less depressed (VALIANT, mean ejection fraction 35%). In nondiabetic renal disease, the combination gave better protection from advancing renal disease, together with a striking reduction in proteinuria reduction.

13. *ARBs, hypertension, and diabetes.* ARBs have been well studied in those with LV hypertrophy and type 2 diabetic nephropathy, with benefits that are largely blood pressure–independent. ARBs were usually combined with a diuretic. When compared with control antihypertensive regimens, ARBs were better at reducing stroke and heart failure, but not coronary heart disease.[90] In VALUE, a very large trial comparing valsartan with the CCB amlodipine in high-risk hypertensives, outcomes were very similar except for less new diabetes with valsartan.

14. *ARBs and reduction of cardiovascular risk.* Cardiovascular protection achieved by ramipril in the HOPE trial and perindopril in EUROPA needs to be repeated with an ARB. A large prevention trial, ON TARGET, will remedy this defect by comparing telmisartan with ramipril.

15. *Less new diabetes.* An important finding in HOPE, and now confirmed in trials with ARBs, is the decreased development of new diabetes. Thus RAAS inhibition may alter the diabetic process itself, perhaps by lessening insulin resistance.

16. *Cautions in black patients.* Monotherapy for hypertension often requires either the addition of a diuretic or a higher dose of the ACE inhibitor or ARBs. Angioedema with ACE inhibitors occurs more commonly in black patients. In heart failure, diuretic cotherapy may explain why ACE inhibitors seem to be as effective in black patients as in others.

17. *Contraindications* to ACE inhibitors and to the ARBs are few. Bilateral renal artery stenosis and pregnancy (a boxed warning for both groups of agents) preclude use. Hypotension and a substantially increased serum creatinine require thorough evaluation before use and careful monitoring after starting the drug. Hyperkalemia is also a risk with both ACE inhibitors and the ARBs.

18. *Aldosterone and spironolactone.* Aldosterone, the final effector of the renin-angiotensin-aldosterone system (RAAS), is increased in heart failure. Its adverse effects include sodium retention, hypokalemia, endothelial dysfunction, and (experimental) myocardial fibrosis. In the definitive RALES heart failure trial on NYHA classes III and IV, the addition of low doses of the aldosterone antagonist, spironolactone, decreased mortality when added to conventional therapy including an ACE inhibitor. In the EPHESUS trial, eplerenone with similar properties to spironolactone but with fewer antiandrogenic side effects reduced the risk of death when added to prior therapy for postinfarct LV dysfunction. Thus eplerenone improved the outcome beyond that of prior proven therapy for heart failure, which was usually with an ACE inhibitor or ARB, β-blocker, and diuretic. Hyperkalemia must be avoided.

REFERENCES

1. White HD. Should all patients with coronary disease receive angiotensin-converting-enzyme inhibitors? *Lancet* 2003;362:755–757.
2. Mann DL, et al. Angiotensin-receptor blockade in acute myocardial infarction—a matter of dose. *N Engl J Med* 2003;349:1963–1965.
3. Francis GS. ACE inhibition in cardiovascular disease. *N Engl J Med* 2000;342: 201–202.
4. White WB, et al. Effects of the selective aldosterone blocker eplerenone versus the calcium antagonist amlodipine in systolic hypertension. *Hypertension* 2003;41: 1021–1026.
5. Matsumoto T, et al. Chymase inhibition prevents cardiac fibrosis and improves diastolic dysfunction in the progression of heart failure. *Circulation* 2003;107:2555–2558.
6. Webster KA, et al. Apoptosis inhibitors for heart disease. *Circulation* 2003;108: 2954–2956.
7. Opie LH, et al. Enhanced angiotensin-II activity in heart failure: reevaluation of the counterregulatory hypothesis of receptor subtypes. *Circ Res* 2001;88:654–658.
8. Levy BI. Can angiotensin-II type 2 receptors have deleterious effects in cardiovascular disease? Implications for therapeutic blockade of the renin-angiotensin system. *Circulation* 2004;109:8–13.
9. Weber KT. Aldosterone and spironolactone in heart failure. *N Engl J Med* 1999;341:783–755.
10. Farquharson CAJ, et al. Spironolactone increases nitric oxide bioactivity, improves endothelial vasodilator dysfunction, and suppresses vascular angiotensin I/angiotensin-II conversion in patients with chronic heart failure. *Circulation* 2000;101:594–597.
11. Domanski MJ, et al. Effect of angiotensin converting enzyme inhibition on sudden cardiac death in patients following acute myocardial infarction. A meta-analysis of randomized clinical trials. *J Am Coll Cardiol* 1999;33:598–604.
12. Tonduangu D, et al. Chronic infusion of bradykinin delays the progression of heart failure and preserves vascular endothelium-mediated vasodilation in conscious dogs. *Circulation* 2003;109:114–119.
13. Emanueli C, et al. Dilated and failing cardiomyopathy in bradykinin B(2) receptor knockout mice. *Circulation* 1999;100:2359–2365.
14. Morris SD, et al. Angiotensin-converting enzyme inhibitors potentiate preconditioning through bradykinin B_2 receptor activation in human heart. *J Am Coll Cardiol* 1997;29:1599–1606.
15. Witherow FN, et al. Bradykinin contributes to the vasodilator effects of chronic angiotensin-converting enzyme inhibition in patients with heart failure. *Circulation* 2001;104:2177–2181.
16. Danser AHJ, et al. Angiotensin-converting enzyme in the human heart. Effect of the deletion/insertion polymorphism. *Circulation* 1995;92:1387–1388.
17. Myerson SG, et al. Left ventricular hypertrophy with exercise and ACE gene insertion/deletion polymorphism. *Circulation* 2001;103:226–230.
18. RESOLVD Study. Comparison of candesartan, enalapril, and their combination in congestive heart failure. Randomized Evaluation of Strategies for Left Ventricular Dysfunction (RESOLVD) Pilot Study. *Circulation* 1999;100:1056–1064.
19. HOPE Study Investigators. Effects of ramipril on cardiovascular and microvascular outcomes in people with diabetes mellitus. Results of the HOPE study and the MICRO-HOPE substudy. *Lancet* 2000;355:253–259.
20. Fox KN. European Trial On Reduction of Cardiac Events with Perindopril in Stable Coronary Artery Disease Investigators: efficacy of perindopril in reduction of cardiovascular events among patients with stable coronary artery disease: Randomized, double-blind, placebo-controlled, multicentre trial (the EUROPA Study). *Lancet* 2003;362:782–788.
21. HOPE Investigators. Effects of an angiotensin-converting enzyme inhibitor, ramipril, on cardiovascular events in high-risk patients. *N Engl J Med* 2000;342:145–153.
22. McEwan JR, et al. The effect of sulindac on the abnormal cough reflex associated with dry cough. *J Pharmacol Exp Ther* 1990;255:161–164.
23. Granger CB, et al. Effects of candesartan in patients with chronic heart failure and reduced left-ventricular systolic function intolerant to angiotensin-converting-enzyme inhibitors: the CHARM-Alternative trial. *Lancet* 2003;362:772–776.
24. RALES Study. For the Randomized Aldactone Evaluation Study Investigators. The effect of spironolactone on morbidity and mortality in patients with severe heart failure. *N Engl J Med* 1999;341:709–717.
25. ALLHAT Collaborative Research Group. Major outcomes in high-risk hypertensive patients randomized to angiotensin-converting enzyme inhibitor or calcium channel blocker vs diuretic. The Antihypertensive and Lipid-Lowering Treatment to Prevent Heart Attack Trial (ALLHAT). *JAMA* 2002;288:2981–2997.
26. Kostis JB, et al. Omapatrilat and enalapril in patients with hypertension: the Omapatrilat Cardiovascular Treatment vs. Enalapril (OCTAVE) trial. *Am J Hypertens* 2004;17:103–111.
27. Messerli FH, et al. Vasopeptidase inhibition and angio-oedema. *Lancet* 2000;356:608–609.
28. Nussberger J, et al. Bradykinin-mediated angioedema. *N Engl J Med* 2002;347:621–622.
29. Slater EE, et al. Clinical profile of angioedema associated with angiotensin converting-enzyme inhibition. *JAMA* 1988;260:967–970.
30. Ruggenenti P, et al. Renoprotective properties of ACE-inhibition in non-diabetic nephropathies with non-nephrotic proteinuria. *Lancet* 1999;354:359–364.
31. Anand IS, et al. Edema of cardiac origin. Studies of body water and sodium, renal function, hemodynamic indexes, and plasma hormones in untreated congestive

cardiac failure. *Circulation* 1989;80:299–305.

32. Pfeffer JM, et al. Influence of chronic captopril therapy on the infarcted left ventricle of the rat. *Circ Res* 1985;57:84–95.

33. SOLVD Investigators. Effect of enalapril on mortality and the development of heart failure in asymptomatic patients with reduced left ventricular ejection fractions. *N Engl J Med* 1992;327:685–691.

34. Flather MD, et al. Long-term ACE-inhibitor therapy in patients with heart failure or left-ventricular dysfunction: a systematic overview of data from individual patients. ACE-Inhibitor Myocardial Infarction Collaborative Group. *Lancet* 2000;355:1575–1581.

35. Sharpe N, et al. Treatment of patients with symptomless left ventricular dysfunction after myocardial infarction. *Lancet* 1988;1:255–259.

36. CIBIS II Study. The Cardiac Insufficiency Bisoprolol Study II (CIBIS-II): a randomised trial. *Lancet* 1999;353:9–13.

37. MERIT-HF Study Group. Effect of metoprolol CR/XL in chronic heart failure: Metoprolol CR/XL Randomized Trial in Congestive Heart Failure (MERIT-HF). *Lancet* 1999;353:2001–2007.

38. Poole-Wilson PA, et al. Comparison of carvedilol and metoprolol on clinical outcomes in patients with chronic heart failure in the Carvedilol Or Metoprolol European Trial (COMET): randomised controlled trial. *Lancet* 2003;362:7–13.

39. Pitt B, et al. Eplerenone, a selective aldosterone blocker in patients with left ventricular dysfunction after myocardial infarction. *N Engl J Med* 2003;348:1309–1321.

40. McMurray JJ, et al. Effects of candesartan in patients with chronic heart failure and reduced left-ventricular systolic function taking angiotensin-converting-enzyme inhibitors: the CHARM-Added trial. *Lancet* 2003;362:767–771.

41. Beilin LJ. Non-steroidal anti-inflammatory drugs and antihypertensive drug therapy. *J Hypertens* 2002;20:849–850.

42. Dzau VJ, et al. Prostaglandins in severe congestive heart failure: relation to activation of the renin-angiotensin system and hyponatremia. *N Engl J Med* 1984;310: 347–352.

43. Teo KK, et al. Effects of long-term treatment with angiotensin-converting-enzyme inhibitors in the presence or absence of aspirin: a systematic review. *Lancet* 2002;360:1037–1043.

44. MacFadyen RJ, et al. Differences in first dose response to ACE inhibition in congestive cardiac failure—a placebo-controlled study. *Br Heart J* 1991;66:206–211.

45. CONSENSUS Trial Study Group. Effects of enalapril on mortality in severe heart failure: Results of the Co-operative North Scandinavian Enalapril Survival Study (CONSENSUS). *N Engl J Med* 1987;316:1429–1435.

46. Packer M, et al. Comparative effects of low doses and high doses of the angiotensin converting-enzyme inhibitor, lisinopril, on morbidity and mortality in chronic heart failure. *Circulation* 1999;100:2312–2318.

47. Nanas JN, et al. Outcome of patients with congestive heart failure treated with standard versus high doses of enalapril: a multicenter study. High Enalapril Dose Study Group. *J Am Coll Cardiol* 2000;36:2090–2095.

48. Friedrich SP, et al. Intracardiac angiotensin-converting enzyme inhibition improves diastolic function in patients with left ventricular hypertrophy due to aortic stenosis. *Circulation* 1994;90:2761–2771.

49. Haber HL, et al. Intracoronary angiotensin-converting enzyme inhibition improves diastolic function in patients with hypertensive left ventricular hypertrophy. *Circulation* 1994;89:2616–2625.

50. Scott AC, et al. Skeletal muscle reflex in heart failure patients: role of hydrogen. *Circulation* 2003;107:300–306.

51. Dalla Libera L, et al. Beneficial effects on skeletal muscle of the angiotensin-II type 1 receptor blocker irbesartan in experimental heart failure. *Circulation* 2001;103: 2195–2200.

52. Sarnak MJ, et al. Anemia as a risk factor for cardiovascular disease in The Atherosclerosis Risk in Communities (ARIC) study. *J Am Coll Cardiol* 2002;40:27–33.

53. Shekelle PG, et al. Efficacy of angiotensin-converting enzyme inhibitors and beta-blockers in the management of left ventricular systolic dysfunction according to race, gender, and diabetic status: a meta-analysis of major clinical trials. *J Am Coll Cardiol* 2003;41:1529–1538.

54. Pitt B. Aldosterone blockade in patients with systolic left ventricular dysfunction. *Circulation* 2003;108:1790–1794.

55. Materson BJ, et al. Single-drug therapy for hypertension in men. A comparison of six antihypertensive agents with placebo. The Department of Veterans Affairs Cooperative Study Group on Antihypertensive Agents. *N Engl J Med* 1993;328: 914–921.

56. Wing LM, et al. A comparison of outcomes with angiotensin-converting-enzyme inhibitors and diuretics for hypertension in the elderly. *N Engl J Med* 2003;348:583–592.

57. Bloom BS. Continuation of initial antihypertensive medication after 1 year of therapy. *Clin Ther* 1998;20:671–681.

58. CAPPP Study Group. Effect of angiotensin-converting-enzyme inhibition compared with conventional therapy on cardiovascular morbidity and mortality in hypertension: the Captopril Prevention Project (CAPPP) randomised trial. *Lancet* 1999;353: 611–616.

59. STOP-2 Study. Randomised trial of old and new antihypertensive drugs in elderly patients: cardiovascular mortality and morbidity in the Swedish Trial in Old Patients with Hypertension-2 study. *Lancet* 1999;354:1751–1756.

60. Vermes E, et al. Enalapril decreases the incidence of atrial fibrillation in patients with left ventricular dysfunction: insight from the Studies Of Left Ventricular Dysfunction (SOLVD) trials. *Circulation* 2003;107:2926–2931.

61. AIRE Study. The effect of ramipril on mortality and morbidity of survivors of acute myocardial infarction with clinical evidence of heart failure. *Lancet* 1993;342: 821–828.

62. TRACE Study. A clinical trial of the angiotensin-converting-enzyme inhibitor trandolapril in patients with left ventricular dysfunction after myocardial infarction. *N Engl J Med* 1995;333:1670–1676.

63. Latini R, et al. Clinical effects of early angiotensin-converting enzyme inhibitor treatment for acute myocardial infarction are similar in the presence and absence of aspirin: systematic overview of individual data from 96,712 randomized patients. Angiotensin-converting Enzyme Inhibitor Myocardial Infarction Collaborative Group. *J Am Coll Cardiol* 2000;35:1801–1807.

64. SMILE Study. For the Survival of Myocardial Infarction Long-Term Evaluation Study Investigators. The effect of the angiotensin-converting-enzyme inhibitor zofenopril on mortality and morbidity after anterior myocardial infarction. *N Engl J Med* 1995;332:80–85.

65. GISSI-3 Study Group. GISSI-3: effects of lisinopril and transdermal glyceryl trinitrate singly and together on 6-week mortality and ventricular function after acute myocardial infarction. *Lancet* 1994;343:1115–1122.

66. Zuanetti G, et al. Effect of ACE inhibitor lisinopril on mortality in diabetic patients with acute myocardial infarction. *Circulation* 1997;96:4239–4245.

67. ACE Inhibitor Myocardial Infarction Collaborative Group. Indications for ACE Inhibitors in the Early Treatment of Acute Myocardial Infarction; Systematic Overview of Individual Data From 100,000 Patients in Randomized Trials. *Circulation* 1998;97:2202–2212.

68. Galcera-Tomas J, et al. Effects of early use of atenolol or captopril on infarct size and ventricular volume: A double-blind comparison in patients with anterior acute myocardial infarction. *Circulation* 2001;103:813–819.

69. SAVE Study. Effect of captopril on mortality and morbidity in patients with left ventricular dysfunction after myocardial infarction. Results of the Survival and Ventricular Enlargement trial. *N Engl J Med* 1992;327:669–677.

70. AIREX Study. On behalf of the AIREX Study Investigators. Follow-up study of patients randomly allocated ramipril or placebo for heart failure after acute myocardial infarction: AIRE Extension (AIREX) Study. *Lancet* 1997;349:1493–1497.

71. Torp-Pedersen C, et al. For the TRACE Study Group. Effect of ACE inhibitor trandolapril on life expectancy of patients with reduced left ventricular function after acute myocardial infarction. *Lancet* 1999;354:9–12.

72. Pretorius M, et al. Angiotensin-converting enzyme inhibition alters the fibrinolytic response to cardiopulmonary bypass. *Circulation* 2003;108:3079–3083.

73. Prasad A, et al. Anti-ischemic effects of angiotensin- converting enzyme inhibition in hypertension. *J Am Coll Cardiol* 2001;38:1116–1122.

74. Pepine CJ, et al. Effects of angiotensin-converting enzyme inhibition on transient ischemia: the Quinapril Anti-Ischemia and Symptoms of Angina Reduction (QUASAR) trial. *J Am Coll Cardiol* 2003;42:2049–2059.

75. Vijan S, et al. Treatment of hypertension in type 2 diabetes mellitus: blood pressure goals, choice of agents, and setting priorities in diabetes care. *Ann Intern Med* 2003;138:593–602.

76. European Society of Hypertension Guidelines Committee. European Society of Cardiology guidelines for the management of arterial hypertension. *J Hypertens* 2003;21:1011–1053.

77. Opie LH, et al. Diabetic nephropathy. Can renoprotection be extrapolated to cardiovascular protection? (Editorial). *Circulation* 2002;106:643–645.

78. MICRO-HOPE Study. Effects of ramipril on cardiovascular and microvascular outcomes in people with diabetes mellitus: results of the HOPE study and the MICRO-HOPE substudy. *Lancet* 2000;355:253–259.

79. Lazarus JM, et al. For the Modification of Diet in Renal Disease Study Group. Achievement and safety of a low blood pressure goal in chronic renal disease. *Hypertension* 1997;29:641–650.

80. Giatras I, et al. For the Angiotensin-Converting-Enzyme Inhibition and Progressive Renal Disease Study Group. Effect of angiotensin-converting enzyme inhibitors on the progression of nondiabetic renal disease: a meta-analysis of randomized trials. *Ann Intern Med* 1997;127:337–345.

81. GISEN Study Group. (Gruppo Italiano di Studi Epidemiologici in Nefrologia). Renal functions and requirement for dialysis in chronic nephropathy patients on long-term ramipril: REIN follow-up trial. *Lancet* 1998;352:1252–1256.

82. Agodoa LY, et al. For the African American Study of Kidney Disease and Hypertension (AASK) Group. Effect of ramipril vs amlodipine on renal outcomes in hypertensive nephrosclerosis. *JAMA* 2001;285:2719–2728.

83. Pfeffer MA, et al. Valsartan, captopril or both in myocardial infarction complicated by heart failure, left ventricular dysfunction or both. *N Engl J Med* 2003;349:1893–1906.

84. Jong P, et al. Effect of enalapril on 12-year survival and life expectancy in patients with left ventricular systolic dysfunction: a follow-up study. *Lancet* 2003;361:1843–1848.

85. SOLVD Investigators. Effect of enalpril in patients with reduced left ventricular ejection fractions and congestive heart failure. *N Engl J Med* 1991;325:293–302.

86. PROGRESS Collaborative Group. Randomised trial of a perindopril-based blood-pressure-lowering regimen among 6105 individuals with previous stroke or transient ischaemic attack. *Lancet* 2001;358:1033–1041.

87. Dahlof B, et al. Prevention of cardiovascular events with an antihypertensive regimen of amlodipine adding perindopril as required versus atenolol adding bendroflumethiazide as required, in the Anglo-Scandinavian Cardiac Outcomes Trial-Blood Pressure Lowering Arm (ASCOT-BPLA): a multicentre randomised controlled trial. Lancet. 2000;366:895-906.

   Cushman DW, et al. Differentiation of angiotensin-converting enzyme (ACE) inhibitors by their selective inhibition of ACE in physiologically important target organs. *Am J Hypertens* 1989;2:294–306.

89. Birkenhäger WH, et al. Non-peptide angiotensin type 1 receptor antagonists in the treatment of hypertension. *J Hypertens* 1999;17:873–881.

90. BP Trialists. Effects of different blood-pressure lowering regimens on major cardiovascular events: results of prospectively-designed overviews of randomised trials. *Lancet* 2003;362:1527–1535.

91. Dahlöf B, et al. For the LIFE Study Group. Cardiovascular morbidity and mortality in the Losartan Intervention For Endpoint reduction in hypertension study (LIFE): a randomised trial against atenolol. *Lancet* 2002;359:995–1003.

91a. Julius S, et al. Outcomes in hypertensive patients at high cardiovascular risk treated with regimens based on valsartan or amlodipine: the VALUE randomised trial. *Lancet* 2004;363:2022–2031.

92. Opie LH. Renoprotection by angiotensin-receptor blockers and ACE inhibitors in hypertension. *Lancet* 2001;358:1829–1231.

93. Lewis E, et al. For the Collaborative Study Group. The effect of angiotensin-converting enzyme inhibition on diabetic nephropathy. *N Engl J Med* 1993;329:1456–1462.

94. Lindholm LH, et al. Risk of new-onset diabetes in the Losartan Intervention For Endpoint reduction in hypertension study. *J Hypertens* 2002;20:1879–1886.

95. Lindholm LH, et al. Metabolic outcome during 1 year in newly detected hypertensives: results of the Antihypertensive Treatment and Lipid Profile in a North of Sweden Efficacy Evaluation (ALPINE study). *J Hypertens* 2003;21:1563–1574.

96. Pfeffer MA, et al. Effects of candesartan on mortality and morbidity in patients with chronic heart failure: the CHARM-overall programme. *Lancet* 2003;362:777–781.

97. Kajstura J, et al. Angiotensin-II induces apoptosis of adult ventricular myocytes in vitro. *J Mol Cell Cardiol* 1997;29:859–870.

98. Tsutsumi Y, et al. Angiotensin-II type 2 receptor overexpression activates the vascular kinin system and causes vasodilation. *J Clin Invest* 1999;104:925–935.

99. Schulz R, et al. AT1-receptor blockade in experimental myocardial ischemia/reperfusion. *Clin Nephrol* 2003;60 Suppl 1:S67–S74.

100. Takai S, et al. Chymase-dependent angiotensin-II formation in human vascular tissue. *Circulation* 1999;100:654–658.

101. Nickenig G, et al. Insulin induces upregulation of vascular AT_1 receptor gene expression by postranscriptional mechanisms. *Circulation* 1998;98:2543–2460.

102. Nickenig G, et al. Upregulation of vascular angiotensin-II receptor gene expression by low-density lipoprotein in vascular smooth muscle cells. *Circulation* 1997;95:473–478.

103. Cohn JN, et al. For the Valsartan Heart Failure Trial Investigators. A randomized trial of the angiotensin-receptor blocker valsartan in chronic heart failure. *N Engl J Med* 2001;345:1667–1675.

104. Hamroff G, et al. Addition of angiotensin-II receptor blockade to maximal angiotensin-converting enzyme inhibition improves exercise capacity in patients with severe congestive heart failure. *Circulation* 1999;99:990–992.

105. Nakao N, et al. Combination treatment of angiotensin-II receptor blocker and angiotensin-converting-enzyme inhibitor in non-diabetic renal disease (COOPERATE): a randomised controlled trial. *Lancet* 2003;361:117–124.

106. Owens P, et al. Comparison of antihypertensive and metabolic effects of losartan and losartan in combination with hydrochlorothiazide—a randomized controlled trial. *J Hypertens* 2000;18:339–345.

107. ELITE II Study. Effect of losartan compared with captopril on mortality in patients with symptomatic heart failure: randomised trial—the Losartan Heart Failure Survival Study ELITE II. *Lancet* 2000;355:1582–1587.

108. Dickstein K, et al. Effects of losartan and captopril on mortality and morbidity in high-risk patients after acute myocardial infarction: the OPTIMAAL randomised trial. Optimal Trial in Myocardial Infarction with Angiotensin-II Antagonist Losartan. *Lancet* 2002;360:752–760.

109. Brenner BM, et al. For the RENAAL Study Investigators. Effects of losartan on renal and cardiovascular outcomes in patients with type 2 diabetes and nephropathy. *N Engl J Med* 2001;345:861–869.

110. Lindholm LH, et al. For the LIFE Study Group. Cardiovascular morbidity and mortality in patients with diabetes in the Losartan Intervention For Endpoint reduction in hypertension study (LIFE): a randomised trial against atenolol. *Lancet* 2002;359:1004–1010.

111. Kjeldsen SE, et al. For the LIFE Study Group. Effects of losartan on cardiovascular morbidity and mortality in patients with isolated systolic hypertension and left ventricular hypertrophy. *JAMA* 2002;288:1491–1498.

112. Lacourciere Y, et al. For the Candesartan/Losartan study investigators. A comparison of the efficacy and duration of action of candesartan cilexetil and losartan as assessed by clinic and ambulatory blood pressure after a missed dose, in truly hypertensive patients. A placebo-controlled, forced titration study. *Am J Hypertens* 1999;12:1181–1187.

113. Parving H-H, et al. For the Irbesartan in Patients with Type 2 Diabetes and Microalbuminuria Study Group. The effect of irbesartan on the development of diabetic nephropathy in patients with type 2 diabetes. *N Engl J Med* 2001;345:870–878.

114. Lewis EJ, et al. Renoprotective effect of the angiotensin-receptor antagonist irbesartan in patients with nephropathy due to type 2 diabetes. *N Engl J Med* 2001;345:851–860.

115. VALUE Trial Group. The Valsartan Antihypertensive Long-term Use Evaluation (VALUE) trial of cardiovascular events in hypertension. Rationale and design. *Blood Pressure* 1998;7:176–183.

116. Lee TH. "Me-too" products–friend or foe? *N Engl J Med* 2004;350:211–212.

117. Douglas JG, et al. Management of high blood pressure in African Americans: consensus statement of the Hypertension in African Americans Working Group

International Society on Hypertension in Blacks. *Arch Intern Med* 2003;163:525–541.

118. Silvestre JS, et al. Activation of cardiac aldosterone production in rat myocardial infarction: effect of angiotensin-II receptor blockade and role in cardiac fibrosis. *Circulation* 1999;99:2694–2701.

119. Zannad F, et al. Limitation of excessive extracellular matrix turnover may contribute to survival benefit of spironolactone therapy in patients with congestive heart failure. Insights from the Randomized Aldactone Evaluation Study (RALES). *Circulation* 2000;102:2700–2706.

120. Flack JM, et al. Efficacy and tolerability of eplerenone and losartan in hypertensive black and white patients. *J Am Coll Cardiol* 2003;41:1148–1155.

121. Pitt B, et al. Effects of eplerenone, enalapril, and eplerenone/enalapril in patients with essential hypertension and left ventricular hypertrophy: the 4E-left ventricular hypertrophy study. *Circulation* 2003;108:1831–1838.

122. Grandi AM, et al. Aldosterone antagonist improves diastolic function in essential hypertension. *Hypertension* 2002;40:647–652.

123. Nikolaidis LA, et al. Angiotensin-converting enzyme inhibitors improve coronary flow reserve in dilated cardiomyopathy by a bradykinin-mediated, nitric oxide-dependent mechanism. *Circulation* 2002;105:2785–2790.

124. V-HeFT II Study. A comparison of enalapril with hydralazine-isosorbide dinitrate in the treatment of chronic congestive cardiac failure. *N Engl J Med* 1991;325:303–310.

125. JNC VII. The Seventh Report of the Joint National Committee on Prevention, Detection, Evaluation and Treatment of High Blood Pressure. *JAMA* 2003;289:2560–2572.

126. Dzau V, et al. Resolved and unresolved issues in the prevention and treatment of coronary artery disease. *Am Heart J* 1991;221:1244–1263.

6

Digitalis, Acute Inotropes, and Inotropic Dilators. Acute and Chronic Heart Failure

Philip A. Poole-Wilson • Lionel H. Opie

"The very essence of cardiovascular practice is the recognition of early heart failure."

Sir Thomas Lewis, 1933[1]

CHRONIC VERSUS ACUTE HEART FAILURE

Heart failure is a clinical condition in which an abnormality of cardiac contraction and/or relaxation results in the common symptoms of exertional shortness of breath and tiredness. Despite this simple definition, to establish the presence and cause of heart failure is often challenging (Fig. 6-1). The condition is common (prevalence 1% to 3% in populations, increasing with age to 10%), debilitating, detectable, and treatable, and it has a major economic impact on public health systems. The prognosis is poor depending on severity at the time of presentation; 50% of patients are dead within 4 years.

Heart failure has been recognized and described for many centuries. As a consequence numerous words or phrases have become established in clinical practice. These include older terms such as forward and backward failure, high- and low-output failure, right and left heart failure. More useful and current terminology includes acute and chronic heart failure, systolic (big heart and reduced ejection fraction) and diastolic (near normal size heart or ejection fraction) heart failure, and adjectives such as overt, treated, compensated, relapsing, congestive, or undulating.

A clinically useful approach is to consider three recognizable clinical conditions. Acute heart failure is characterized by the recent onset of severe shortness of breath. The term is almost synonymous with pulmonary edema. Cardiogenic shock is shock due to a cardiac cause and is a condition recognizable by evidence of peripheral constriction (cold peripheries, confusion, sweating), anuria or oliguria, and a low systolic blood pressure (less than 90 mmHg). Sometimes the phrase "acute heart failure" is used to encompass both pulmonary edema and cardiogenic shock. The third condition is chronic heart failure, which in the untreated state is dominated by the symptoms and signs associated with the retention and distribution around the body of salt and water.

Chronic Heart Failure

Chronic heart failure differs from acute failure in the aims of therapy. In acute heart failure, the short-term aim is to provide immediate symptomatic relief and to rescue the patient from imminent cardiorespiratory death by optimizing the hemodynamic status. The emphasis is on agents given intravenously. In chronic heart failure, the objectives are to prevent progressive damage to the myocardium (prevention), to prevent or reverse further enlargement of the heart (reverse remodeling), to improve the quality of life by relief of symptoms, and to prolong life. Reduction of hospitalization is an

DIAGNOSIS AND INVESTIGATION OF HF

P-Wison 2005

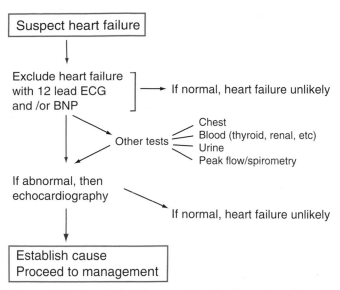

Figure 6-1 Overall clinical approach to the diagnosis and investigation of heart failure *(HF). BNP* = brain natriuretic peptide.

important goal for health providers because that is the major determinant of cost relating to the management of heart failure. The origin of symptoms in chronic heart failure is still not well understood but, in contrast to acute heart failure, is not directly and simply related to the elevated left atrial pressure. Successive pivotal trials have now established, first, the disabling nature of conventionally treated congestive heart failure (CHF) if left to run its natural course, and, second, that certain agents can reduce but not prevent the increased mortality. The most effective drugs act largely by modulating the neurohumoral responses in heart failure (Fig. 6-2). The key drugs are angiotensin-converting enzyme (ACE) inhibitors, β-blockers, aldosterone inhibitors (spironolactone and eplerenone), and angiotensin receptor blockers (ARBs). Diuretics provide symptomatic relief from fluid overload. A second group of drugs comprises agents that have positive inotropic effects and generally increase cell cyclic AMP and calcium levels, which tend to increase mortality. Most of these agents increase mortality in chronic heart failure, probably because of worsening myocardial damage and promotion of apoptosis. Digitalis has characteristics of both groups, because it both inhibits the neurohumoral response and has a positive inotropic effect. These properties might explain why it has an overall neutral effect on mortality.

Acute Heart Failure

In *cardiogenic shock* the major goals are load reduction, preservation of cardiac function, and maintenance of an optimal blood pressure so as to promote renal perfusion. Preload reduction by urgent reduction of pulmonary capillary pressure and right atrial filling pressure is sought along with a positive inotropic effect. Depending on the blood pressure, the afterload might either have to be reduced by vasodilation, or sometimes increased by peripheral vasoconstriction. These aims can be achieved by using a variety of intravenous inotropes, including dopamine, dobutamine, milrinone, and others. Some of these, such as high-dose dopamine and norepinephrine, cause α-mediated vasoconstriction to increase the blood pressure in shock-like states. The inotropic-dilators, such as milrinone, and low-dose

Progressive heart failure, NYHA classes

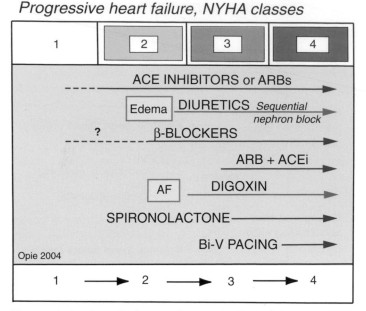

Figure 6-2 Schematic therapy of progressive heart failure. Note early use of ACE inhibitors, and increasingly early use of β-blockers. The role of diuretics is fundamental in relief of edema and fluid retention, using the principle of sequential nephron block. *AF* = atrial fibrillation. *ARB + ACEi* = combination of these agents, as used in some trials with benefit. However, this combination is controversial. *Bi-V* = biventricular pacing, also called cardiac resynchronization therapy. NYHA = New York Heart Association class of severity of heart failure. (*Figure © LH Opie, 2005.*)

dopamine, have a prominent vasodilator component to their inotropic action that is desired if the blood pressure is relatively well maintained.

In *acute heart failure* the symptom of shortness of breath is directly related to the high left atrial pressure. Treatment is aimed at immediate reduction of left atrial pressure (preload). Diuretics, morphine (antianxiolytic), and nitrates are used expeditiously. Intravenous natriuretic peptides are now being investigated (nesiritide).

DIGITALIS COMPOUNDS: DIGOXIN

Although digoxin is only a weak positive inotropic drug, it does have a unique profile of properties (Fig. 6-3). Besides its inotropic effect, it slows the ventricular rate, especially in atrial fibrillation, which allows better ventricular filling. Its use is therefore standard practice in CHF with atrial fibrillation. Digoxin also decreases the sympathetic drive generated by the failing circulation, which provides a rationale for its use in CHF in sinus rhythm. Nonetheless, this use remains controversial, especially since a trial on 6800 patients failed to show any mortality benefit for digoxin,[2] so that its use in sinus rhythm remains optional.[3] A subset of patients in this trial showed no benefit in terms of quality of life or symptoms, which further questions the indication for the use of digoxin in patients in sinus rhythm. The optimal use of digoxin requires a thorough knowledge of the multiple factors governing its efficacy and toxicity, including numerous drug interactions. Because the effects of digoxin in the acutely ill patient with hypoxia and electrolyte disturbances are often difficult to predict and because of lack of evidence of efficacy, digoxin is now seldom used in acute heart failure.

The combined inotropic-bradycardic action of digitalis is unique when compared to the many sympathomimetic inotropes that all tend

INOTROPIC, VAGAL AND SYMPATHETIC EFFECTS OF DIGOXIN

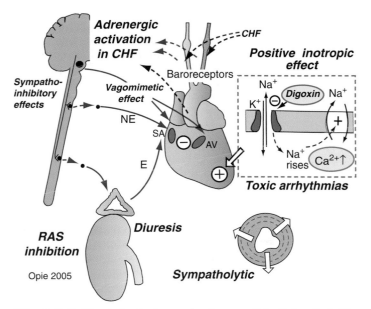

Figure 6-3 Digoxin has both neural and myocardial cellular effects. The inotropic effect of digoxin is due to inhibition of the sodium pump in myocardial cells. Slowing of the heart rate and inhibition of the atrioventricular *(AV)* node by vagal stimulation and the decreased sympathetic nerve discharge are important therapeutic benefits. Toxic arrhythmias are less well understood, but may be caused by calcium-dependent afterpotentials. *CHF* = congestive heart failure; *E* = epinephrine; *NE* = norepinephrine; *RAS* = renin-angiotensin system; *SA* = sinoatrial node. (*Figure © LH Opie, 2005.*).

to cause tachycardia. Digitalis, whatever its defects, remains the only inotrope available for use in the treatment of chronic heart failure, despite the narrow therapeutic-toxic margin and the numerous drug interactions, and despite the current uncertainty regarding the dose and blood levels required to obtain an optimal effect.

Pharmacologic Properties of Digoxin

All cardiac glycosides share an aglycone ring wherein the pharmacologic activity resides, usually combined with one to four molecules of sugar that modify the pharmacokinetic properties. Digoxin is a polar compound with an OH group binding to the steroid nucleus, whereas digitoxin is nonpolar with lesser central nervous system penetration.

Sodium Pump Inhibition Sodium pump inhibition explains the myocardial cellular effect of digitalis. As the sodium pump (Na/K-ATPase) is inhibited, there is a transient increase in intracellular sodium close to the sarcolemma, which in turn promotes calcium influx by the sodium-calcium exchange mechanism. The end result is an increased cytosolic calcium ion concentration with enhanced myocardial contractility (Fig. 6-3), and the theoretical risk of increased arrhythmias. However, digoxin may act as an inotrope at lower doses and blood levels than those that have been regarded as standard.[4-7]

Autonomic and Renin-Angiotensin Effects Sinus slowing and atrioventricular (AV) nodal inhibition results from *parasympathetic activation*. The extent of the inhibitory effect on the AV node depends partly on the degree of vagal tone, which varies from person to person. A modest direct depression of nodal tissue may account for those effects of digitalis still found after vagal blockade. Part of the toxic symptoms of digitalis may be explained by parasympathomimetic effects, such as nausea, vomiting, and anorexia. *Sympathetic inhibition* may play an important role in the effects of digitalis in CHF. Digitalis inhibits sympathetic nerve discharge, an effect that occurs before any observed hemodynamic changes.[5] *Renin release* from the kidney is inhibited because digoxin decreases the activity of the renal sodium pump with a natriuretic effect. Less renin release should lead to vasodilation to help offset the direct vasoconstrictor mechanism of digoxin (see next paragraph).

Hemodynamic Effects Hemodynamic effects of intravenous digoxin in heart failure were first described in a classic paper by McMichael and Sharpey-Schafer in 1944,[8] who showed that acute digitalization improved cardiac output in patients with heart failure. The fall in the venous pressure is probably best explained by a decreased sympathetic drive. The direct effect of digoxin on peripheral veins and arteries is mild vasoconstriction, because intracellular calcium increases. Likewise there is coronary constriction. The action of digoxin on AV conduction, which it slows, and on the AV refractory period, which it prolongs, is primarily dependent on increased vagal tone and only to a minor extent on the direct effect of digoxin.

Pharmacokinetics of Digoxin (Table 6-1) The serum half-life is 1.5 days. About one third of the body stores are lost daily, mostly as unchanged digoxin by the kidneys. About 30% is excreted by nonrenal routes (stools, hepatic metabolism) in those with normal renal function. In digitalized subjects, about half of the digoxin is bound to skeletal muscle receptors, accounting (with blood) for most of the volume of distribution. The "fit" between digitalis and the receptor is much less "tight" for skeletal muscle than for the myocardium, which remains the major site of action. In approximately 10% of patients, *intestinal flora* convert digoxin to an inactive reduction product, dihydrodigoxin. In such patients the blood level stays low unless the gut flora are inhibited by antibiotics such as erythromycin or tetracycline. Multiple pharmacokinetic factors influence the blood level obtained with a given dose of digoxin (Tables 6-2 and 6-3) and the sensitivity to digoxin (Table 6-4). In *renal impairment*, excretion is decreased and the maintenance dose is lower. The loading dose may also be lower (see next section).

Digoxin Use: Changes in Clinical Practice

Indications for Digitalis The most solid indication for digitalis is still the combination of chronic CHF with chronic atrial fibrillation. Here its

Table 6-1 Digoxin Pharmacokinetics

1. 75% of oral dose rapidly absorbed; rest inactivated in lower gut to digoxin reduction products by bacteria
2. Circulates in blood, unbound to plasma proteins; previous "therapeutic level" 1–2 ng/mL, current level 0.5–1.5 ng/ml; blood half-life about 36 h
3. Binds to tissue receptors in heart and skeletal muscle
4. Lipid-soluble; brain penetration
5. Most of absorbed digoxin excreted unchanged in urine (tubular excretion and glomerular filtration). About 30% undergoes nonrenal clearance, more in renal failure
6. In chronic renal failure, reduced volume of distribution
7. With small lean body mass, reduced total binding to skeletal muscle

Table 6-2 | **Causes of Abnormally Low Serum Digoxin Level***

Dose Too Low or Not Taken

Poor Absorption

Malabsorption, high bran diet
Drug interference: cholestyramine, sulfasalazine, neomycin, para-
aminosalicylic acid, kaolin-pectin, rifampin (= rifampicin)
Hyperthyroidism (additional mechanisms possible)
Enhanced intestinal conversion to inactive metabolites

Enhanced Renal Secretion

Improved GFR as vasodilator therapy enhances renal blood flow

*Here defined as levels below 0.5 ng/ml or 0.6 nmol/L.[11]

Table 6-3 | **Drug Interactions and Other Causes of High Serum Digoxin Levels**

Excess Initial Dose for Body Mass (small lean body mass)

Decreased Renal Excretion

Severe hypokalemia (<3 mEq/L)
Concurrent cardiac drugs (quinidine, verapamil, amiodarone)
Depressed renal blood flow (congestive heart failure, β-blockers)
Depressed GFR (elderly patients, renal disease)

Decreased Nonrenal Clearance

Antiarrhythmic drugs (quinidine, verapamil, amiodarone, propafenone)
Calcium channel blockers (verapamil and possibly others)

Decreased Conversion in Gut to Digoxin Reduction Products

In unusual patients, antibiotics can inhibit bacteria that convert digoxin
to inactive reduction products (erythromycin, tetracycline)

Table 6-4 | **Factors Altering Sensitivity to Digoxin at Apparently Therapeutic Levels**

Physiologic Effects

Enhanced vagal tone (increased digoxin effect on SA and AV nodes)
Enhanced sympathetic tone (opposite to vagal effect)

Systemic Factors or Disorders

Renal failure (reduced volume of distribution and excretion)
Low lean body mass (reduced binding to skeletal muscle)
Chronic pulmonary disease (hypoxia, acid-base changes)
Myxedema (? prolonged half-life)
Acute hypoxemia (sensitizes to digitalis arrhythmias)

Electrolyte Disorders

Hypokalemia (most common; sensitizes to toxic effects)
Hyperkalemia (protects from digitalis arrhythmias)
Hypomagnesemia (caused by chronic diuretics; sensitizes to toxic effects)
Hypercalcemia (increases sensitivity to digitalis)
Hypocalcemia (decreases sensitivity)

Cardiac Disorders

Acute myocardial infarction (may cause increased sensitivity)
Acute rheumatic or viral carditis (danger of conduction block)
Thyrotoxic heart disease (decreased sensitivity)

Concomitant Drug Therapy

Diuretics with K+ loss (increased sensitivity via hypokalemia)
Drugs with added effects on SA or AV nodes (verapamil, diltiazem,
β-blockers, clonidine, methyldopa, or amiodarone)

dosage and effects are still judged clinically. Digoxin toxicity must be avoided. In *CHF with sinus rhythm*, digitalis has gone through four phases. First, it was regarded with the diuretics as essential first-line therapy. Then reports on ineffectiveness or development of tolerance came in, so that its use declined, especially in the United Kingdom. Thereafter, the hemodynamic benefits of digitalis were reestablished as a result of several small hemodynamic studies and the two major withdrawal studies.[9,10] Even more recently the limited benefits found in the large DIG trial[2,11] and the very narrow therapeutic-toxic window[7] have cast major doubts on the ideal dose and blood levels. These problems have relegated digoxin to an optional extra in the management of CHF, given in lower doses than before (such as 0.125 mg daily)[6] and to obtain symptomatic rather than mortality benefit.[3,7]

In *chronic atrial fibrillation without heart failure* digoxin is no longer the drug of first choice. It may, however, still be used (1) prior to cardioversion, even though it may delay recovery from tachycardia-induced atrial remodeling,[12] and (2) in chronic atrial fibrillation in combination with verapamil, diltiazem, or β-blocking drugs to control the ventricular rate during exercise. Note the verapamil-digoxin interaction (Table 6-3). In *chronic atrial fibrillation with heart failure*, a logical combination is with a β-blocker that not only slows the ventricular rate but also improves exercise tolerance and the ejection fraction.[13]

Outmoded Indications for Digoxin Digoxin is no longer used in *paroxysmal atrial fibrillation*, because it neither controls the ventricular rate nor terminates a paroxysm. Drug control of paroxysmal atrial fibrillation has shifted from digoxin to more specific antiarrhythmics such as flecainide, sotalol, amiodarone, and dofetiltide (see Chapter 8). Once used in *acute supraventricular tachycardias*, digoxin has been superseded by more modern approaches (see Chapter 8). In *mitral stenosis with sinus rhythm*, prophylactic digoxin is also no longer appropriate. Rather, earlier operative intervention is often required. *Acute left ventricular (LV) failure* is generally treated by intravenous diuretics, by preload reduction by nitrates, and by acute ACE inhibition. If an inotropic effect is desired, then more potent inotropes are selected, such as dopamine, dobutamine, or milrinone, so that digitalis is outmoded unless initiated as part of longer term chronic therapy.

Doses and Blood Levels of Digoxin There is general agreement that the therapeutic-toxic window of digoxin is narrow. Previously, the ideal blood level was pragmatically regarded as 1 to 2 ng/mL (1.3 to 2.6 nmol/L). Currently lower doses and lower blood levels are finding strong spokesmen. Overall, the problem is that there have been no well-designed studies prospectively linking digoxin dose to blood levels to clinical outcome. Of note, low doses (0.125 mg daily) with a low blood level (mean: 0.8 ng/ml) provide as much hemodyamic benefit as standard doses (0.25 mg daily, mean blood level 1.5 ng/ml) without impairing the autonomic effect as measured by the heart rate variability.[4] Digoxin withdrawal studies show that such low doses are as good as the higher doses in maintaining LV function.[9,14,15] Decisive data come from a retrospective analysis of the large DIG trial on 3782 heart failure patients followed up for 3 years.[11] All-cause mortality was modestly decreased albeit, by only 6% in the tertile with digoxin levels in the previously "low" range, 0.5 to 0.8 ng/ml or 0.6 to 1.0 nmol/L. The next tertile of digoxin levels (0.9 to 1.1 ng/mL) had no effect on mortality, whereas higher levels (1.2 ng/mL or more) were associated with a mortality increase of 12%.[11] The hypothesis is that digoxin has bidirectional effects on mortality, with the "turnaround" level being about 1.0 ng/mL,[7] giving a practical therapeutic range of 0.5 to 1.0 ng/mL (Fig. 6-4) and certainly no higher. Although this conclusion is based on imperfect data and is strictly speaking only hypothesis generating,[11] we are unlikely to obtain more decisive data in the

K+ and TOXIC DIGOXIN LEVELS

Data points (●) from Shapiro, 1979

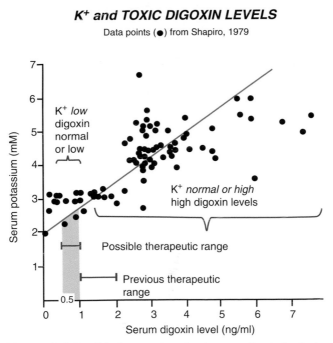

Figure 6-4 Possible therapeutic and toxic serum digoxin levels. As the serum potassium falls the heart is sensitized to the arrhythmias of digitalis toxicity. Conversely, as the serum potassium rises, a higher serum digoxin level is tolerated. Note current lower "therapeutic" levels of digoxin.[11] There are no good prospective data linking digoxin levels to outcome. (*Potassium data modified from Shapiro W. Am J Cardiol 1978;41:852–859, with permission.*)

near future. To achieve the previous "therapeutic" but now potentially toxic levels of 1.0 to 2.0 ng/ml, various nomograms have been designed to calculate the dose, taking into account lean body mass and renal function. Clearly these calculations will give too high a dose by present standards.

Digitalization First check renal function and then consider the age of the patient. In the past, the aim of digitalization was to achieve clinical benefit, not easy to assess in the absence of atrial fibrillation when the apical heart rate was the guide. Therefore the alternate aim was to achieve therapeutic blood levels, while avoiding the toxic range of more than 2 ng/ml. Currently the more relaxed trend toward a pragmatically lower digoxin dose means that although dosage is still commonly initiated at 0.25 mg per day, a lower dose of 0.125 mg daily may be more appropriate to achieve lower blood levels,[6] and even lower doses may be indicated if the patient is older than 70 years of age or if there is renal impairment.[3] To aim for "the highest possible dose tolerated" is no longer acceptable practice, being potentially dangerous. *Blood digoxin levels* are still valuable to allow for variable gastrointestinal (GI) absorption, variable cardiac responses, and possible drug interactions. Steady-state plasma and tissue concentrations are achieved in 5 to 7 days. The blood digoxin levels oscillate, so that a *single evening dose* is given to allow a steady-state situation for blood digoxin assays in the morning is advised; timing in relation to meals is not important. *Loading doses*, such as 0.5 mg three times a day for 1 day, are still sometimes given for severely decompensated patients. *Rapid digitalization*, now very seldom used, can be achieved by a combination of intravenous digoxin (0.5 mg IV) and oral digoxin (0.25 mg, one or two doses) to a total of 0.75 to 1.0 mg.

Digitalis Contraindications

Contraindications Contraindications are many: (1) *Hypertrophic obstructive cardiomyopathy* (hypertrophic subaortic stenosis, asymmetrical septal hypertrophy) is a contraindication (unless there is atrial fibrillation and severe myocardial failure), because the inotropic effect can worsen outflow obstruction. (2) The possibility of *digitalis toxicity* is a frequent contraindication, pending a full history of digitalis dosage, renal function tests, and measurement of serum digoxin. (3) In some cases of *Wolff-Parkinson-White (WPW) syndrome* with atrial fibrillation, digitalization may accelerate anterograde conduction over the bypass tract to precipitate ventricular tachycardia or ventricular fibrillation (see Fig. 8-2). (4) Significant *AV nodal heart block*. Intermittent complete heart block or second-degree AV block or sick sinus syndrome may be worsened by digitalis, especially if there is a history of Stokes-Adams attacks or when conduction is likely to be unstable as in acute myocardial infarction (AMI) or acute myocarditis. (5) *Diastolic dysfunction*, seen most notably with concentric ventricular hypertrophy as in hypertension or aortic stenosis, and associated with the paradox of a normal or high ejection fraction, does not respond to digitalis.

Relative Contraindications (1) If a poor response can be expected, as when low-output states are caused by valvular stenosis or chronic pericarditis; (2) in high-output states including chronic cor pulmonale and thyrotoxicosis; (3) when atrial fibrillation occurs without heart failure or when atrial fibrillation is caused by thyrotoxicosis; (4) all conditions increasing digitalis sensitivity to apparently therapeutic levels such as hypokalemia (Fig. 6-4), chronic pulmonary disease, myxedema, acute hypoxemia; (5) postinfarct because of the risk of increased mortality (see p. 158); (6) renal failure—a lower dose, monitoring of plasma potassium, and a watch for digitalis toxicity are needed; (7) sinus bradycardia or sick sinus syndrome—occasional patients will show a marked fall in sinus rate or sinus pauses, especially during cotherapy with other drugs inhibiting the sinus node, such as β-blockers, diltiazem, verapamil, reserpine, methyldopa, and clonidine; (8) cotherapy with other drugs inhibiting AV conduction (verapamil, diltiazem, β-blockers, amiodarone); here intravenous digoxin may be hazardous; (9) cotherapy with drugs altering digoxin levels; (10) heart failure accompanying acute glomerulonephritis because renal excretion of digoxin is impaired; and (11) severe myocarditis, which may predispose to digoxin-induced arrhythmias and decreased digoxin effect.

Clinical States Altering Digitalis Activity

Digoxin in the Elderly In the elderly, the etiology of CHF is often complex and multifactorial, requiring astute clinical diagnostic skills to detect any reversible cause. As in younger patients, digoxin is indicated, especially for chronic atrial fibrillation combined with CHF and, second, for significant systolic failure that is otherwise optimally treated. The *pharmacokinetics* of digoxin in the elderly have been well studied. Digoxin absorption is delayed but not decreased. A decreased skeletal muscle and lean body mass cause increased digoxin levels (Table 6-4). Digoxin half-life may be prolonged up to 73 hours in the elderly, depending on the decrease in renal function. There is no solid evidence of any alteration in myocardial sensitivity or in the response to digoxin in older individuals. The *dose of digoxin* in the elderly is up to and often lower than 0.125 mg daily, such as 0.125 mg every second day with a check of blood levels (Fig. 6-4) and special care with renal impairment.

Digoxin and Renal Function *The most important determinant of the daily digoxin dosage in all age groups is renal function* (creatinine clearance or glomerular filtration rate, GFR). The clinician usually relies on measurement of the serum creatinine. However, serum creatinine may be normal in an elderly patient with a GFR that is half normal if there is a marked decrease in muscle mass, because the amount of creatinine released daily is diminished. Even the GFR provides only a rough estimate of the renal excretion of digoxin, because it is excreted both by the glomerulus and by the tubules. In *severe renal insufficiency*, there is a decrease in the volume of distribution of digoxin, so that it is not exact to use a nomogram to estimate the maintenance dose based on creatinine clearance. One practical policy is to start with a maintenance dose of less than 0.125 mg/day in patients with severe renal insufficiency and then to rely on serum digoxin levels for dose adjustment.

Digoxin and Pulmonary Heart Disease Not only is digoxin not beneficial in patients with right heart failure due to cor pulmonale, but it may also be especially hazardous with sensitivity to digoxin intoxication because of hypoxia, electrolyte disturbances, and sympathetic discharge.

Digoxin and Myocardial Infarction Acute intravenous digoxin is not given in *early phase* AMI, especially because it constricts epicardial coronary arteries and experimentally increases infarct size. When *atrial fibrillation* develops with a rapid ventricular response, consider heart failure and treat cautiously by esmolol or verapamil or diltiazem to reduce the ventricular rate, or if needed, cardiovert.

Drug Interactions with Digoxin

The number of drug interactions is large (Table 6-3). Although there are no rules to guide the clinician, it is of interest that several of the offending drugs are antiarrhythmics, including verapamil. The *quinidine-digoxin* interaction is best known. The concomitant administration of quinidine causes the blood digoxin level approximately to double, probably by reducing both renal and extrarenal clearance. *Quinine*, an agent sometimes used in the therapy of muscle cramps, acts likewise. The *verapamil-digoxin* interaction is equally important, with blood digoxin levels rising by about 50% to 75%. *Amiodarone* and *propafenone* (see Chapter 8) also elevate serum digoxin levels. Other antiarrhythmics, including procainamide, have no interaction with digoxin (Table 6-5). *Diuretics* may induce hypokalemia which (1) sensitizes the heart to digoxin toxicity and (2) shuts off the tubular secretion of digoxin when the plasma potassium falls to below 2 to 3 mEq/L.

Digitalis Toxicity

The typical patient with digitalis toxicity (Table 6-6) is elderly with advanced heart disease and atrial fibrillation with abnormal renal function. Hypokalemia is common (Fig. 6-4). Digitalis toxicity should, however, be considered in any patient receiving digoxin or other digitalis compounds who presents with a new GI, ocular, or central nervous system complaint, or in whom a new arrhythmia or

Table 6-5	Antiarrhythmic Drugs That Have No Pharmacokinetic Interactions with Digoxin
Class IA agents:	procainamide, disopyramide
Class IB agents:	lidocaine, phenytoin, tocainide, mexiletine
Class II agents:	β-blockade, unless renal blood flow critical
Class III agent:	sotalol (but not amiodarone); ibutlide, dofetiltide
Class IV agent:	diltiazem (modest elevation compared with verapamil)

DIGITALIS TOXICITY: Ca^{2+} OVERLOAD
Opie 2004

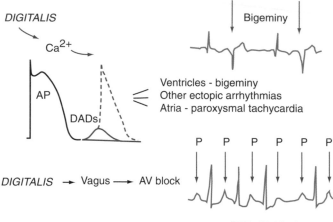

Figure 6-5 The cellular basis of the arrhythmias of digitalis toxicity lies in calcium overload, as a result of excess inhibition of the sodium pump (see Fig. 6-3). The result is the formation of delayed afterdepolarizations *(DADs)* and risk of ventricular ectopy, typically bigeminy, or atrial arrhythmias such as paroxysmal atrial tachycardia *(PAT)*. Added excess vagal stimulation (Fig. 6-3) causes the typical pattern of PAT with block, as shown above. *(Figure © LH Opie, 2005.)*

Table 6-6	Features of Digitalis Toxicity
System	**Symptoms and Signs**
Gastrointestinal	Anorexia, nausea, vomiting, diarrhea
Neurologic	Malaise, fatigue, confusion, facial pain, insomnia, depression, vertigo, colored vision (green or yellow halos around lights)
Cardiologic	Palpitations, arrhythmias, syncope
Blood	High digoxin level; may be normal level with low potassium; check magnesium, urea, creatinine

AV conduction disturbance develops. Symptoms do not necessarily precede serious cardiac arrhythmias. The *cellular mechanism* of digitalis toxicity resides in part in (1) intracellular calcium overload that predisposes to calcium-dependent delayed afterdepolarizations which may develop into ventricular automaticity (Fig. 6-5); (2) excess vagal stimulation, predisposing to sinus bradycardia and AV block; and (3) an added "direct" depressive effect of digoxin on nodal tissue.

Typical Digitalis Arrhythmias These are largely explained by increased vagal tone and include AV block, unexplained sinus bradycardia, and atrial fibrillation with a ventricular response of less than 50/minute. Digoxin toxicity also increases automaticity in junctional and His-Purkinje tissue. Thus, accelerated atrial, junctional or ventricular arrhythmias may result and when combined with AV nodal block are highly suggestive of digitalis toxicity (Fig. 6-5). Bidirectional tachycardia is rare but typical. Classically, increased ventricular ectopic beats give the pattern of bigeminy. When cotherapy elevates digoxin levels, the features of toxicity may depend on the agent added. With quinidine, tachyarrhythmias become more likely; amiodarone and verapamil seem to repress the ventricular arrhythmias of digoxin toxicity, so that bradycardia and AV block are more likely.

Diagnosis of Digoxin Toxicity The diagnosis of digoxin toxicity is confirmed if the arrhythmias resolve when the drug is discontinued, and/or if the digoxin blood level is inappropriately high for the patient in the presence of suspicious clinical features. Provided that hypokalemia is excluded (Fig. 6-4), a low plasma digoxin level strongly suggests that an arrhythmia or conduction disturbance is not due to digoxin toxicity. Occasionally, intravenous digoxin antibodies are given for diagnosis of suspected digoxin toxicity when blood levels are not diagnostic or the clinical problem is too complex to solve otherwise.

Treatment of Digoxin Toxicity Much depends on the clinical severity. With only suggestive symptoms, *withdrawal of digoxin* is sufficient while confirmation by elevated plasma levels is awaited. With dangerous arrhythmias and a low plasma potassium, potassium chloride may be infused intravenously very cautiously as 30 to 40 mEq in 20 to 50 ml of saline at 0.5 to 1 mEq/minute into a large vein through a plastic catheter (infiltration of potassium solution can cause tissue necrosis and infusion into small veins causes local irritation and pain). *Oral potassium* (4 to 6 g of potassium chloride, 50 to 80 mEq) may be given orally in divided doses when arrhythmias are not urgent (e.g., premature ventricular contractions). Potassium is contraindicated if AV conduction block or hyperkalemia are present, because potassium further increases AV block. *Activated charcoal* (50 to 100 g) is used to enhance GI clearance of digoxin. *Cholestyramine* has a similar but less powerful effect.

Antiarrhythmics for Digoxin Toxicity Lidocaine is usually chosen for ventricular ectopy because it does not impair the AV conduction that is frequently present. *Phenytoin*, in addition, reverses the high-degree AV block, possibly acting by a central mechanism. The dose is 100 mg intravenously every 5 minutes to a total of 1000 mg or until side effects appear. Quinidine and amiodarone must be avoided because they displace digoxin from binding sites to increase blood digoxin levels. Disopyramide can have a marked negative inotropic effect. β-Blockers should be avoided because of added nodal depression. *Interacting drugs* need attention. Any drugs elevating the blood digoxin level should be stopped (verapamil, quinidine), as also should β-blockade (added AV or sinus nodal inhibition). On the other hand, because of its very long half-life, there is little point in stopping amiodarone. Temporary transvenous *ventricular pacing* may be required for marked sinus bradycardia or advanced heart block not responsive to atropine.

Digoxin-Specific Antibodies (Digibind) These can be strikingly effective therapy for life-threatening digoxin intoxication, especially when there is severe ventricular tachycardia or significant hyperkalemia (>5.5 mEq/L). To calculate dose, work out total body digoxin load from the blood level; each vial binds about 0.5 mg of digoxin.

Current Position of Digoxin in the Therapy of CHF

Digoxin is often used in the treatment of heart failure with chronic atrial fibrillation. In heart failure in sinus rhythm, digoxin has slipped from those that are mandatory drugs, which are those that are known to prolong life, to being optional except when heart failure is combined with atrial fibrillation. In the essential category are ACE inhibitors, β-blockers, ARBs, and aldosterone blockers. The current trend is toward lower digoxin doses that might be safer, and achieve any proposed benefit with less risk of digoxin toxicity. The ideal blood levels remain unknown, but an aim of about 0.5 to 1 ng/mL or 0.6 to 1.2 nmol/L (much lower than before) seems reasonable.

ACUTE INOTROPES: SYMPATHOMIMETICS AND OTHERS

Physiologically, the basis of the acute inotropic response to an increased adrenergic drive is the rapid increase in the tissue levels of the second messenger, cyclic AMP. Pharmacologically, acute inotropic support uses the same principles, either by administration of exogenous catecholamines, which stimulate the β-receptor, or by inhibition of the breakdown of cyclic AMP by phosphodiesterase (PDE) inhibitors (Fig. 6-6). To give acute support to the failing circulation may require temporary peripheral vasoconstriction by α-adrenergic stimulation. Hence there are a variety of catecholamine-like agents used for acute heart failure, depending on the combination of acute inotropic stimulation, acute vasodilation, and acute vasoconstriction that may be required (Table 6-7). In addition, in acute heart failure, intravenous furosemide and nitrates counter pulmonary congestion.

Adrenergic Receptors and Inotropic Effects

Norepinephrine *Norepinephrine* is the endogenous catecholamine that is synthesized and stored in granules in adrenergic nerve endings in the myocardium. When sympathetic nerves to the heart are activated, norepinephrine is released from its stores and stimulates specific *β_1-adrenergic receptors* (see Fig. 1-1). Most of the released norepinephrine is subsequently taken up by the same adrenergic nerve endings and stored for renewed release. Smaller amounts are metabolized. *Epinephrine*, released from the adrenal glands, is a mixed β_1 and β_2-stimulant with high-dose α-effects.

Pathophysiological Role of β-Receptors Stimulation of the *β_1-receptors* increases the rate of discharge of the sinoatrial node, thereby

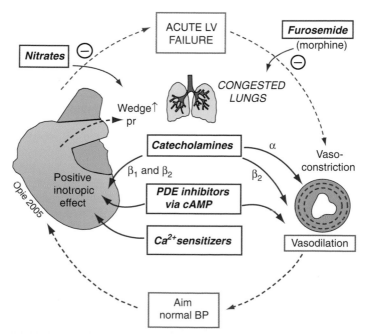

Figure 6-6 Some principles of therapy for acute LV failure. Note opposing effects of (1) vasoconstriction resulting from α-adrenergic effects (norepinephrine, high doses of epinephrine or dopamine) and (2) vasodilation resulting from vascular cyclic AMP elevation from β_2-effects or phosphodiesterase (PDE) inhibition (Fig. 6-9). (*Figure © LH Opie, 2005.*)

Table 6-7 Sympathomimetic Inotropes for Acute Cardiac Failure Therapy

Drugs and Mediating Receptors	Dobutamine β1 > β2 > α	Dopamine Dopaminergic >β; High dose α	Norepinephrine β1 > α > β2	Epinephrine β1 = β2 > α	Isoproterenol β1 > β2	Milrinone PDE Inhibitor	Phenylephrine α-Agonist
Dose infusion μg/kg/min	2–15	2–5 renal effect 5–10 inotropic 10–20 SVR ↑	0.01–0.03 max. 0.1	0.01–0.03 max. 0.1–0.3	0.01–0.1	Bolus 50–75 (10 min) Drip 0.375–0.75	0.2–0.3
Elim $t\frac{1}{2}$ min	2.4	2.0	3.0	2.0	2.0	150	20
Inotropic effect	↑↑	↑↑	↑	↑↑	↑↑↑	↑↑	0
Arteriolar vasodilation	↑	↑↑	0	↑	↑	↑↑	0, ↓
Vasoconstriction	High dose ↑	High dose ↑↑	↑↑	High dose ↑ ↑↑	0	0	↑↑↑
Chronotropic effect	↑	0, ↑	↑	0, ↑	↑↑↑	0	0, ↓
Blood pressure effect	↑	High dose ↑	↑	0	↑	0 →	↑↑↑
Diuretic effect (direct)	0	↑↑	↓	0	0	0 →	0 →
Arrhythmia risk	↑↑	High dose ↑	↑	↑↑↑	↑↑↑	↑	0

↑ = increase; ↓ = decrease; 0 = no change. Elim $t\frac{1}{2}$ = elimination half life; SVR = systemic vascular resistance.

163

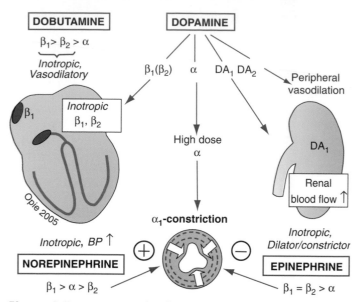

Figure 6-7 Receptor-specific effects of physiologic and pharmacologic catecholamines. For concepts regarding adrenergic receptor stimulation by dobutamine, see Ruffolo.[50] For norepinephrine, see Bristow.[51] (*Figure © LH Opie, 2005.*)

increasing heart rate and AV conduction, and the force and speed of contraction of atrial and ventricular myocardium. β_1-stimulation also enhances the rate of relaxation of the myocardium (see Fig. 1-2). Norepinephrine has vasoconstrictive effects that result from stimulation of the vascular α-receptors, so that the blood pressure rises. Hence the positive inotropic effect of norepinephrine (Fig. 6-7) is accompanied by an elevation of systolic and diastolic blood pressure. *β_2-Adrenergic receptors* convey another type of β-mediated sympathomimetic effect, namely that causing dilation of the smooth muscles of the blood vessels, bronchi, and uterus. A population of *β_2-receptors* is found in the human heart but not in most other animal species. The number is about 25% but in heart failure because of the selective downregulation of *β_1-receptors*, can be as high as 40% to 50%. In the normal heart, stimulation of the *β_2-adrenergic receptors* has effects similar to those of the β_1-receptors mediating more stimulation of adenylate cyclase, that is, the coupling is tighter. These receptors also mediate protective antiapoptotic signals (see Fig. 1-7). This is one hypothetical mode of lessening the progression of mycocyte loss.

Cardiovascular Therapeutic Effects of Adrenergic Agents

Adrenergic Effects on Blood Pressure In the case of norepinephrine, the net effect is blood pressure elevation (dominant peripheral α-effects), whereas in the case of epinephrine at physiological doses, the vasodilatory effects of β_2-stimulation offset the blood pressure elevating effects of α-stimulation. The net effect of epinephrine is an elevation only of systolic blood pressure (increased stroke volume) with a fall of diastolic blood pressure (β_2-peripheral dilation). Only at high pharmacological doses of epinephrine does α-constriction elevate diastolic blood pressure.

β-Adrenergic Stimulation of the Failing Heart Sympathomimetic agents could thus benefit the acutely failing heart: β_1-stimulation by an inotropic effect, β_2-stimulation by afterload reduction (peripheral arterial vasodilation), and α-stimulation by restoring pressure in hypotensive states (Table 6-7). Experimental work unfortunately

shows that catecholamine stimulation as exemplified by norepineph-rine infusion should be used with caution in the low output state of AMI. β_1-Effects may precipitate arrhythmias and tachycardia, which can potentially increase ischemia, while excessive α-effects increase the afterload as the blood pressure rises beyond what is required for adequate perfusion. Although β_2-activation achieves beneficial vasodi-lation and also mediates some inotropic effect, such stimulation also causes hypokalemia with enhanced risk of arrhythmias. A further and serious problem is that prolonged or vigorous β_1-stimulation may lead to or increase receptor downgrading with a diminished inotropic response (see Fig. 1-8). Catecholamine toxicity leads to myocyte breakdown and death. These are the reasons why sympathomimetics are used only in short-term treatment of acute heart failure.

α-Adrenergic Effects If the blood pressure is low, as in cardiogenic shock, a crucial decision is whether it is desired to increase the blood pressure solely by inotropic support or by a combination of inotropic and peripheral vasoconstrictory effects, or only by peripheral vaso-constriction. Although the latter aim can be achieved by using pure *α-stimulants*, such as *phenylephrine* (5 to 20 mg in 500 mL, slow infu-sion) or *methoxamine* (3 to 10 mg at 1 mg/min), this option is not logical, because heart failure itself automatically invokes reflex adrenergic vasoconstriction. Both these α-stimulants may be useful in anesthetic hypotension. Occasionally phenylephrine is still used in primary vasodilatory conditions, such as *septic shock*. The real therapeutic aim in the latter condition is inhibition of excess vaso-dilatory nitric oxide.

Combined Inotropic and Vasoconstrictory Effects These are often required, as may, for example, be achieved by using high-dose dopamine. Fur-thermore, bearing in mind that there are often defects in the rate of formation of cyclic AMP in chronically failing hearts, when there is acute-on-chronic heart failure, then a logical combination becomes dopamine plus a PDE inhibitor such as milrinone. If only inotropic stimulation is required, dobutamine is the agent of choice, with, however, the risk of dropping the diastolic blood pressure by its peripheral β_2 effect. If inotropic stimulation plus peripheral vaso-dilation is required, then low dose dopamine or milrinone is appropriate.

Mixed Adrenergic Intravenous Inotropes These agents ($\beta > \alpha$-adrenergic stimulation) have as their common property the stimulation of both β- and α-adrenergic receptors to a varying degree. α-Adrenergic stim-ulation also results in some modest positive inotropic response in the human heart, probably of greater importance when α-receptors are relatively upgraded as in severe CHF. Included in this group of mixed adrenergic agents is dobutamine, previously considered as highly selective for β_1-receptors, but now thought also to stimulate β_2- and α-receptors (Table 6-7).

Dobutamine

Dobutamine (*Dobutrex*), a synthetic analog of dopamine, is a β-adren-ergic stimulating agent ($\beta_1 > \beta_2 > \alpha$). Its major characteristic is a potent inotropic effect (Fig. 6-7). However its β_2 stimulatory effect may lead to hypotension. Sometimes the latter leads to a fall in diastolic pres-sure with a reflex tachycardia. Furthermore, long-term mortality may be increased.[16] Therefore prior enthusiasm for this agent is cooling, despite short-term hemodynamic benefit[16] and the unexpected finding that it reduces rather than increases cardiac sympathetic activity in heart failure patients.[17] To avoid hypotension, a logical combination (without evidence-based outcome data) is that of dobutamine with vasoconstrictor dopamine.

Pharmacokinetics, Dose, and Indications An infusion is rapidly cleared (half-life 2.4 minutes). The standard intravenous dose is 2.5 to 10 µg/kg/minute, occasionally up to 40 µg/kg/minute. The drug can be infused for up to 72 hours with monitoring. There is no oral preparation. *Indications* are acute-on-chronic refractory heart failure; severe acute myocardial failure (AMI, after cardiac surgery); cardiogenic shock; and excess β-blockade.

Dobutamine Use, Side Effects, and Precautions The ideal candidate for dobutamine therapy is the patient who has severely depressed LV function with a low cardiac index and elevated LV filling pressure, but in whom extreme hypotension is not present (mean arterial blood pressure <70 mmHg but no clinical shock) (see later, Fig. 6-10). The potential disadvantages of dobutamine are (1) that in severe CHF the β-receptors may be downgraded or therapeutically blocked so that dobutamine may not be as effective as anticipated,[17] (2) blood pressure may decrease or stay unchanged, and not increase, and (3) there may be risk of serious arrhythmias.[16] Although there may be less tachycardia and arrhythmias than with isoproterenol, all inotropic agents increasing cytosolic calcium have risk of enhanced arrhythmias. Tolerance to the inotropic effect may develop after prolonged infusion. *Precautions* are: dilute in sterile water or dextrose or saline, not in alkaline solutions. Use within 24 hours. Hemodynamic or careful clinical monitoring of patient required. Check blood potassium (may fall) to minimize arrhythmias.

Dopamine (Intropin)

Dopamine is a catecholamine-like agent used for therapy of severe heart failure and cardiogenic shock. Physiologically it is both the precursor of norepinephrine and releases norepinephrine from the stores in the nerve endings in the heart (Fig. 6-7). However, in the periphery this effect is overridden by the activity of the prejunctional dopaminergic DA_2-receptors, inhibiting norepinephrine release and thereby helping to vasodilate. Therefore, overall dopamine stimulates the heart by both β- and α-adrenergic responses and causes vasodilation through dopamine receptors. Theoretically, dopamine has the valuable property in severe CHF or shock of specifically increasing blood flow to the renal, mesenteric, coronary, and cerebral beds by activating the specific postjunctional dopamine DA_1-receptors. However, the concept of the therapeutic "renal dose" is now outdated (see p. 166). At high doses dopamine causes α-receptor stimulation with peripheral vasoconstriction; the peripheral resistance increases and renal blood flow falls. The dose should therefore be kept as low as possible to achieve the desired ends. Sometimes a combination of dopamine and vasodilator therapy or dopamine with dobutamine is better than increasing the dose of dopamine into the vasoconstrictor range unless the latter effect is specifically required despite its problems.

Properties and Use of Dopamine Dopamine, a "flexible molecule," also fits into many receptors to cause direct β_1- and β_2-receptor stimulation, as well as α-stimulation. The latter explains why in high doses dopamine causes significant vasoconstriction. By increasing renal blood flow, dopamine may induce diuresis or it may potentiate the effects of furosemide. *Pharmacokinetics:* Dopamine is inactive orally. Intravenous dopamine is metabolized within minutes by dopamine β-hydroxylase and monoamine oxidase. *Dose and indications.* In refractory cardiac failure, dopamine can be given only intravenously, which restricts its use to short-term treatment. The dose starts at 0.5 to 1 µg/kg/minute and is raised until an acceptable urinary flow, blood pressure, or heart rate is achieved; vasoconstriction begins at about 10 µg/kg/minute and becomes marked at higher doses, then calling for an added α-blocking agent or sodium nitroprusside. In a few patients vasoconstriction can begin at doses as low as 5 µg/kg/minute. In cardiogenic shock or AMI, 5 µg/kg/minute of dopamine is enough to give a maximum increase in stroke volume, while renal flow reaches a peak at 7.5 µg/kg/minute, and arrhythmias may appear at 10 µg/kg/minute. In septic shock, dopamine has an inotropic effect and increases urine volume. Dopamine is widely used for acute myocardial failure after cardiac surgery.

Is there a "renoprotective" dose? Dopamine is sometimes given for renal protection or for diuresis in critically ill patients at a typical dose of 0.5 to 2.5 µg/kg/minute. In an intensive care setting, patients at risk of acute renal failure were not endowed with any special renal protection, so that there is "no justification" for the renoprotective concept.[18] Furthermore, there are undesirable side effects such as depression of ventilation and increased pulmonary shunting in hypoxic patients.[19] The result is blunting of conscious discomfort, not a problem during mechanical ventilation but the weaning phase becomes more difficult. In those not ventilated, simple supplemental oxygen might save the day.[19] *Is contrast-dye nephropathy* prevented by "renal" dose dopamine? Results have not been consistent and overall disappointing.[20] *Intermittent outpatient dopamine* for chronic heart failure does not work[3] and may do harm.

Precautions, Side Effects, and Interactions Dopamine must not be diluted in alkaline solutions. Blood pressure, electrocardiogram, and urinary flow are monitored constantly with intermittent measurements of cardiac output and pulmonary wedge pressure if possible. For oliguria, first correct hypovolemia; try furosemide. Dopamine is contraindicated in ventricular arrhythmias, and in pheochromocytoma. Use with care in aortic stenosis. Extravasation can cause sloughing, prevented by infusing the drug into a large vein through a plastic catheter, and treated by local infiltration with phentolamine. If the patient has recently taken a monoamine-oxidase (MAO) inhibitor, the rate of dopamine metabolism by the tissue will fall and *the dose should be cut to one tenth* of the usual.

Comparison of Dopamine and Dobutamine Dopamine is the preferred inotrope in the patient who requires both a pressor effect (high-dose α-effect) and increase in cardiac output, and who does not have marked tachycardia or ventricular irritability. In the latter situation the sympatholytic effect of dobutamine may be of some benefit.[17] Dopamine is especially beneficial when renal blood flow is impaired in severe CHF. In cardiogenic shock, infusion of equal concentrations of dopamine and dobutamine may afford more advantages than either drug singly. The key to the effective use of these (and all intravenous inotropes) is careful monitoring of the hemodynamic response in the individual patient.

Epinephrine (Adrenaline)

Epinephrine gives mixed β1-β2-stimulation with some added α-mediated effects at a high dose (Table 6-7). A low physiologic infusion rate (<0.01 µg/kg/minute) decreases blood pressure (vasodilator effect), whereas >0.2 µg/kg/minute increases peripheral resistance and blood pressure (combined inotropic and vasoconstrictor effects). It is used chiefly when combined inotropic/chronotropic stimulation is urgently desired as in cardiac arrest. Then the added α-stimulatory effect of high-dose epinephrine helps to maintain the blood pressure and overcomes the peripheral vasodilation achieved by β2-receptor stimulation. The acute *dose* is 0.5 mg subcutaneously or intramuscularly (0.5 ml of 1 in 1000), or 0.5 to 1.0 mg into the central veins, or 0.1 to 0.2 mg intracardiac. The *terminal half-life* is 2 minutes. *Side effects* include tachycardia, arrhythmias, anxiety, headaches, cold extremities, cerebral hemorrhage, and pulmonary edema. *Contraindications* include late pregnancy because of risk of inducing uterine contractions.

Norepinephrine (Noradrenaline)

Norepinephrine is given in an *intravenous dose* of 8 to 12 µg/minute with a terminal half-life of 3 minutes. This catecholamine has prominent β_1- and α-effects with less β_2-stimulation. Norepinephrine chiefly stimulates α-receptors in the periphery (with more marked α-effects than epinephrine) and β-receptors in the heart. Logically, norepinephrine should be of most use when a shock-like state is accompanied by peripheral vasodilation (*"warm shock"*). In the future, drugs inhibiting the formation of vasodilatory nitric oxide will probably be of greater use in such patients. *Side effects* of norepinephrine include headache, tachycardia, bradycardia, and hypertension. Note the risk of necrosis with extravasation. *Combination therapy* with PDE inhibitors helps to avoid the hypotensive effects of the PDE inhibitors. *Contraindications* include late pregnancy (see Epinephrine) and preexisting excess vasoconstriction.

Isoproterenol (Isoprenaline)

This relatively pure β-stimulant ($\beta_1 > \beta_2$) is still sometimes used. Its cardiovascular effects closely resemble those of exercise including a positive inotropic and vasodilatory effect. Theoretically, it is most suited to situations where the myocardium is poorly contractile and the heart rate slow, yet the peripheral resistance high as, for example, after cardiac surgery in patients with prior β-blockade. Another ideal use is in β-blocker overdose. The intravenous dose is 0.5 to 10 µg/minute, the plasma half-life is about 2 minutes, and the major problem lies in the risk of tachycardia and arrhythmias. Furthermore, it may drop the diastolic blood pressure by its β_2-vasodilator stimulation. Other side effects are headache, tremor, and sweating. Contraindications include myocardial ischemia, which can be worsened, and arrhythmias.

β_2-Agonists

In healthy volunteers, β_2-receptors mediate chronotropic, inotropic, and vasodilator responses. Although not well tested in CHF where there is known to be cardiac β_2-receptor uncoupling, some evidence suggests clinical benefit in patients already treated by diuretics and digoxin. The drugs used are basically bronchodilators (terbutaline; albuterol = salbutamol) and should therefore theoretically be ideal for the combination of chronic obstructive airways disease and CHF. By inducing hypokalemia and prolonging the QT-interval, β_2-agonists may increase the risk of arrhythmias.

Calcium Sensitizers

Here the principle is that there is no attempt to increase cell calcium, the common mechanism of action of the conventional inotropes with the inevitable risk of arrhythmias. Rather the contractile apparatus is sensitized to the prevailing level of calcium. Theoretically these agents should increase contractile force without the risk of calcium-induced arrhythmias. This expectation has not been met in the case of several members of this group that also have PDE inhibitory properties with arrhythmogenic risks. *Levosimendan* is licensed in some European countries but under consideration in the United States. It sensitizes troponin C to calcium, without impairing diastolic relaxation.[21] In addition it has vasodilatory effects mediated by opening of vascular ATP-sensitive potassium channels.[21] In the important LIDO study on 103 patients in severe low-output heart failure, levosimendan (infused at 0.1 µg/kg/minute for 24 hours after a loading dose of 24 µg/kg over

10 min) compared well with dobutamine (5 to 10 µg/kg/minute) in that hemodynamic improvement was accompanied by reduced mortality up to 180 days.[21] No placebo group was included so that the difference could have been due to harmful effects of dobutamine. An oral form is under development.

AGENTS WITH BOTH INOTROPIC AND VASODILATOR PROPERTIES ("INODILATORS")

Although "inodilation" is a term coined by Opie in 1989,[22] the rationale goes back at least to 1978 when Stemple and colleagues[23] combined the advantages of the vasodilator effects of nitroprusside with the inotropic effect of dopamine, thereby reducing both afterload and preload (Fig. 6-8). Recent recognition of the sympatholytic properties of digoxin should strictly speaking lead to its inclusion in the group of inodilators. Nonetheless, it is the PDE inhibitors that are the prototypical agents (Fig. 6-9).

Phosphodiesterase-III Inhibitors

These agents, epitomized by milrinone, inhibit the breakdown of cyclic AMP in cardiac and peripheral vascular smooth muscle, resulting in augmented myocardial contractility and peripheral arterial and venous vasodilation (Fig. 6-9). For ill-understood reasons, these effects occur with relatively little change in heart rate or blood pressure. The added dilator component may explain relative conservation of the myocardial oxygen consumption. Nonetheless, the increased levels of myocardial cyclic AMP may predispose to ventricular arrhythmias, which could explain the findings in the Milrinone-Digoxin trial in which milrinone was no better than digoxin and led to an increase in ventricular arrhythmias.[24] The only inotropic dilator currently licensed in the United States is milrinone, while both milrinone and enoximone are available in the United Kingdom.

Milrinone Milrinone (*Primacor*) is approved for intravenous use in the United States and the United Kingdom. Its pharmacologic mechanism of action is by PDE-III inhibition, with a prominent vasodilator component. The package insert gives a prominent warning that there is no

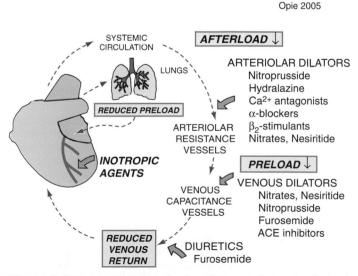

ARTERIOLAR vs VENOUS VASODILATORS

Opie 2005

Figure 6-8 Comparative sites of action of agents reducing the afterload, or reducing the preload, and of inotropic agents. (*Figure © LH Opie, 2005.*)

INOTROPIC DILATORS

Opie 2004

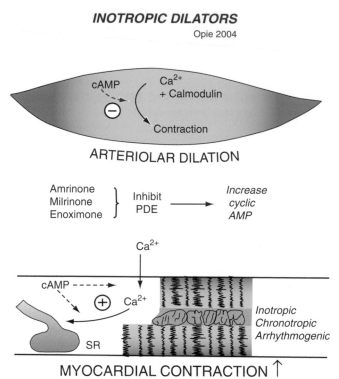

Figure 6-9 Inotropic dilators ("inodilators") have as their mechanism of action an increase of cyclic AMP in vascular smooth muscle *(top)* and in myocardium *(bottom)*. PDE = phosphodiesterase. *(Figure © LH Opie, 2005.)*

evidence for efficacy or safety when given for longer than 48 hours. The further warning is that long-term oral use increased ventricular arrhythmias[24] and mortality.[14] In the large OPTIME-CHF trial on 949 patients with acute exacerbations of heart failure on a background of chronic heart failure, milrinone gave no additional benefit beyond placebo yet caused more complications such as new atrial fibrillation and sustained hypotension, without any overall mortality benefit.[25] A later analysis of the same study revealed a trend to outcome benefit in the nonischemic but not in the ischemic patients.[26] There is no evidence that long-term continuous or intermittent infusions may impart substantial benefit without potentially serious hazards. However, a logical new use is in patients with acute-on-chronic heart failure, already receiving β-blockade, who need acute inotropic support that by-passes the β-receptor.

Indications and doses are as follows. Milrinone is licensed only for intravenous use in patients with acute heart failure who are closely monitored, with facilities to treat any acute life-threatening ventricular arrhythmias that may arise. There is no experience with infusions of longer than 48 hours. A slow intravenous injection (over 10 minutes, diluted before use, 50 μg/kg) is followed by an intravenous infusion at a rate of 0.375 to 0.750 μg/kg/minute, usually for up to 12 hours following surgery or up to 48 hours in acute heart failure; the maximum daily dose is 1.13 mg/kg. Reduce the dose in renal failure according to the creatinine clearance (see package insert). For example, a clearance of 20 mL/minute/1.73 m^2 gives an infusion rate of 0.28 μg/kg/minute. *Contraindications* are acute myocardial infarction, tight aortic stenosis, or hypertrophic obstructive subaortic stenosis. *Short-term inotropic support* by milrinone on top of the otherwise optimal management of exacerbations of chronic heart failure cannot be recommended unless there is clear clinical need for inotropes or pressor agents.

Combination therapy and drug interactions are as follows. Milrinone gives added hemodynamic benefit to patients already receiving ACE inhibitors, with, however, a high risk of vasodilatory side effects. Milrinone may be combined with modest doses of dobutamine, enhancing the inotropic effects while lowering filling pressures. When the blood pressure is low, milrinone could logically be combined with high-dose dopamine. There appear to be few or no adverse drug interactions.

Enoximone This investigational agent, not available in the United States, is licensed as *Perfan* for intravenous use in the United Kingdom (loading dose: 90 µg/kg/minute over 10 to 30 minutes, then 5 to 20 µg/kg/minute, decrease doses in renal failure). Although licensed for CHF where cardiac output is reduced and filling pressures increase, in practice it should ideally be used against acute not chronic heart failure or in bridging situations such as for patients awaiting transplantation. It seems that enoximone has not overcome the common problem of PDE inhibitors, namely enhancement of cyclic AMP levels and hence the risk of serious arrhythmias. The latter might explain why enoximone increased mortality in severe heart failure, while the central stimulatory effects of cyclic AMP might explain why physical mobility and quality of life improved.[27] This unexpected paradox triggered a debate, not yet resolved, of whether it is more important to improve the quality or quantity of life in chronic severe end-stage heart failure.

LOAD REDUCTION AND VASODILATION
Principles of Load Reduction

Vasodilation, once a specialized procedure, is now commonplace in the therapy of CHF and hypertension, as the peripheral circulation has become one of the prime sites of cardiac drug action. Vasodilators may be classified according to the site of action in the circulation (Fig. 6-8). Preload reducers (predominantly venodilators) may be separated from those reducing primarily the afterload (predominantly arteriolar dilators), while mixed agents act on both pre- and afterload and are combined venoarteriolar dilators. ACE inhibitors can be regarded as specialized vasodilators that have many other additional properties (see Chapter 5). Whereas other vasodilators, especially the arteriolar dilators, reflexly activate the renin-angiotensin axis, ACE inhibitors both vasodilate and inhibit this system, besides having sympatholytic properties.

Preload Reduction Normally as the preload (the LV filling pressure) increases so also does the peak LV systolic pressure, and the cardiac output rises (ascending limb of the Frank-Starling curve). In diseased hearts the increase in cardiac output is much less than normal, and the output fails to rise and may even fall as the filling pressure rises (the apparent descending limb of Frank-Starling curve). However, the optimal filling pressure for the diseased heart is very variable, not always being higher than normal. Reduction of the preload is generally but not always useful. Clinically, the major drugs reducing the preload in CHF are (1) furosemide by its diuretic effect and (2) the nitrates that dilate the systemic veins to reduce the venous return and thus the filling pressure in both the right and left heart chambers.

Afterload Reduction The therapeutic aim is reduction of the peripheral vascular resistance to lessen the load on the heart, improved renal function, and better skeletal muscle perfusion. Reduction of the systemic (= peripheral) vascular resistance is not the same as blood pressure reduction, because in CHF a compensatory increase in the cardiac output tends to maintain the arterial pressure during afterload reduction. Specific afterload reducers are few and limited in practice to two.

First, hydralazine is a nonspecific agent whose cellular mode of action is still undecided, although it may well act as a potassium channel opener. Second, the CCBs are also afterload reducers and widely used in hypertension. They often have a negative inotropic effect, thereby restricting their use in CHF, in which they are as a group contraindicated. Amlodipine may be an exception with, however, severe restrictions (see Chapter 3).

Combined Preload and Afterload Reduction Sodium nitroprusside, used for very severe hypertension or CHF, must be given intravenously under close supervision and careful monitoring. The *α-adrenergic blockers* give combined pre- and afterload reduction, the latter explaining their antihypertensive effect. Theoretically, they should also work in CHF but do not. Rather, as a group, they increase the incidence of heart failure when given as monotherapy for hypertension (see Chapter 7, p. 204). Of the two combined α-β-blockers, labetalol and carvedilol, only the latter is well tested in heart failure (Chapter 1, p. 16). The β-blocking component of these drugs should be able to inhibit β-mediated myocardial toxicity resulting from neuroadrenergic activation in heart failure, and the α-blocking component to reduce peripheral vasoconstriction.

Nitroprusside: The Prototype Balanced Vasodilator Nitroprusside is a donor of nitric oxide (NO) that vasodilates by formation of cyclic GMP in vascular tissue (see Fig. 2-2). Intravenous sodium nitroprusside (*Nipride, Nitropress*) remains the reference vasodilator for severe acute low output left-sided heart failure provided that the arterial pressure is reasonable, because it acts rapidly and has a balanced effect, dilating both arterioles and veins (Fig. 6-8). Nitroprusside, an ultrarapid agent, seems particularly useful for increasing LV stroke work in acute severe refractory heart failure caused by mitral or aortic regurgitation. Hemodynamic and clinical improvements are also observed in patients with severe pump failure complicating AMI, in heart failure after cardiac surgery, and in patients with acute exacerbation of chronic heart failure. Because of the need for careful continuous monitoring and its light sensitivity, and the severe risk of cyanide toxicity,[28] nitroprusside is being replaced in severe acute-on-chronic heart failure by nitrates or by the inotropic dilators such as milrinone, and in hypertensive crises by intravenous nicardipine or enalaprilat or fenoldopam or labetalol (see Table 7-6). Thus this agent is now used much less than previously.

Properties, Precautions, and Cyanide Toxicity With infusion of nitroprusside, the hemodynamic response (direct vasodilation) starts within minutes and stops equally quickly. Nitroprusside given intravenously is converted to cyanmethemoglobin and free cyanide in the red cells; the free cyanide is then converted to thiocyanate in the liver and is cleared by the kidneys (half-life 7 days). Extravasation must be avoided. The solution in normal saline (avoid alkaline solutions) must be freshly made and then shielded from light during infusion; it should be discarded when 4 hours old, or before if discolored. *Toxicity* is a special problem with nitroprusside especially when given at high doses or for long periods especially if there is liver or renal failure to limit cyanide metabolism and excretion of end products. Cyanide accumulation can kill cells by inhibition of oxidative metabolism, which leads to anaerobic metabolism with lactic acidosis. This sequence is potentially fatal. However, the latter may be a terminal event more related to circulatory failure.[28] The clinical picture of *cyanide toxicity* is very variable and goes from abdominal pain to unexplained death. Nervous system features are prominent and include changed mental status, unexplained encephalopathy, focal lesions, convulsions (cyanide apoplexy), and even brain death.[28] Cyanide toxicity is more common than often thought and can be avoided by (1) keeping the infusion dose as low and as short as possible, and no longer than 10 minutes at top dose in the treatment of severe hypertension; (2) maintaining clinical suspicion; (3) giving concomitant sodium thiosulfate,[28] and (4) searching for indirect evidence of toxicity such as increasing blood lactate and blood thiocyanate levels. Using the latter, it is sometimes permissible to go up to 3 days of low-dose nitroprusside when using this agent as a bridge to a mechanical assist device or to transplantation (see Indications). However, thiocyanate levels only indirectly reflect cyanide toxicity and give imperfect guidance. *Thiocyanate toxicity* is another hazard (toxic thiocyanate level 100 µg/mL). Thiocyanate is relatively nontoxic, but can become so in the presence of renal failure, giving a variety of GI and central nervous features, some of which overlap with cyanide toxicity.

Nitroprusside: Doses, Indications, and Contraindications The usual dose is 0.5 to 10 µg/kg/minute, but infusion at the maximal rate should *never* last for more than 10 minutes. The package insert gives a boxed warning that except when used briefly or at very low rates (<2 µg/kg/minute), that toxic cyanide can reach potentially lethal levels. The infusion rate needs careful titration against the blood pressure, which must be continuously monitored to avoid excess hypotension, which can be fatal. When treating severe hypertension, the package insert warns that if the blood pressure has not been adequately controlled after 10 minutes of infusion at the maximal rate, the drug should be stopped immediately. Conversely, nitroprusside must not be abruptly withdrawn during the treatment of heart failure because of the danger of rebound hypertension.

Indications include the following situations: (1) severe acute-on-chronic heart failure especially with regurgitant valve disease, to "rescue" the patient or to act as a bridge to transplantation or to a mechanical assist device; (2) in hypertensive crises (see Table 7-6); (3) in dissecting aneurysm; (4) for controlled hypotension in anesthesia (maximum dose 1.5 µg/kg/minute); and (5) after coronary bypass surgery, when patients frequently have reactive hypertension as they are removed from hypothermia, so that nitroprusside or nitrates may be given for 24 hours provided that hypotension is no problem. *Contraindications* are as follows: Preexisting hypotension (systolic <90 mmHg, diastolic <60 mmHg). All vasodilators are contraindicated in severe obstructive valvular heart disease (aortic or mitral or pulmonic stenosis, or obstructive cardiomyopathy). Unexpectedly, carefully monitored nitroprusside can improve cardiac output in very tight aortic stenosis with severe heart failure, acting as a bridge to valve replacement and showing that an increased total vascular resistance contributes to the load on the suffering left ventricle.[29] AMI is not a contraindication, provided that excess hypotension is avoided. Nitroprusside is contraindicated in hepatic or renal failure because clearance of toxic metabolites is depressed.

Side Effects of Nitroprusside Besides cyanide toxicity, these are as follows. Overvigorous treatment may cause an excessive drop in LV end-diastolic pressure, severe hypotension, and myocardial ischemia. Fatigue, nausea, vomiting, and disorientation caused by toxicity tend to arise, especially when treatment continues for more than 48 hours. In patients with renal failure, thiocyanate accumulates with high-dose infusions and may produce hypothyroidism after prolonged therapy. Hypoxia may result from increased ventilation-perfusion mismatch with pulmonary vasodilation.

Treatment of Cyanide Toxicity First, be vigilant to avoid it. Keep infusion rate low. Discontinue the infusion once the diagnosis is suspected (blood thiocyanate levels are only an indirect guide). Give sodium nitrite 3% solution at less than 2.5 ml/minute to total dose of 10 to 15 ml/minute, followed by an injection of sodium thiosulfate, 12.5 g in 50 ml of 5% dextrose water over 10 minutes. Repeat if needed at half these doses.

Nitrates

Nitrates are now used in the therapy of both acute and chronic heart failure (see Chapter 2). They work increasing vasodilatory vascular cyclic GMP. Their major effect is venous rather than arteriolar dilation, thus being most suited to patients with raised pulmonary wedge pressure and clinical features of pulmonary congestion. Nitrates produce a "pharmacologic phlebotomy." Intravenous nitrates are usually chosen above nitroprusside for acute pulmonary edema of myocardial infarction, because of the extensive experience with nitrates in large trials. The only favorable experience with long-term nitrate therapy is for chronic heart failure, in combination with hydralazine and before the era of ACE inhibitors and β-blockade (see Chapter 2). Besides acting as vasodilators, nitrates may oppose the harmful growth promoting effects of norepinephrine, raised in CHF, on cardiac mycocytes and fibroblasts.[30] However, this possible benefit, mediated by cyclic GMP, has not been translated into clinical practice.

Nesiritide

This agent (Natrecor) represents a new drug class, being a recombinant preparation of the human B-type natriuretic peptide (hBNP). This is identical to the endogenous hormone produced by the ventricles in response to increased wall stress and volume overload. It acts on guanylate cyclase in a similar way to nitric oxide (see Fig. 2-2), and therefore is a venous and arterial vasodilator. However, it has a greater effect than nitroglycerine in reducing right atrial pressure, pulmonary capillary wedge pressure, and cardiac index.[31] Nesiritide, when added to standard therapy by intravenous and/or oral diuretics, gave greater relief of dyspnea than did nitroglycerin.[31] Compared with dobutamine, nesiritide was required for a shorter period and gave a lower 6-month mortality, so that there was an overall saving in health costs.[32] Nesiritide is indicated for the intravenous treatment of patients with acutely decompensated congestive heart failure with dyspnea at rest or minimal activity. The dose is 2 μg/kg bolus, followed by an intravenous continuous infusion of 0.01 μg/kg/minute that may be increased up to a maximum of 0.03 μg/kg/minute with the rate-limiting side effect being hypotension. There is no experience with infusions for longer than 48 hours. There is no information about the possibility that tolerance might develop as in the case of nitroglycerine.

Hydralazine

Hydralazine is predominantly an arteriolar dilator. Its mechanism of action is not well understood. It causes a marked reactive increase in cardiac output with little or no decrease in pulmonary wedge or right atrial pressures. Hydralazine is particularly effective in patients with mitral regurgitation when it increases forward stroke volume and decreases regurgitant volume. It has also been tested in heart failure of ischemic or myopathic etiology.[33]

Pharmacokinetics and Use Hydralazine is rapidly absorbed from the gut (peak concentration 1 to 2 hours). It is metabolized via acetylation in the liver with subsequent excretion in the urine. The plasma half-life is 2 to 8 hours, but the hypotensive effect is longer lasting, possibly because of hydralazine binding to the arterial wall. In severe renal failure, the dosage should be reduced. Patients with fast acetylation rates need a dose about 25% higher than those with slow rates. Lupus syndrome is more likely to develop in slow acetylators. In *chronic LV failure*, in the Ve-HeFT trials, the dose of hydralazine combined with isosorbide dinitrate was 150 to 300 mg daily in four divided doses.[33] Hydralazine may potentiate nitrates by retarding the development of nitrate tolerance (see Chapter 2). The role of hydralazine alone in heart failure patients already treated by diuretics, ACE inhibitors, and other effective agents is not clear and not recommended.[3] Note that the FDA approves neither isosorbide dinitrate nor hydralazine nor the combination for treatment of CHF. In *hypertension*, hydralazine is still used where cost is important, often with diuretics and a β-blocker. The usual dose is 50 to 75 mg every 6 to 8 hours, but two divided doses a day are equally effective. Sometimes it is still given intravenously for severe hypertension without cardiac complications (see Table 7-6), as in pregnancy. *Side effects* include fluid retention (renin release) that may necessitate diuretic therapy. In hypertension, the tachycardia may be limited by concurrent β-blockade. The lupus syndrome is rare with doses below 200 mg a day or with total doses below 100 g. Patients on higher doses or prolonged therapy should be checked for antinuclear factors. In CHF, reflex tachycardia is unusual, perhaps because reflex arcs are blunted. Polyneuropathy (usually responsive to pyridoxine) and drug fever are rare side effects.

Adenosine

Adenosine is a purine nucleoside clinically used for its antiarrhythmic (see Chapter 8) and vasodilatory properties. Adenosine receptor stimulation lessens cyclic AMP, and hyperpolarizes the sarcolemma by increasing potassium conductance, thereby giving the effect against supraventricular tachycardias (see Fig. 8-7). Adenosine also indirectly blocks the inward calcium current. Physiologically, adenosine is formed from the breakdown of ATP to AMP (adenosine monophosphate) and the further breakdown of AMP to adenosine. It is transported into vascular smooth muscle cells by a specific adenosine transport system to act as a potent vasodilator. Adenosine is then either degraded by deamination or is rephosphorylated to reform AMP. As a *vasodilator*, it induces and maintains hypotension during surgery.[34] The two risks of such vasodilation are coronary "steal" (it increases coronary blood flow to the nonischemic myocardium) and cerebral vascular dilation, the latter precluding its use in those with intracranial hypertension.

Adenosine Use and Dosage Adenosine must be administered intravenously. It is very rapidly metabolized with a plasma half-life of seconds (see Chapter 8, p. 248). Besides its licensed indications as *Adenocard* in the treatment and diagnosis of supraventricular tachycardias, it is used in anesthesia for inducing hypotension or control of hypertensive episodes as a continuous intravenous infusion of 50 to 350 μg/kg/minute. Intravenous injections of adenosine, licensed as *Adenoscan* in the United States are used during thallium-201 and sestamibi cardiac imaging to assess coronary flow reserve in patients who cannot exercise. The dose is 140 μg/kg/minute for 6 min, to a total of 0.84 mg/kg. The thallium is injected at the mid-point of the adenosine infusion. Adenosine is also used to induce wall motion abnormalities, thereby diagnosing myocardial regions at risk for ischemia.

Drug Interactions with Adenosine Pharmacodynamic interactions may occur with other inhibitors of the sinus and AV nodes, such as β-blockers or verapamil or diltiazem, or with other vasodilators. *Methylxanthines*, including *theophylline* and *aminophylline*, competitively inhibit the adenosine receptors. *Dipyridamole* blocks the cellular uptake of adenosine and thus prolongs its effect. Some calcium blockers, including *verapamil, nitrendipine,* and *nifedipine,* inhibit the transport of adenosine into cells and may thereby potentiate its actions. *Benzodiazepines* reduce adenosine deaminase activity to potentiate adenosine.

Other Vasodilators

Enalaprilat This, the active form of enalapril, may be given intravenously to patients with severe hypertension (see Table 7-6).

Neutral Endopeptidase (NEP) Inhibitors Here the prototype drug is *omapatrilat*, already extensively tested in heart failure and in hypertension. However, due to the high incidence of angioedema, especially in black patients, it failed to achieve a license for hypertension in the United States. Omapatrilat and other endopeptidase inhibitors such as candoxatril[35] decrease the degradation of ANP and BNP, and improve hemodynamic and renal function in CHF. These powerful drugs are also ACE inhibitors. Their clinical use is limited by the relatively high rate of angioedema (Chapter 5, p. 115).

Dopamine-Receptor Stimulators *Fenoldopam* is a dopamine agonist (DA_1) able to reduce blood pressure in severe hypertension with a sodium diuresis in contrast to nitroprusside, which causes sodium retention. However, tachycardia is a prominent side effect. It is licensed for use in severe or malignant hypertension (see Table 7-6). Another dopamine agonist, *ibopamine*, was tested for chronic oral use in heart failure, but was withdrawn because of increased mortality.

THERAPY OF ACUTE HEART FAILURE

Acute LV failure (acute pulmonary oedema) is a complex situation often requiring multiple drugs acting at various sites, depending on the overall hemodynamic status (Fig. 6-10). The immediate treatment is upright sitting posture, oxygen, intravenous loop diuretics and morphine with or without an antiemetic. Nitrates or nesiritide may also be used in the relief of pulmonary edema. This treatment frequently achieves dramatic short-term benefits to save the patient from drowning in his own secretions. Subsequently sympathomimetic inotropes and inotropic dilators may provide limited further benefit. But there is little or no evidence that they give long-term benefit. Rather mortality may be increased (see section on Milrinone). Such drugs are best used as a means of temporarily supporting the failing heart, or as a bridge to an LV assist device or transplantation.[36] Inotropes or inodilators are indicated when the blood pressure is low and renal perfusion is reduced. An important choice, largely depending on the blood pressure and the peripheral perfusion (Fig. 6-10), is whether to give an agent increasing or decreasing the peripheral vascular resistance. Once acute intervention has stabilized the patient, the cause of the acute shock-like condition and/or the acute deterioration must be established. Thereafter, the management is that of chronic heart failure.

Logic for Combined Inotropic and/or Vasodilator Support There are several reasons for combining agents with different inotropic mechanisms. First, the β-stimulants such as dobutamine may become progressively ineffective over many hours, probably due to increasing β-receptor downregulation. Hence the addition of a PDE inhibitor that bypasses the β-receptor, to increase cyclic AMP is logical, especially in the presence of preexisting β-blockade.[36] Second, a frequent combination is that of dopamine to maintain the blood pressure with dobutamine to give inotropic support. Of note, *calcium sensitizers* such as levosimendan may displace β-stimulants from their prime position as inotropes of choice for acute heart failure.[36] Regarding vasodilators, nitroprusside, nitroglycerin or nesiritide may be combined with other agents to optimize the hemodynamic benefit. Prior β-blockade therapy should probably not be stopped during an acute exacerbation of heart fialure.[37] Maintaining an adequate ventricular filling pressure is essential with these combined therapies and invasive monitoring is required.

THERAPY OF CHRONIC SEVERE HEART FAILURE

When the acute phase is over, the patient is often left with chronic severe heart failure that requires a different management policy. That policy is almost the same as in patients presenting initially with

SHOCK, HYPOTENSION, PULMONARY EDEMA

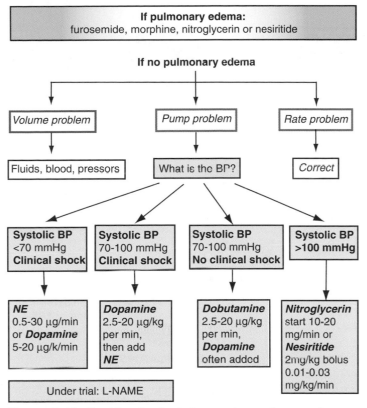

Figure 6-10 Algorithm for shock, hypotension, and acute pulmonary edema. Note important role of clinical judgment and decision making in management. For details of approach, see statement of American Heart Association Emergency Cardiac Care Committee, *JAMA* 1992;268:2199–2241. For nesiritide, see *JAMA* 2002;287;1531.

chronic heart failure. The diagnosis must be established with certainty, the etiology determined, concomitant disease identified, and an assessment of symptom severity and prognosis made (Fig. 6-1). Symptomatic therapy is aimed at achieving optimal diuresis to treat or prevent sodium and water retention. The disadvantageous neurohumoral response is inhibited by ACE inhibition, angiotensin receptor blockers, β-blockade, and aldosterone inhibitors (spironolactone) (Fig. 6-2). Digoxin may be used for the control of heart rate in atrial fibrillation and might contribute in sinus rhythm by acting as a sympathoinhibitory agent. Drugs should be used in the doses effective in the major trials.

Current Trends

Although the myocardium might be largely destroyed, symptomatic improvement is still possible using a judicious mixture of diuretics, ACE inhibition, β-adrenergic blockade, aldosterone blockers, digoxin, ARBs, and vasodilators (Fig. 6-11). Overall the strategy is to rest the feeble myocardium and to avoid stimulation. Drugs that improve prognosis are the ACE inhibitors, β-blockers, and aldosterone blockers, while diuretics relieve fluid retention and dyspnea, and yet others may be harmful (Table 6-8). Recent trends are, first, increasing use of the angiotensin receptor blockers (ARBs), often instead of ACE inhibitors; second, increasing mechanical intervention for severe heart failure, including biventricular pacing (cardiac resynchroniza-

MAXIMAL THERAPY FOR SEVERE CHF

Opie 2004

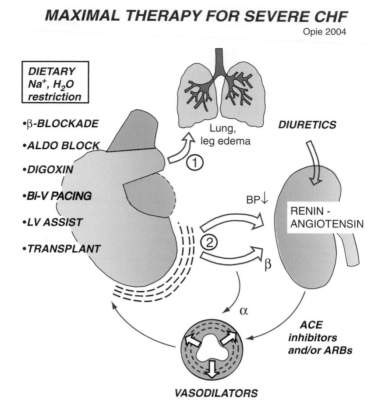

Figure 6-11 Principles of maximum therapy for CHF. Diuretics are given for back pressure into the lungs with edema (1) yet stimulate the renin-angiotensin system. Poor LV function also activates this system (2) by a low blood pressure with decreased renal perfusion and/or by reflex β-adrenergic *(β)* baroreceptor activation. Vasoconstriction results from formation of angiotensin-II *(AII)* and/or from α-adrenergic activity. Logically, ACE inhibitors or ARBs are an integral part of the therapy, as are β-blockers. Aldosterone *(Aldo)* blockers are essential. Digoxin is required when there is atrial fibrillation. Biventricular pacing *(Bi-V)*, also called CRT, is especially used when there is delayed conduction *(long QRS)*. LV assist devices are regarded as a bridge to transplantation. *(Figure © LH Opie, 2005.)*

tion therapy, CRT),[38] left ventricular assist devices (LVADs), and implantable cardioverter defibrillators (ICDs, see Fig. 8-10).

Uncertainty Regarding Role of ARBs

There is strong evidence for the use of an ARB in ACE inhibitor-intolerant patients. That policy is based on the findings of the ELITE II (losartan), Val-HeFT (valsartan), and CHARM-ALTERNATIVE (candesartan) trials as discussed in Chapter 5. In addition, three large trials have reported on the use of angiotensin receptor blockers (ARBs) in chronic heart failure and two for heart failure during or soon after an acute myocardial infarction. These trials are, respectively, ELITE II, Val-HeFT, CHARM, OPTIMAAL, and VALIANT (see Chapter 5). None of the trials showed an ARB to be worse than an ACE inhibitor but there were many differences relating to power of the studies, drug used, formulation of the drug, and whether the ARB was tested against an ACE inhibitor or against placebo on top of an ACE inhibitor. At the same time two large studies with added aldosterone blockers, spironolactone, or eplerenone, the RALES (chronic heart failure) and EPHESUS (heart failure post-MI) studies, showed a substantial reduction of mortality. Thus there are now three ways in which the renin-angiotensin-aldosterone pathway may be inhibited: an ACE inhibitor, an ARB, or

Table 6-8	Heart Failure; Drugs That Reduce Mortality, Improve Symptoms, or Might Harm

Reduce Mortality; Must Try to Use

1. ACE inhibitors
2. β-Blockers
3. Spironolactone or eplerenone

Improve Symptoms; Use According to Clinical Judgment

1. Diuretics
2. Digoxin (low dose)
3. Nitrates

May Be Harmful; Use Cautiously After Due Consideration

1. Inotropes and inotropic dilators
2. Antiarrhythmics, except β-blockers and amiodarone
3. Calcium channel blockers
4. High-dose digoxin

Table drawn up in collaboration with P.J. Commerford.

aldosterone blockade. There is a danger of polypharmacy. Which combination of drugs is best for which patient is very uncertain. The most difficult question relates to a patient already treated with diuretics, an ACE inhibitor, and a β-blocker. Should an ARB, an aldosterone antagonist, or both be added? Whereas in VALIANT it was not beneficial,[39] in the CHARM-added study the ARB-ACE inhibitor combination was.[40] One difference may lie in the intensity of the heart failure, the majority in CHARM being in class III, whereas in VALIANT most were in classes I and II. Hypothetically, those with more severe heart failure and a higher use of diuretics would be expected to have greater renin-angiotensin activation, and hence more response to the ARB-ACE inhibitor combination.

Choice of β-Blocker

A second area of uncertainty has arisen with regard to the selection of a β-blocker. The COMET trial tested the hypothesis that carvedilol (a nonselective β-blocker) was superior to the cardioselective blocker metoprolol tartrate in the treatment of chronic heart failure.[41] The study showed a large reduction of mortality with carvedilol in contrast to metoprolol. Does this major difference reflect the short-acting formulation of metoprolol and the dose that was used, or the benefits of added β_2-blockade due to carvedilol? The issue of what would have happened had carvedilol been compared to the long-acting formulation of metoprolol in the doses that are licensed for heart failure in the United States, will never be solved. In the presence of asthma, the more cardioselective metoprolol may be chosen. Otherwise there are several arguments for carvedilol. It is licensed in the United States for a large number of indications related to various stages of heart failure, including post-MI LV dysfunction, mild heart failure, moderate heart failure, and severe heart failure. There were few problems upon the careful addition of carvedilol to class IV patients already treated by a diuretic and an ACE inhibitor or ARB, provided that there was no clinical fluid retention.[42] In addition, carvedilol decreases systemic and cardiac norepinephrine spillover, an effect not shared by short-acting metoprolol, and possibly explained by inhibition of presynaptic β_2-receptors.[43]

Maximum Therapy of Congestive Heart Failure

General measures and lifestyle include mild salt restriction (avoid excessive intake of salt) and, in the presence of poor renal perfusion, water restriction. Anemia, if present, warrants therapy. Although periodic bed rest may be required to achieve optimal diuresis (the patient returning to bed for 1 to 2 hours of supine rest after taking the diuretic), in principle physical activity should be maintained and, if possible, an exercise rehabilitation program undertaken for which there is strong evidence.[44] One of the most cost-effective of the new approaches to CHF is *home-based intervention* by a cardiac nurse, which reduces hospitalization and improves event-free survival.[45] Such home nursing visits give advice and support and oversee drug therapy, often very complex in advanced heart failure. Advice should be given on flu immunization, alcohol consumption, cessation of smoking, sexual activity, diet, drug interactions, exercise, flying, lifestyle, and risk factors.

Diuretic doses must be carefully adjusted to steer the course between optimal relief of edema and excess diuresis with ionic disturbances and prerenal azotemia. In the elderly, excess use of diuretics can lead to tiredness and fatigue. Following the principle of sequential nephron blockade (see Fig. 4-2), combination diuretic therapy will often be required and is usually more comfortable for patients. In those unusual patients who have severe heart failure with major restriction of the GFR (below 15 to 20 ml/minute), high doses of furosemide alone or more often combined with a thiazide diuretic are used. Metolazone is a powerful diuretic used in difficult resistant cases. Potassium sparers are often combined with those diuretics that do not spare potassium. In diuretic-resistant patients, first check for interacting drugs, especially nonsteroidal anti-inflammatory drugs (NSAIDs) (see Fig. 4-4). Oral furosemide has variable absorption characteristics and occasionally the patient may benefit by a change to the better absorbed torsemide.[46] Intermittent low-dose dopamine infusions are not normally recommended but might occasionally help to improve renal blood flow and to initiate a diuresis. Nesiritide can also be used in this situation.

ACE inhibitors. The key concept is that ACE inhibitors should be used or at least considered for use in all patients. They should be titrated upwards to the doses used in clinical trials unless hypotension or symptoms such as dizziness manifest themselves. When an ACE inhibitor is introduced for the first time to a patient already receiving high-dose diuretics (and therefore with intense renin-angiotensin activation), the diuretic dose must first be reduced and care taken to minimize or avoid first-dose hypotension. When an ACE inhibitor is truly not tolerated because of, for example, severe coughing, first ensure that worsening heart failure is not the cause of the cough, and then change to an angiotensin receptor blocker (ARB) on the basis of five large trials (ELITE-2, CHARM, Val-HeFT, OPTIMAAL and VALIANT; see Chapter 5).

β-Blockers have reduced mortality substantially. The specific agents tested are: bisoprolol (CIBIS II), metoprolol succinate (MERIT-HF), and carvedilol (COPERNICUS), with doses as given in Table 1-2. As a consequence all patients with chronic heart failure and an enlarged heart should be considered for treatment with a β-blocker. The patient should be hemodynamically stable when treatment is initiated. That usually means that the treatment is begun not in hospital but in a heart failure unit. β-Blockade is not a "rescue" treatment for more severe heart failure. Even class IV patients can be tried on a β-blocker, specifically carvedilol.[42] It is essential to start with a very low dose of the β-blocker, to set aside those patients reacting adversely, and then to titrate the dose upwards slowly and steadily over many weeks. Incremental increases of dose should not be undertaken in less than 2 weeks. There is no hurry. Some physicians strive to reach the target dose in trials; others are cautious. Once the heart rate is reduced by about ten beats, the patient is clearly β-blocked to some degree.

Spironolactone reduces mortality in class III and IV patients otherwise optimally treated. The drug is being widely used in class II patients although there is no formal trial in such patients. EPHESUS has shown an important mortality benefit with *eplerenone* (a new aldosterone inhibitor) in patients with heart failure related to acute myocardial infarction (see Chapter 5). Eplerenone causes less gynecomastia than spironolactone. With either agent, plasma potassium needs careful monitoring to avoid potentially lethal hyperkalemia, and this therapy is not substantiated for those with renal failure.

Angiotensin-II receptor blockers (ARBs) are now being widely used in patients who are, for whatever reason, intolerable of ACE inhibitors. Whether patients should receive an ARB in addition to an ACE inhibitor is controversial. There is also no trial or any accepted policy giving guidance as to whether an ARB should be added to therapy before, after, or with an aldosterone antagonist.

Digoxin, as considered in detail in this chapter, is no longer regarded as an essential drug but rather an optional choice, often given in lower doses than before, on the grounds that it may reduce hospitalization. Its many drug interactions and contradictions also limit its use. Amazingly, after more than 200 years of use, the optimal serum level is still not known, though falling all the time. Digoxin still has a place in heart failure with atrial fibrillation, especially in combination with β-blockade, where optimal inhibition of the AV node and improved LV function is required.

Antiarrhythmics may be required. Ventricular tachyarrhythmias are a major cause of fatalities in CHF. It is important to avoid predisposing factors such as hypokalemia, digoxin excess, or chronic use of PDE inhibitors. Class I agents should be avoided. Long-term amiodarone may be considered in a low dose, and where there are facilities and there are good indications, an implantable cardioverter defibrillator (ICD) may be chosen, as outlined in Chapter 8. Atrial fibrillation is a common and serious problem, and requires one of two policies: either conversion to sinus rhythm and thereafter probably low-dose amiodarone, or rate control both at rest and during exercise (see Chapter 11, p. 376).

Short-term inotropic support by sympathomimetics or inotropic dilators cannot be lightly undertaken. Yet milrinone or others may give dramatic relief as a rescue operation, when inotropic support is essential. In patients with exacerbation of heart failure, and not needing urgent inotropic or pressor support, there may be modest benefit in those with nonischemic at the risk of adverse effects.[25,26] There is no role for intermittent outpatient infusions of dopamine or dobutamine. An apparently paradoxical use for PDE inhibition is in severe heart failure, in patients who cannot tolerate β-blockade, where the inotropic support acts as a bridge to the introduction of a β-blocker.[47] Larger trials are now testing this proposal.[36]

Vasodilator therapy. In patients who remain symptomatic despite full therapy (diuretics, ACE inhibitors, β-blockers, spironolactone, ARBs, and probably digoxin) isosorbide dinitrate with hydralazine is worth trying.

Novel drugs. Those that should work but have been disappointing include (1) endothelin antagonists, which unload the heart by vasodilation and improve coronary endothelial integrity, and (2) cytokine antagonists, including etanercept which decoys tumor necrosis factor-α (TNF-α) from its receptor. *Pentoxyfylline* is a complex agent that decreases the synthesis of TNF-α and improves the ejection fraction, yet it also has PDE activity and outcome data are missing. Vasopressin (ADH, antidiuretic hormone) antagonists are logical.[47a] New diuretics include the adenosine (A_1) receptor antagonists[48] that protect against the decline in renal function found with standard diuretics, such as furosemide. At a molecular level it should be possible to modulate the adverse effects of myocyte death by apoptosis. Of these, the only agents that are already available and licensed, albeit not for use in CHF, are pentoxyfylline and etanercept.

Cardiac resynchronization therapy (CRT) and implantable cardioverter defibrillators (ICDs) are being increasingly used in patients with heart failure. Both devices have been shown to reduce mortality in large clinical trials or in meta-analyses, but several important trials have not yet reported. The precise indications are still controversial. CRT is usually considered when there is QRS prolongation as a sign of impaired intraventricular conduction, but may also help when the QRS is narrow. These treatments may be life-saving but are expensive, which raises severe problems in relation to national medical budgets.

Cardiac surgery must be considered when valve defects are present, or there is clear evidence of myocardial ischemia, or a remodeling procedure is indicated. Mechanical assist devices may bridge the gap between the decision to transplant and the availability of a donor heart. Mechanical assist devices are being considered for lifetime treatment. Nonetheless, the prognosis in such patients given modern medical management may be more favorable than previously anticipated. For example, there is only one formal trial of assist devices (REMATCH).[49] In it, the device was better than medical therapy in prolonging survival over 2 years. But only 20% to 24% of patients were given β-blockers, a percentage that today would be regarded as unacceptable.

Cardiac transplantation is a measure of last resort. The number of procedures is falling partly because of the lack of donors and the improvement of medical therapy. The indications are now more stringent than previously. There are no controlled trials of transplantation.

S U M M A R Y

1. *Heart failure is a complex potentially fatal condition,* which includes acute heart failure, often needing therapy by intravenous furosemide and short-term inotropes, and chronic heart failure that requires neurohumoral antagonism by ACE inhibitors (or ARBs), β-blockers, and aldosterone blockers, besides diuretics.

2. *Digoxin becomes optional.* In the past, digoxin was standard therapy in congestive heart failure, at a time when inotropic therapy was regarded as desirable. A major problem is that the ideal dose and blood levels are not known, though clearly lower than before. Its use in patients already optimally treated by mortality-reducing drugs such as β-blockers, ACE inhibitors, and aldosterone blockers has never been tested. A small mortality benefit may exist at blood levels below 1.0 ng/mL, converting to a 12% mortality increase at higher blood levels (previously regarded as therapeutic). Thus the therapeutic-toxic window is small. There are also many contraindications to the use of digoxin and many interacting drugs. All these problems make digoxin a difficult drug to use correctly. The strongest indication for digoxin remains the combination of atrial fibrillation and congestive heart failure. Otherwise, in our view, digoxin is now relegated to an optional extra in the management of CHF, given chiefly to obtain symptomatic benefit, and requiring careful dosing.

3. *Acute heart failure with pulmonary edema* is treated with oxygen, intravenous diuretics, morphine, and an antiemetic. Nitrates and (where available) levosimendan are alternative therapies. Nesiritide is a vasodilatory natriuretic peptide.

4. *Cardiogenic shock with or without pulmonary edema.* β-Receptor stimulatory inotropes are often used in the acute therapy of severe heart failure but these drugs may further damage the myocardium. The problem of β-receptor downregulation may require added PDE inhibition. Available drugs are dobutamine and dopamine. Calcium sensitizing drugs may have a role not yet clearly defined.

5. *Inotropic-dilators (PDE inhibitors).* Although these are no longer used in oral form, the intravenous preparations with their inotropic and vasodilator effects should be especially useful in patients with β-receptor downgrading, as in severe CHF or during prolonged therapy with dobutamine or other $β_1$-stimulants, or after chronic β-blockade. Thus milrinone has a limited place in the management of short-term therapy of heart failure.

6. *Load reduction and vasodilators.* These are often chosen in severe acute heart failure, especially when the blood pressure is relatively well maintained, to relieve the burden on the failing myocardium. Such agents include furosemide, nitrates, nesiritide, and nitroprusside. They may be carefully combined with agents that give inotropic or pressure support such as dobutamine or dopamine.

7. *Current approaches to chronic heart failure.* The four major new approaches to the management of CHF are, first, inhibition of the β-adrenergic response by β-blockers initially given in very low doses; second, inhibition of aldosterone effects by spironolactone or eplerenone; and, third the use of ARBs. General measures include intense monitoring of the patient at home by visits from a cardiac nurse and exercise training. Mechanical and electrical devices (ICDs, CRT, and mechanical assist devices) are under evaluation but increasingly used with substantial trial support.

8. *The future therapy of heart failure.* It is dangerous to be a prophet. Some small advances may emerge from further neurohumoral inhibition with novel vasopressin inhibitors. Inhibitors or stimulants of the many growth pathways could be advantageous. Stem cell therapy is likely to become feasible. Further developments in mechanical devices are certain to happen. Ultimately heart failure is a biological problem and the solution will lie in the prevention of the causes of the disorder and in the ability to replace or repair the myocardial cells using gene therapy or stem cell regeneration. What is not in doubt is that the pharmacological therapy of congestive heart failure is a topic characterized by increasing innovation and excitement.

REFERENCES

1. Lewis T. *Diseases of the Heart.* 1933, London: Macmillan.
2. Digitalis Investigation Group. The effect of digoxin on mortality and morbidity in patients with heart failure. *N Engl J Med* 1997;336:525–533.
3. Packer M, et al. Consensus recommendations for the management of chronic heart failure. *Am J Cardiol* 1999;83 (2A):1A–38A.
4. Slatton M, et al. Does digoxin provide additional hemodynamic and autonomic benefit at higher doses in patients with mild to moderate heart failure and normal sinus rythm? *J Am Coll Cardiol* 1997;29:1206–1213.
5. Hauptman P, et al. Digitalis. *Circulation* 1999;99:1265–1270.
6. Gheorghiade M, et al. Digoxin in the management of cardiovascular disorders. *Circulation* 2004;109:2959–2964.
7. Eichhorn EJ, et al. Digoxin—new perspective on an old drug. *N Engl J Med* 2002;347: 1394–1395.
8. McMichael J, et al. The action of intravenous digoxin in man. *Q J Med* 1944;13: 123–135.
9. PROVED Study. Randomised study assessing the effects of digoxin withdrawal in patients with mild to moderate chronic congestive heart failure. Results of the PROVED trial. *J Am Coll Cardiol* 1993;22:955–962.
10. RADIANCE Study. Withdrawal of digoxin from patients with chronic heart failure treated with angiotensin-converting enzyme inhibitors. *N Engl J Med* 1993;329:1–7.
11. Rathore SS, et al. Association of serum digoxin concentration and outcomes in patients with heart failure. *JAMA* 2003;289:871–878.
12. Tieleman R, et al. Digoxin delays recovery from tachycardia-induced electrical remodeling of the atria. *Circulation* 1999;100:1836–1842.
13. Khand AU, et al. Carvedilol alone or in combination with digoxin for the management of atrial fibrillation in patients with heart failure? *J Am Coll Cardiol* 2003;42:1944–1951.
14. PROMISE Study. Effect of oral milrinone on mortality in severe chronic heart failure. *N Engl J Med* 1991;325:1468–1475.
15. Adams KF, Jr., et al. Clinical benefits of low serum digoxin concentrations in heart failure. *J Am Coll Cardiol* 2002;39:946–953.
16. O'Connor CM, et al. Continuous intravenous dobutamine is associated with an increased risk of death in patients with advanced heart failure: insights from the Flolan International Randomized Survival Trial (FIRST). *Am Heart J* 1999;138:78–86.

17. Al-Hesayen A, et al. The effects of dobutamine on cardiac sympathetic activity in patients with congestive heart failure. *J Am Coll Cardiol* 2002;39:1269–1274.

18. Galley HF. Renal-dose dopamine: will the message now get through? *Lancet* 2000;356:2112.

19. Johnson R. Low-dose dopamine and oxygen transport by the lung. *Circulation* 1998;98:97–99.

20. Gare M, et al. The renal effect of low-dose dopamine in high-risk patients undergoing coronary angiography. *J Am Coll Cardiol* 1999;34:1682–1688.

21. Follath F, et al. Efficacy and safety of intravenous levosimendan compared with dobutamine in severe low-output heart failure (the LIDO study): a randomised double-blind trial. *Lancet* 2002;360:196–202.

22. Opie LH. Inodilators. *Lancet* 1986;1:1336.

23. Stemple DR, et al. Combined nitroprusside-dopamine therapy in severe chronic congestive heart failure. Dose-related hemodynamic advantages over single drug infusions. *Am J Cardiol* 1978;42:267–275.

24. DiBianco R, et al. A comparison of oral milrinone, digoxin, and their combination in the treatment of patients with chronic heart failure. *N Engl J Med* 1989;320: 677–683.

25. Cuffe MS, et al. Short-term intravenous milrinone for acute exacerbation of chronic heart failure. *JAMA* 2002;287:1541–1547.

26. Felker GM, et al. Heart failure etiology and response to milrinone in decompensated heart failure: results from the OPTIME-CHF study. *J Am Coll Cardiol* 2003;41: 997–1003.

27. Cowley AJ, et al. On behalf of the Enoximome Investigators. Treatment of severe heart failure: quantity or quality of life? A trial of enoximone. *Br Heart J* 1994;72:226–230.

28. Robin ED, et al. Nitroprusside-related cyanide poisoning. Time (long past due) for urgent, effective interventions. *Chest* 1992;102:1842–1845.

29. Khot UN, et al. Nitroprusside in critically ill patients with left ventricular dysfunction and aortic stenosis. *N Engl J Med* 2003;348:1756–1763.

30. Calderone A, et al. Nitric oxide, atrial natriuretic peptide, and cyclic GMP inhibit the growth-promoting effects of norepinephrine in cardiac myocytes. *J Clin Invest* 1998;101:812–818.

31. VMAC Investigators. Intravenous nesiritide vs nitroglycerin for treatment of decompensated congestive heart failure. *JAMA* 2002;287:1531–1540.

32. Silver MA, et al. Effect of nesiritide versus dobutamine on short-term outcomes in the treatment of patients with acutely decompensated heart failure. *J Am Coll Cardiol* 2002;39:798–803.

33. Cohn J, et al. Effect of vasodilator therapy on mortality in chronic congestive heart failure. Results of Veterans Administration Cooperative Study. *N Engl J Med* 1986;1986:1547–1552.

34. Owall A, et al. Clinical experience with adenosine for controlled hypotension during cerebral aneurysm surgery. *Anesth Analg* 1987;66:229–234.

35. Westheim AS, et al. Hemodynamic and neuroendocrine effects for candoxatril and frusemide in mild stable chronic heart failure. *J Am Coll Cardiol* 1999;34:794–801.

36. Felker GM, et al. Inotropic therapy for heart failure: an evidence-based approach. *Am Heart J* 2001;142:393–401.

37. Gattis WA, et al. Clinical outcomes in patients on beta-blocker therapy admitted with worsening chronic heart failure. *Am J Cardiol* 2003;91:169–174.

38. Bradley DJ, et al. Cardiac resynchronization and death from progressive heart failure. *JAMA* 2003;289:730–740.

39. Pfeffer MA, et al. Valsartan, captopril or both in myocardial infarction complicated by heart failure, left ventricular dysfunction or both. *N Engl J Med* 2003;349: 1893–1906.

40. McMurray JJ, et al. Effects of candesartan in patients with chronic heart failure and reduced left-ventricular systolic function taking angiotensin-converting-enzyme inhibitors: the CHARM-Added trial. *Lancet* 2003;362:767–771.

41. Poole-Wilson PA, et al. Comparison of carvedilol and metoprolol on clinical outcomes in patients with chronic heart failure in the Carvedilol Or Metoprolol European Trial (COMET): randomised controlled trial. *Lancet* 2003;362:7–13.

42. Krum H, et al. Effects of initiating carvedilol in patients with severe chronic heart failure: results from the COPERNICUS Study *JAMA* 2003;289:712–718.

43. Azevedo ER, et al. Nonselective versus selective β-adrenergic receptor blockade in congestive heart failure. *Circulation* 2001;104:2194–2199.

44. ExTraMATCH Collaborative. Exercise training meta-analysis of trials in patients with chronic heart failure (ExTraMATCH). *Br Med J* 2004;328:189.

45. Stewart S, et al. Effects of a multidisciplinary, home based intervention on unplanned readmissions and survival among patients with chronic congestive heart failure: a randomised controlled study. *Lancet* 1999;354:1077–1083.

46. Brater D. Pharmacology of diuretics. *Am J Med Sci* 2000;319:38–50.

47. Shakar SF, et al. Combined oral positive inotropic and beta-blocker therapy for treatment of refractory class IV heart failure. *J Am Coll Cardiol* 1998;31:1336–1340.

47a. Gheorghiade M, et al. Effects of tolvaptan, a vasopressin antagonist, in patients hospitalized with worsening heart failure. *JAMA* 2004;291:1963–1971.

48. Gottlieb SS, et al. BG9719 (CVT-124), an A1 adenosine receptor antagonist, protects against the decline in renal function observed with diuretic therapy. *Circulation* 2002;105:1348–1353.

49. REMATCH Study Group. Long-term use of a left ventricular assist device for end-stage heart failure. *N Engl J Med* 2001;345:1435–1443.

50. Ruffolo R. The mechanism of action of dobutamine. *Ann Intern Med* 1984;100: 313–314.

51. Bristow M. Changes in myocardial and vascular receptors in heart failure. *J Am Coll Cardiol* 1993;22 (Suppl A):61A–71A.

7

Antihypertensive Drugs

Norman M. Kaplan • Lionel H. Opie

> "Treatment with any commonly-used regimen reduces the risk of total major cardiovascular events, and the larger reductions in blood pressure produce larger reduction in risk."
>
> BP LOWERING TREATMENT TRIALISTS, 2003[1]

The blood pressure (BP) is the product of the cardiac output (CO) and the peripheral vascular resistance (PVR):

$$BP = CO \times PVR$$

Hence all antihypertensive drugs must act either by reducing the CO (β-blockers and diuretics) or the peripheral vascular resistance (all the others, and perhaps a late effect of β-blockade). Diuretics act chiefly by volume depletion, thereby reducing the CO, and also as indirect vasodilators. Most of the antihypertensive drugs, including diuretics, β-blockers, angiotensin-converting enzyme (ACE) inhibitors, angiotensin-II receptor blockers (ARBs), and calcium channel blockers (CCBs), but excluding the centrally active agents and ganglion blockers, have other uses and are therefore discussed elsewhere in this book. Despite the host of potential agents, the therapy of hypertension is usually simple, as many patients have minimally or moderately elevated pressures that usually respond adequately to lifestyle modification and to one, two or, at the most, three drugs (Table 7-1). Recently the BP goals have dropped, especially in those with diabetes, renal disease, or target organ damage, thereby increasing the requirement for combination therapy. Asymptomatic patients, however, often will not stay on therapy, particularly if it makes them feel weak, sleepy, forgetful, or impotent. In this regard, the ACE inhibitors and especially the ARBs seem very well tolerated. Fortunately, with most currently used modern antihypertensive agents, the quality of life improves rather than deteriorates.[2,3] A small proportion of patients have resistant hypertension that responds only to multiple therapies after excluding poor compliance or secondary cause. It must constantly be considered that hypertension is usually multifactorial in etiology, that different drugs act by different mechanisms (Fig. 7-1), and that the aim is to match the drug to the patient.

PRINCIPLES OF TREATMENT

The Decision to Treat: Nondrug Therapy for ALL

Before any drug therapy is begun, the persistence of the patient's hypertension should be ascertained by multiple measurements over at least a few weeks, preferably at home and at work, unless the pressure is so high as to mandate immediate therapy. Nondrug therapies should be standard in all hypertensive patients, particularly weight reduction for obese patients and moderate dietary *sodium restriction* from the usual level of about 10 g per day down to about 5 g sodium chloride (85 mmol) or 2.0 g sodium (88 mmol), which will reduce the BP by about 7/4 mmHg in hypertensive individuals, according to a meta-analysis of 28 trials.[4] If this change were applied to a whole population, there would be an expected 14% reduction in stroke deaths. In the DASH-sodium study, further sodium chloride restriction to about 4 g per day (urinary sodium of 65 mmol/day) enhanced

185

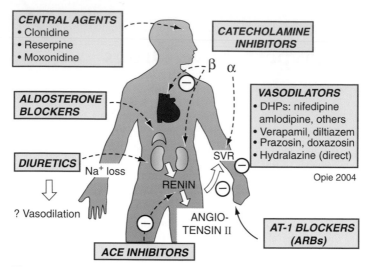

Figure 7-1 Different types of antihypertensive agents act at different sites. Because hypertension is frequently multifactorial in origin, it may be difficult to find the ideal drug for a given patient and drug combinations are often used. *ARBs* = angiotensin receptor blockers; *AT-1* = angiotensin II subtype 1; *DHPs* = dihydropyridines; *SVR* = systemic vascular resistance. (*Figure © LH Opie, 2005.*)

Table 7-1 Specifics About Some Orally Effective Antihypertensives

Drug	Registered Trade Name (in USA)	Dose Range (mg/day)	Doses/Day

For diuretics (see Tables 4-3, 4-5, 4-6), **β-blockers** (see Table 1-3), **combined α-β-blockers** (see Table 1-3), **ACE inhibitors** (see Table 5-4), **angiotensin receptor blockers (ARBs)** (see Table 5-12), **calcium antagonists (CCBs)** (see Tables 3-2, 3-5)

α-Blockers			
Prazosin	Minipress	2.0–20.0	2
Terazosin	Hytrin	1–20	1
Doxazosin	Cardura	1–16	1
Direct Vasodilators			
Hydralazine	Apresoline	50–200	2–3
Minoxidil	Loniten	5–40	1
Nonreceptor Adrenergic Inhibitors			
Reserpine	Serpasil	0.05–0.25	1
Rauwolfia root	Raudixin	50–100	1
Centrally Active			
Methyldopa	Aldomet	500–1500	2
Clonidine	Catapres	0.5–1.5	2–3
Clonidine transdermal	Catapres-TTX	1 patch	(Once weekly)
Guanabenz	Wytensin	8–64	2
Guanfacine	Tenex	1–3	1
Peripheral			
Guanethidine	Ismelin	10–150	1
Guanadrel	Hylorel	10–75	2

the BP-lowering benefits of the high-fruit, high-vegetable DASH-diet to give a total reduction of about 7 mmHg lower than the standard diet. This degree of BP fall is about the same as that achieved with an effective antihypertensive agent. Thus the *ideal diet* is low in calories, rich in fresh rather than processed foods, and high in fruits and vegetables (and hence high in potassium) besides being low in fat and sodium.[5] *Weight loss* reduces BP, improves the quality of life, and specifically benefits those with left ventricular hypertrophy.[6] Multifactorial intervention with both weight loss and sodium restriction should be used before drug therapy is instituted, especially in the elderly and in those with marginal BP elevations.[7] Other measures include increased *aerobic exercise*,[8] cessation of smoking, and moderation of alcohol. Smoking is an independent risk factor for coronary heart disease and stroke, besides increasing the risk of malignant hypertension (via accelerated renal artery damage).

Ideal BP Levels A radical change in approach to modestly or even minimally elevated BP has resulted from a 12-year follow up of subjects in the Framingham Heart Study[9] and from a mega-meta analysis on one million adults.[10] Any increase in BP above 115/75 mmHg increases cardiovascular risk which doubles with every rise of 20/10 mmHg.[10] The previously normal and high-normal BP ranges of 120 to 139 mmHg systolic and 80 to 89 mmHg diastolic are now considered *prehypertensive*, with calls for active lifestyle changes to avoid moving into the overtly hypertensive category, which remains 140/90 mmHg or more.[11,12] Increased longevity means that these stricter views have led to more active antihypertensive intervention at lower BP levels; sometimes this even involves giving drugs where there are no solid trial data such as in those below 140/90 mmHg, where only lifestyle modification is presently appropriate. Lifestyle management also remains the first-line approach for diastolic pressures of 90 to 95 mmHg or even higher, depending on the risk factor profile (Table 7-2). However, seeing that cardiovascular risk starts at only 115/75 mmHg, and considering the shocking statistic that middle-aged American adults have a 90% lifetime risk of developing hypertension,[13] the real recommendation should be "lifestyle modification for all."

When in doubt about a marginal BP level, multiple out-of-the-office readings should be obtained, either by inexpensive *home BP* devices or by *ambulatory BP monitoring*. As hypertension is merely one of several risk factors for coronary artery disease or stroke, it makes sense to treat at lower BP values in smokers or diabetic individuals, or in the presence of higher blood cholesterols or angina or left ventricular hypertrophy (LVH). Conversely, in very low risk groups (nonsmoking middle-aged white women) there may not be much advantage in drug treatment of mild to moderate hypertension. Consequently, risk factor stratification is now advised in all expert guidelines.

Risk Factors The efficacy of antihypertensive treatment depends not only on the control of the BP, but also on the control of coexisting risk factors, especially those for coronary heart disease, which is the major cause of mortality in hypertension (Fig. 7-2). Whereas in low-risk groups, many hundreds of patients must be treated to prevent one stroke, in very high risk groups, such as the elderly, only 20 to 25 patients need to be treated for 1 year to prevent one cardiovascular event, including stroke. To aid the assessment of risk factors, there are the well-known Framingham tables and several websites including *www.chdrisk.com*, and others. Explaining the exact risk over 10 years to a specific patient often helps in achieving a desirable lifestyle and reaching BP goals. Here the new European guidelines show color-coded tables, with the highest risk of 10-year fatality being in red and the lowest in green.[14] The patient can readily grasp that reaching a specific BP goal means moving from a "bad" color, say orange, to a better one, say yellow, with less risk of stroke or heart attack. However, none of the available risk calculations factor in the "new boy on the block," C-reactive protein (CRP), that together with a high BP can increase risk more than threefold.[15]

Systolic versus Diastolic versus Pulse Pressure Although all recommendations for treatment in the past were based on a cutoff diastolic BP

Table 7-2 Risk Stratification in Treatment of Hypertension

Other Risk Factors and Disease History	Blood Pressure (mmHg)				
	Normal SBP 120–129 or DBP 80–84	High Normal SBP 130–139 or DBP 85–89	Grade 1 SBP 140–159 or DBP 90–99	Grade 2 SBP 160–179 or DBP 100–109	Grade 3 SBP ≥ 180 or DBP ≥ 110
No other risk factors	Average risk	Average risk	<15% 10-yr risk	15–20% 10-yr risk	20–30% 10-yr risk
One or two risk factors	<15% 10-yr risk	<15% 10-yr risk	15–20% 10-yr risk	15–20% 10-yr risk	>30% 10-yr risk
Three or more risk factors or TOD or diabetes mellitus	15–20% 10-yr risk	20–30% 10-yr risk	20–30% 10-yr risk	20–30% 10-yr risk	>30% 10-yr risk
Associated clinical conditions	20–30% 10-yr risk	>30% 10-yr risk	>30% 10-yr risk	>30% 10-yr risk	>30% 10-yr risk

Based on and modified from recommendations of European Societies of Cardiology and Hypertension.[21] 10-year risk of cardiovascular disease according to Framingham criteria.

Risk factors for coronary heart disease (note slight differences from ATP III in Chapter 10): blood pressure as above; cholesterol level >250 mg/dL, LDL > 155 mg/dL, HDL-cholesterol <40 mg/dL in men, <48 mg/dL in women; family history of premature CHD; smoking; age (men > 55, women > 65), abdominal obesity, C-reactive protein ≥1 mg/dL.

TOD, target organ damage: left ventricular hypertrophy; ultrasound evidence of arterial disease, increased serum creatinine up to 1.5 mg/dL (133 μmol/L) in males, slightly lower in females, microalbuminuria up to 300 mg/24 h.

Associated clinical conditions: cerebrovascular disease including transient ischemic attack (TIA); angina or myocardial infarction; congestive heart failure; renal impairment; proteinuria; peripheral vascular disease; advanced retinopathy.

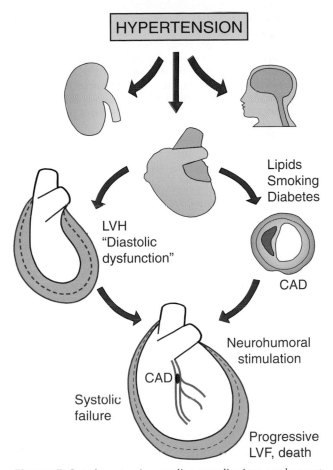

Figure 7-2 In hypertension, cardiac complications are the most common cause of death. Hypertension also kills by renal and cerebral complications. The two major cardiac events are left ventricular hypertrophy *(LVH)* and promotion of coronary artery disease *(CAD)*. The end result of LVH and CAD is left ventricular systolic failure *(LVF)* which, if progresses, can lead to death. *(Figure © LH Opie, 2005.)*

level, there are two important new developments. First, the BP level must be seen as part of an overall risk profile. Second, systolic levels should be considered, particularly in the elderly. At all ages, there are even more predictive of risk than are diastolic values[16] and JNC VII states that systolic BP is a "much more important" cardiovascular risk factor than the diastolic in those older than 50 years.[11,12] A wide pulse pressure, largely reflecting a high systolic level, may be the most accurate predictor of all.[17]

Overall Aims of Treatment

Reducing cardiovascular risk is the sole aim of therapy. Because the majority of patients with mild to moderate hypertension are entirely asymptomatic, it is essential to emphasize the value of lowering of BP in achieving this goal. A practical approach stresses the importance of lifestyle changes for all and gears the number of drugs to be used to the BP goal that in turn depends on risk assessment, target organ damage, and associated diseases. At least in some individuals drug treatment may impair the quality of life or induce adverse changes in blood chemistry and blood lipids. Ideally all abnormalities associated with hypertension, including shortened life expectancy, should be reverted to normal. Although overall cardiovascular mortality has been reduced by therapy, primarily through a decrease in stroke mortality, the excess risks for coronary disease associated with elevated BP have not been fully removed by reduction of the pressure to levels seen in untreated people. There are several possibilities including (1) the multifactorial nature of coronary heart disease, (2) the short duration of treatment, (3) the lack of adequate 24-hour control of BP, (4) the metabolic side effects or other hazards of the drugs used, and (5) overtreatment in susceptible patients. Some trials have suggested a *J-shaped curve* indicating an increase of coronary complications in patients whose diastolic BP was reduced to 85 mmHg or lower. The HOT trial attempted to disprove the presence of a J-curve.[18] Despite a less than desired separation of BP in the three groups assigned to reach a diastolic of 90, 85, or 80 mmHg, the lowest incidence of endpoints was seen at a DBP of 83 mmHg and a small but apparent increase in cardiovascular mortality occurred when the DBP was lowered below 70 mmHg. In diabetic persons the situation may be different. In the HOT study, significantly less total mortality was noted in the 1501 high-risk diabetic hypertensive individuals whose DBP was titrated with the aim of reduction to below 80 mmHg. As to the systolic goal of therapy, the lowest cardiovascular mortality in the HOT study was at a SBP of 139 mmHg. In other studies of elderly individuals with isolated systolic hypertension, a decrease of diastolic pressure to below 65 mmHg increased the risk of stroke and coronary heart disease.[19] Therefore, caution and careful monitoring remain advisable.

Choice of Initial and Subsequent Drugs For many years, a great deal of attention, energy, and money have been spent in deciding which drug is the best choice for initial therapy and which combination is best for eventual therapy. The issue is still debated: for initial therapy the US Seventh Joint National Committee[11,20] advocates a low-dose thiazide diuretic for most patients whereas the European Hypertension Society[21] recommends whatever class seems most appropriate for the patient, while the World Health Organization[22] states that any class may be used but a diuretic is preferred. Thus two out of the three major guidelines give a low-dose diuretic as the first choice for most uncomplicated patients and certainly when cost comes into the equation. When, however, the relatively rich Europeans are considered, with well-financed social security programs, then the new angiotensin receptor blockers (ARBs) that are virtually symptom-free are increasingly chosen, especially because in several comparative studies they have had the edge over other drug groups.[1] However, some major outcome studies are still awaited. Note that the ARBs were usually combined with low-dose diuretics, again showing the strong trend toward combination therapy.

As to the eventual therapy needed to reach the lower goals of BP now advocated by all experts, there is agreement to add whatever is appropriate for the individual patient, that is, a *"compelling"* indication[11,20] or a *"favored choice,"*[21] to a diuretic and to add additional drugs from other classes to reach the goal.

Whereas the details vary somewhat, the tabulation of the 2003 European guidelines fits most situations very nicely (Table 7-3). All classes have their place, even α-blockers, which were maligned by the rigid construction of the ALLHAT trial.[23] Not unexpectedly, peripheral edema developed after substitution of a low dose of an α-blocker for a diuretic or ACE inhibitor in patients with incipient heart failure.[24]

If these various guidelines are followed, the use of low-dose diuretic therapy should markedly increase. On the other hand, the β-blockers will probably be used less overall but more in those patients who need them because of myocardial infarction or heart failure. CCBs have

Table 7-3 Guidelines for Selecting Drug Treatment for Hypertension

Class of Drug	Favored Indications	Possible Indications	Compelling Contraindications	Possible Contraindications
Diuretics (low-dose thiazides)	Congestive heart failure; Elderly hypertensive patients; Systolic hypertension; African origin subjects	Obesity	Gout	Pregnancy; Dyslipidemia; Metabolic syndrome; Sexually active men
Diuretics (loop)	Congestive heart failure; Renal failure		Hypokalemia	
Diuretics (antialdo)	Congestive heart failure; Postinfarct; Aldosteronism (1° or 2°)	Refractory hypertension	Hyperkalemia; Renal failure	Diabetic renal disease
β-Blockers	Angina; Tachyarrhythmias; Post-MI Heart failure (up-titrate)	Pregnancy; Diabetes	Asthma; severe COPD Heart block*	Metabolic syndrome; Athletes and exercising patients; Erectile dysfunction; Peripheral vascular disease
ACE inhibitors	Left ventricular dysfunction or failure; Postinfarct; Nephropathy, type 1; Diabetic or nondiabetic proteinuria	CV protection (BP already controlled); type 2 nephropathy	Pregnancy; Hyperkalemia; Bilateral renal artery stenosis	Severe cough; Severe aortic stenosis
Angiotensin-II antagonists (ARBs)	ACE inhibitor cough; Diabetes type 2 nephropathy including microalbuminuria; LVH; Heart failure	Postinfarct	Pregnancy; Bilateral renal artery stenosis Hyperkalemia	Severe aortic stenosis
Calcium antagonists (CCBs)	Angina, effort; Elderly patients; Systolic hypertension; Supraventricular tachycardias‡; Carotid atherosclerosis	Peripheral vascular disease; Diabetes; African origin; Pregnancy	Heart block†; Clinical heart failure (possible exception: amlodipine, but needs care)	Early heart failure

*Grade 2 or 3 atrioventricular block.
†Grade 2 or 3 atrioventricular block with verapamil or diltiazem.
‡Verapamil or diltiazem.
ACE = angiotensin converting enzyme; Aldo = aldosterone; CV = cardiovascular; COPD = chronic obstructive pulmonary disease.
Modified from the report of the European Societies.²¹

been proved safe in the ALLHAT trial[23] whereas ACE inhibitors received bad marks when used in blacks[23] but better marks when used in elderly Caucasians.[25] But in both these studies the ACE inhibitors could not be combined with their natural partners, the diuretics. ARBs, the fastest growing class, are better than comparators with regards to stroke, heart failure, and major cardiovascular events,[1] and may also be the best in type 2 diabetic persons.[26] However, in hypertension there are no good comparative head-to-head outcome studies with their cheaper siblings, the ACE inhibitors. In fact, ARBs are no better than ACE inhibitors in heart failure[27] or in postinfarct patients.[28]

One old drug, spironolactone, has been revitalized for use in heart failure[29] and a congener that provides more selective aldosterone blockade, eplerenone, will probably become a major player, not only for heart failure[30] but for all types of hypertension if not priced too high.[31] Meanwhile reserpine is used only where its low cost is important, as no marketing is being expended in its favor.

Metabolic Syndrome A complex interrelation between hypertension, obesity, and maturity onset diabetes may be explained by *insulin-resistance* as the common denominator (Fig. 7-3). The fear is that high doses of diuretics and β-blockers, separately or especially together, may further impair insulin sensitivity with risk of overt diabetes and/or lipid abnormalities.[32] In contrast, other classes of antihypertensives, such as ACE inhibitors, ARBs, and α-blockers, improve insulin sensitivity. A CCB or ACE inhibitor or ARB is less likely than a diuretic or β-blocker to induce new diabetes.[33] Thus, these categories are also logical first-choice agents, in particular for the large number of obese hypertensive people with the metabolic syndrome (Table 7-4).

Relative Efficacy As seen in Table 7-3, certain drugs are favored in certain patients, that is, diuretics and CCBs in blacks and the elderly, and ACE inhibitors or ARBs in diabetic persons with nephropathy. Moreover, all drugs have certain limitations and contraindications. However, it should be noted that in the overall hypertensive population,

INSULIN RESISTANCE

Opie 2004

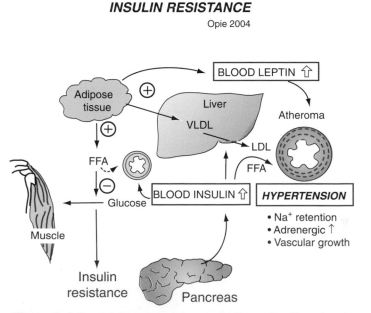

Figure 7-3 Proposed sequence of events leading to insulin resistance; based on inhibition of uptake of glucose by circulating free fatty acids *(FFA)*. Hypothetically, FFA promote insulin resistance[III] and insulin upregulates vascular AT-I receptors.[112] (*Figure © LH Opie, 2005.*)

BP MANAGEMENT

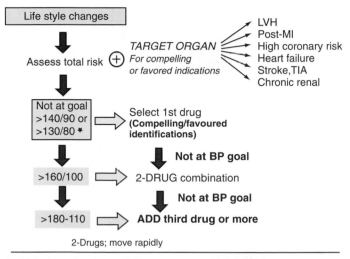

Figure 7-4 Proposed simplified treatment algorithm for hypertension, based on JNC 7[11,12] and European Society recommendations.[21]

Table 7-4 | Definition of the Metabolic Syndrome

Risk Factor	Defining Level	Level, Metric Units
*Abdominal obesity**		
Men	>40 in.	>102 cm
Women	>35 in.	>88 cm
Triglycerides	≥150 mg/dL	≥1.7 mmol/L
HDL-cholesterol		
Men	<40 mg/dL	<1.1 mmol/L
Women	<50 mg/dL	<1.3 mmol/L
Fasting glucose	≥110 mg/dL	≥6.1 mmol/L
Blood pressure	≥130/85 mmHg	≥130/85 mmHg

*Waist measurement for abdominal obesity.

the response rate, that is, BP lowered to below 140/90 mmHg, to each of the five major groups of agents may be no more than 30% to 40% depending on the severity of the hypertension and the drug chosen, so that combination therapy (Fig. 7-4) is usually required in addition to lifestyle modification. Finally, financial considerations may be crucial. Diuretics, reserpine, and hydralazine are inexpensive, as are generic β-blockers, ACE inhibitors, and verapamil. Other agents can be much more expensive.

DIURETICS FOR HYPERTENSION

Diuretics have been the basis of several impressive trials, many in elderly patients, in which hard end-points have been reduced. Diuretics are widely recommended as first-line therapy. They are better at reducing coronary heart disease, heart failure, stroke, and cardiovascular and total mortality than placebo, and in at least one of these end points they are better than β-blockers, calcium channel blockers, ACE inhibitors (but equal to the ARBs), and α-blockers.[34] Diuretics are inexpensive. Thus it is not surprising that they are still widely used either as monotherapy (Fig. 7-5) or in combination

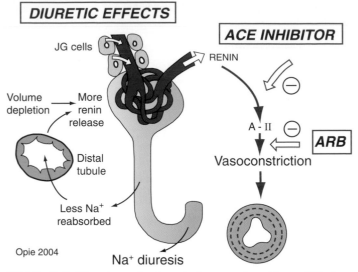

Figure 7-5 Diuretic mechanisms in hypertension. Note self-limiting sequence whereby sodium loss and volume depletion stimulate renin release to promote vasoconstriction. The latter effect is alleviated by concurrent therapy with an ACE inhibitor or an angiotensin receptor blocker *(ARB)*. JG = juxtaglomerular. *(Figure © LH Opie, 2005.)*

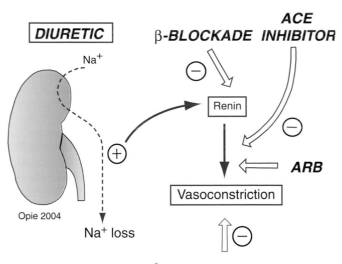

Figure 7-6 Diuretics, basically acting by sodium loss, cause a reactive increase in circulating renin that results in angiotensin-mediated vasoconstriction to offset the hypotensive effect. Diuretics therefore combine well with β-blockers, which inhibit the release of renin, with ACE inhibitors that inhibit the formation of angiotensin-II, with angiotensin receptor blockers *(ARBs)*, and with calcium antagonists *(CCBs)*, which directly oppose diuretic-induced vasoconstriction. Of these combinations, that of diuretic and ACE inhibitor is particularly well tested. ACE inhibitors lessen the metabolic side effects of diuretics. *(Figure © LH Opie, 2005.)*

(Fig. 7-6). They combine particularly well with β-blockers or with ACE inhibitors and ARBs. However, the dihydropyridine (DHP) CCBs have inherent diuretic properties, making this combination less effective. The vascular complications that are more directly related to the height of the BP per se (strokes and congestive heart failure) have been reduced, more so than that of the most common cause of disease and death among hypertensive persons, namely coronary heart disease.[35] Hypothetically, metabolic side effects from the high doses of diuretics used in earlier trials, particularly on lipids and insulin sensitivity,[32] as well as potassium and magnesium depletion, and increased uric acid levels,[33] may in part explain why death from coronary disease has not decreased as much as it should have. For example, a serum potassium of 3.5 mmol/L or below increased cardiovascular events by about four times over a mean follow-up of 6.7 years.[36] Also on the debit side, impotence is a relatively frequent side effect.[37] Furthermore, the response in younger whites (under 60 years) is poor.[38] There may also be a slight risk of increased renal cell carcinoma, especially in women, that may discourage diuretic use in young women.

A persistent problem with the concept of low-dose diuretic therapy is that there are no good comparative studies between the different diuretics, their "low" doses, and outcomes. However, the available evidence suggests that the following are low doses that nonetheless are effectively and safely antihypertensive in mild-to-moderate hypertension: hydrochlorothiazide 12.5 mg, chlorthalidone 12.5 to 15 mg, and bendrofluazide 1.25 mg.[39] If chlorthalidone is about 1.5 to 2 times as potent as hydrochlorothiazide, as indirect evidence suggests,[40] then these comparisons suggest an advantage for chlorthalidone.

Diuretic Dose: Hydrochlorothiazide Although a single morning dose of 12.5 mg of *hydrochlorothiazide* or its equivalent will provide a 10 mmHg fall in the BP of most uncomplicated hypertensive persons within several weeks, even that dose is probably too high in combination therapies. Higher doses such as 25 mg increase the risk of diabetes.[41] Lower doses (6.25 mg hydrochlorothiazide) are equally effective when combined with β-blockade or ACE inhibition or an ARB. Such low doses of hydrochlorothiazide may require several weeks to act. Low-dose thiazides may be combined with all other classes, although the DHP CCBs have their own diuretic capacity. Alternatively, salt restriction may be the secret in making low-dose hydrochlorothiazide work. The advantage of low-dose hydrochlorothiazide (or its equivalent in other diuretics) is that adverse metabolic and lipid effects are minimized or completely avoided. Nevertheless, even 12.5 mg of hydrochlorothiazide may still induce potassium wastage, and hypokalemia. Strictly speaking, we do not know that the low doses of diuretics currently used really result in patient benefit except in the elderly where low-dose chlorthalidone (12.5 mg) was chosen as initial therapy in the SHEP study.[42] Even there, in many patients the dose was doubled and a β-blocker added. Logically, the lower the dose of diuretic, the fewer the metabolic side effects, whereas (within limits) the antihypertensive potency may still be adequately expressed.

Chlorthalidone Chlorthalidone 15 mg daily was used in the TOMH study[43] in patients with very mild hypertension. Combined with weight loss and other measures, it was as effectively antihypertensive as other groups of agents. It gave an unexpectedly good quality of life (despite the doubling of impotence) and at the end of 4 years blood cholesterol changes (elevated at 1 year) had reverted to normal.[43] Chlorthalidone 12.5 mg daily was the first-line treatment in the study on systolic hypertension in the elderly SHEP study.[42] Thereafter the dose was doubled in about one third and atenolol was added, if needed, to control BP. In SHEP, after 4.5 years, total stroke was reduced by 36%. On the debit side, the higher dose increased the risk of hypokalemia with loss of cardiovascular benefit.[44] In ALLHAT, chlorthalidone at a dose of 12.5 to 25 mg was considered the best overall drug versus the CCB amlodipine or the ACE inhibitor lisinopril but at the cost of increased diabetes and hypokalemia.[23]

Bendrofluazide Bendrofluazide, a standard thiazide in the United Kingdom, once given at 10 mg a day in a large trial, is effective over 24 hours at a daily dose of only 1.25 mg.[45]

Other Diuretics The modified thiazide *indapamide (Lozol, Natrilix)* may be more lipid neutral and is promoted in some countries as a vasodilating diuretic. The previous standard dose of 2.5 mg once daily has been dropped by the manufacturers to 1.5 mg daily in a sustained release formulation. Yet the potassium may fall, and the blood glucose and uric acid rise, as warned in the package insert. Indapamide induces regression of LV hypertrophy and may be better than enalapril 20 mg once daily.[46] *Metolazone (Zaroxolyn)*, another modified thiazide, can induce diuresis even with severe renal insufficiency and its effect lasts for 24 hours.

Of the *loop diuretics*, furosemide is not ideal as it is short acting and needs to be given twice a day to be adequately antihypertensive. The more recently introduced *torsemide (Demadex)* is particularly well studied in hypertension. Some reports have suggested that torasemide is free of metabolic and lipid side effects yet antihypertensive when used in the subdiuretic dose of 2.5 mg once daily.[47] At the higher daily doses registered for hypertension in the United States, namely 5 to 10 mg, it becomes natriuretic with greater risk of metabolic changes.

Aldosterone Antagonists Based on the RALES trial (see Chapter 5), spironolactone is finding wider use in hypertensive persons with congestive heart failure provided that serum potassium is carefully monitored. Eplerenone *(Inspra)* is a more specific congener with much less risk of gynecomastia. Besides improving survival of post-myocardial infarction (post-MI) heart failure, eplerenone is now being marketed for hypertension, either alone or in combination with other agents, with, however, strict warnings about contraindications that include hyperkalemia above 5.5 mEq/L, a reduced creatinine clearance ≤30 mL/min, type 2 diabetes with early renal involvement, and the use of other K-retaining agents or K-supplements *(www.pfizer.com/download/uspi_inspra.pdf)*. There is a special argument for these agents in primary aldosteronism but also in those subjects with resistant hypertension.[48]

Other Potassium-Sparing Diuretics These may add a few cents to the cost but save a good deal more by the prevention of diuretic-induced hypokalemia and hypomagnesemia. The risk of torsades-related sudden death should also be reduced.[49] To be effectively antihypertensive, the potassium-sparing agents are combined with another diuretic, generally a thiazide. Fixed-dose combinations of triamterene *(Dyazide, Maxzide)* or amiloride *(Moduretic)* with hydrochlorothiazide are usually chosen. The general problem is that the thiazide dose is too high. The dose of hydrochlorothiazide in one tablet of Dyazide is 25 mg, but only about half is absorbed. Maxzide contains 25 or 50 mg hydrochlorothiazide. Standard Moduretic contains 50 mg (far too much), but in Europe, a "mini-Moduretic" *(Moduret)* with half the standard thiazide dose is now marketed to overcome this objection. However, even these doses are probably too high. *Aldactazide* combines 25 mg of spironolactone with 25 mg thiazide.

Combinations of Diuretics with Other Antihypertensives Diuretics may add to the effect of all other types of antihypertensives (Table 7-5). Combination with ACE inhibition or an ARB is particularly logical (see Chapter 5). A number of well-designed factorial studies have varied the dose of hydrochlorothiazide from 6.25 mg to 25 mg and studied the interaction with a β-blocker,[50] or diltiazem,[51] or an ACE inhibitor.[52] In general, somewhat greater antihypertensive effects were obtained with 25 mg hydrochlorothiazide, yet the difference between the high and the low doses of thiazide were negligible when the alternate agent

Table 7-5 Combination Drugs for Hypertension

Drug Combination	Trade Name
β-Blockers and Diuretics	
Atenolol 50 or 100 mg/chlorthalidone 25 mg	Tenoretic
Bisoprolol 2.5, 5, or 10 mg/hydrochlorothiazide 6.25 mg	Ziac*
Metoprolol tartrate 50 or 100 mg/hydrochlorothiazide 25 or 50 mg	Lopressor HCT
Nadolol 40 or 80 mg/bendroflumethiazide 5 mg	Corzide
Propranolol LA 40 or 80 mg/hydrochlorothiazide 25 mg	Inderide
Timolol 10 mg/hydrochlorothiazide 25 mg	Timolide
ACE Inhibitors and Diuretics	
Benazepril 5, 10, 20 mg/hydrochlorothiazide 6.25, 12.5, or 25 mg	Lotensin HCT
Captopril 25 or 50 mg/hydrochlorothiazide 15 or 25 mg	Capozide*
Enalapril 5 or 10 mg/hydrochlorothiazide 12.5 or 25 mg	Vaseretic
Lisinopril 10 or 20 mg/hydrochlorothiazide 12.5 or 25 mg	Prinzide; Zestoretic
Moexipril 7.5 or 15 mg/hydrochlorothiazide 12.5 or 25 mg	Uniretic
Quinapril 10 or 20 mg/hydrochlorothiazide 12.5 or 25 mg	Accuretic
Angiotensin-II Receptor Antagonists and Diuretics	
Candesartan 16 or 32 mg/hydrochlorothiazide 12.5 or 25 mg	Atacand HCT
Eprosartan 600 mg/hydrochlorothiazide 12.5 or 25 mg	Teveten HCT
Irbesartan 75 or 150 mg, hydrochlorothiazide 12.5 mg	Avalide
Losartan 50, 100 mg/hydrochlorothiazide 12.5 or 25 mg	Hyzaar
Telmisartan 40 or 80 mg/hydrochlorothiazide 12.5 mg	Micardis HCT
Valsartan 80 or 160 mg/hydrochlorothiazide 12.5 mg	Diovan HCT
CCBs and ACE Inhibitors	
Amlodipine 2.5 or 5 or 10 mg/benazepril 10 or 20 mg	Lotrel
Verapamil (extended release) 180 or 240 mg/trandolapril 1, 2 or 4 mg	Tarka
Felodipine 5 mg/enalapril 5 mg	Lexxel
Diuretic Combinations	
Triamterene 37.5, 50 or 75 mg/hydrochlorothiazide 25 or 50 mg	Dyazide, Maxide
Spironolactone 25 or 50 mg/hydrochlorothiazide 25 or 50 mg	Aldactazide
Amiloride 5 mg/hydrochlorothiazide 50 mg	Moduretic

Modified from JNC 7 with one error (Aldactone) corrected.[11,12]
*Approved for initial therapy in the United States.

was given at higher doses. Thus there is a good argument for starting combination therapy with 6.25 mg hydrochlorothiazide, a dose that effectively avoids hypokalemia.

Diuretics: Conclusions Despite reservations about metabolic side effects such as increased diabetes at higher doses, truly low-dose diuretics remain the preferred initial treatment, especially in the elderly, the obese, and in black patients. Compared with placebo, low-dose diuretics reduce stroke and coronary disease in the elderly and achieve outcome benefit, including mortality reduction, in patients with mild to moderate hypertension.[35] Diuretics appear to work particularly well in elderly blacks while being much less effective in younger whites.[38]

Two large positive outcome studies with diuretics have been in the elderly, with the mean age well above 60 years even at the start of the trial.[23,42] Of note, in these and other trials the diuretic dose was often uptitrated whereas a better course would probably be to keep the dose low and to add a second agent. For example, in obese individuals, diuretic therapy should first be combined with weight reduction. Then, in view of the association of obesity with insulin insensitivity, the next step would be to add an ACE inhibitor or ARB rather than increasing the diuretic dose.

β-BLOCKERS FOR HYPERTENSION

β-Blockade (Fig. 7-7) was previously recommended by the American Joint National Committee for first-line therapy as an alternate to diuretics,[53] but this favored status has been lost in JNC VII, which is not surprising considering the relative lack of good outcome data in well-designed trials, and poor results when compared with diuretics in the elderly. Thus in the British Medical Research Council trial in the elderly, diuretics reduced mortality from coronary heart disease, whereas β-blockers did not.[54] A subsequent meta-analysis confirmed that in older hypertensives, β-blockers gave poor results.[55] Nonetheless, β-blockers have strengths, having as "compelling indications" heart failure, post-MI, high coronary risk, and diabetes mellitus in JNC VII.[11,12] The European recommendations omit "high coronary risk," and add angina pectoris, pregnancy, and tachyarrhythmias (Table 7-4). First principles but no solid trial data state that β-blockade would be particularly suitable for patients with "increased adrenergic drive," often betrayed by a resting tachycardia and other features for the anxiety syndrome. In young hypertensive individuals, the cardiac output is high and the systemic vascular resistance not increased, so

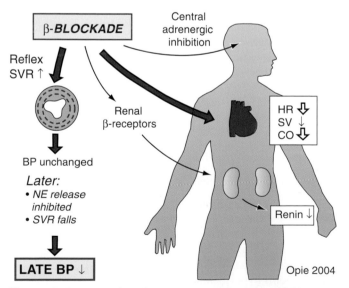

Figure 7-7 Proposed antihypertensive mechanisms of β-blockade. An early fall in heart rate *(HR)*, stroke volume *(SV)*, and cardiac output *(CO)* does not lead to a corresponding fall in blood pressure because of baroreflex-mediated increased peripheral α-adrenergic vasoconstriction, with a rise in systemic vascular resistance. Within a few days β-blockade of prejunctional receptors on the terminal neuron with consequent inhibition of release of norepinephrine *(NE)*, which may explain why the SVR falls to normal. The blood pressure now falls. In the case of vasodilatory β-blockers, with added α-blockade, there is an early decrease in SVR and a rapid fall in BP.[113] *(Figure © LH Opie, 2005.)*

that here too β-blockade should theoretically be ideal treatment, although no formal studies can prove this point.

In black patients, vasodilation or sodium loss seems to be the key to successful treatment; hence, logical first choices are diuretics, or the vasodilatory β-blockers labetalol or carvedilol, or centrally active agents or vasodilators apart from the ACE inhibitors or ARBs. In general, black patients have low renin values and so do the elderly; thus, the ineffectiveness of β-blockers and ACE inhibitors in elderly black males[38] is explicable.

Dosage It is best to start with a low dose to lessen the chances of initial fatigue, which is probably due in part to the fall in cardiac output. A low dose, in the elderly, lessens the risk of excess bradycardia. Today, standard doses are what used to be termed low. For example, with propranolol there is little, if any, additional antihypertensive effect with doses above 80 mg/day, given either once or twice per day.[56] If the response to ordinary doses of a β-blocker is inadequate, a higher dose may sometimes work but, more generally, it is easier to change to another category of agent or to undertake combination therapy.

Side Effects In addition to inducing fatigue and reducing exercise capacity, β-blockers impair insulin sensitivity and were the only class of agents associated with a significant increase in the incidence of diabetes.[57] They should not be given to patients with bronchospastic disease and only cautiously to those with chronic obstructive pulmonary disease.[58] They may mask hypoglycemia in diabetic individuals on insulin, with sweating the only unhidden manifestation.

Pharmacokinetics Dose adjustment is more likely to be required with more lipid-soluble (lipophilic) agents, which have a high "first-pass" liver metabolism that may result in active metabolites: the rate of formation will depend on liver blood flow and function. The ideal β-blocker for hypertension would be long-acting, cardioselective (see Fig. 1-9), and usually effective in a standard dose. Simple pharmacokinetics may be an added advantage (no liver metabolism, little protein binding, no lipid solubility, and no active metabolites). Sometimes added vasodilation should be an advantage, as in the elderly or in black patients. The ideal drug would also be "lipid neutral" as claimed for some agents (see Table 10-4). In practice, once-a-day therapy is satisfactory with many β-blockers, but it is important to check early morning predrug BP to ensure 24-hour coverage (as with all agents). Combinations of β-blockers with one or another agent from all other classes have been successful in the therapy of hypertension. Nonetheless, combination with another drug suppressing the renin-angiotensin system, such as an ACE inhibitor or an ARB, is not logical nor did it work well in ALLHAT. *Diuretics plus β-blockers*, in combination (Table 7-5), should ideally contain no more than 12.5 mg hydrochlorothiazide, 1.25 mg bendrofluazide, or a similar low dose of another diuretic. Bisoprolol 2.5 to 10 mg plus only 6.25 mg hydrochlorothiazide (*Ziac*) is available in the United States and licensed for initial therapy.

Meta-analysis When compared with placebo, β-blockers reduce stroke and heart failure, but without benefit on other major outcomes such as coronary heart disease, cardiovascular or total mortality.[35] Compared with low-dose diuretics, β-blockers increased cardiovascular events.[34] These results may reflect the small number of well-designed placebo controlled outcome trials with β-blockers.

CALCIUM CHANNEL BLOCKERS

Calcium channel blockers (CCBs, calcium antagonists) compare well in their antihypertensive effect with diuretics or β-blockers. CCBs act primarily to reduce peripheral vascular resistance, aided by at least an initial diuretic effect, especially in the case of the dihydropyridines (DHPs). No negative inotropic effect can be detected in patients with initially normal myocardial function. Regarding the effects on plasma catecholamines, DHPs must be distinguished from non-DHPs such as verapamil and diltiazem. As a group, DHPs reflexly stimulate the adrenergic system to increase plasma catecholamines modestly,[59] with a borderline elevation of plasma renin activity caused by the counterregulatory effect (Fig. 7-8). Non-DHPs tend to decrease catecholamine levels. There are several long-term outcome studies available with CCBs in hypertension, including the Syst-Eur study with nitrendipine,[60] the STOP-2 study with felodipine or isradipine,[61] the INSIGHT study with long acting nifedipine,[33] the ALLHAT and VALUE studies with amlodipine (Table 3-6),[23] and two recent studies with verapamil, CONVINCE[62] and INVEST.[41] The general message is that CCBs are safe and effective.[1] CCBs are particularly effective in elderly patients and are equally effective in blacks as in nonblacks. They act independently of sodium intake. CCBs may be selected as initial monotherapy, especially if there are other indications for these agents such as angina pectoris or Raynaud's phenomenon or supraventricular tachycardia (non-DHPs). Several formulations are now available providing 24-hour BP coverage with once-daily dosing. The long-acting DHP nitrendipine provided better protection from all cardiovascular endpoints in the diabetic hypertensive individuals than in the non-diabetic individuals enrolled in the Syst-Eur trial.[63] Moreover, CCB-treated diabetics in the Syst-Eur trial did significantly better than the diuretic-treated diabetic persons in the SHEP trial.

CCBs Compared with Diuretics CCBs are more expensive than diuretics (also advocated for elderly or black patients); however, CCBs cause

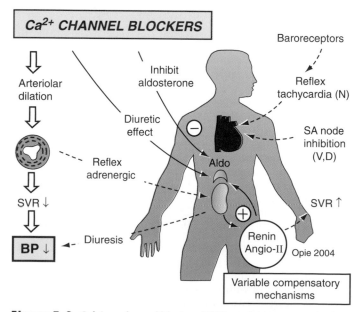

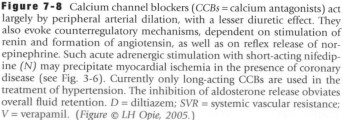

Figure 7-8 Calcium channel blockers (*CCBs* = calcium antagonists) act largely by peripheral arterial dilation, with a lesser diuretic effect. They also evoke counterregulatory mechanisms, dependent on stimulation of renin and formation of angiotensin, as well as on reflex release of norepinephrine. Such acute adrenergic stimulation with short-acting nifedipine (*N*) may precipitate myocardial ischemia in the presence of coronary disease (see Fig. 3-6). Currently only long-acting CCBs are used in the treatment of hypertension. The inhibition of aldosterone release obviates overall fluid retention. *D* = diltiazem; *SVR* = systemic vascular resistance; *V* = verapamil. (*Figure* © *LH Opie, 2005.*)

no metabolic disturbances in potassium, glucose, uric acid, or lipid metabolism.[23] Patients on CCBs do not require intermittent blood chemistry checks. In a study on South African black hypertensive persons, a CCB regime was better able to reduce DBP below 90 mmHg than hydrochlorothiazide 12.5 to 25 mg.[64] There is no evidence that CCBs cause impairment of renal function. On the contrary, in ALLHAT indices of renal function were better preserved in the CCB group.[23]

CCBs Compared with β-Blockers CCBs cause less fatigue and little or no interference with normal cardiovascular dynamics, especially during exercise. CCBs have fewer contraindications and can, for example, be used safely in asthmatic persons. CCBs cause little or no interference with diabetic control and are not contraindicated in peripheral vascular disease. DHPs may be used in the presence of bradycardia and are not inhibitory on the AV node in clinical doses. Caution is advised with DHPs post-infarction, especially in the absence of β-blockade. Verapamil is, however, licensed in some European countries for postinfarct protection in the absence of heart failure when β-blockers are contraindicated. In African-Americans verapamil was better than a β-blocker in slowing the progress of diabetic nephropathy.[65]

CCBs Compared to ACE Inhibitors With equal antihypertensive efficacy, CCB-based therapy provides better protection against stroke than does ACE-inhibitor based therapy[23] but is clearly less protection against heart failure.[1] In the black hypertensives with renal insufficiency in the AASK trial, those with microalbuminuria had an initial increase in GFR on amlodipine and a subsequent equal fall in GFR as did those on ramipril or metoprolol.[66] Those with macroalbuminuria did better on the ACE inhibitor or β-blocker. In the ALLHAT trial, amlodipine was equally protective as was lisinopril (both compared to chlorthalidone) against renal damage and heart attacks with better protection against stroke in the black participants.[23] In INVEST, verapamil-trandolapril compared well on coronary outcomes with atenolol-hydrochlorothiazide.[41] For other CCB-ACE inhibitor combinations, see Table 7-5. For comparison with ARBs, see p. 203.

Meta-analysis of Outcome Studies with CCBs Taking together the available studies in 2003, CCBs compared with placebo reduced stroke, coronary heart disease, major cardiovascular events, and cardiovascular death with, however, a trend to increased heart failure.[1] Compared with conventional therapy by diuretics and/or β-blockers, CCBs had the same effect on cardiovascular death and total mortality, increased heart failure, with a strong trend to decreased stroke. In addition, there was a lower rate of new diabetes with CCBs than with conventional therapy.[23]

Safety Issues The questions relating to the long-term safety of CCBs have been resolved in that higher doses of short-acting agents may cause ischemic events, probably by precipitously lowering the BP, whereas long-acting CCBs do not cause ischemia, cancer, or gastrointestinal bleeding or any other serious problem.

ACE INHIBITORS FOR HYPERTENSION

ACE inhibitors (Fig. 7-9), once reserved for refractory hypertension, especially when renal in origin, have become the primary agents for many hypertensives. ACE inhibitors have minimal side effects (cough and rarely angioedema), simplicity of use, a flat dose-response curve, and virtual absence of contraindications except for bilateral renal artery stenosis and pregnancy. By reducing the intraglomerular pressure they occasionally cause the serum creatinine to rise significantly and may precipitate hyperkalemia, especially in the presence of pre-existing renal dysfunction or when combined with potassium-retaining diuretics such as spironolactone. They readily combine with other modalities of treatment and are well accepted by the

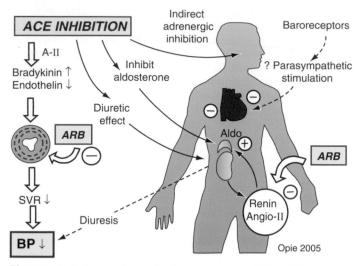

Figure 7-9 Proposed mechanisms whereby ACE inhibitors and angiotensin receptor blockers *(ARBs)* may have their antihypertensive effects. Note that the major effect is on the peripheral arterioles causing vasodilation and a fall in the systemic vascular resistance *(SVR)*, also called the peripheral vascular resistance. Indirect inhibition of adrenergic activity also promotes arteriolar dilation. Decreased angiotensin-II *(A-II)* levels may also act by increased formation of bradykinin and decreased formation of endothelin, as well as by inhibition of central effects of angiotensin-II with indirect adrenergic inhibition, thereby differing from the vasodilation induced by CCBs (see Fig. 7-8). Parasympathetic activity is also stimulated. *Aldo* = aldosterone. *(Figure © LH Opie, 2005.)*

elderly. Furthermore, a strong case has been made for their preferential use in diabetic hypertensive patients, in postinfarction follow-up, and in renal failure. The HOPE study[67] emphasizes their role in cardiovascular protection in high-risk patients. Captopril was the first ACE inhibitor, but multiple others are now available. All are antihypertensive, with few practical differences, except for duration of action (Table 5-4).

In *mild to moderate hypertension*, ACE inhibitors can be used as monotherapy, even in low-renin patients, or in combination with other standard agents. For monotherapy, moderate dietary salt restriction is especially important.[68] The reason why only a variable percentage of mild to moderate hypertensives respond to monotherapy with ACE inhibition may be differences in the sodium intake and the relative activity in the renin-angiotensin mechanism.

Meta-analysis of Outcome Studies As summarized by the Blood Pressure Trialists[1] in trials up to 2003, ACE inhibitor based therapy was better than placebo against stroke, coronary heart disease, heart failure, major cardiovascular events, cardiovascular death, and total mortality. When compared to diuretic ± β-blocker based therapy, ACE inhibitor therapy was exactly equal though there was a trend toward lesser benefit in stroke. When compared to CCB-based therapy, ACE inhibitor therapy was equivalent for coronary heart disease, cardiovascular death, and total mortality; clearly better for prevention of heart failure; and marginally worse for prevention of stroke.

Coronary Disease and ACE Inhibitors In the HOPE trial of patients at high risk of coronary heart disease, the addition of ramipril provided substantial cardioprotection.[67,68] However, uncertainty exists as to whether this was related to the extra antihypertensive effect provided by the ACE-inhibitor, especially throughout the night.[70] Note that the ramipril was given as 10 mg at night. In the PROGRESS trial of patients with cerebral vascular disease, the ACE inhibitor (perindopril) alone did little, but when given with a diuretic (indapamide) provided excellent protection against recurrent stroke.[71] In the EUROPA study, perindopril given in a high dose of 8 mg to patients with established coronary disease but with other otherwise relatively low risk, gave substantial cardiovascular protection especially by reducing myocardial infarction. Here, too, there was substantial BP reduction. In addition, a large body of experimental evidence supports the notion that there are direct vascular protective effects.

Renal Disease and ACE Inhibitors In *renovascular hypertension*, where circulating renin is high and a critical part of the hypertensive mechanism, ACE inhibition is logical first-line therapy. Because the hypotensive response may be dramatic, a low test dose is essential. Captopril 6.25 mg acts quickest and is shortest in its duration of action. With standard doses of captopril or enalapril, the GFR falls acutely largely to recover in cases of unilateral, but not bilateral, disease. However, blood flow to the stenotic kidney may remain depressed after removal of the angiotensin-II support, and progressive ischemic atrophy is possible. Careful follow-up of renal blood flow and function is required. Angioplasty or surgery is likely preferable to chronic medical therapy, especially in those with bilateral disease.

In *acute severe hypertension*, sublingual (chewed) captopril rapidly brings down the BP, but it is not clear how bilateral renal artery stenosis can be excluded quickly enough to make the speed of action of captopril an important benefit. Furthermore, the safety of such sudden falls of BP in the presence of possible renal impairment (always a risk in severe hypertension) has not been evaluated.

In *diabetic hypertensive patients* enrolled in the UKPDS trial, the ACE inhibitor captopril was no better than β-blockade.[72] However, with diabetic nephropathy, that is, proteinuria, ACE-inhibitors and ARBs provide preferential dilation of the renal efferent arterials, immediately reducing intraglomerular pressure and thereby providing long-term protection against progressive glomerulosclerosis.[73] On the other hand, CCBs (particularly the DHPs) also dilate afferent arterials, increasing intraglomerular blood flow and sometimes promoting proteinuria (for a metaanalysis, see ref 18, Chapter 3).

In *nondiabetic chronic nephropathy*, the majority with hypertension, the ACE inhibitor ramipril slowed the progression to end-stage when compared with placebo plus conventional antihypertensive agents.[74] The impressive aspect of this study is that the benefit of ramipril was obtained apparently independently of any BP reduction. In the AASK trial of nondiabetic proteinurics, ramipril was more protective than amlodipine.[75]

Special Groups of Patients In *elderly hypertensive patients*, ACE inhibitors were originally thought not to work so well because of the trend to a low renin status in that group. Three large outcome studies have now documented the efficacy and outcome benefit of therapy based on ACE inhibition in elderly whites.[25,61] In *elderly black hypertensive men*, captopril was no better than placebo,[38] perhaps because there were two factors (ethnic group and age), both predisposing to a low-renin state. Similarly, in the ALLHAT trial lisinopril did not protect the *black patients* against stroke,[23] probably because the trial design did not allow combination with a diuretic. In *hypertension with heart failure*, ACE inhibitors with diuretics have been automatic first-line therapy. This choice is not challenged by the impressive benefits of β-blockade in heart failure, because the latter therapy has always been added to preexisting ACE inhibition and diuretic therapy. In *pregnancy hypertension*, ACE inhibitors are totally contraindicated because fetal growth impaired.

Combinations with ACE Inhibitors ACE inhibitors are often combined with *thiazide diuretics* to enhance hypotensive effects (see Fig. 7-3 and Table 7-5), and to lessen metabolic side effects. This combination is logical because diuretics increase renin, the effects of which are antagonized by ACE inhibitors. Combinations of several ACE inhibitors with diuretics are now available. The ideal thiazide dose should not exceed 12.5 mg hydrochlorothiazide and 6.25 mg may be enough. Such addition of a thiazide is better for lowering the blood pressure than increasing the dose of the ACE inhibitor. When combined with potassium-retaining thiazide diuretics (*Dyazide, Moduretic, Maxzide*), and especially spironolactone or eplerenone, there is a *risk of hyperkalemia* because ACE inhibitors decrease aldosterone secretion and hence retain potassium (Fig. 7-9). Nonetheless, in the RALES heart failure study, low-dose spironolactone was added to ACE inhibition and diuretic with little hyperkalemia, yet these patients were carefully monitored and the dose of ACE inhibitor reduced if necessary.[29] *ACE inhibition plus β-blockade* is theoretically not a combination of choice because both agents have an ultimate antirenin effect. *ACE inhibitors plus CCBs* are now increasingly used in the therapy of hypertension. This combination attacks both the renin-angiotensin system and the increased peripheral vascular resistance. There may be specific renal benefits, especially with verapamil. The ACE inhibitor reduces the ankle edema of the DHPs and the latter reduces the cough of the ACE inhibitor. Both types of agents are free of metabolic and central nervous system side effects. Large-scale studies on the combination will soon become available (ASCOT study).

ACE Inhibitors: Summary In addition to BP lowering, the overall evidence is that these agents also confer vascular protection, especially in diabetic individuals and in renal disease. ACE inhibitors combine well with diuretics and CCBs, and have relatively infrequent side effects.

ANGIOTENSIN-II RECEPTOR BLOCKERS (ARBs)

Angiotensin-II subtype 1 (AT-1) blockers act on the specific receptor for angiotensin-II that has a highly adverse role in promoting cardiovascular pathology (see Table 5-1). The prototype, losartan, has now been joined by many others (Tables 5-10 and 7-5). ARBs are being used more and more for hypertension and for heart failure, although the latter is not yet a registered indication in the United States. In hypertension (Fig. 7-9) they have thus far shown the capacity to reduce BP with consistently few side effects and, in particular, the absence or lower incidence of ACE-inhibitor side effects such as cough and angioedema, the latter rare but potentially fatal. In hypertension, there is increasing evidence of their capacity to reduce hard end-points.[1] ARBs are superior to β-blockade in patients with left ventricular hypertrophy[76] and to alternate therapies in type 2 diabetic persons with nephropathy[26] but not better than ACE inhibitors in heart failure[77] or in postinfarct patients.[78] VALUE is an important study on 15,245 high-risk hypertensive subjects, comparing valsartan with the CCB amlodipine on outcome measures. The CCB gave a more rapid and persistent antihypertensive effect, and protected better against MI and stroke, but the ARB reduced heart failure and new onset diabetes.[78a] ON TARGET is an extremely large HOPE-style study that still has to run for several years. It is the only large study directly comparing an ARB with an ACE inhibitor, and tests the hypothesis that the ARB telmisartan is as good as or better than ramipril in conferring cardiovascular protection on high-risk cardiovascular groups (Table 5-12). The theoretical advantages and disadvantages of the ARBs versus the ACE inhibitors have been evaluated earlier (Table 5-10). Besides combining as well with diuretics (Table 7-5) as do the ACE inhibitors, another popular combination is ARB plus CCB, which gives a better lipid outcome and a lesser incidence of metabolic syndrome and new diabetes than a diuretic plus β-blocker combination.[32]

Current and Future Role of ARBs in Hypertension While awaiting ON TAR
one view is that the ARBs block the same renin-angiotensin system
do the ACE inhibitors, with much the same effects but at greater co
Thus, an ACE inhibitor would remain preferable with an ARB subst.
tuted only if ACE-intolerance develops. Another view is that ARBs have
an excellent record in comparative studies showing better cardiovascular outcome benefit,[1] virtually without the major side effects of ACE
inhibitors, and provide symptom-free control of hypertension. It must,
however, be acknowledged that the better outcomes are largely driven
by studies on specialized subgroups of hypertensive individuals, namely
those with left ventricular hypertrophy or type 2 diabetic nephropathy,[1]
two conditions that two major guidelines already recognize as compelling or favored indications for ARBs.[21,22] As the new trials with ARBs
come in there is bound to be increasing pressure for registration of new
indications beyond hypertension and increasing use of these agents.
Thus losartan is already registered for prevention of stroke in the United
States for patients with left ventricular hypertrophy and valsartan is
under evaluation for postinfarct protection.

α-ADRENERGIC BLOCKERS

Of the α_1-receptor blockers, *prazosin (Minipress)*, *terazosin (Hytrin)*,
and *doxazosin (Cardura)* are available in the United States. Their advantages are freedom from metabolic or lipid side effects and a more
appropriate physiologic action than β-blockers in lowering peripheral
resistance. Some patients develop troublesome side effects: drowsiness, diarrhea, postural hypotension, and occasional tachycardia. Tolerance, related to fluid retention, may develop during chronic therapy
with α_1-blockers, requiring increased doses or added diuretics. Fluid
retention may explain why the doxazosin arm of the ALLHAT study
was terminated because of an excess of heart failure, compared with
reference diuretic.[23] Thus, these agents now have a lesser place in
initial monotherapy. Nonetheless, in the TOMH studies[43] on mild
hypertension, doxazosin 2 mg/day given over 4 years and combined
with hygienic measures reduced the BP as much as agents from other
groups. The quality of life improved as much as with placebo, though
not quite as much as with acebutolol; blood cholesterol fell, and the
incidence of impotence was lowest in the doxazosin group.[37,79]

Thus, despite the disappointing ALLHAT result, α-blockers may still
be chosen, especially in those with features of the metabolic syndrome
or in the many men with benign prostatic hypertrophy, in whom α-
blockers provide symptomatic relief.[80] α-Blockers combine well with
β-blockers or diuretics. Combination with CCBs may give an excess
hypotensive response, by eliminating two of the three major vasoconstrictive mechanisms, the remaining one being angiotensin-
mediated. Little is known of α-blockers plus ACE inhibitors.
Phenoxybenzamine and phentolamine are combined α_1- and α_2-
blockers used only for *pheochromocytoma*.

DIRECT VASODILATORS

Hydralazine used to be a standard third drug, its benefits enhanced
and side effects lessened by concomitant use of a diuretic and an
adrenergic inhibitor. Being inexpensive, hydralazine is still widely
used in the Third World. Elsewhere, fear of lupus (especially with continued doses above 200 mg daily) and lack of evidence for regression
of left ventricular hypertrophy has led to its replacement by the CCBs
vasodilators. *Minoxidil* is a potent long-acting vasodilator acting on
potassium channel. In addition to inciting intense renal sodium
ntion that requires large doses of loop diuretics to overcome, it
causes profuse hirsutism, so its use is usually limited to men
evere refractory hypertension or renal insufficiency (it dilates
rterioles). Occasionally minoxidil causes pericarditis. In one
mass increased by 30%.

CENTRAL ADRENERGIC INHIBITORS

The centrally acting agents, *reserpine* is easiest to use in a low dose 0.05 mg/day, which provides almost all of its antihypertensive action with fewer side effects than higher doses. Onset and offset of action are slow and measured in weeks. When cost is crucial, reserpine and diuretics are the cheapest combination. *Methyldopa*, still widely used despite adverse central symptoms and potentially serious hepatic and blood side effects, acts like clonidine on central α_2-receptors, usually without slowing the heart rate. *Clonidine, guanabenz,* and *guanfacine* provide all of the benefits of methyldopa with none of the rare but serious autoimmune reactions (as with methyldopa, sedation is frequent). In the VA study[38] clonidine 0.2 to 0.6 mg/day was among the more effective of the agents tested. It worked equally well in younger and older age groups and in blacks and whites. The major disadvantage was the highest incidence of drug intolerance (14%). A *transdermal form of clonidine (Catapres-TTS)* provides once-a-week therapy likely minimizing the risks of clonidine-withdrawal. *Guanabenz* resembles clonidine but may cause less fluid retention and reduces serum cholesterol by 5% to 10%. *Guanfacine* is a similar agent that can be given once daily. *Imidazole receptor blockers* are available in Europe, but not in the United States.

PATIENT PROFILING

Ideally, the antihypertensive drug should be matched to the patient, as follows.

Hypertensive Patients with Lipidemias For patients with established lipidemias, a statin will be needed, particularly in view of the impressive coronary and stroke protection with 10 mg atorvastatin in the ASCOT-LLA trial where the mean cholesterol level was only modestly elevated (see Chapter 10). Although higher doses of *diuretics* previously used increased plasma cholesterol, with modern low-dose treatment the problem is less.[81] When more subtle indices of dyslipidemias are taken, such as the ratio of apolipoprotein B to A, then diuretics remain at a disadvantage, at least versus ARB therapy.[82] The diuretic dose should be as low as possible, while maintaining antihypertensive efficacy. Regarding *β-blockade*, many clinicians assume that the protection β-blockers provide against recurrent heart attacks may serve to prevent initial coronary events in hypertensive individuals, but the evidence is not clear-cut.[35] In general, β-blockers tend to raise serum triglycerides, to lower HDL-cholesterol levels, and to impair insulin sensitivity. Long-term β-blockade may precipitate type 2 diabetes,[57] which is both a cardiovascular risk and predisposes to lipidemias. β-Blockers with ISA may decrease rather than increase the serum total and LDL-cholesterol.[79] By contrast to the potential problems raised by diuretics and β-blockers, the *α-blockers* clearly improve the blood lipid profile, whereas the ACE inhibitors, ARBs, and CCBs are "lipid neutral" in most studies. All of these agents also allow a better exercise performance than β-blockers.

Hypertensive Patients with Angina The only antianginal antihypertensive agents are β-blockers and CCBs. Diuretics, α-blockers, ACE inhibitors, and ARBs do not have direct antianginal effects, although indirect improvements in the myocardial oxygen balance by regression of left ventricular hypertrophy and/or reduction of BP should benefit. In the HOPE study on patients at high cardiovascular risk, ACE inhibitor reduced the risk of myocardial infarction by 20% and that of worsening angina by 11% (Table 5-9).

Postinfarct Hypertensive Patients In patients with hypertension often drops the BP, which may then creep back in the post months. There has been no adequate prospective study to d the best treatment of postinfarct hypertension but β-blockers, ACE inhibitors or ARBs, and aldosterone blockers that are indicated post-MI should also handle the hypertension.

Hypertension in Elderly Patients Multiple trials have documented even better protection against stroke and other outcome measures by treatment of the elderly than reported in the middle-aged.[83] Thus, an equivalent BP reduction will produce a greater benefit in the elderly than in younger patients, especially if there are other risk factors such as diabetes mellitus.[63] Dementia was delayed in two studies.[84,85]

Which age groups should be treated? Most studies chose people 65 to 74 years of age. However, benefits were also found in 6 trials in 824 hypertensive individuals, 80 years of age and over, although mortality was not reduced.[86]

Which are the BP limits? There is compelling evidence to suggest that sustained systolic BP elevations above 160 mmHg require treatment,[83] and that the systolic rather than the diastolic pressure is of greater importance in this age group. Therefore *isolated systolic hypertension* (with diastolic BP below 90) is now very actively treated. In the presence of end-organ damage, including abnormalities of the thoracic or abdominal aorta, and/or diabetes, BP values above 140 mmHg should be taken as reason for active therapy. Less commonly, there is *isolated diastolic hypertension* with sustained diastolic BP values of 90 mmHg and systolic values that are not elevated. These levels should be treated as in younger patients.

Are lifestyle changes still possible? Again, whenever possible, treatment includes nonpharmacological measures as in younger patients, including exercise training. Even walking sharpens cognitive skills in the elderly patients.[87] Elderly women are especially salt-sensitive. Besides salt restriction, increased dietary potassium may be protective.[88] The combination of salt restriction and loss of weight is especially desirable.[89]

How low to go? To avoid tissue underperfusion, low initial doses of drugs may be followed by a cautious increase. Indiscriminate reduction of diastolic BP below a certain optimal value, perhaps around 80 mmHg, may actually increase mortality.[90] This is the so-called *J-shaped curve* (see this chapter, p. 189), perhaps of particular significance in hypertensive men with myocardial ischemia or left ventricular hypertrophy.

Which drugs should be chosen for the elderly hypertensive patient? Low-dose *diuretics* remain the first-line drug choice in the elderly, because they were used in the SHEP study[42] and several other major trials and perhaps, equally important, because they help to prevent osteoporosis (see Chapter 4) and dementia,[85] conditions that are often disabling in the elderly.

Calcium channel blockers able to reduce morbidity and mortality in the elderly, the agents used being nitrendipine in Syst-Eur,[60] and Syst-China[91] and nifedipine in elderly Chinese hypertensive patients,[92] all being long-acting dihydropyridines. Amlodipine was equal to a diuretic or an ACE inhibitor in coronary protection in the ALLHAT trial.[23]

β-Blockers are at a disadvantage compared with diuretics in the elderly.[55] But β-blockade combined with diuretics[93] can reduce overall and stroke mortality. Risks of β-blockade in the elderly include excess sinus or AV node inhibition and a decreased cardiac output, which in the senescent heart could more readily precipitate failure.

ACE inhibitors are also often used in the elderly. The STOP-2 trial provides evidence that they are as good as conventional treatment and perhaps better than CCBs,[61] and in the men in the Australian trial, better than a diuretic.[45] Logically, ACE inhibitors are more effective with dietary salt restriction, or low-dose diuretics, or both. ACE inhibitors improve insulin sensitivity in the elderly, which may help protect from adverse metabolic effects of concurrent diuretics. So far SCOPE has been the only study with an ARB in the elderly,[94] but most of the patients in LIFE, ALLHAT and VALUE were elderly.

Combination treatment is often required, as was the case in nearly two thirds of elderly hypertensive patients in ALLHAT.[23] β-Blockers plus diuretics, ACE inhibitor plus diuretics, and CCBs plus β-blockers all seem to work equally well, using mortality and cardiovascular events as outcome measures.[61]

Black Patients An important view is that African-American hypertensive patients represent a unique population, usually underrepresented in major clinical trials except for ALLHAT.[95] In ALLHAT, the risk for stroke was greater with the ACE inhibitor lisinopril but the control of BP was poorer, probably owing to the trial design that prohibited the combination of the ACE inhibitor with a diuretic.[23] Of note, angioedema in African-Americans was much more common with lisinopril (0.7%) than with chlorthalidone (<0.1%). Black patients respond better to monotherapy with a diuretic or to a CCB than to monotherapy with an ACE inhibitor or ARB or β-blocker. The common denominator might be the low renin status of elderly black patients taken as a group. Overall evidence suggests that combination with diuretic increases sensitivity to a β-blocker or an ACE inhibitor or an ARB likely because the diuretic increases renin. In a direct comparison, CCB therapy was more effective than a low-dose diuretic as first-line therapy in South African black patients,[64] perhaps because sodium intake was not controlled.

Smokers It is imperative that the patient stops smoking. Smoking, besides being an independent risk factor for coronary artery disease and for stroke (the latter often forgotten), also interacts adversely with hypertension. First, smoking helps to promote renovascular and malignant hypertension. Second, smoking damages the vascular endothelium, the integrity of which is now thought to be important in maintaining a normal BP and erectile function. Third, heavy smoking results in a sustained rise in BP or intense swings to high systolic values, as revealed by ambulatory measurements.[96] Apparently normal casual office BP values while the patient is not smoking mask the adverse effects of smoking on the BP.

Obese Hypertensive Patients The characteristics of obesity hypertension are an increased plasma volume, a high cardiac output (explicable by Starling's law), and a low peripheral vascular resistance. The basic mechanisms are complex but include an increased tubular reabsorption of sodium and increased sympathetic outflow. Weight reduction, although a laudable and crucial goal, which in itself reduces the BP and improves the quality of life, is not easy to achieve and may require multiple visits to the dietician and group counseling as well as increased exercise. Nonetheless, even small degrees of weight loss, if maintained, will help to keep BP down. For every 1-kg weight loss there is a BP reduction of about 1 mmHg.[97]

Because of the association between insulin resistance and obesity, and the potential adverse effects of high doses of diuretics on insulin, the dose of diuretic should be kept low. Vigorous dietary restriction of calories, salt, and fat is able to improve blood lipid profiles and insulin sensitivity in the obese so that such measures should be combined with low-dose diuretic. Left ventricular hypertrophy is a particular hazard, which obesity and insulin resistance promote independently of the BP. Regarding further drug choice, in the absence of good trial data, a logical selection would be an agent that is metabolically neutral and known to combine well with a diuretic such as an ACE inhibitor or an ARB.

Diabetic or Prediabetic Hypertensive Patients In diabetic patients, the BP aims are lower than in nondiabetic individuals. JNC VII recommends a goal BP of 130/80 mmHg. In diabetic patients with isolated systolic hypertension, the systolic BP should drop to about 140 mmHg.[63] Again, treatment starts with lifestyle modification including control of hyperglycemia. Both diabetes (type 2; maturity onset; non-insulin-dependent) and hypertension are associated with insulin resistance. Both high-dose thiazides and β-blockers can impair insulin sensitivity in nondiabetic hypertensive patients. Therefore, it makes sense to avoid high-dose diuretics and β-blockers in the therapy of those prone to diabetes by a personal or family history or in non-insulin-dependent diabetic patients. Rather, there are arguments for the use of ACE inhibition or an ARB.[33,98]

CCBs generally leave diabetic control unaltered and in the Syst-Eur trial the long-acting DHP nitrendipine protected the diabetic patients better than did the diuretic in SHEP.[63] ACE inhibitors also work. Although there is no conclusive evidence that such "metabolic management" is beneficial for hypertensive type 2 diabetic or for prediabetic patients, the approach is nonetheless logical, because defects in glucose metabolism and insulin resistance develop over many years into overt diabetes. This sequence probably accounts for the increased development of type 2 diabetes in hypertensive patients treated with β-blockers.[57] Therapy-induced new diabetes has a serious prognosis.[98a]

Diabetic Patients with Nephropathy In type 1 diabetic nephropathy, ACE inhibitors have repeatedly been shown to reduce proteinuria and protect against progressive glomerular sclerosis and loss of renal function.[98] In type 2 diabetic nephropathy, four trials with ARBs have shown similar renal protection.[98] Evidence-based guidelines therefore suggest ACE inhibitors for type 1 and ARBs for type 2 diabetic renal disease.[21] The strong likelihood that ACE-inhibitors would be as effective in type 2 patients if they had been tested and their proven healing benefits means that in practice ACE inhibitors will be used whenever ARBs cannot be afforded.

Taking together the available information on those with only micro-albuminuria and those with overt nephropathy, ARBs or ACE inhibitors emerge as the preferable class of drug to control hypertension in diabetic patients. They will, however, often have to be combined with other drugs including diuretics, β-blockers, and CCBs. Because of the serious long-term significance of microalbuminuria and because increased BP is a major risk factor for renal protein leakage in diabetic patients, the cornerstone to the management of diabetic hypertensive patients is to reduce the BP to below 130/80 mmHg.

Exercising Hypertensive Patients Low to moderate intensity aerobic exercise training lowers the resting BP, so that increased exercise is part of lifestyle modification in the treatment of hypertension. Lack of exercise is an independent risk factor for coronary heart disease. Exercise training helps to delay the onset of type 2 diabetes,[99] protects the coronary endothelium,[100] and increases HDL-cholesterol. The benefits of exercise also extend to the elderly. When, besides lifestyle modification and exercise, drug treatment is required, then the best category of drug might be that which leaves the increased cardiac output of exercise unchanged while blunting the simultaneous BP rise. This goal is best attained by the ACE inhibitors or ARBs or by CCBs (especially the dihydropyridines). β-Blockade, in contrast, limits the cardiac output by decreasing the heart rate, even in the case of vasodilatory β-blockers. Furthermore, β-blockade tends to decrease HDL-cholesterol despite exercise training.

Pregnancy Hypertension The best tested drug is methyldopa (category B; see Table 11-9). ACE inhibitors and ARBs are totally contraindicated.

SPECIFIC AIMS OF ANTIHYPERTENSIVE THERAPY

Regression of Left Ventricular Hypertrophy (LVH) Preferably diagnosed by echocardiography, LVH is increasingly seen as an important adverse complication of hypertension. Apart from being an independent cardiovascular risk factor, LVH is associated with abnormalities of diastolic function, which can result in dyspnea or even overt left ventricular failure. An important point is that regression of the BP does not rapidly result in decreased LVH. Although several important retrospective analyses support the concept that the most effective agents in achieving left ventricular regression are those that interrupt the growth pathways that make myocytes hypertrophy such as the ACE inhibitors or CCBs, rather than diuretics or β-blockers, in the multi-center VA trial extending over 1 year, hydrochlorothiazide was the best of six agents.[101] The best policy in relation to LVH is therefore not clear. The LIFE study (see Table 5-12) gave a decisive advantage to the ARB, losartan, versus a β-blocker, atenolol,[76] explicable by interruption of the growth-promoting effect of angiotensin-II by losartan. Among the lifestyle measures, reduction of obesity and salt intake may be especially important. Logically, because increased myocardial stretch following systemic hypertension is at least one factor provoking protein synthesis, meticulous BP control over 24 hours would seem important. Of interest is the concept that it is not only the daytime BP that governs LVH, but also the absence of a normal nocturnal BP fall. Furthermore, prolonged treatment, up to 3 years, may be required to achieve full regression.[102]

Atrial Fibrillation LV hypertrophy caused by hypertension predisposes to left atrial enlargement and thus to atrial fibrillation. Control of ventricular rate is one viable strategy, as achieved by a number of antihypertensive drugs: verapamil, diltiazem, and β-blockers. Going further back, LVH itself must be tackled by strict control of the BP, with good arguments for starting with an ARB followed by the addition of a diuretic.[76] A further argument is that an ARB, irbesartan, helped to lessen postcardioversion left atrial stunning.[103] For *hypertension with atrial fibrillation*, the aim is again to reduce the BP to low values (say 130/80 mmHg) to prevent further left atrial enlargement, while verapamil or diltiazem or β-blockade may have a special role.

Early Morning BP Rise The highest BP found soon after rising and in the early morning hours is strongly associated with sudden death, AMI, and stroke. Logically, there has been a drive for the use of ultra-long–acting agents to blunt this early morning rise. In reality, the optimal management of early morning hypertension is still not clear and only one comparative prospective trial addressed this point. The drug used was time-released verapamil, *Covera HS*, which showed no benefit of the CCB over β-blocker–based therapy[62] (see Table 3-6). However, this trial was prematurely terminated. Presently, the ideal policy, especially in those at risk of cardiac complications, is to achieve a normal BP in the morning, a normal BP at night, and a normal diurnal rhythm, all as measured by ambulatory BP monitors.

Ventricular Arrhythmias Although often associated with LVH, ventricular ectopic activity seems relatively harmless and does not warn of sudden cardiac death. Rather, persistent and significant ventricular tachycardia may reflect accompanying coronary artery disease. Severe life-threatening arrhythmias in high-risk hypertensives may require class III agents, such as the β-blocker sotalol or amiodarone (see Chapter 8), taking care to avoid diuretic-induced hypokalemia with risk of torsades.

Prevention of Erectile Dysfunction Sexual dysfunction, especially in men, has been reported with almost every antihypertensive drug, probably a consequence of reduction of blood flow through genital vessels already having endothelial damage from the ravages of smoking, hypercholesterolemia, and diabetes. In addition, erectile dysfunction can reflect early systemic vascular disease even in the absence of overt cardiovascular disease.[104] Any diuretic therapy should be phased out; it is this category of drugs that most consistently causes impotence.[37] Next come the β-blockers. CCBs as a group seem less prone to give sexual problems. Several studies show the superiority of ACE inhibition or ARBs in maintenance or even improvement of male sexual function when compared with β-blockade.[105] In the TOMH study, the incidence of impotence fell only in those receiving the α-blocker doxasozin.[37] When needed, sildenafil or one of its successors (see Fig. 2-3) can be used in hypertensive patients without angina and therefore not taking nitrates.

Optimal Intellectual Activity In general, antihypertensives with the exception of centrally active agents such as clonidine should be free of central side effects. Nevertheless, β-blockers may have subtle effects on the intellect. Although propranolol is the major culprit, even the lipid-insoluble agent atenolol is not blameless. To be totally sure of unimpaired intellectual activity, CCBs or ACE inhibitors or ARBs seem to be the agents of choice.

Overall Quality of life (QOL) In general, all categories of antihypertensive agents improve the quality of life except for propranolol and methyldopa, and probably other centrally active agents such as clonidine.[2] Caution is advised in the interpretation of QOL studies since dropouts from adverse effects are not included. Nonetheless impaired exercise capacity or lessened sexual performance, both as with β-blockers, clearly are bad news for the active male hypertensive patient. Conversely, a sufferer from anxiety-driven hypertension and tachycardia can achieve dramatic subjective relief from β-blocker.

Cost-Effectiveness In the *Third World* and often elsewhere, expensive drugs are a luxury, and the principles of choice are governed by economic necessity. Much can be said for low-dose thiazide diuretics as initial therapy, followed by reserpine. Low-dose thiazides are relatively free of metabolic side effects. The cost of reserpine is extremely low, it is effectively antihypertensive, and it is relatively free from significant hemodynamic or subjective side effects. A diuretic-based therapy is also logical in black patients, and sensitizes the patient to β-blocker or ACE inhibitor therapy. When compliance is relatively limited by educational handicaps, the very long biologic half-life of reserpine, with catecholamine depletion lasting for many weeks, could be a major advantage. Furthermore, a cheap vasodilator (hydralazine) can readily be combined with diuretic-reserpine as the next step to give a "poor man's" equivalent of the ACE inhibitor/ARB plus diuretic plus CCB combination.

ACUTE SEVERE HYPERTENSION

First, it is important to consider whether the patient is suffering from a hypertensive urgency (BP very high, must come down but not necessarily rapidly) or emergency (complicated by acute heart failure or papilledema or hypertensive encephalopathy), before choosing any of the drugs listed in Tables 7-6 and 7-7. For urgent therapy, careful use of rapidly acting oral therapy agents such as furosemide and captopril is appropriate for initiation, with other agents added under tight supervision. For a true emergency, hospitalization is essential with careful administration of one of several agents (Tables 7-6 and 7-7). Some time ago, the choice used to fall on an intravenous agent, then sublingual nifedipine became standard therapy, since it consistently reduced systolic and diastolic BP by about 20% within 20 to 30 minutes. Such a rapid reduction of hypertension may, however, have adverse end organ effects on brain and heart.[106] *Thus, it is prudent to consider whether rapid pressure reduction is really desirable in the presence of cerebral symptoms or symptoms of myocardial ischemia.* Also of note, the short-acting form of nifedipine is not licensed for hypertension in the United States. Therefore, carefully titrated *intravenous nicardipine or labetalol* is preferable. A new choice is intravenous fenoldopam, a dopamine DA_1-selective agent.[107] This has the advantage of improving renal blood flow, and the disadvantage of causing a reflex tachycardia. For acute LV failure, enalaprilat or sublingual captopril is first choice (Table 7-6), together with a loop diuretic. For acute coronary syndromes, intravenous nitroglycerin is first choice, often with esmolol.

Nitroprusside and other parenteral agents are still used extensively. These all require careful monitoring to avoid overshoot. Nitroprusside reduces preload and afterload and has the risk of rebound hypertension. The package insert warns against continuing a high dose infusion for more than 10 minutes if the BP does not drop, because of the danger of cyanide toxicity (see Chapter 6, p. 171). *Labetalol* does not cause tachycardia and gives a smooth dose-related fall in BP; the side effects of β-blockade, such as bronchospasm, may be countered by the added α-blockade of labetalol. Diazoxide is best avoided. Hydralazine and dihydralazine may cause tachycardia and are also best avoided, especially in angina, unless there is concomitant therapy with a β-blocker.

In *acute stroke with hypertension*, the benefits of BP reduction remain conjectural, and most neurologists would reduce the BP only if the diastolic level exceeds 120 mmHg.[108]

RESISTANT HYPERTENSION

When confronted with the occasional patient who appears to be refractory to all known forms of therapy, the following points are worth considering: (1) Is the patient really compliant with the therapy? (2) Exclude white coat hypertension. Are the BP values taken in the doctor's office really representative of those with which the patient lives? (There can be striking differences.) (3) Has the patient developed some complications such as atherosclerotic renal artery stenosis or renal failure? (4) Has the patient increased salt or alcohol intake, or taken sympathomimetic agents or nonsteroidal anti-inflammatory agents or one of the new COX-2 inhibitors? (5) Are there temporary psychological stresses? (6) Could a cause of secondary hypertension be inapparent? For example, a high aldosterone/renin ratio[109] may be a clue to inapparent hyperaldosteronism that requires either replacing the thiazide by an aldosterone antagonist, or a combination of the two.[48] Then, finally, is the therapy really maximal, particularly regarding the diuretic dose, because overfilling of dilated vasculature by reactive sodium retention may also preclude a fall in the peripheral resistance? (Note that the concept of low-dose diuretic therapy must be abandoned at this stage.)

Logically, truly *refractory hypertension* means that the peripheral vascular resistance or the cardiac output or both has failed to fall. Generally, the emphasis should be on vasodilator therapy, acting on every conceivable mechanism: calcium antagonism, α-blockade, ACE inhibition, angiotensin receptor blockade, K^+ channel-induced vasodilation by *minoxidil*, and high-dose diuretics. Severe hypertension often has a volume-dependent component and reactive sodium retention often accompanies the fall in BP induced by vasodilatory drugs and especially minoxidil; therefore the addition of more diuretics, particularly the loop agents, is an important component of maximal therapy. Of the loop diuretics, the new agent torsemide is registered for once daily use in hypertension. Of the others, metolazone is equally effective as torsemide and even more certain to provide 24-hour efficacy.

The *ganglion blockers* (*guanethidine* and *guandrel*), now decidedly ou͡ of fashion because of frequent orthostatic hypotension and interfe͡

Table 7-6 Drugs Used in Hypertensive Urgencies and Emergencies

Clinical Requirement	Mechanism of Antihypertensive Effect	Drug Choice	Dose
Urgent reduction of severe acute hypertension	NO donor	Sodium nitroprusside infusion (care: cyanide toxicity)	0.3–2 µg/kg/min (careful monitoring)
Hypertension plus ischemia (± poor LV)	NO donor	Nitroglycerin infusion	5–100 µg/min (no PVC tubing)
Hypertension plus ischemia plus tachycardia	β-blocker (especially if good LV) α-β-blocker	Esmolol bolus or infusion Labetalol bolus or infusion	50–250 µg/kg/min 2–10 mg; 2.5–30 µg/kg/min
Hypertension plus heart failure	ACE inhibitor (avoid negative inotropic drugs)	Enalaprilat (iv); Captopril (s-l)	0.5–5 mg bolus; 12.5–25 mg s-l
Hypertension without cardiac complications	Vasodilators including those that increase heart rate	Hydralazine Nifedipine (see text)[†] Nicardipine: Infusion	5–10 mg boluses 5–10 mg s-l (care) 5–15 mg/hr (NB 0.1 mg/ml)
Severe or malignant hypertension, also with poor renal function	Dopamine (DA-1) agonist; avoid with β-blockers	Fenoldopam*	0.2–0.5 µg/kg/min
Hypertension plus pheochromocytoma	α-β- or combined α-β-blocker (avoid pure β-blocker)	Phentolamine Labetalol: Bolus : Infusion	1–4 mg boluses 2–10 mg 2.5–30 µg/kg/min

*Licensed as Corlopam for use in severe or malignant hypertension in the United States; for detailed infusion rates, see package insert. Note tachycardia as side effect must not be treated by β-blockade (package insert).

[†]Not licensed in the United States; note cautions in text.

iv = intravenous, LV = left ventricle, s-l = sublingual.

Table 7-7 Preferred Parenteral Drugs for Specific Hypertensive Emergencies (in Order of Preference)

Emergency	Preferred	Avoid (Reason)
Hypertensive encephalopathy	Labetalol Nicardipine Nitroprusside	Methyldopa (sedation) Diazoxide (fall in cerebral blood flow), Reserpine (sedation)
Accelerated-malignant hypertension	Labetalol* Fenoldopam† Enalaprilat† Nicardipine†	Methyldopa (sedation)
Left ventricular failure	Enalaprilat Nitroglycerin Nitroprusside	Labetalol, esmolol, and other β-blockers ($\downarrow$CO)
Coronary insufficiency	Nitroglycerin Esmolol Nicardipine	Hydralazine ($\uparrow$ CO), Diazoxide ($\uparrow$ CO), Nitroprusside (coronary steal)
Dissecting aortic aneurysm	Esmolol Nitroprusside	Hydralazine ($\uparrow$ CO), Diazoxide ($\uparrow$ CO),
Catecholamine excess	Labetalol α plus β-blockers	All others (less specific)
Postoperative	Labetalol Nitroglycerin Nicardipine	

*Licensed for severe hypertension.
†Licensed for hypertension.
‡Licensed for malignant hypertension.
§Dose 0.5 to 5 mg/min as intravenous infusion; onset 1 to 5 min; S/E: general autonomic blockade.
CO = cardiac output.

ence with sexual activity, should therefore be reserved for the last resort.

SUMMARY

1. *Major advances* since the last edition of this book are as follows. First, the BP goals have become lower, but strongly related to the degree of risk. Therefore, risk factor stratification is now an important part of the evaluation of hypertension. Blood lipid profiles should always be undertaken and clinical examination should establish target organ damage prior to multifactorial lifestyle intervention.

2. *Elderly persons and diabetic individuals* have emerged as two major high-risk groups. In the elderly, treatment of hypertension and systolic hypertension reduces stroke, cardiovascular events, and all-cause mortality. In diabetic persons, BP should ideally be reduced to 130/80 mmHg in addition to provision of statin therapy.

3. *As agents of first choice,* the Joint National Committee in the United States recommends low-dose diuretics for uncomplicated hypertension in patients lacking specific indications for other agents, because diuretics reduce a variety of important endpoints, including all-cause mortality. By contrast, the European Society of Hypertension proposes that any of five categories of drugs should be suitable, namely low-dose diuretics, β-blockers, CCBs, ACE inhibitors, or angiotensin receptor blockers (ARBs). It may be expected that treatment of mild hypertension by any of these five types of agents, together with lifestyle modification, will result in a rather similar reduction of BP and an improvement of quality of life with few adverse effects for any specific agent.

4. *In diabetic patients,* ACE inhibitors or ARBs are almost always the first choice. Diuretics, CCBs, and β-blockers may all be needed to bring down the BP to the low levels required.

5. *In the elderly,* agents that have been primarily used in trials are low-dose diuretics and long-acting dihydropyridine calcium blockers.

6. *In coronary disease* in hypertensive patients, optimal management should help achieve the control of both BP and blood lipids, thereby hopefully helping to reduce coronary mortality. No particular group of antihypertensive agents seems particularly effective in reducing coronary mortality. By contrast, statins are achieving increasing success.

7. *In severe emergency hypertension,* selection should be made from the available intravenous agents according to the characteristics of the patient. For those with severe hypertension but no acute target organ damage, fast-acting oral agents such as furosemide and captopril should be used.

8. *In refractory hypertension,* it is important to ensure compliance, to exclude a secondary cause including aldosteronism, to think of white-coat hypertension, and then only to increase the medication.

9. *General approach.* We recommend a patient-guided approach together with a consideration of the major outcome trials and guidelines as the most appropriate way to treat hypertension.

REFERENCES

1. BP Trialists. Effects of different blood-pressure lowering regimens on major cardiovascular events: results of prospectively-designed overviews of randomised trials. *Lancet* 2003;362:1527–1535.
2. Beto JA, et al. Quality of life in treatment of hypertension. A meta-analysis of clinical trials. *Am J Hypertens* 1992;5:125–133.
3. PROGRESS Collaborative Group. Effects of blood pressure lowering with perindopril and indapamide therapy on dementia and cognitive decline in patients with cerebrovascular disease. *Arch Intern Med* 2003;163:1069–1075.
4. He FJ, et al. Effect of modest salt reduction on blood pressure: a meta-analysis of randomized trials. Implications for public health. *J Hum Hypertens* 2002;16:761–770.
5. Sacks FM, et al. For the DASH-Sodium Collaborative Research Group. Effects on blood pressure of reduced dietary sodium and the Dietary Approaches to Stop Hypertension (DASH) diet. *N Engl J Med* 2001;344:3–10.
6. Schillaci G, et al. Effect of body weight changes on 24-hour blood pressure and left ventricular mass in hypertension: a 4-year follow up. *Am J Hypertens* 2003;16:634–639.
7. Appel LJ, et al. Effects of comprehensive lifestyle modification on blood pressure control: main results of the PREMIER clinical trial. *JAMA* 2003;289:2083–2093.
8. Tanasescu M, et al. Physical activity in relation to cardiovascular disease and total mortality among men with type 2 diabetes. *Circulation* 2003;107:2435–2439.
9. Vasan RS, et al. Impact of high-normal blood pressure on the risk of cardiovascular disease. *N Engl J Med* 2001;345:1291–1297.
10. Lewington S, et al. Age-specific relevance of usual blood pressure to vascular mortality: a meta-analysis of individual data for one million adults in 61 prospective studies. *Lancet* 2002;360:1903–1913.
11. Chobanian AV, et al. The Seventh Report of the Joint National Committee on Prevention, Detection, Evaluation, and Treatment of High Blood Pressure: the JNC 7 report. *Hypertension* 2003;42:1206–1252.
12. Chobanian AV, et al. The Seventh Report of the Joint National Committee on Prevention, Detection, Evaluation and Treatment of High Blood Pressure. *JAMA* 2003;289:2560–2572.
13. Vasan RS, et al. Residual lifetime risk for developing hypertension in middle-aged women and men: The Framingham Heart Study. *JAMA* 2002;287:1003–1010.
14. De Backer G, et al. European guidelines on cardiovascular disease and prevention in clinical practice. *Atherosclerosis* 2003;171:145–155.
15. Blake GJ, et al. Blood pressure, C-reactive protein, and risk of future cardiovascular events. *Circulation* 2003;108:2993-2999.
16. Benetos A, et al. Prognostic value of systolic and diastolic blood pressure in treated hypertensive men. *Arch Intern Med* 2002;162:577–581.
17. Izzo JJ, et al. Clinical advisory statement: importance of systolic blood pressure in older Americans. *Hypertension* 2000;35:1021–1024.
18. HOT Study. Effects of intensive blood-pressure lowering and low-dose aspirin in patients with hypertension: principal results of the Hypertension Optimal Treatment (HOT) randomised trial. *Lancet* 1998;351:1755–1762.
19. Somes GW, et al. The role of diastolic blood pressure when treating isolated systolic hypertension. *Arch Intern Med* 1999;159:2004–2009.
20. JNC VII. The Seventh Report of the Joint National Committee on Prevention, Detection, Evaluation and Treatment of High Blood Pressure. *JAMA* 2003;289:2560–2572.
21. European Society of Hypertension Guidelines Committee. European Society of Cardiology guidelines for the management of arterial hypertension. *J Hypertens* 2003;21:1011–1053.

22. WHO/ISH Writing Group. 2003 World Health Organisation (WHO)/ International Society of Hypertension (ISH) statement on management of hypertension. *J Hypertens* 2003;21:1983–1992.

23. ALLHAT Collaborative Research Group. Major outcomes in high-risk hypertensive patients randomized to angiotensin-converting enzyme inhibitor or calcium channel blocker vs diuretic. The Antihypertensive and Lipid-Lowering Treatment to Prevent Heart Attack Trial (ALLHAT). *JAMA* 2002;288:2981–2997.

24. Kaplan NM. Treatment of hypertension: lifestyle modifications. In: Kaplan's Clinical Hypertension, Kaplan NM, ed. Philadelphia: Lippincott Williams & Wilkins; 2002:206–236.

25. Wing LM, et al. A comparison of outcomes with angiotensin-converting-enzyme inhibitors and diuretics for hypertension in the elderly. *N Engl J Med* 2003;348: 583–592.

26. Berl T, et al. Cardiovascular outcomes in the Irbesartan diabetic nephropathy trial of patients with type 2 diabetes and overt nephropathy. *Ann Intern Med* 2003;138: 542–549.

27. Pitt B, et al. Effect of losartan compared with captopril on mortality in patients with symptomatic heart failure: randomised trial—the Losartan Heart Failure Survival Study ELITE II. *Lancet* 2000;355:1582–1587.

28. Pfeffer MA, et al. Valsartan, captopril or both in myocardial infarction complicated by heart failure, left ventricular dysfunction or both. *N Engl J Med* 2003;349: 1893–1906.

29. RALES Study, et al. For the Randomized Aldactone Evaluation Study Investigators. The effect of spironolactone on morbidity and mortality in patients with severe heart failure. *N Engl J Med* 1999;341:709–717.

30. Pitt B, et al. Eplerenone, a selective aldosterone blocker in patients with left ventricular dysfunction after myocardial infarction. *N Engl J Med* 2003;348: 1309–1321.

31. White WB, et al. Effects of the selective aldosterone blocker eplerenone versus the calcium antagonist amlodipine in systolic hypertension. *Hypertension* 2003;41: 1021–1026.

32. Lindholm LH, et al. Metabolic outcome during 1 year in newly detected hypertensives: results of the Antihypertensive Treatment and Lipid Profile in a North of Sweden Efficacy Evaluation (ALPINE study). *J Hypertens* 2003;21:1563–1574.

33. Opie LH, Schall R. Old antihypertensives and new diabetics. *J Hypertens* 2004; 22:1453–1458.

34. Psaty BM, et al. Health outcomes associated with various antihypertensive therapies used as first-line agents. *JAMA* 2003;289:2534–2544.

35. Psaty BM, et al. Health outcomes associated with antihypertensive therapies uses as first-line agents. A systemic review and meta-analysis. *JAMA* 1997;277:739–745.

36. Cohen HW, et al. High and low serum potassium associated with cardiovascular events in diuretic-treated patients. *J Hypertens* 2001;19:1315–1323.

37. Grimm RH, et al. Long-term effects on sexual function of five antihypertensive drugs and nutritional hygienic treatment in hypertensive men and women. Treatment of Mild Hypertension Study (TOMHS). *Hypertension* 1997;29:8–14.

38. Materson BJ, et al. Single-drug therapy for hypertension in men. A comparison of six antihypertensive agents with placebo. The Department of Veterans Affairs Cooperative Study Group on Antihypertensive Agents. *N Engl J Med* 1993;328: 914–921.

39. Reyes AJ. Diuretics in the therapy of hypertension. *J Hum Hypertens* 2002;16(Suppl 1):S788–3.

40. Carter BL, et al. Hydrochlorothiazide versus chlorthalidone: evidence supporting their interchangeability. *Hypertension* 2004;43:4–9.

41. Pepine CJ, et al. A calcium antagonist vs a non-calcium antagonist hypertension treatment strategy for patients with coronary artery disease. The International Verapamil-Trandolapril Study (INVEST): a randomized controlled trial. *JAMA* 2003;290:2805–2816.

42. SHEP Cooperative Research Group. Prevention of stroke by antihypertensive drug treatment in older persons with isolated systolic hypertension Final results of the Systolic Hypertension in the Elderly Program (SHEP). *JAMA* 1991;265:3255–3264.

43. TOMH Study. Treatment of Mild Hypertension study (TOMH). Final results. *JAMA* 1993;270:713–724.

44. Franse LV, et al. Hypokalemia associated with diuretic use and cardiovascular events in the Systolic Hypertension in the Elderly Program. *Hypertension* 2000;35: 1025–1030.

45. Wiggan MI, et al. Low dose bendrofluazide (1.25 mg) effectively lowers blood pressure over 24 h. Results of a randomized, double-blind, placebo-controlled crossover study. *Am J Hypertens* 1999;12:528–531.

46. Gosse P, et al. On behalf of the LIVE investigators. Regression of left ventricular hypertrophy in hypertensive patients treated with indapamide SR 1.5 mg versus enalapril 20 mg: the LIVE study. *J Hypertens* 2000;18:1465–1475.

47. Baumgart P. Torasemide in comparison with thiazides in the treatment of hypertension. *Cardiovasc Drugs Ther* 1993;7(Suppl 1):63–68.

48. Nishizaka M, et al. Efficacy of low-dose spinronolactone in subjects with resistant hypertension. *Am J Hypertens* 2003;16:925–930.

49. Siscovick DS, et al. Diuretic therapy for hypertension and the risk of primary cardiac arrest. *N Engl J Med* 1994;330:1852–1857.

50. Frishman WH, et al. A multifactorial trial design to assess combination therapy in hypertension. *Arch Intern Med* 1994;154:1461–1468.

51. Thulin T, et al. Diltiazem compared with metoprolol as add-on-therapies to diuretics in hypertension. *J Hum Hypertens* 1991;5:107–114.

52. Elliott WJ, et al. Equivalent antihypertensive effects of combination therapy using diuretic + calcium antagonist compared with diuretic + ACE inhibitor. *J Hum Hypertens* 1990;4:717–723.

53. JNC VI. Joint National Committee on Prevention, Detection, Evaluation and Treatment of High Blood Pressure. The Sixth Report of the Joint National Committee on Prevention, Detection, Evaluation and Treatment of High Blood Pressure. *Arch Intern Med* 1997;157:2413–2446.

54. MRC Working Party. Medical Research Council trial of treatment of hypertension in older adults: principal results. *Br Med J* 1992;304:405–412.

55. Messerli FH, et al. Are beta-blockers efficacious as first-line therapy for hypertension in the elderly? A systematic review. *JAMA* 1998;279:1903–1907.

56. Serlin MJ, et al. Propranolol in the control of blood pressure. *Clin Phamacol Ther* 1980;27:586–592.

57. Gress TW, et al. For the Atherosclerosis Risk in Communities Study. Hypertension and antihypertensives therapy as risk factors for type 2 diabetes mellitus. *N Engl J Med* 2000;342:905–912.

58. Salpeter SR, et al. Cardioselective beta-blockers in patients with reactive airway disease: a meta-analysis. *Ann Intern Med* 2002;137:715–725.

59. Grossman EH, et al. Effect of calcium antagonists on plasma norepinephrine levels, heart rate and blood pressure. *Am J Cardiol* 1997;80:1453–1458.

60. Syst-Eur Trial. Randomised double-blind comparison of placebo and active treatment for older patients with isolated systolic hypertension (Syst-Eur Trial). *Lancet* 1997;350:757–764.

61. STOP-2 Study. Randomised trial of old and new antihypertensive drugs in elderly patients: cardiovascular mortality and morbidity in the Swedish Trial in Old Patients with Hypertension-2 study. *Lancet* 1999;354:1751–1756.

62. Black HR, et al. Principal results of the Controlled Onset Verapamil Investigation of Cardiovascular End Points (CONVINCE) trial. *JAMA* 2003;289:2073–2082.

63. Tuomilehto J, et al. Effects of calcium-channel blockade in older patients with diabetes and systolic hypertension. *N Engl J Med* 1999;340:677–684.

64. Sareli P, et al. Efficacy of different drug classes used to initiate antihypertensive treatment in black subjects: results of a randomized trial in Johannesburg, South Africa. *Arch Intern Med* 2001;161:965–971.

65. Bakris GL, et al. Effect of calcium channel or β-blockade on the progression of diabetic nephropathy in African Americans. *Hypertension* 1997;29:744–750.

66. Wright JT Jr, et al. For the African American Study of Kidney Disease and Hypertension Study Group (AASK). Effect of blood pressure lowering and antihypertensive drug class on progression of hypertensive kidney disease. *JAMA* 2002:2421–2431.

67. HOPE Investigators. Effects of an angiotensin-converting enzyme inhibitor, ramipril, on cardiovascular events in high-risk patients. *N Engl J Med* 2000;342:145–153.

68. Chrysant SG, et al. Effects of isradipine or enalapril on blood pressure in salt-sensitive hypertensives during low and high dietary salt intake. MIST II Trial Investigators. *Am J Hypertens* 2000;13:1180–1188.

69. HOPE Study Investigators. Effects of ramipril on cardiovascular and microvascular outcomes in people with diabetes mellitus. Results of the HOPE study and the MICRO-HOPE substudy. *Lancet* 2000;355:253–259.

70. Svensson P, et al. Comparative effects of ramipril on ambulatory and office blood pressures: a HOPE substudy. *Hypertension* 2001;38:E28–32.

71. PROGRESS Collaborative Group. Randomised trial of a perindopril-based blood-pressure-lowering regimen among 6105 individuals with previous stroke or transient ischaemic attack. *Lancet* 2001;358:1033–1041.

72. UKPDS 39. UK Prospective Diabetes Study Group. Efficacy of atenolol and captopril in reducing risk of macrovascular and microvascular complications in type 2 diabetes: UKPDS 39. *Br Med J* 1998;317:713–720.

73. Bakris GL, et al. For National Kidney Foundation, Hypertension and Diabetes Executive Committees Working Group. Preserving renal function in adults with hypertension and diabetes. *J Am J Kidney Dis* 2000;36:646–661.

74. REIN Study. On behalf of the Gruppo Italiano di Studi Epidemiologici in Nefrologia (GISEN) Study. Renal function and requirements for dialysis in chronic nephropathy patients on long-term ramipril: REIN follow up trial. *Lancet* 1998;352:1252–1256.

75. Antonios T, et al. A diuretic is more effective than a β-blocker in hypertensive patients not controlled on amlodipine and lisinopril. *Hypertension* 1996;27: 1325–1328.

76. LIFE Study Group. Cardiovascular morbidity and mortality in the Losartan Intervention For Endpoint reduction in hypertension study (LIFE): a randomised trial against atenolol. *Lancet* 2002;359:995–1003.

77. ELITE II Study. Effect of losartan compared with captopril on mortality in patients with symptomatic heart failure: randomised trial—the Losartan Heart Failure Survival Study ELITE II. *Lancet* 2000;355:1582–1587.

78. Pfeffer MA, et al. Effects of candesartan on mortality and morbidity in patients with chronic heart failure: the CHARM-overall programme. *Lancet* 2003;362:777–781.

78a. Julius S, et al. Outcomes in hypertensive patients at high cardiovascular risk treated with regimens based on valsartan or amlodipine: the VALUE randomised trial. *Lancet* 2004;363:2022–2031.

79. Grimm RH, et al. For the Treatment of Mild Hypertension Study (TOMHS) Research Group. Long-term effects on plasma lipids of diet and drugs to treat hypertension. *JAMA* 1996;275:1549–1556.

80. McConnell JD, et al. The long-term effect of doxazosin, finasteride, and combination therapy on the clinical progression of benign prostatic hyperplasia. *N Engl J Med* 2003;349:2387–2398.

81. Moser M. Why are physicians not prescribing diuretics more frequently in the management of hypertension? *JAMA* 1998;279:1813–1816.
82. Lindholm LH. Major benefits from cholesterol-lowering in patients with diabetes. *Lancet* 2003;361:2000.
83. Staessen JA, et al. Risks of untreated and treated isolated systolic hypertension in the elderly: meta-analysis of outcome trials. *Lancet* 2000;355:865–872.
84. Forette F, et al. For the Syst-Eur Investigators. The prevention of dementia with antihypertensive treatment. *Arch Intern Med* 2002;162:2046–2052.
85. Guo Z, et al. Occurrence and progression of dementia in a community population aged 75 years and older. *Arch Neurol* 1999;56:991–996.
86. Gueyffier F. Antihypertensive drugs in very old people: a subgroup meta-analysis of randomised controlled trials. *Lancet* 1999;353:793–796.
87. Larkin M. Walking sharpens some cognitive skills in elderly. *Lancet* 1999;354:401.
88. He FJ, et al. Potassium intake and blood pressure. *Am Heart J* 1999;12:849–851.
89. Whelton PK, et al. For the TONE Collaborative Group. Sodium reduction and weight loss in the treatment of hypertension in older persons. A randomized controlled Trial for Nonpharmacologic interventions in the Elderly (TONE). *JAMA* 1998;279: 839–846.
90. Boutitie F, et al. For the INDANA Project Steering Committee. *Ann Intern Med* 2002;136:438–448.
91. Syst-China Collaborative Group. Comparison of active treatment and placebo in older Chinese patients with isolated systolic hypertension. *J Hypertens* 1998;16:1823–1829.
92. Gong L, et al. Shanghai Trial of Nifedipine in the Elderly (STONE). *J Hypertens* 1996;14:1237–1245.
93. STOP Study. Morbidity and mortality in the Swedish Trial in Old Patients with Hypertension (STOP-Hypertension). *Lancet* 1991;338:1281–1285.
94. SCOPE Study, et al. The Study on Cognition and Prognosis in the Elderly (SCOPE): principal results of a randomised double-blind intervention trial. *J Hypertens* 2003;21:875–886.
95. Douglas JG, et al. Management of high blood pressure in African Americans: consensus statement of the Hypertension in African Americans Working Group of the International Society on Hypertension in Blacks. *Arch Intern Med* 2003;163:525–541.
96. Minami J, et al. Is it time to regard cigarette smoking as a risk factor in the development of sustained hypertension? *Am J Hypertens* 1999;12:948–949.
97. Neter JE, et al. Influence of weight reduction on blood pressure: a meta-analysis of randomized controlled trials. *Hypertension* 2003;42:878–884.
98. Vijan S, et al. Treatment of hypertension in type 2 diabetes mellitus: blood pressure goals, choice of agents, and setting priorities in diabetes care. *Ann Intern Med* 2003;138:593–602.
98a. Verdecchia P, et al. Adverse prognostic significance of new diabetes in treated hypertensive subjects. *Hypertension* 2004;43:963–969.
99. Diabetes Prevention Program Research Group. Reduction in the incidence of type 2 diabetes with lifestyle intervention and metformin. *N Engl J Med* 2002;346:393.
100. Hambrecht R, et al. Effect of exercise on coronary endothelial function in patients with coronary artery disease. *N Engl J Med* 2000;342:454–460.
101. Gottdiener JS, et al. Effect of single-drug therapy on reduction of left ventricular mass in mild to moderate hypertension. *Circulation* 1997;95:2007–2014.
102. Franz I-W, et al. Time course of complete normalization of left ventricular hypertrophy during long-term antihypertensive therapy with angiotensin converting enzyme inhibitors. *Am J Hypertens* 1998;11:631–639.
103. Madrid A, et al. Use of irbesartan to maintain sinus rhythm in patients with long-lasting persistent atrial fibrillation: a prospective and randomized study. *Circulation* 2002;106:331–336.
104. Kaiser DR, et al. Impaired brachial artery endothelium-dependent and -independent vasodilation in men with erectile dysfunction and no other clinical cardiovascular disease. *J Am Coll Cardiol* 2004;43:179–184.
105. Fogari R, et al. Sexual activity in hypertensive men treated with valsartan or carvedilol: a crossover study. *Am J Hypertens* 2001;14:27–31.
106. Grossman E, et al. Should a moratorium be placed on sublingual nifedipine capsules given for hypertensive emergencies and pseudoemergencies. *JAMA* 1996;276:1328–1331.
107. Oparil S, et al. Fenoldopam: a new parenteral antihypertensive. *Am J Hypertens* 1999;12:653–664.
108. Chalmers J, et al. International Society of Hypertension (ISH): statements on blood pressure and stroke. *J Hypertens* 2003;21:649–650.
109. Schwartz GL, et al. Screening for primary aldosteronism: implications of an increased plasma aldosterone/renin ratio. *Clinical Chemistry* 2002;48:1919–1923.
110. National Cholesterol Education Program Expert Panel. Detection, evaluation and treatment of high blood cholesterol in adults. (Adult Treatment Panel III). *Circulation* 2002;106:3143–3421.
111. Boden G. Role of fatty acids in the pathogensis of insulin resistance and NIDDM. *Diabetes* 1996;45:3–10.
112. Nickenig G, et al. Insulin induces upregulation of vascular AT_1 receptor gene expression by postranscriptional mechanisms. *Circulation* 1998;98:2543–2460.
113. Lund-Johansen P, et al. Acute and chronic hemodynamic effects of drugs with different actions on adrenergic receptors: a comparison between alpha blockers and different types of beta blockers with and without vasodilating effect. *Cardiovasc Drugs Ther* 1991;5:605–615.

Antiarrhythmic Drugs and Strategies

John P. DiMarco • Bernard J. Gersh • Lionel H. Opie

"Devices and radiofrequency ablation have revolutionized the therapy of life-threatening and highly symptomatic arrhythmias."

AUTHORS OF THIS CHAPTER, 2004

Section A   ANTIARRHYTHMIC DRUGS

Arrhythmias require treatment either for alleviating significant symptoms or for prolonging survival. The wisdom of treating arrhythmias "prophylactically" has been severely questioned by a large trial (Cardiac Arrhythmia Suppression Trial)[1] and by a meta-analysis of nearly 100,000 patients with acute myocardial infarction (AMI) treated with antiarrhythmic drugs.[2] Although it is chiefly the class III and class I (and especially the class IC agents) that are proarrhythmic, the principle raised is important. Arrhythmias should be treated by drugs whose prophylactic power outweighs the adverse effects, as may be the case for β-blockers and amiodarone. The latter is now regarded as "one of the leading antiarrhythmic drugs because of proven efficacy and safety,"[3] yet serious side effects still constrain its wider use,[4] so that the search for the perfect antiarrhythmic drug continues. In the meantime, β-blockers and amiodarone are the agents that cover many situations. Expanding technologies and the imperfections of current antiarrhythmic drugs have led to an explosion in the use of devices and ablative techniques for both supraventricular and ventricular arrhythmias.

Classification There are four established classes of antiarrhythmic action (Table 8-1). In life-threatening arrhythmias, the strong trend is away from class I agents to class III agents and now to devices. The original classification now incorporates ionic mechanisms and receptors as the basis of the more complex Sicilian Gambit system for antiarrhythmic drug classification (Fig. 8-1).[5] Another descriptive division is into those drugs used only in the therapy of supraventricular tachycardias (Table 8-2) and those used chiefly against ventricular tachycardias (Table 8-3). Currently, there is no evidence that class I agents reduce death, there is such evidence favoring β-blockers especially in ischemic heart disease, and there is increasing evidence that amiodarone is effective against a wide spectrum of arrhythmias, but being inferior to implantable cardioverter defibrillators (ICDs) in the highest risk patients.[6]

CLASS IA: QUINIDINE AND SIMILAR COMPOUNDS

Historically, quinidine was the first antiarrhythmic drug used, and its classification as a class IA agent (the others being disopyramide and procainamide) might suggest excellent effects with superiority to other agents. That is not so, and now that the defects and dangers of quinidine are better understood, it is used less and less. Class I agents are those that act chiefly by inhibiting the fast sodium channel with depression of phase 0 of the action potential. In addition, they prolong the action potential duration and thereby have a mild class III action (Fig. 8-1). Such compounds can cause proarrhythmic

Table 8-1 Antiarrhythmic Drug Classes

Class	Channel Effects	Repolarization Time	Drug Examples
1A	Sodium block Effect ++	Prolongs	Quinidine Disopyramide Procainamide
1B	Sodium block Effect +	Shortens	Lidocaine Phenytoin Mexiletine Tocainide
1C	Sodium block Effect +++	Unchanged	Flecainide Propafenone
II	I_f, a pacemaker and depolarizing current; indirect Ca^{2+} channel block	Unchanged	β-Blockers (excluding sotalol that also has class III effects)
III	Repolarizing K^+ currents	Markedly prolongs	Amiodarone Sotalol Ibutilide Dofetilide
IV	AV nodal Ca^{2+} block	Unchanged	Verapamil Diltiazem
IV-like	K^+ channel opener (hyperpolarization)	Unchanged	Adenosine

+ = inhibitory effect; ++ = markedly inhibitory effect; +++ = very major inhibitory effect.

complications by prolonging the QT-interval in certain genetically predisposed individuals or by depressing conduction and promoting reentry. There are no large-scale outcome trials to suggest that quinidine or other class I agents decrease mortality; rather there is indirect evidence that suggests increased or at best neutral mortality.

Quinidine

The proarrhythmic and noncardiac side effects of quinidine together with its potential for drug interactions have led to a dramatic reduction in its use, even though the alternatives are not without their own problems. Nevertheless quinidine remains the historical prototype of class I agents.

Basic Electrophysiology Quinidine has a wide spectrum of activity against reentrant as well as ectopic atrial and ventricular tachyarrhythmias. It slows conduction and increases refractoriness in the retrograde fast pathway limb of AV nodal tachycardias and over the accessory pathway. Quinidine also slows the ventricular response to atrial fibrillation in Wolff-Parkinson-White (WPW) syndrome (Fig. 8-2). Regarding *receptor effects*, quinidine inhibits peripheral and myocardial α-adrenergic receptors, explaining the hypotension seen with intravenous administration. Furthermore, quinidine inhibits muscarinic receptors to increase sympathetic tone by this vagolytic effect. Thus it may cause sinus tachycardia and facilitate AV conduction to increase the ventricular rate in atrial flutter or fibrillation. Increased sympathetic tone may explain part of the proarrhythmic effect. *Pharmacokinetics and therapeutic levels* are shown in Table 8-3.

Indications and Doses The attempted pharmacological conversion of atrial flutter or fibrillation by quinidine has almost totally been replaced by class III agents such as amiodarone or sotalol, or the newer agents ibutilide and dofetilide, with, however, increasing use of

Text continued on p. 224

Table 8-2 Antiarrhythmic Drugs Used Only in Therapy of Supraventricular Arrhythmias

Agent	Dose	Pharmacokinetics and Metabolism	Side Effects and Contraindications	Interactions and Precautions
Adenosine (class IV-like)	For paroxysmal SVT, initial dose 6 mg by rapid IV. If the dose ineffective within 1–2 min, 12 mg may be given and if necessary, 12 mg after a further 1–2 min. A dose of 0.0375 to 0.25 mg per kg body weight is reported to be effective in children.	$t_{1/2}$ = 10–30 sec. Rapidly taken by active transport system into erythrocytes and vascular endothelial cells (major route of elimination) where it is metabolized to inosine and adenosine monophosphate.	Usually transient and include nausea, light-headedness, headache, flushing, provocation of chest pain, sinus or AV nodal inhibition, bradycardia, and with large dose infusion, rare side effects hypotension, tachycardia, bronchospasm. Contraindication in asthma, second- or third-degree AV block, sick sinus syndrome.	**Caution:** In atrial flutter, adenosine may precipitate 1:1 conduction Dipyridamole inhibits the breakdown of adenosine, therefore dose of adenosine should be reduced. Methylxanthines (caffeine, theophylline) antagonize the interaction of adenosine with its receptors.
Verapamil (class IV)	5–10 mg by slow IV push (over 2–3 min), which can be repeated with 10 mg in 10–15 min if tolerated. In USA a second dose of 10 mg given after 10 min if required. Oral dose: 120–480 mg daily in 3 to 4 divided doses.	$t_{1/2}$ 2–8 h after an oral dose or after IV administration. After repeated oral doses this increases to 4.5–12 h. Verapamil acts within 5 min of IV administration and 1–2 h after oral administration with a peak plasma level after 1–2 h. Approximately 90% absorbed from the GI tract with intersubject variation and considerable first-pass metabolism in the liver (CYP1A2) and the bioavailability is only about 20%.	Contraindicated in hypotension, cardiogenic shock, marked bradycardia, second- or third-degree AV block, WPW syndrome, wide complex tachycardia, VT and uncompensated heart failure. Also in sick sinus syndrome without a pacemaker	Decreased serum concentrations of phenobarbital, phenytoin, sulfinpyrazone, and rifampin. Increased serum concentrations of digoxin, quinidine, carbamazepine, and cyclosporin. Increased toxicity with rifampin and cimetidine. Dose reduced if impaired liver function.
Diltiazem (class IV)	Initial dose 0.25 mg/kg over 2 min, ECG, BP monitoring. Further dose of 0.35 mg/kg after 15 min if required. For AF or flutter, initial infusion of 5–10 mg/h, may increase by 5 mg/h up to 15 mg/h, up to 24 h.	$t_{1/2}$ = 3–5 h (longer in the elderly). After absorption diltiazem extensively metabolized by cytochrome P450 with bioavailability of about 40% with considerable interindividual variation. 80% bound to plasma protein. No effect of renal or hepatic dysfunction on plasma concentration of diltiazem.	AV block, bradycardia and rarely asystole or sinus arrest. C/I in sick sinus syndrome, preexisting second- or third-degree heart block, wide QRS tachycardia, marked, bradycardia or LV failure.	Risk of bradycardia, AV block with amiodarone, β-blockers, digoxin and mefloquine. Blood diltiazem may ↑ with cimetidine and ↓ with inducers: barbiturates, phenytoin, and rifampin. Reduce doses of carbamazepine, cyclosporine. Digoxin level variable, may ↑, watch AV node.

Drug	Dose	Side effects / contraindications	Interactions
Esmolol (class II)	IV 500 µg/kg/min loading dose over 1 min before each titration/maintenance step. Use steps of 50, 100, 150, and 200 µg/kg/min over 4 min each, stopping at the desired therapeutic effect.	$t_{1/2}$ = 9 min. Following an initial bolus and infusion, onset of action occurs within 2 min and a 90% steady-state level is reached within 5 min. Following discontinuation full recovery from β-blockade properties occur at 18–30 min. Esmolol metabolized in red blood cells without renal or hepatic metabolism.	Hypotension, peripheral ischemia, confusion, thrombophlebitis, and skin necrosis from extravasation, bradycardia, bronchospasm. Contraindicated in severe bradycardia, heart block (>1º), cardiogenic shock and overt heart failure.	Interactions with catecholamine depleting drugs. Can increase digoxin blood levels and prolong the action of succinylcholine
Ibutilide (class III)	IV infusion: 1 mg over 10 min, (under 60 kg: 0.01 mg/kg). If needed, repeat after 10 min	Initial distribution $t_{1/2}$ is 1.5 min. Elimination $t_{1/2}$ averages 6 h (range 2–12 h). Efficacy is usually within 40 min.	Nausea, headache, hypotension, bundle branch block, AV nodal block, bradycardia, torsades de pointes, sustained monomorphic VT, tachycardia, ventricular extrasystoles. Avoid concurrent therapy with class I or III agents. Care with amiodarone or sotalol. C/I: previous torsades de pointes, decompensated heart failure	Interactions with class IA and other class III antiarrhythmic drugs which prolong the QT interval (e.g., antipsychotics, antidepressants, macrolide antibiotics, and some antihistamines). Check QT (Fig. 8–4). Correct hypokalemia and hypomagnesemia
Dofetilide (class III)	Dose 125–500 µg, must be individualized* twice daily. Check QT 2–3 h after dose, if QTc is >15% or >500 msec, reduce dose. If QTc >500 msec, stop	Oral peak plasma concentration in 2.5 h and a steady state within 48 h. 50% excreted by kidneys unchanged.	Torsades de pointes in 3% of patients which can be reduced by ensuring normal serum K, avoiding dofetilide or reducing the dose if abnormal renal function, bradycardia, or baseline QT↑. Avoid with other drugs increasing QT: C/I: previous torsades, creatinine clearance <20 ml/min	Increased blood levels with ketoconazole, verapamil, cimetidine, or inhibitors of cytochrome CYP3 A4 including macrolide antibiotics, protease inhibitors such as ritonavir. Other precautions as above.

C/I = contraindication
Table modified from previous editions.
*See section on Dofetilide, page 246.

Table 8-3 Antiarrhythmic Drugs Used in Therapy of Ventricular Arrhythmias

Agent	Dose	Pharmacokinetics and Metabolism	Side Effects and Contraindications	Interactions and Precautions
Quinidine (class 1A)	Orally 1.2–1.6 g/day in divided doses, 4- to 12-hourly depending on preparation. **Not recommended**	$t^1/_2$ 7–9 h. Level: 2.3–5 μg/mL. Hepatic hydroxylation. Reduce dose in liver disease.	Many side effects including diarrhea, nausea; torsades de pointes and hypotension. Vagolytic. Monitor QRS, QT, plasma K	Increases digoxin level. Enzyme inducers; cimetidine; Class III agents (torsades); diuretics. Warfarin (risk of bleeding).
Procainamide (class 1A)	IV 100 mg bolus over 2 min up to 25 mg/min to 1 g in first h; then 2–6 mg/min. Oral 1 g, then up to 500 mg 3 hourly	$t^1/_2$ 3.5 h. Level 4–10 μg/mL. Plasma metabolism to NAPA. Rapid renal elimination.	Hypotension with IV dose. Limit oral use to 6 months (lupus). Torsades de pointes rare.	No digoxin interaction. Class III agents (torsades).
Disopyramide (class 1A)	Oral dose 100–200 mg 6-hourly. Loading dose 300 mg (less if CHF).	$t^1/_2$ 8 h. Level 3–6 μg/mL; toxic >7 μg/mL. Hepatic metabolism (50%), unchanged urinary excretion (50%).	Prominent vagolytic (urinary retention, dry mouth) and negative inotropic effects. Hypotension, torsades, congestive heart failure	No digoxin interaction; Class III agents (torsades).
Lidocaine (class 1B)	IV 75–200 mg; then 2–4 mg/min for 24–30 h. (No oral use).	Effect of single bolus lasts only few min, then $t^1/_2$ about 2 h. Rapid hepatic metabolism. Level 1.4–5.0 μg/mL; toxic >9 μg/mL.	Reduce dose by half if liver blood flow low (shock, β-blockade, cirrhosis, cimetidine, severe heart failure). High-dose CNS effects	β-Blockers decrease hepatic blood flow and increase blood levels. Cimetidine (decreased hepatic metabolism of L).
Mexiletine (class 1B)	*IV 100–250 mg at 25 mg/min, then 250 mg over next h, then 125 mg over next 2 h, then 30 mg/h. Oral 100–400 mg 8-hourly; loading dose 400 mg.	$t^1/_2$ 10–17 h. Level 1–2 μg/mL. Hepatic metabolism, inactive metabolites.	CNS, GI side effects. Bradycardia, hypotension especially during cotherapy.	Hepatic enzyme inducers†; disopyramide and β-blockade; increases the theophylline levels.

Drug	Dose	Pharmacokinetics	Side effects	Interactions/Precautions
Phenytoin (class IB)	IV 10–15 mg/kg over 1 h. Oral 1 g; 500 mg for 2 days; then 400–600 mg daily.	$t^1/_2$ 24 h. Level 10–18 µg/mL. Hepatic metabolism. Hepatic or renal disease requires reduced doses.	Hypotension, vertigo, dysarthria, lethargy, gingivitis, macrocytic anemia, lupus, pulmonary infiltrates.	Hepatic enzyme inducers.[†]
Flecainide (class IC)	*IV 1–2 mg/kg over 10 min, then 0.15–0.25 mg/kg/h. Oral 100–400 mg 2 times daily. Hospitalize.	$t^1/_2$ 13–19 h. Hepatic $^2/_3$; $^1/_3$ renal excretion unchanged. Keep trough level below 1.0 µg/mL	QRS prolongation. Proarrhythmia. Depressed LV function. CNS side effects. Increased incidence of death postinfarct.	Many, especially added inhibition of conduction and nodal tissue.
Moricizine (class IC)	200–300 mg 3 times daily.	$t^1/_2$ 6–13 h. Numerous hepatic metabolites; long-lasting.	Proarrhythmia especially if preexisting congestive heart failure. QRS prolongation. Modest negative inotropic effect. GI side effects. Proarrhythmia.	Little experience in hepatic or renal failure.
Propafenone (class IC)	*IV 2 mg/kg then 2 mg/min. Oral 150–300 mg 3 times daily.	$t^1/_2$ variable 2–10 h, up to 32 h in nonmetabolizers. Level 0.2–3.0 µg/mL. Variable hepatic metabolism (P-450 deficiency slows).		Digoxin level increased. Hepatic enzyme inducers.[†]
Sotalol (class III)	160–480 mg daily, occasionally higher in two divided doses.	$t^1/_2$ 12 h. Not metabolized. Hydrophilic. Renal loss.	Myocardial depression, sinus bradycardia, AV block. Torsades if hypokalemic.	Added risk of torsades with IA agents or diuretics. Decrease dose in renal failure.
Amiodarone (class III)	Oral loading dose 1200–1600 mg daily; maintenance 200–400 mg daily, sometimes less. IV 150 mg over 10 min, then 360 mg over 6 h, then 540 mg over remaining 18 h, then 0.5 mg/min	$t^1/_2$ 25–110 days. Level 1.0–2.5 µg/mL. Hepatic metabolism. Lipid soluble with extensive distribution in body. Excretion by skin, biliary tract, lachrymal glands.	Complex dose-dependent side effects including pulmonary fibrosis. QT-prolongation. Torsades uncommon.	Class IA agents predispose to torsades. β-blockers predispose to nodal depression, yet give better therapeutic effects.
Bretylium tosylate (class III) **seldom used**	IV 5–10 mg/kg, lifting arm, repeat to max 30 mg/kg, then IV 1–2 mg/min or IM 5–10 mg/kg 8-hourly at varying sites (local necrosis).	$t^1/_2$ 7–9 h. Level 0.5–1.0 µg/mL.	IV: hypotension. Initial sympathomimetic effects.	Decrease dose in renal failure.

*Not licensed for intravenous use in the United States, doses taken from British National Formulary (March 2004).
[†]Hepatic enzyme inducers = barbiturates, phenytoin, rifampin, St. John's wort, which induce hepatic enzymes thereby decreasing blood levels of the drug.
IM = intramuscular; IV = intravenous; level = therapeutic blood level; $t^1/_2$ = plasma half-life.
Compiled by L H Opie and modified from previous editions.

CLASSES OF ANTIARRYTHMIC DRUGS
Opie 2004

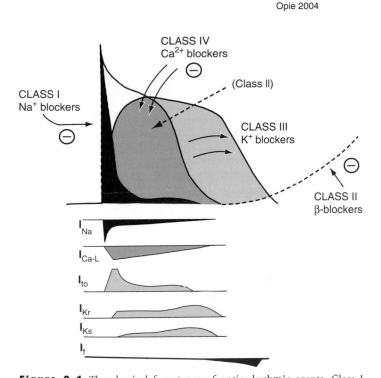

Figure 8-1 The classical four types of antiarrhythmic agents. Class I agents decrease phase zero of the rapid depolarization of the action potential (rapid sodium channel). Class II agents, β-blocking drugs, have complex actions including inhibition of spontaneous depolarization (phase 4) and indirect closure of calcium channels, which are less likely to be in the "open" state when not phosphorylated by cyclic AMP. Class III agents block the outward potassium channels to prolong the action potential duration and hence refractoriness. Class IV agents, verapamil and diltiazem, and the indirect calcium antagonist adenosine, all inhibit the inward calcium channel which is most prominent in nodal tissue, particularly the AV node. Most antiarrhythmic drugs have more than one action. In the lower panel are shown the major currents on which antiarrhythmics act, according to the Sicilian gambit.[5] Ca-L = long-lasting calcium; I = current; I_f = inward funny current; K_r = rapid component of repolarizing potassium current; K_s = slow component; Na = sodium; to = transient outward.

cardioversion. Post-cardioversion, quinidine helps to maintain sinus rhythm but at the cost of a threefold increase in the odds of death.[7] Conventionally, the patient is hospitalized and monitored for 72 hours when the proarrhythmic effects may be most evident, including an early increase in premature ventricular contractions. Traditionally, a test dose of 0.2 g of quinidine sulfate is given to check for drug idiosyncrasy, including cardiovascular collapse, although such serious side effects are seldom seen. Then sustained oral therapy is started. Conventional dosing is 300 mg or 400 mg quinidine sulfate four times daily or every 6 hours with a usual total dose of 1.2 to 1.6 g/day with a maximum of 2 g in 24 hours. Long-acting quinidine preparations (similar dose limits) are quinidine gluconate (multiples of 330 mg or 325 mg) and quinidine polygalacturonate (multiples of 275 mg 8- to 12-hourly). The systemic availability is nearly equivalent for the above doses of these three preparations.

Precautions Quinidine toxicity including idiosyncrasy is best prevented by a test dose and by serial measurements of QRS-duration and QT-

AV NODAL RE-ENTRY VERSUS WPW
Opie 2004

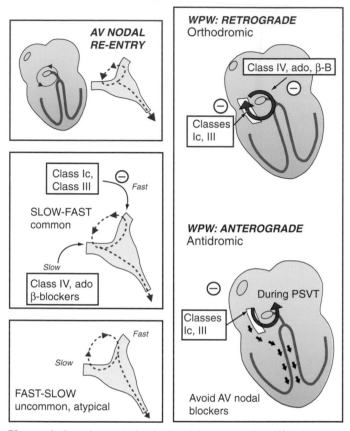

Figure 8-2 Atrioventricular *(AV)* nodal reentry and Wolff-Parkinson-White (WPW) or preexcitation syndrome. The *left panel* shows AV nodal reentry without WPW. The common pattern is slow-fast *(middle panel)* while fast-slow conduction *(bottom right)* is uncommon. The slow and fast fibers of the AV node are artificially separated for diagrammatic purposes. The *right panel* shows WPW with the bypass tract as a white band. During paroxysmal supraventricular tachycardia (PSVT), when antero-grade conduction occurs over the AV node and retrograde conduction most commonly through the accessory pathway, the QRS pattern should be normal (orthodromic SVT, *top right*). Less commonly, the accessory pathway is used as the anterograde limb and the AV node (or a second accessory pathway) is the retrograde limb (antidromic SVT, *bottom right*). The QRS pattern shows the pattern of full preexcitation. In such preexcited atrial tachycardias, agents that block the AV node may enhance conduction over the accessory pathway to the ventricles (red downward arrows) leading to rapid ventricular rates that predispose to ventricular fibrillation. Sites of action of various classes of antiarrhythmics are indicated. *Ado* = adenosine. *β-B* = β-blocker. (*Figure © LH Opie, 2005.*)

interval on the ECG. Conduction delay and proarrhythmic effects are potentially serious. The dose should be reduced or therapy reassessed if the QRS duration widens by 50% (or 25% in the presence of intra-ventricular conduction defects), or if the total QRS duration exceeds 140 milliseconds, or if QT or QTU prolongation occurs beyond 500 milliseconds. These guidelines, although reasonable, are not well documented. Besides monitoring QRS- and QT-intervals throughout, hypokalemia must be avoided because it predisposes to torsades de pointes, which is the probable explanation of quinidine syncope. In patients with the sick sinus syndrome, a direct depressant effect of quinidine may be seen (Table 8-4); in others nodal depression is overridden by the vagolytic effect. *Drug interactions* are many (Table 8-5) and an additional reason for not using quinidine.

Side Effects Serious side effects may develop soon after the first dose if there is idiosyncrasy, or gradually from cumulative overdosage. Most common are diarrhea (33%), nausea (18%), headache (13%), and dizziness (8%) with a high rate of discontinuation (15%).[8] Long-term tolerance in those without early side effects is excellent. *Hypersensitivity* reactions to quinidine include fever, skin rash, angioedema, thrombocytopenia, agranulocytosis, hepatitis, and lupus erythematosus. Proarrhythmic side effects may increase mortality.

Contraindications Quinidine is contraindicated when ventricular tachyarrhythmias are associated with or caused by QT prolongation or if there is prior therapy with drugs (cardiac or non-cardiac) known to predispose to torsades de pointes. Caution is required with a preexisting prolonged QT-interval or preexisting QRS prolongation or clinical congestive heart failure (CHF), with low initial doses and close monitoring. Other relative contraindications are sick sinus syndrome, bundle branch block, myasthenia gravis, and severe liver failure (altered pharmacokinetics); also ulcerative colitis and regional enteritis. Watch for numerous drug interactions. Periodic blood counts are advisable during long-term therapy.

Treatment of Acute Quinidine Toxicity Stop quinidine, reduce plasma potassium if elevated, and acidify urine to encourage excretion. Torsades de pointes or severely disorganized conduction may require correction of potassium level, magnesium sulfate infusion, cardioversion, or temporary atrial or ventricular overdrive pacing.

Conclusions on Quinidine In view of numerous side effects, drug interactions, cautions, and contraindications, as well as lack of positive outcome data, quinidine is very far from an ideal antiarrhythmic agent. *We do not recommend its use.*

Procainamide

Procainamide (Pronestyl) is generally effective against a wide variety of supraventricular and ventricular arrhythmias, including ventricular tachycardia (VT). As in the case of quinidine, no effect on mortality or survival has been shown. Although usually given orally, intravenous procainamide may be tried if lidocaine fails. The oral use is limited by a short half-life and the long-term danger of the lupus syndrome. In contrast, other side effects are less than with quinidine (GI, QRS prolongation or torsades, hypotension) and there is no interaction with digoxin.

Basic Pharmacology Procainamide is a class IA agent, like quinidine, but does not prolong the QT-interval to the same extent (Table 8-4). Procainamide has less interaction with muscarinic receptors than does quinidine. There is direct sympathetic inhibition, so, that vasodilation occurs through a mechanism different from that with quinidine. Regarding pharmacokinetics, side effects, cautions, and drug interactions, see Tables 8-3 and 8-5.

Dose and Indications An oral loading dose of procainamide (1 g) is followed by up to 500 mg 3-hourly. A slow-release preparation of procainamide (*Procanbid*) appears to allow 12-hourly dosing intervals at a dose of about 25 mg/kg every 12 hours. The bolus dose against ventricular tachycardia is 10 mg/kg at an injection rate of 100 mg/minute.[9] The dose for intravenous infusion is 100 mg over 2 minutes, then up to 25 mg/minute to a maximum of 1 g in the first hour, then 2 to 6 mg/minute. Like other class IA agents, procainamide is also effective

Table 8-4 Effects and Side Effects of Some Ventricular Antiarrhythmic Agents on Electrophysiology and Hemodynamics

Agent	Sinus Node	Sinus Rate	A-HIS	PR	AV Block	H-P	WPW	QRS	QT	Serious Hemodynamic Effects	Risk of Torsades	Risk of Monomorphic VT
Quinidine	↓	↑	0	0/→	0	→	↓A/R	↑↑	↑↑	IV use	++	0, +
Procainamide	0	0/↑	0/↓	0/→	Avoid	→	↓A/R	0/→	↑	IV hypotension	+	0, +
Disopyramide	→↓	←	0	0/→	0	0/↓	↓A/R	↑	↑	IV ↓↓↓	+	0, +
Lidocaine	0	0	0/↓	0	0	0	↓/0	0	0	Toxic doses	0	0
Phenytoin	0	0	↑/0	0	Lessens	0	↓/0	0	↓	IV hypotension	0, +	0, +
Mexiletine	0	0	↑/0	0	↓/0	↓/0	↓/0	0/→	0	Toxic doses	0, +	0, +
Flecainide	0/↓	0	↓↓↓	↑	Avoid	↓↓	↓A/R	↑↑	↑ (via QRS)	IV ↓↓	0	+++
Propafenone	0/↓	0	→	↑	Avoid	↓↓	↓A/R	↑	0	IV↓	0	+++
Sotalol	↓↓	↓↓	→	↑	Avoid	0	A/R	0	↑↑	IV use	++	0, +
Amiodarone	↓	↓	→	0/→	Avoid	0/↓	A/R	0	↑↑	IV use	+/−	0, +

A = antegrade; A-His = Atria-His conduction; H-P = His-Purkinje conduction; IV = intravenous; LV = left ventricle; R = retrograde; WPW = Wolff-Parkinson-White syndrome accessory pathways; ↑ = increases; → = prolongs; ← = shortens.
Compiled by L H Opie and modified from previous editions.

Table 8-5	Interactions (Kinetic and Dynamic) of Antiarrhythmic Drugs	
Drug	**Interaction with**	**Result**
Quinidine (*not recommended*)	Digoxin	Increased digoxin level
	Other Class 1 antiarrhythmics	Added negative inotropic effect and/or depressed conduction
	β-Blockers, verapamil	Enhanced hypotension, negative inotropic effect
	Amiodarone	Risk of torsades; increased quinidine levels
	Sotalol	Risk of torsades
	Diuretics	If hypokalemia, risk of torsades
	Verapamil	Increased quinidine level
	Nifedipine	Decreased quinidine level
	Warfarin	Enhanced anticoagulation
	Cimetidine	Increased blood levels
	Enzyme inducers	Decreased blood levels
Procainamide	Cimetidine	Decreases renal clearance
	Class III agents, diuretics	Torsades
Disopyramide	Other Class 1 antiarrhythmics	Depressed conduction. Torsades
	Amiodarone, sotalol	Enhanced hypotension
	β-blockers, verapamil	Increased anticholinergic effect
	Anticholinergics	
	Pyridostigmine	Decreased anticholinergic effect
Lidocaine	β-Blockers, cimetidine, Halothane	Reduced liver blood flow (increased blood levels)
	Enzyme inducers	Decreased blood levels
Tocainide	None known	—
Mexiletine	Enzyme inducers	Decreased mexiletine levels
	Disopyramide, β-blockers,	Negative inotropic potential
	Theophylline	Theophylline levels increased
Flecainide	Major kinetic interaction with amiodarone	Increase of blood F levels; half-dose
	Added negative inotropic effects (β-blockers, quinidine, disopyramide)	As above
	Added HV conduction depression (quinidine, procainamide)	Conduction block
Propafenone	As for flecainide (but amiodarone interaction not reported); digoxin; warfarin	Enhanced SA, AV and myocardial; Depression, digoxin level increased; anticoagulant effect enhanced
Sotalol	Diuretics, Class 1A agents, amiodarone, tricyclics, phenothiazines (Fig. 8-4)	Risk of torsades; avoid hypokalemia
Amiodarone	As for sotalol	Risk of torsades
	Digoxin	Increased digoxin levels
	Phenytoin	Double interaction, see text
	Flecainide	Increased flecainide levels
	Warfarin	Increased warfarin effect
Ibutilide	All agents increasing QT	Risk of torsades

Table continued on opposite page

Table 8-5	Interactions (Kinetic and Dynamic) of Antiarrhythmic Drugs— *Continued*	
Drug	**Interaction with**	**Result**
Dofetilide	All agents increasing QT interval	Risk of torsades
	Liver interactions with verapamil, cimetidine, ketoconazole, trimethoprim	Increased dofetilide blood level, more risk of torsades
Verapamil Diltiazem	β-Blockers, excess digoxin, myocardial depressants, quinidine	Increased myocardial or nodal depression
Adenosine	Dipyridamole Methylxanthines (caffeine, theophylline)	Adenosine catabolism inhibited; much inhibited; much increased half-life; reduce A dose; Inhibit receptor; decreased drug effects

Enzyme inducers = hepatic enzyme inducers, i.e., barbiturates, phenytoin, rifampin.
For references, see Table 8-4 in previous edition.

against supraventricular tachyarrhythmias including those of the WPW syndrome. It is frequently used as an initial attempt at pharmacologic cardioversion of atrial fibrillation of recent onset, although less effective than intravenous ibutilide.[10] In sustained ventricular tachycardia, procainamide is more effective than lidocaine at the cost of QRS and QT widening.[9]

Side Effects and Contraindications During chronic oral therapy, almost one fifth of patients experience early side effects (rash, fever) and the majority have late side effects (arthralgia, rash).[11] Despite the efficacy of procainamide the risk of lupus (likeliest in slow acetylators) is about one third of those patients treated for longer than 6 months. Agranulocytosis may be a late side effect of procainamide, especially with the slow-release preparation. Hypotension, QRS and QT widening are common side effects with intravenous administration.[9,10] Heart block may develop or increase. In atrial fibrillation or flutter the ventricular rate may increase as the atrial rate slows, so that concomitant digitalization is advisable. The vagolytic effect of procainamide is much weaker than that of quinidine. Proarrhythmic effects, including torsades de pointes, may be dose-related. Regarding *contraindications*, these are shock, myasthenia gravis (see quinidine), heart block, and severe renal or cardiac failure.

Conclusions: Procainamide This agent has a wide spectrum of antiarrhythmic activity, yet without serious side effects except for hypotension and QRS and QT widening, making this an attractive class I agent for intravenous use. Side effects limit oral use except for short periods, as when postoperative atrial fibrillation complicates cardiac surgery.

CLASS IB: LIDOCAINE AND SIMILAR COMPOUNDS

As a group, class IB agents inhibit the fast sodium current (typical class I effect) while shortening the action potential duration in nondiseased tissue. The former has the more powerful effect, while the latter might actually predispose to arrhythmias, but ensures that QT prolongation does not occur. Class IB agents act selectively on diseased or ischemic tissue, where they are thought to promote conduction block, thereby interrupting reentry circuits. They have a particular affinity for binding with inactivated sodium channels with rapid onset-offset kinetics, which may be why such drugs are ineffective in atrial arrhythmias, because the action potential duration is so short.

Lidocaine

Lidocaine (Xylocaine; Xylocard) has become the standard intravenous agent for suppression of serious ventricular arrhythmias associated with AMI and with cardiac surgery. The concept of prophylactic lidocaine to prevent VT and ventricular fibrillation (VF) in AMI is now outmoded.[12,13] This intravenous drug has no role in the control of chronic recurrent ventricular arrhythmias. Lidocaine acts preferentially on the ischemic myocardium and is more effective in the presence of a high external potassium concentration. Therefore, hypokalemia must be corrected for maximum efficacy (also for other class I agents). Lidocaine has no value in treating supraventricular tachyarrhythmias.

Pharmacokinetics The bulk of an intravenous dose of lidocaine is rapidly deethylated by liver microsomes (Table 8-3). The two critical factors governing lidocaine metabolism and hence its efficacy are liver blood flow (decreased in old age and by heart failure, β-blockade, and cimetidine) and liver microsomal activity (enzyme inducers). Because lidocaine is so rapidly distributed within minutes after an initial intravenous loading dose, there must be a subsequent infusion or repetitive doses to maintain therapeutic blood levels (Fig. 8-3). Lidocaine

LIDOCAINE KINETICS

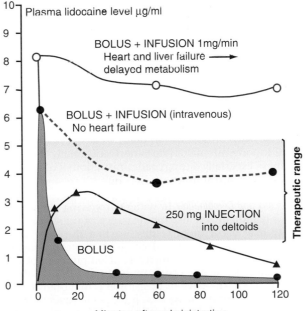

Figure 8-3 Lidocaine kinetics. To achieve and to maintain an adequate blood level of lidocaine requires an initial bolus followed by an infusion. For an intramuscular injection to give sustained high blood levels may require a dose of 400 mg. Note that in the presence of cardiac or liver failure, delayed metabolism increases the blood level with danger of toxic effects. (*Figure © LH Opie, 2005.*)

metabolites circulate in high concentrations and may contribute to toxic and therapeutic actions. After prolonged infusions, the half-life may be longer (up to 24 hours) because of redistribution from poorly perfused tissues.

Dose A constant infusion would take 5 to 9 hours to achieve therapeutic levels (1.4 to 5.0 µg/ml), so standard therapy includes a loading dose of 75 to 100 mg intravenously, followed after 30 minutes by a second loading dose, or 400 mg intramuscularly. Thereafter lidocaine is infused at 2 to 4 mg/minute for 24 to 30 hours, aiming at 3 mg/minute, which prevents VF but may cause serious side effects in about 15% of patients, in half of whom the lidocaine dose may have to be reduced. Poor liver blood flow (low cardiac output or β-blockade), liver disease, or cimetidine or halothane therapy calls for halved dosage. The dose should also be decreased for elderly patients in whom toxicity develops more frequently and after 12 to 24 hours of infusion.

Clinical Use 1. *Should lidocaine be administered routinely to all patients with AMI?* The question has been asked for at least 25 years. Increasingly the answer is no. Recent evidence from more than 20 randomized trials and 4 meta-analyses have shown that lidocaine reduces VF but adversely affects mortality rates, presumably because of bradyarrhythmias and asystole.[13,14] Therefore lidocaine should not routinely be used in AMI. In view of these findings, lidocaine is no longer considered as a standard treatment in patients with AMI, but is reserved for those patients who have already experienced VF. 2. *Should lidocaine be used routinely before attempted defibrillation of ventricular tachyarrhythmias?* The answer is no—any benefits are cancelled by the greater delays involved in achieving defibrillation. 3. *When can it be used?* When tachyarrhythmias or very frequent premature ventricular contractions (PVCs) seriously interfere with hemodynamic status in patients with AMI (especially when already β-blocked) and during cardiac surgery or general anesthesia. 4. *When should lidocaine not be used?* Prophylactically or when there is bradycardia or bradycardia plus ventricular tachyarrhythmias, when atropine (or pacing) and not lidocaine is required.

Side Effects Lidocaine is generally free of hemodynamic side effects, even in patients with congestive heart failure, and it seldom impairs nodal function or conduction (Table 8-4). The higher infusion rate of 3 to 4 mg/minute may result in drowsiness, numbness, speech disturbances, and dizziness, especially in patients older than 60 years of age. Minor adverse neural reactions can occur in about half the patients, even with 2 to 3 mg/minute of lidocaine. Occasionally there is sinoatrial (SA) arrest, especially during coadministration of other drugs that potentially depress nodal function.

Drug Interactions and Combination In patients receiving cimetidine, propranolol, or halothane, the hepatic clearance of lidocaine is reduced and toxicity may occur more readily, so that the dose should be reduced. With hepatic enzyme inducers (barbiturates, phenytoin, and rifampin) the dose needs to be increased. Combination of lidocaine with early β-blockade is not a contraindication, although there is no reported experience. The obvious precaution is that bradyarrhythmias may become more common because β-blockade reduces liver blood flow. Hence a standard dose of lidocaine would have potentially more side effects, including sinus node inhibition.

Lidocaine Failure If lidocaine apparently fails, is there hypokalemia? Are there technical errors? Is the drug really called for or should β-blockade rather be used? If none of these factors are present, a blood level is taken (if available) and the infusion rate can be increased cautiously until development of the central nervous system effects (confusion, slurred speech). Alternatively or concomitantly, procainamide is tried before resorting to class III agents, such as intravenous amiodarone.

Conclusions: Lidocaine Lidocaine remains a reasonable initial therapy for treatment of sustained ventricular tachycardia, predominantly because of ease of use and a low incidence of hemodynamic side effects and drug interactions. However, the efficacy of lidocaine is relatively low (15% to 20%) compared with other class I antiarrhythmic drugs (procainamide—approximately 80%). Thus the use of lidocaine allows about a fifth of monomorphic ventricular tachycardias to be terminated and suppressed with virtually no risk of side effects.

Phenytoin (Diphenylhydantoin)

Phenytoin (Dilantin, Epanutin) has four specific uses. First, in digitalis-toxic arrhythmias, it maintains AV conduction or even enhances it, especially in the presence of hypokalemia; it also inhibits delayed afterdepolarizations. Second, phenytoin is effective against the ventricular arrhythmias occurring after congenital heart surgery. Third, phenytoin is used in the congenital prolonged QT syndrome when β-blockade alone has failed; here, reliable comparative studies have not been done. Why phenytoin is so effective in the ventricular arrhythmias of young children is not known. Fourth, occasionally in patients with epilepsy and arrhythmias its dual action comes to the fore. The oral maintenance dose is 300 to 600 mg/day (4 to 8 mg/kg/day in children). The long half-life allows once daily dosage with, however, the risk of serious side effects including dysarthria, pulmonary infiltrates, lupus, gingivitis, and macrocytic anemia. Phenytoin is an inducer of hepatic enzymes and therefore alters the dose requirements of many other drugs used in cardiology, including the antiarrhythmic drugs quinidine, lidocaine, and mexiletine.

CLASS IC: AGENTS

These agents have acquired a particularly bad reputation as a result of the proarrhythmic effects seen in CAST (Cardiac Arrhythmia Suppression Trial)[1] (flecainide) and the CASH (Cardiac Arrest Study Hamburg) studies[15] (propafenone). As a group they have three major electrophysiological effects. First, they are powerful inhibitors of the fast sodium channel causing a marked depression of the upstroke of the cardiac action potential. In addition they may variably prolong the action potential duration by delaying inactivation of the slow sodium channel[16] and inhibition of the rapid repolarizing current (I_{Kr})[17] which may explain their marked inhibitory effect on His-Purkinje conduction with QRS widening. Class IC agents are all potent antiarrhythmics used largely in the control of paroxysmal supraventricular and ventricular tachyarrhythmias resistant to other drugs. Their markedly depressant effect on conduction, together with prolongation of the action potential duration, may explain the development of electrical heterogeneity and proarrhythmias. In addition, faster heart rates, increased sympathetic activity, and diseased or ischemic myocardium all contribute to the proarrhythmic effects of these drugs.[18] These drugs must therefore be avoided in patients with structural heart disease. In others, they are widely used to prevent recurrences of atrial fibrillation. Here the evidence is strong for propafenone and moderate for flecainide.[19] They have to compete with sotalol (limited to severe cases because of the danger of torsades de pointes) and with amiodarone, more effective than sotalol or class I agents[20] at the cost of serious side effects.

Flecainide

Flecainide (Tambocor) is effective for the treatment of both supraventricular and ventricular arrhythmias. Its associated proarrhythmic potential limits its use, especially in the presence of structural heart disease because poor LV function exaggerates the proarrhythmic effects. The negative inotropic effect also limits its use in ischemic heart disease or dilated cardiomyopathy. The drug should be started under careful observation, using a gradually increasing low oral dose with regular electrocardiograms to assess QRS complex duration and occasionally serum levels. Once steady-state treatment has been reached (usually five times the half-life of the drug), it is advisable to perform a 24-hour Holter analysis or a symptom limited exercise stress test to detect potential arrhythmias during maximum effort.[21] For pharmacokinetics, side effects, and drug interactions see Tables 8-3 to 8-5.

Indications are (1) life-threatening sustained ventricular tachycardia where the benefit outweighs the proarrhythmic risks, and (2) paroxysmal supraventricular tachycardia including WPW arrhythmias, and paroxysmal atrial flutter or fibrillation, always only in patients without structural heart disease. For maintenance of sinus rhythm after cardioversion of atrial fibrillation, it is moderately successful.[19] Flecainide is *contraindicated* in patients with structural heart disease because of the risk of proarrhythmia, and in patients with right bundle branch block and left anterior hemiblock unless a pacemaker is implanted (package insert). It is also contraindicated in the sick sinus syndrome, when the left ventricle is depressed, and in the postinfarct state. There is a boxed warning in the package insert against use in chronic sustained atrial fibrillation.

Cardiac proarrhythmic effects of flecainide include aggravation of ventricular arrhythmias and threat of sudden death as in the CAST study.[1] The proarrhythmic effect is related to nonuniform slowing of conduction. Monitoring the QRS-interval is logical but "safe limits" are not established. Furthermore, as shown in the CAST study,[1] late proarrhythmic effects can occur. In patients with preexisting sinus node or AV conduction problems, there may be worsening of arrhythmia. Flecainide increases the endocardial pacing threshold. Atrial proarrhythmic effects are of two varieties. As the atrial rate falls the ventricular rate might rise. Therefore if prescribed for prevention of atrial flutter or fibrillation, this drug should probably be coadministered with digitalis, β-blocker, or verapamil to avoid accelerated AV conduction (package insert). Second, ventricular arrhythmias may be precipitated.

Propafenone

Propafenone (Rythmol in the United States, Arythmol in the United Kingdom, Rytmonorm in rest of Europe) has a spectrum of activity and some side effects that resemble those of other class IC agents, including the proarrhythmic effect. In the CASH study, propafenone was withdrawn from one arm because of increased total mortality and cardiac arrest recurrence.[15] Propafenone is regarded as relatively safe in suppressing supraventricular arrhythmias including those of the WPW syndrome and recurrent atrial fibrillation,[22] always bearing in mind the need first to eliminate structural heart disease.

Pharmacology In keeping with its class IC effects, propafenone blocks the fast inward sodium channel, has a potent membrane stabilizing activity, and increases PR and QRS times without effect on the QT-interval. It also has mild β-blocking and calcium (L-type channel) antagonist properties. For pharmacokinetics, side effects, drug interactions, and combinations, see Tables 8-3 to 8-5. Note that in 7% of whites, the hepatic cytochrome isoenzyme, P-450 2D6, is genetically absent, so that propafenone breakdown is much slower.

Dose This is 150 to 300 mg three times daily, up to a total of 1200 mg daily with some patients needing four times doses and some only two.

The UK trial[22] compared 300 mg twice with three times daily; the latter was both more effective and gave more adverse effects. Marked interindividual variations in its metabolism mean that the dose must be individualized.

Indications for Propafenone In the United States (only oral form), these are: (1) life-threatening ventricular arrhythmias and (2) suppression of supraventricular arrhythmias, including those of the WPW syndrome and recurrent atrial flutter or fibrillation.[12,23] These must be in the absence of structural heart disease (risk of proarrhythmia). There is strong evidence in favor of propafenone in acute conversion of atrial fibrillation and for maintenance of sinus rhythm.[19] *Intravenous propafenone* (not licensed in the United Kingdom or the United States) followed by oral propafenone, is as effective as amiodarone in the conversion of chronic atrial fibrillation.[24] *Propafenone "on-demand,"* also called the "pill in the pocket," may be tried for paroxysmal atrial fibrillation though not licensed for this purpose, after a trial under strict observation. Propafenone 600 mg orally is taken with the onset of a paroxysm, and then 300 mg 8 hours later; most attacks are aborted.[25] *Relative contraindications* include preexisting sinus, AV or bundle branch abnormalities, or depressed LV function. Patients with asthma and bronchospastic disease including chronic bronchitis should not, in general, be given propafenone (package insert). Propafenone has mild β-blocking properties, especially when the dose exceeds 450 mg daily. It is estimated that the β-blockade effect is approximately 1/40 that of propranolol.[26]

LESSER USED CLASS 1 AGENTS
Mexiletine

Mexiletine (Mexitil), like lidocaine is a class 1B agent that is used chiefly against ventricular arrhythmias. Unlike lidocaine, it can be given orally. There are several arguments favoring it as one of several reasonable choices for ventricular arrhythmias requiring therapy: (1) Efficacy comparable to quinidine; (2) little or no hemodynamic depression; (3) no QT prolongation; and (4) no vagolytic effects. However, frequent GI and central nervous side effects limit the dose and possible therapeutic benefit. As in the case of other class 1B agents, there are no data to prove reduced mortality. For pharmacokinetics, doses, side effects, and contraindications, see Table 8-3. For drug interactions and combination therapy, see Table 8-5.

The major approved indication is treatment of life-threatening ventricular arrhythmias. In practice, its chief use at present is as an adjunct. For example, it may be often added to amiodarone in patients with an ICD in place and frequent recurrences of ventricular tachycardia. Mexiletine 300 mg 8-hourly is as effective as procainamide. A similar dose of mexiletine can be combined with quinidine (about 1 g daily) with a lower incidence of side effects and better antiarrhythmic action than with higher doses of either agent alone. In a major clinical trial on postinfarct patients, mexiletine reduced Holter-monitored arrhythmias in the first 6 months without improved mortality over 1 year; in fact, mortality strongly tended to increase.[27] The mechanism cannot be via torsades de pointes, because mexilitene (like other class 1B and 1C agents) does not prolong the QT-interval. In LQT3 (a genetic variety of long-QT syndrome) mexiletine via its sodium-channel blocking activity, shortens the prolonged QT-interval and reduces QT-interval dispersion.[28]

Disopyramide

Disopyramide is a class 1A antiarrhythmic agent, electrophysiologically like quinidine, with a similar antiarrhythmic profile. Like quinidine, it prolongs the QRS- and QT-intervals, the latter involving risk of torsades. Like quinidine, it improves AV nodal conduction because of its anticholinergic action. Unlike quinidine, it has strong trial data in its favor for maintenance of sinus rhythm after conversion of atrial fibrillation.[19] Another crucial difference lies in the side effect profile. Disopyramide causes fewer GI problems, yet much stronger anticholinergic side effects such as urinary retention. Disopyramide inhibits the muscarinic receptors 40 times more effectively than does quinidine. Thus, there is a relative increase of sympathetic activity, masking the direct depressant effects of disopyramide on the sinus node and conduction tissue. A prominent and largely unexplained side effect of disopyramide is the negative inotropic effect, so marked that disopyramide is also used in the therapy of hypertrophic obstructive cardiomyopathy and neurocardiogenic syncope, presumably because it interferes with excitation contraction coupling. For specifics on pharmacokinetics, doses, indications, side effects, cautions, and contraindications see Tables 8-3 to 8-5. To reduce the anticholinergic side effects of disopyramide, cholinesterase activity may be inhibited by pyridostigmine bromide (Mestinon Timespan, 90 to 180 mg three times daily) or bethanechol (Urecholine).

Moricizine

Moricizine (Ethmozine) is a phenothiazine derivative, originally from the previous Soviet Union and approved in the United States (but rarely used) for management of documented ventricular life-threatening arrhythmias. Electrophysiologically, it has both class IB and class IC properties (Table 8-4). Moricizine was evaluated in the CAST-II study for possible benefit in postinfarct ventricular premature systoles in which the flecainide and encainide arms of the CAST study were stopped.[29] Moricizine was ineffective as well as harmful. It induced more cardiac arrests within the first 2 weeks of initiation of therapy.

CLASS II AGENTS: β-ADRENERGIC ANTAGONISTS

Whereas class I agents are increasingly suspect from the long-term point of view, β-blockers have an excellent record in reducing post-MI mortality.[2,30] These agents act on: (1) the current I_f, now recognized as an important pacemaker current that also promotes proarrhythmic depolarization in damaged heart tissue; and (2) the inward calcium current, I_{Ca-L} (Fig. 8-1) which is indirectly inhibited as the level of tissue cyclic AMP falls. The general arguments for β-blockade include (1) the role of tachycardia in precipitating some arrhythmias, especially those based on triggered activity; (2) the increased sympathetic activity in patients with sustained VT and in patients with AMI; (3) the fundamental role of the second messenger of β-adrenergic activity, cyclic AMP, in the causation of ischemia-related VF; and (4) the associated antihypertensive and anti-ischemic effects of these drugs. The mechanism of benefit of β-blockade in postinfarct patients is uncertain, but is likely to be multifactorial and probably antiarrhythmic in part.[30]

Indications Antiarrhythmic therapy by β-blockade is indicated for the following: It is used especially for inappropriate or unwanted sinus tachycardia, for paroxysmal atrial tachycardia provoked by emotion or exercise, for exercise-induced ventricular arrhythmias, in the arrhythmias of pheochromocytoma (combined with α-blockade to avoid hypertensive crises), in the hereditary prolonged QT syndrome, in heart failure,[31] and sometimes in the arrhythmias of mitral valve prolapse. A common denominator to most of these indications is increased sympathetic β-adrenergic activity. In patients with stable controlled heart failure, β-blockers reduce all-cause, cardiovascular, and sudden death mortality rates.[31-33] β-Blockers are also effective as monotherapy in severe recurrent VT not obviously ischemic in origin, and empirical β-blocker therapy seems as good as electrophysiological guided therapy with class I or class III agents. β-Blocker therapy improved survival in patients with ventricular fibrillation or symptomatic ventricular tachycardia not treated by specific antiarrhythmics in the AVID trial.[34] β-Blockers in combination with amiodarone have a synergistic effect to significantly reduce cardiac mortality.[35]

Which β-Blocker for Arrhythmias? The antiarrhythmic activity of the various β-blockers is reasonably uniform, the critical property being that of β_1-adrenergic blockade,[31] without any major role for associated properties such as membrane depression (local anesthetic action), cardioselectivity, and intrinsic sympathomimetic activity (see Figs. 1-9 and 1-10). These additional properties have no major influence on the antiarrhythmic potency. *Esmolol*, a selective β1 antagonist, has a half-life of 9 minutes with full recovery from its β-blockade properties at 18 to 30 minutes.[36] Esmolol is quickly metabolized in red blood cells, independently of renal and hepatic function. Because of its short half-life, esmolol can be useful in situations where there are relative contraindications or concerns about the use of a β-blocker. For instance, in a patient with a supraventricular tachycardia, fast atrial fibrillation or atrial flutter, and associated chronic obstructive airway disease or moderate left ventricular dysfunction, esmolol would be advantageous as a therapeutic intervention.

In the United States, the β-blockers licensed for antiarrhythmic activity include propranolol, sotalol, and acebutolol. The latter is attractive because of its cardioselectivity, its favorable or neutral effect on the blood lipid profile (see Chapter 10), and its specific benefit in one large postinfarct survival trial. However, the potential capacity of acebutolol to suppress serious ventricular arrhythmias has never been shown in a large trial. Metoprolol 25 to 100 mg twice daily, not licensed for this purpose in the United States, was the agent chosen when empirical β-blockade was compared with electrophysiologic guided antiarrhythmic therapy for the treatment of ventricular tachyarrhythmias. Both sotalol (class II and III activities) and metoprolol (class II) reduce the recurrence of ventricular tachyarrhythmias and inappropriate discharges following ICD implantation.[37,38] In the Cardiac Arrest Study Hamburg (CASH) study, amiodarone was compared to metoprolol, propafenone, and ICDs.[15] ICDs were best. While the propafenone arm was stopped prematurely because of excess mortality compared to other therapies, patients on metoprolol had a survival equivalent to that of those treated with amiodarone.

The drawback to β-blockade antiarrhythmic therapy continues to be the many patients with absolute or relative contraindications including pulmonary problems, conduction defects, or overt untreated severe heart failure. A large meta-analysis[39] showed that a mortality reduction of up to 40% could still be achieved despite such relative contraindications. It is important to recognize that mild to moderate LV dysfunction, already treated by ACE inhibitors and diuretics, is no longer an absolute contraindication, but rather a strong indication for β-blockers, especially if there is symptomatic heart failure (class II and III). Another drawback is that the efficacy of β-blockers against symptomatic ventricular arrhythmias is less certain. *At present, β-blockers are the closest to an ideal class of antiarrhythmic agents for general use because of their broad spectrum of activity and established safety record.* Furthermore, the use of β-blockers in combination with other antiarrhythmic agents may have a synergistic role and can reduce the proarrhythmic effects seen with some of these agents.

MIXED CLASS III AGENTS: AMIODARONE AND SOTALOL

As the evidence for increased mortality in several patient groups with class I agents mounts, attention has shifted to class III agents. In the

ESVEM trial[40] sotalol was better than six class I antiarrhythmic agents. Amiodarone, in contrast to class I agents, exerts a favorable effect on a variety of serious arrhythmias.[41] Both amiodarone and sotalol are mixed, not pure, class III agents, a quality that may be of crucial importance.

The *intrinsic problem* with class III agents is that these compounds act by lengthening the action potential duration and hence the effective refractory period, and must inevitably prolong the QT-interval to be effective. In the presence of added hypokalemia, hypomagnesemia, or bradycardia, QT prolongation may predispose to torsades de pointes. This may especially occur with agents such as sotalol that simultaneously cause bradycardia and prolong the action potential duration. By acting only on the repolarization phase of the action potential, class III agents should leave conduction unchanged. However, amiodarone and sotalol all have additional properties that modify conduction— amiodarone being a significant sodium channel inhibitor and sotalol a β-blocker. Amiodarone makes the action potential pattern more uniform throughout the myocardium, thereby opposing electrophysiologic heterogeneity that underlies some serious ventricular arrhythmias. The efficacy of amiodarone exceeds that of other antiarrhythmic compounds including sotalol. Furthermore, the incidence of torsades with amiodarone is much lower than expected from its class III effects. Yet amiodarone has a host of multisystem potentially serious side effects that sotalol does not.

Amiodarone

Amiodarone (Cordarone) is a unique "wide spectrum" antiarrhythmic agent, chiefly class III but with also powerful class I activity and ancillary class II and class IV activity. In general, the status of this drug has changed from that of a "last ditch" agent to one that is increasingly used when life-threatening arrhythmias are being treated. Its established antiarrhythmic benefits and potential for *mortality reduction*[3] need to be balanced against, first, the slow onset of action of oral therapy that may require large oral loading doses. Second, the many serious side effects, especially pulmonary infiltrates and thyroid problems, dictate that there must be a fine balance between the maximum antiarrhythmic effect of the drug and the potential for the side effects. Third, there are a large number of potentially serious drug interactions, some of which predispose to torsades de pointes, which is nonetheless rare when amiodarone is used as a single agent. In recurrent atrial fibrillation, low-dose amiodarone may be strikingly effective with little risk of side effects.[20] Otherwise, the use of amiodarone in as low a dose as possible should be restricted to selected patients with refractory ventricular arrhythmias especially in the post-MI group. For those with severe heart failure, an ICD is preferred (see p. 267).

Electrophysiology Amiodarone is a complex antiarrhythmic agent, predominantly class III, that shares at least some of the properties of each of the other three electrophysiologic classes of antiarrhythmics. The class III activity means that amiodarone lengthens the effective refractory period by prolonging the action potential duration in all cardiac tissues, including bypass tracts. It also has a powerful class I antiarrhythmic effect inhibiting inactivated sodium channels at high stimulation frequencies. Amiodarone noncompetitively blocks α- and β-adrenergic receptors (class II effect), this effect is additive to competitive receptor inhibition by β-blockers.[3] The weak calcium antagonist (class IV) effect might explain bradycardia and AV nodal inhibition and the relatively low incidence of torsades de pointes. Furthermore, there are relatively weak coronary and peripheral vasodilator actions.

Pharmacokinetics The pharmacokinetics of this highly lipid soluble drug differ markedly from other cardiovascular agents.[3] After variable (30% to 50%) and slow GI absorption, amiodarone is very slowly eliminated with a half-life of about 25 to 110 days. The onset of action after oral administration is delayed and a steady-state drug effect (*amiodaronization*) may not be established for several months unless large loading doses are used. Even when given intravenously, its full electrophysiologic effect is delayed,[42] although major benefit can be achieved within minutes as shown by its effect on shock-resistant ventricular fibrillation.[43] Amiodarone is lipid-soluble and extensively distributed in the body and highly concentrated in many tissues, especially in the liver and lungs. It undergoes extensive hepatic metabolism to the pharmacologically active metabolite, desethyl-amiodarone. A correlation between the clinical effects and serum concentrations of the drug or its metabolite has not been clearly shown, although there is a direct relation between the oral dose and the plasma concentration, and between metabolite concentration and some late effects, such as that on the ventricular functional refractory period. The therapeutic level, not well defined, may be between 1.0 and 2.5 mg/ml, almost all of which (95%) is protein bound. Higher levels are associated with increased toxicity.[3] Amiodarone is not excreted by the kidneys but rather by the lachrymal glands, the skin, and the biliary tract.

Dose When reasonably rapid control of an arrhythmia is needed, the initial loading regimen is up to 1600 mg daily in two to four divided doses usually given for 7 to 14 days, which is then reduced to 400 to 800 mg/day for a further 1 to 3 weeks. Practice varies widely however, with loading doses of as low as 600 mg daily being used in less urgent settings. Maintenance doses vary, but for high dose therapy 400 mg or occasionally more is employed. The loading dose is essential because of the slow onset of full action with a delay of about 10 days. By using a loading dose, sustained ventricular tachycardia can be controlled after a mean interval of 5 days. Either way the ECG needs to be monitored regularly (sinus bradycardia). Downward dose adjustment may be required during prolonged therapy to avoid development of side effects while maintaining optimal antiarrhythmic effect. Maintenance doses for atrial flutter or fibrillation are generally lower (200 mg daily or less) than those needed for serious ventricular arrhythmias. *Intravenous amiodarone* (approved in the United States) may be used for intractable arrhythmias. Start with 150 mg/10 minutes, then 360 mg over the 6 next hours, then 540 mg over the remaining 24 hours, to give a total of 1000 mg over 24 hours, or for atrial fibrillation in AMI or after cardiac surgery (see next section), 5 mg/kg over 20 minutes, 500 to 1000 mg over 24 hours, then orally, and then 0.5 mg/minute. Deliver by volumetric infusion pump. Higher intravenous loading doses are more likely to give hypotension. For shock-resistant cardiac arrest, the intravenous dose is 5 mg/kg of estimated body weight, with a further dose of 2.5 mg/kg if the VF persists after a further shock.[43]

Indications In the United States, the license is only for recurrent VF or hemodynamically unstable VT after adequate doses of other ventricular antiarrhythmics have been tested or are not tolerated, because its use is accompanied by substantial toxicity. Nonetheless, amiodarone is now more widely used especially in lower, relatively nontoxic doses. In the prophylactic control of *life-threatening ventricular tachyarrhythmias* (especially post-MI and in association with congestive cardiac failure), or after cardiac surgery,[44] amiodarone is generally regarded as one of the most effective agents available. Strictly controlled studies, such as EMIAT (European Myocardial Infarction Amiodarone Trial), and CAMIAT (Canadian Amiodarone Myocardial Infarction Arrhythmia Trial), and the meta-analyses based on these and other studies (ECMA—EMIAT/CAMIAT Meta-Analysis, and ATMA—Amiodarone Trials Meta-Analysis) are all available.[45] The results show that arrhythmia related deaths are very significantly reduced (about 30% reduction), whereas total mortality is only marginally reduced (12% reduction). A possibility is that patients prevented from dying of arrhythmic deaths could then die from reinfarction or heart failure.

Intravenous amiodarone is indicated for the initiation of treatment and prophylaxis of frequently recurring ventricular fibrillation or destabilizing ventricular tachycardia and those refractory to other therapies. When oral amiodarone cannot be used, then the intravenous form is also indicated. *Caution*: risk of hypotension with intravenous amiodarone. Generally intravenous amiodarone is used for 48 to 96 hours while oral amiodarone is instituted. In the ARREST study (amiodarone for resuscitation after out-of-hospital cardiac ARREST) amiodarone was better than placebo (44% versus 34%, $P = 0.03$) in reducing immediate mortality.[46] Similar data were obtained when amiodarone was compared with lidocaine for shock-resistant ventricular fibrillation.[43] For the acute conversion of chronic atrial fibrillation, intravenous amiodarone is as effective as intravenous propafenone,[24] both having strong evidence in their favor.[19]

In *preventing recurrences of paroxysmal atrial fibrillation or flutter*, amiodarone is highly effective.[19,20] Sinus rhythm was maintained more successfully with low-dose amiodarone (80% at 1 year), than with either sotalol or class I agents. Note that this benefit of low-dose amiodarone (standard dose 200 mg/day) was obtained at the cost of a low incidence of side effects, such as the virtual absence of torsades, and only 2% of pulmonary fibrosis.[20] Nonetheless, amiodarone is not licensed for supraventricular arrhythmias in the United States. *Contraindications* to amiodarone are severe sinus node dysfunction with marked sinus bradycardia or syncope, second- or third-degree heart block, known hypersensitivity, cardiogenic shock, and probably severe chronic lung disease.

Major Trials with Amiodarone Over the last few years, several important trials relating to the use of amiodarone in a range of clinical situations have clarified the major role of this multifunctional drug in atrial fibrillation,[20] in ventricular arrhythmias,[41,45,47,48] and in cardiac arrest.[43] The relative merits of amiodarone versus *implantable cardioverter defibrillators (ICDs)* have also been explored.[41,49] EMIAT and CAMIAT compared amiodarone to placebo in post-MI patients with reduced ejection fraction (EMIAT) or complex ventricular ectopy.[47,48] Both trials demonstrated reductions in arrhythmic death and resuscitated VF, but the reduction in overall mortality did not reach statistical significance. Subanalyses suggested an important *favorable interaction of amiodarone therapy with β-blockers*.[35] Trials examining primary or secondary prevention of arrhythmic cardiac death with ICDs have usually used amiodarone as the comparator for "conventional therapy." Although ICDs have been shown to be superior in several trials, though not in AMIOVERT,[41] the two therapies are probably best regarded as complementary rather than alternatives. In the Canadian trial (Table 8-6), ICDs were superior to amiodarone only in patients in the highest risk quartile.[6] In *heart failure*, based on prospective randomized trials in patients with heart failure (GESICA and CHF-STAT),[50,51] as well as a meta-analysis of the amiodarone trials,[45] a number of conclusions can be drawn. First, unlike other antiarrhythmic drugs, amiodarone appears reasonably safe with little or no associated increase in mortality, and a low risk of proarrhythmia even when administered to patients with heart failure. Second, apart from the GESICA trial, amiodarone effects on mortality in heart failure have been only borderline[45] or, in a decisive very large trial, no different from placebo (SCD-HeFT, Table 8-6). Therefore, *we do not recommend prophylactic amiodarone therapy in all patients with LV dysfunction*.

Cardiac Side Effects and Torsades de Pointes Amiodarone may inhibit the SA or AV node (about 2% to 5%), which can be serious in those with

Table 8-6 Key Trials with Antiarrhythmics or Devices for Ventricular Arrhythmias

Drug Class or Device	Acronym	Hypothesis	Key Results
IC	CAST (Cardiac Arrhythmia Suppression Trial)[1] Steinbeck[154]	PVC suppression gives benefit	Mortality doubled in treatment group
II		EPS guided versus empiric β-blockade with metoprolol	Equal benefits; EPS not needed
I, III (Sotalol)	ESVEM (Electrophysiological Study Versus ECG Monitoring, 1993)[55]	Which drug class is better? Which selection method is better?	Sotalol better than 6 Class I agents; Holter = EPS
III	EMIAT (European Myocardial Infarct Amiodarone Trial, 1997)[47]	Amiodarone can reduce sudden death in post-MI with low ejection fraction	Arrhythmia deaths decreased, total deaths unchanged
III	CAMIAT (Canadian Acute Myocardial Infarction Amiodarone Trial)[48]	Post AMI with frequent VPS or nonsustained VT—? reduced mortality	Sudden death and mortality reduced
ICD	MADIT (Multicenter Automatic Defibrillator Implantation Trial)[146]	ICD in high-risk patients (coronary artery disease + NSVT on EPS) would improve beyond drugs	Mortality reduced by half, trial stopped
ICD	AVID (Antiarrhythmic Versus Implantable Defibrillators)[133]	Resuscitated VF or VT (with low ejection fraction) better on ICD	26–31% mortality reduction with ICD; trial terminated
ICD	MUSTT (Multicenter Unsustained Tachycardia Trial)[155]	EPS guided therapy can reduce death in survivors of AMI	Cardiac arrest or death from arrhythmia reduced by 27% in ICD group
ICD	CIDS (Canadian Implantable Defibrillator Study)[6]	ICD vs. amiodarone: effects on VF; cardiac arrest or sustained VT; all-cause deaths	ICD better than amiodarone only in highest risk patients; 50% less risk with ICD
ICD	MADIT-2[147]	ICD in post-MI LV failure; EF ≤30%	All cause mortality reduced by 31% by ICD
ICD	DEFINITE (Defibrillators in non-ischemic cadiomyopathy)[149]	Dilated cardiomyopathy, optimal medical therapy, EF ≤35%	Arrhythmic mortality reduced by 74%
ICD, III (Amiodarone)	SCD-HeFT (Sudden Cardiac Death-Heart Failure Trial)[150]	Heart failure, ICD or amiodarone better than placebo	Total mortality reduced by 23% by ICD, no effect of amiodarone

EF = ejection fraction; EPS = electrophysiological stimulation; ICD = implanted cardioverter defibrillator; NSVT = nonsustained ventricular tachycardia; PVC = premature ventricular complex; VF = ventricular fibrillation; VT = ventricular tachycardia.

241

prior sinus node dysfunction or heart block. It is probably a safe drug from the hemodynamic point of view. Only 1.6% required discontinuation of amiodarone because of bradycardia in a meta-analysis.[3] In heart failure, torsades de pointes is relatively rare with amiodarone (approximately 0.5% or less),[3] yet special care needs to be taken in CHF to avoid hypokalemia and digoxin toxicity.

Pulmonary Side Effects In higher doses, there is an unusual spectrum of toxicity, the most serious being pneumonitis, potentially leading to pulmonary fibrosis and occurring in 10% to 17% at doses of about 400 mg/day, and by which may be fatal in 10% of those affected (package insert). Yet the condition may be overdiagnosed.[3] Meta-analysis of double-blind amiodarone trials suggests that there is an absolute risk of 1% of pulmonary toxicity per year, with some fatal cases. Of note, pulmonary toxicity may be dose-related, and very rarely occurs with the low doses of about 200 mg daily, used for prevention of recurrent atrial fibrillation.[4,52] Pulmonary complications usually regress if recognized early and if amiodarone is discontinued, and the patient kept alive by symptomatic therapy, which may include steroids.

Thyroid Side Effects Amiodarone also has a complex effect on the metabolism of thyroid hormones (it contains iodine and shares a structural similarity to thyroxin), the main action being to inhibit the peripheral conversion of T4 to T3 with a rise in the serum level of T4 and a small fall in the level of T3; serum reverse T3 is increased as a function of the dose and duration of amiodarone therapy. In most patients, thyroid function is not altered by amiodarone. In about 6% hypothyroidism may develop during the first year of treatment, but hyperthyroidism only in 0.9%[3]; the exact incidence varies geographically. Hyperthyroidism may precipitate arrhythmia breakthrough and should be excluded if new arrhythmias appear during amiodarone therapy. At a moderate dose of amiodarone (200 to 400 mg daily), there may be biochemically documented but clinically silent alterations in thyroid function in 10% of patients. Besides clinical vigilance, biannual thyroid function tests, of which the most useful are the TSH and the serum T4, are recommended.

Other Extracardiac Side Effects Regarding the CNS side effects, proximal muscle weakness, peripheral neuropathy, and neural symptoms (headache, ataxia, tremors, impaired memory, dyssomnia, bad dreams) occur with variable incidence. Peripheral neuropathy occurred in 0.6% per year in the meta-analysis.[3] *GI side effects* were uncommon in the GESICA study.[50] Yet nausea can occur in 25% of patients with CHF, even at a dose of only 200 mg daily. Increased plasma levels of liver function enzymes may occur in 10% to 20% of all patients. These effects usually resolve with dose reduction. *Testicular dysfunction* may be a side effect, detected by increased gonadotropin levels in patients on long-term amiodarone. *Less serious side effects* are as follows: Corneal microdeposits develop in nearly all adult patients given prolonged amiodarone. Symptoms and impairment of visual acuity are rare and respond to reduced dosage. Macular degeneration rarely occurs during therapy without proof of a causal relationship. In more than 10% of patients, a photosensitive slate-gray or bluish skin discoloration develops after prolonged therapy, usually exceeding 18 months. Avoid exposure to sun and use a sunscreen ointment with UVA and UVB protection. The pigmentation regresses slowly on drug withdrawal.

Dose-Dependency of Side Effects A full and comprehensive meta-analysis of the side effects of amiodarone showed that even low doses may not be free of adverse effects.[4] At a mean dose of 152 to 330 mg/day, drug withdrawal because of side effects was 1.5 times more common than with placebo.[4] Specifically, however, low-dose amiodarone was not associated with torsades.

Drug Interactions The most serious interaction is an additive proarrhythmic effect with other drugs prolonging the QT-interval, such as class IA antiarrhythmic agents, phenothiazines, tricyclic antidepressants, thiazide diuretics, and sotalol. Combination with sotalol should not be given unless an ICD is in place. Amiodarone may increase quinidine and procainamide levels (these combinations are not advised). With phenytoin, there is a double drug interaction. Amiodarone increases phenytoin levels while at the same time phenytoin enhances the conversion of amiodarone to desethylamiodarone. *A serious and common interaction* is with warfarin. Amiodarone prolongs the prothrombin time and may cause bleeding in patients on warfarin, perhaps by a hepatic interaction; decrease warfarin by about one third and retest the INR. Amiodarone increases the plasma digoxin concentration, predisposing to digitalis toxic effects (not arrhythmias because amiodarone protects); decrease digoxin by about half and remeasure digoxin levels. Amiodarone, by virtue of its weak β-blocking and calcium antagonist effect, tends to inhibit nodal activity and may therefore interact adversely with β-blocking agents and calcium antagonists. However, the antiarrhythmic efficacy of amiodarone is generally increased by coprescription with β-blocking drugs.[35]

Precautions During long-term amiodarone therapy, routine toxicity screening is required.[3] Check baseline pulmonary, thyroid, and liver function tests and plasma electrolytes. To initiate therapy, there is some controversy about the need for hospitalization, which is required for life-threatening VT/VF. For recurrences of atrial fibrillation (not licensed in the United States), low-dose therapy can be initiated on an outpatient basis. If amiodarone is added to an ICD, then the defibrillation threshold is usually increased and must be rechecked prior to discharge from hospital. During chronic therapy the ECG and Holter recordings are monitored and periodic (6 months or annual) chest radiographs or respiratory function tests are performed, and thyroid and liver function tests (6 months) are required. Keep the dose as low as possible.

Sotalol

Sotalol (Betapace in the United States, Sotacor in Europe) was first licensed in the United States for control of severe ventricular arrhythmias. It is now licensed as Betapace AF for maintenance of sinus rhythm in patients with recurrent atrial fibrillation or atrial flutter, who are symptomatic. Although less effective than amiodarone[20,41] sotalol is chosen, particularly when amiodarone toxicity is feared. As a mixed class II and class III agent, it also has all the beneficial actions of the β-blocker. Inevitably, it is also susceptible to the "Achilles' heel" of all class III agents, namely torsades de pointes.

Electrophysiology Sotalol is a racemic mixture of dextro- and levo isomers, and these differ very considerably in their electrophysiological effects. Although these agents have comparable class III activity, the class II activity arises from l-sotalol.[53] The pure class III investigational agent d-sotalol increased mortality in postinfarct patients with a low ejection fraction in the SWORD study.[54] This result suggests that the class III activity, perhaps acting through torsades, can detract from the positive β-blocking qualities of the standard dl-sotalol. In practice, class III activity is not evident at low doses (<160 mg/day) of the racemic drug. In humans, class II effects are sinus and AV node depression. Class III effects are prolongation of the action potential in atrial and ventricular tissue and prolonged atrial and ventricular refractory periods, as well as inhibition of conduction along any bypass tract in both directions. APD prolongation with, possibly, enhanced calcium entry may explain why it causes proarrhythmic afterdepolarizations and why the negative inotropic effect is less than expected. It is a noncardioselective, water-soluble (hydrophilic), non-protein-bound agent, excreted solely by the kidneys, with a plasma half-life of 12 hours (USA package insert). Dosing every 12 hours gives trough concentrations half of those of the peak values.

Indications   Because of its combined class II and class III properties, sotalol is theoretically active against a wide variety of arrhythmias, including sinus tachycardia, paroxysmal supraventricular tachycardia, WPW arrhythmias with either antegrade or retrograde conduction, recurrence of atrial fibrillation,[19] ischemic ventricular arrhythmias, and recurrent sustained ventricular tachycardia or fibrillation. In ventricular arrhythmias, the major outcome study with sotalol was the ESVEM trial[55] in which this drug in a mean dose of about 400 mg daily was better at decreasing death and ventricular arrhythmias than any of six class I agents. The major indication was sustained monomorphic ventricular tachycardia (or ventricular fibrillation) induced in an electrophysiologic study. Of the wide indications, the major current use is in maintenance of sinus rhythm after cardioversion for atrial fibrillation,[19] when sotalol is as about as effective as flecainide or propafenone with the advantage that it can be given to patients with structural heart disease whereas the other two cannot; however, the efficacy of all three is outclassed by amiodarone.[20,52]

Dose   For atrial fibrillation and atrial flutter, currently in sinus rhythm, the detailed package insert indicates that 320 mg/day (two doses) may give the ideal ratio between effects and side effects (torsades). The latter risk is 0.3% at 320 mg/day, but goes up to 3.2% at higher doses when used for atrial fibrillation or flutter (USA package insert). For ventricular arrhythmias, the dose range is 160 to 640 mg/day given in two divided doses. Keeping the daily dose at 320 mg or lower (as recommended for atrial fibrillation recurrences) lessens side effects, including torsades de pointes. Yet doses of 320 to 480 mg may be needed to prevent recurrent VT or VF. When given in two divided doses, steady-state plasma concentrations are reached in 2 to 3 days. In patients with renal impairment or in the elderly, or when there are risk factors for proarrhythmia, the dose should be reduced and the dosing interval increased.

Side Effects   These are those of β-blockade, including fatigue (20%) and bradycardia (13%), added to which is the risk of torsades de pointes. Being a nonselective β-blocker, bronchospasm may be precipitated. For drug interactions see Tables 8-3 and 8-5.

Precautions and Contraindications   For the initial treatment in patients with recurrent atrial fibrillation or flutter, the patient should be hospitalized and monitored for 3 days while the dose is increased (package insert). The drug should be avoided in patients with serious conduction defects, including sick sinus syndrome, second- or third-degree AV block (unless there is a pacemaker), in bronchospastic disease, and when there are evident risks of proarrhythmia. Asthma is a contraindication and bronchospastic disease a strong caution (sotalol is a nonselective β-blocker). The drug is contraindicated in patients with reduced creatinine clearance, below 40 ml/minute (renal excretion). *Torsades de pointes* is more likely when the sotalol dose is high, exceeding 320 mg/day, or when there is bradycardia, or when the baseline QT exceeds 450 milliseconds (package insert), or in severe LV failure, or in the female gender or in the congenital long-QT syndrome. Cotherapy with class IA drugs, amiodarone or other drugs prolonging the QT-interval is avoided (Fig. 8-4). In pregnancy, the drug is category B. It is not teratogenic but does cross the placenta and may depress fetal vital functions. Sotalol is also excreted in mother's milk.

PURE CLASS III AGENTS: IBUTILIDE AND DOFETILIDE

The effectiveness of class III antiarrhythmic drugs such as amiodarone and sotalol has prompted the development of class III agents with

LONG QT WITH RISK OF TORSADES

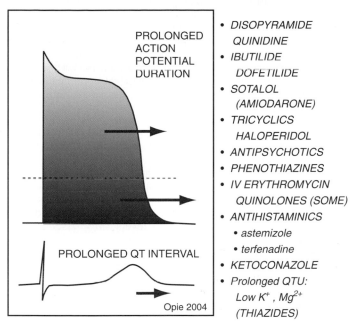

- DISOPYRAMIDE
  QUINIDINE
- IBUTILIDE
  DOFETILIDE
- SOTALOL
  (AMIODARONE)
- TRICYCLICS
  HALOPERIDOL
- ANTIPSYCHOTICS
- PHENOTHIAZINES
- IV ERYTHROMYCIN
  QUINOLONES (SOME)
- ANTIHISTAMINICS
  - astemizole
  - terfenadine
- KETOCONAZOLE
- Prolonged QTU:
  Low K^+, Mg^{2+}
  (THIAZIDES)

Figure 8-4 Therapeutic agents, including antiarrhythmics that may cause QT prolongation. Hypokalemia causes QTU not QT prolongation. Some antiarrhythmic agents act at least in part chiefly by prolonging the action potential duration, such as amiodarone and sotalol. QT prolongation is therefore an integral part of their therapeutic benefit. On the other hand, QT or QTU prolongation, especially in the presence of hypokalemia or hypomagnesemia or when there is cotherapy with one of the other agents prolonging the QT-interval, may precipitate torsades de pointes. (*Figure © LH Opie, 2005.*)

similar efficacy but that lack the systemic side effects of conventional class III agents. Two such drugs, ibutilide and dofetilide, have recently been approved and introduced into clinical practice. The efficacy of ibutilide and dofetilide in the conversion of atrial flutter is noteworthy because, prior to their introduction, drugs have not been found to be efficacious in the cardioversion of atrial flutter.

Ibutilide

Ibutilide (Corvert) is a methanesulfonamide derivative, which prolongs repolarization by inhibition of the delayed rectifier potassium current (I_{kr}) and by selective enhancement of the slow inward sodium current. Ibutilide has no known negative inotropic effects.

Pharmacokinetics Ibutilide is available only as an intravenous preparation because it undergoes extensive first-pass metabolism when administered orally. The pharmacokinetics of ibutilide are linear and are independent of dose, age, sex, and left ventricular function. Its extracellular distribution is extensive, and its systemic clearance is high. The elimination half-life is variable, 2 to 12 hours (mean of 6), reflecting considerable individual variation.[56]

Efficacy of Ibutilide This drug is efficacious in the termination of atrial fibrillation (AF) and flutter with both single and repeated intravenous infusions.[56] It is as effective as amiodarone in cardioversion of atrial fibrillation.[19,57] In patients who had persistent AF or atrial flutter, ibutilide had a conversion efficacy of 44% for a single dose and 49% for a second dose.[58] The mean termination time was 27 minutes after the start of the infusion. Efficacy was higher in atrial flutter than in AF. The efficacy of ibutilide in the cardioversion of atrial flutter is related to an effect on the variability of the cycle length of the tachycardia.[59] Like sotalol, ibutilide exhibits the phenomenon of reverse use dependence in that prolongation of refractoriness becomes less pronounced at higher tachycardia rates. *After cardiac surgery* ibutilide has a dose-dependent effect in conversion of atrial arrhythmias with 57% conversion at a dose of 10 mg.[60] Ibutilide pretreatment facilitates DC cardioversion of AF, but must be followed with 3 to 4 hours of ECG monitoring to exclude torsades.[61]

Adverse Effects QT- and QT_c-interval prolongation is a consistent feature in patients treated with ibutilide. QT prolongation is dose-dependent, maximal at the end of the infusion, and returns to baseline within 2 to 4 hours following infusion.[56] It is thus likely that the chief mechanism accounting for the antiarrhythmic action of ibutilide (prolongation of repolarization) accounts for its proarrhythmic effect as well. *Torsades de pointes* (polymorphic ventricular tachycardia with QT prolongation) is the most significant adverse effect associated with ibutilide therapy in about 4.3%.[62] Cardioversion is required in almost 2% of patients.[62] In LV failure the incidence of torsade is higher at about 6% (package insert). In addition, nonsustained monomorphic VT may occur in nearly 5% of patients.[62] Torsades tends to occur during or shortly after the infusion period (within 1 hour).[62] Patients should be monitored for at least 4 hours after the start of the ibutilide infusion. Plasma concentrations of ibutilide do not predict those at risk of VT, with a higher incidence in patients with heart failure, those with bradycardia, nonwhite subjects, women, and in those given the drug for atrial flutter rather than for AF.[56,62] In general, to avoid proarrhythmia, higher doses of ibutilide and rapid infusion are avoided, the drug is not given to those with preexisting QT prolongation or advanced or unstable heart disease, and the serum K^+ must be >4 mmol/l. Theoretically, other cardiac and noncardiac drugs, which prolong the QT interval, may increase the likelihood of torsade. However, one study, prior therapy with sotalol or amiodarone did not appear to provoke torsades.[61]

Dose The efficacy of ibutilide is dose-related. The recommended dose for treatment of atrial arrhythmias is 1 mg administered by intravenous infusion over 10 minutes. If the arrhythmia is not terminated within 10 minutes after the end of the first infusion, the infusion may be repeated. For patients under 60 kg, the dose should be 0.01 mg/kg. The drug must be administered under continuous cardiac monitoring, also for 4 hours after an infusion, and with resuscitation facilities available.

Drug Interactions Apart from the proposed interaction with sotalol, amiodarone and other drugs prolonging the QT-interval, there are no known drug interactions of ibutilide.

Dofetilide

Like ibutilide, dofetilide (Tikosyn) is a methanesulfonamide drug. Dofetilide prolongs the action potential duration (APD) and QT_c in a concentration-related manner. However, unlike ibutilide, dofetilide has no effect on the early fast inward Na^+ current and exerts its effect solely by inhibition of the rapid component of the delayed rectifier potassium current I_{Kr}. Like ibutilide and sotalol, dofetilide exhibits the phenomenon of reverse use dependence. Dofetilide has mild negative chronotropic effects, is devoid of negative inotropic activity and may be mildly positively inotropic. Whereas ibutilide is given only intravenously, dofetilide is given only orally.

Pharmacokinetics Dofetilide can be given orally. After oral administration, dofetilide is almost completely (92% to 96%) absorbed, and mean maximal plasma concentrations are achieved roughly 2.5 hours after administration. Twice-daily administration of oral dofetilide results in steady state within 48 hours. Fifty percent of the drug is excreted through the kidneys unchanged and there are no active metabolites.

Efficacy Dofetilide has good efficacy in the cardioversion of AF[19] and is even more effective in the cardioversion of atrial flutter. In addition, dofetilide may also be active against ventricular arrhythmias (not licensed). Dofetilide decreases the ventricular fibrillation threshold in patients undergoing defibrillation testing prior to ICD implantation, and suppresses the inducibility of VT. Dofetilide is as effective as sotalol against inducible VT, with fewer side effects.[63] In patients with depressed left ventricular function both with and without a history of myocardial infarction,[64] dofetilide has a neutral effect on mortality. However, dofetilide reduced the development of new AF, increased the conversion of preexisting AF to sinus rhythm, and improved the maintenance of sinus rhythm in these patients with significant structural heart disease. In this study dofetilide also reduced hospitalization.

Indications (1) Cardioversion of persistent atrial fibrillation or atrial flutter to normal sinus rhythm in patients in whom cardioversion by electrical means is not appropriate and in whom the duration of the arrhythmic episode is less than 6 months. (2) Maintenance of sinus rhythm (after conversion) in patients with persistent AF or atrial flutter. Because dofetilide can cause ventricular arrhythmias, it should be reserved for patients in whom AF/atrial flutter is highly symptomatic and in whom other antiarrhythmic therapy is not appropriate. Dofetilide has stronger evidence in its favor for acute cardioversion of atrial fibrillation than for maintenance thereafter, according to a meta-analysis.[19] An important point in its favor is that it can be given to those with a depressed ejection fraction.

Dose of Dofetilide The package insert warns in bold that the dose must be individualized by the calculated creatinine clearance and the QT_c. There must be continuous ECG monitoring and personnel to manage any serious ventricular arrhythmias. For the complex six-step dosing instructions, see the package insert. The calculated dose could be 125–500μg twice daily. Those with a creatinine clearance of below 20 ml/minute should not be given dofetilide. If the increase in the QT_c is >15%, or if the $QT_{c\,is}$ >500 milliseconds, the dose of dofetilide should be reduced. If at any time after the second dose the QT_c is greater than 500 milliseconds, dofetilide should be discontinued.

Adverse Effects As with ibutilide, the major significant adverse effect is torsades de pointes. In the largest trial of dofetilide reported to date, this complication occurred in 3% of patients.[64] The risk of torsades de pointes can be reduced by normal serum potassium and magnesium levels, and by avoiding the drug (or reducing its dosage according to the manufacturer's algorithm) in patients with abnormal renal function, or with bradycardia, or with baseline QT prolongation. Ideally the baseline QTc should be below 429 milliseconds.[65] In the DIAMOND trial, 80% of torsades occurred within the first 3 days of therapy.[64] Therefore, patients should be closely observed (including continuous ECG monitoring) in hospital for the first 3 days of dofetilide therapy. Two important measures effective against torsade are pre-dose adjustment of renal function and post-dose reduction based on QT_c.

Drug Interactions Drugs that increase levels of dofetilide should not be coadministered. These include ketoconazole and other inhibitors of cytochrome CYP 3A4 including macrolide antibiotics and protease inhibitors such as the antiviral agent ritonavir, verapamil, and cimetidine. Check for QT_c prolongation (hypokalemia), especially with diuretics or chronic diarrhea and the coadministration of drugs that increase the QT_c (Fig. 8-4).

Novel Class III Agents

Azimilide, a novel class III antiarrhythmic agent, blocks both the slowly activating (I_{Ks}) and rapidly activating (I_{Kr}) components of the delayed rectifier potassium current, whereas sotalol, amiodarone, or dofetilide block only I_{Kr}.[66] The advantage of blocking the slow repolarizing K current, I_{Ks}, may be in conditions of tachycardia and sympathetic stimulation, when pure I_{Kr} blockers such as sotalol and amiodarone are less likely to be effective. The ALIVE (Azimilide post-Infarction surVival Evaluation) trial concerns the possible prevention by azimilide of cardiac sudden death in high-risk patients after MI, characterized by depressed LV function and a low heart rate variability.[67] The incidence of serious adverse events, including torsades de pointes and agranulocytosis was low, but mortality was unchanged. By contrast azimilide successfully diminished ventricular tachycardia and fibrillation in patients with an implanted ICD.[68]

Dronedarone is an amiodarone-like drug, thought not to have noncardiac tissue side effects, because it lacks iodine in its structure.[69] It is still in early development. The first large study on 199 patients showed that a dose of 800 mg per day, when given to patients after cardioversion for atrial fibrillation, increased the time to relapse from 5.3 days in the controls to 60 days ($P < 0.001$).[70] Over 6 months there was no evidence of thyroid side effects or of proarrhythmia.

CLASS IV AND CLASS IV-LIKE AGENTS

Verapamil and Diltiazem Calcium channel blockade slows conduction through the AV node, and increases the refractory period of nodal tissue. Because of vascular selectivity, *dihydropyridine* compounds do not have significant electrophysiological effects (Chapter 3). The nondihydropyridine agents *verapamil* and *diltiazem* are similar in their electrophysiological properties. They slow the ventricular response rate in atrial arrhythmias, particularly atrial fibrillation. They can also terminate or prevent reentrant arrhythmias in which the circuit involves the AV node. For the termination of junctional tachycardias, verapamil has now been largely superseded by adenosine.

Rare Use in Ventricular Tachycardia A few unusual forms of ventricular tachycardia respond to verapamil or diltiazem. In idiopathic right ventricular outflow tract tachycardia, verapamil is chosen after β-blockade. Fascicular tachycardias often respond to verapamil and torsades de pointes may terminate following verapamil. In all other ventricular arrhythmias, *these agents are contraindicated* because of their hemodynamic effects and inefficacy. Verapamil must not be administered intravenously to patients who have received either oral or recent intravenous β-blockade. Severe and irreversible electromechanical dissociation may occur.

Intravenous Magnesium Intravenous magnesium weakly blocks the calcium channel, as well as inhibiting sodium and potassium channels. The relative importance of these mechanisms is unknown. It can be used to slow the ventricular rate in atrial fibrillation but is poor at terminating junctional tachycardias. It may be the agent of choice in torsades de pointes.[71] It has an additional use in refractory ventricular fibrillation, probably now superseded by intravenous amiodarone.

Adenosine

Adenosine (Adenocard) has multiple cellular effects, including opening of the adenosine-sensitive inward rectifier potassium channel, with inhibition of the sinus and especially the AV node (Fig. 8-5). It is now the first-line agent for terminating narrow complex paroxysmal supraventricular tachycardias (PSVTs).[72] It is also used in the diagnosis of wide-complex tachycardia of uncertain origin.

ADENOSINE INHIBITION OF AV NODE
Opie 2004

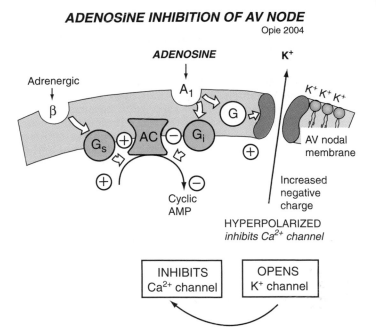

Figure 8-5 Adenosine inhibits the AV node by effects on ion channels. Adenosine acting on the A_1 surface receptor, opens the adenosine-sensitive potassium channel to hyperpolarize and inhibit the AV node and also indirectly to inhibit calcium channel opening. A_1 = adenosine$_1$ receptor; AC = adenylate cyclase; β = β-adrenoreceptor; G = G protein, nonspecific; G_i = inhibitory G protein; G_s = stimulatory G protein. (*Figure © LH Opie, 2005.*)

Dose Adenosine is given as an initial rapid intravenous bolus of 6 mg followed by a saline flush to obtain high concentrations in the heart.[72] If it does not work within 1 to 2 minutes, a 12-mg bolus is given that may be repeated once. At the appropriate dose, the antiarrhythmic effect occurs as soon as the drug reaches the AV node, usually within 15 to 30 seconds. The initial dose needs to be reduced to 3 mg or less in patients taking verapamil, diltiazem, or β-blockers or dipyridamole (see Drug Interactions), or in the elderly who are at risk of sick sinus syndrome. Note the extremely short half-life of 10 to 30 seconds.

Indications The chief indication is for *paroxysmal narrow complex SVT* (usually AV nodal reentry or AV reentry such as in the WPW syndrome or in patients with a concealed accessory pathway). In most cases adenosine has no clinically useful effect on atrial myocardium (see below) but it may unmask occult atrial activity when atrial flutter or atrial tachycardia is not otherwise apparent from the surface electrocardiogram. In *wide-complex tachycardia* of uncertain origin, adenosine can help the management by differentiating between VT or SVT (with aberrant conduction). In the latter case, adenosine is likely to stop the tachycardia, whereas in the case of VT there is unlikely to be any major adverse hemodynamic effect and the tachycardia continues. It may be particularly helpful in VT with retrograde conduction to block the P wave and to show the diagnosis. Thus there is therefore a combined therapeutic-diagnostic test. Occasionally adenosine is effective in *rare forms of idiopathic VT*, such as some types of right ventricular outflow tract VT, dependent on cyclic AMP, and often in the presence of mild V structural abnormalities.[73] Finally intravenous adenosine may be ed to reveal *latent preexcitation* in patients suspected of having the W syndrome.[74] When used for this indication adenosine is admin- ed during sinus rhythm while a mutichannel ECG rhythm strip is ded (ideally all 12 leads) and a normal response occurs if transient high-grade AV block is observed. On the other hand, following adenosine the presence of an anterograde conduction accessory pathway is inferred if there is PR interval shortening/QRS widening without interruption in AV conduction.

Side Effects and Contraindications Those ascribed to the effect of adenosine on the potassium channel are short lived, such as headache (via vasodilation), provocation of chest pain, flushing, and excess sinus or AV nodal inhibition. However, the precipitation of bronchoconstriction in asthmatic patients is of unknown mechanism and can last for 30 minutes. *Transient new arrhythmias* at the time of chemical cardioversion occur in about 65%. Because of a direct effect on atrial and ventricular myocardial refractoriness, the use of adenosine may be associated with a range of *proarrhythmic effects* including atrial and ventricular ectopy, and degeneration of atrial flutter or paroxysmal supraventricular tachycardia into AF.[75] Contraindications are as follows: asthma or history of asthma, second- or third-degree AV block, sick sinus syndrome. Atrial flutter is a relative contraindication, because of the risk of 1:1 conduction and serious tachycardia. *Drug interactions* are as follows. Dipyridamole inhibits the breakdown of adenosine and therefore the dose of adenosine must be markedly reduced in patients receiving dipyridamole. Methylxanthines (caffeine, theophylline) competitively antagonize the interaction of adenosine with its receptors, so that it becomes less effective.

Adenosine versus Verapamil or Diltiazem Adenosine has replaced intravenous verapamil or diltiazem for the rapid termination of narrow QRS complex SVT. It needs to be reemphasized that verapamil or diltiazem, by myocardial depression and peripheral vasodilation can be fatal when given to patients with VT, whereas adenosine with its very transient effects leaves true VT virtually unchanged.

COMBINATION ANTIARRHYTHMIC THERAPY

A combination of antiarrhythmic agents may be used when single drug treatment fails or when the dose must be reduced because of side effects. There are no outcome studies on combination therapy. Retrospective analysis suggests that the combination of β-blockers and amiodarone may improve survival when compared to treatment with either agent alone.[35,47,76]

Some logical "rules"[77-81]:

1. Do not combine agents of the same class or subclasses, or agents with potentially additive side effects, such as the extra risk of arrhythmias with class IA and class IC agents, or the added QT prolongation with class IA agents and sotalol or amiodarone.
2. A logical combination is that of a class I drug that preferentially binds to inactivated sodium channels (class IB), with a drug binding preferentially to activated channels such as a class IA drug, thus explaining the benefits of mexiletine combined with procainamide.
3. Combining β-blockade with sotalol will give excess β-blockade. In contrast, β-blockers and amiodarone combine well.[35]
4. When sotalol followed by amiodarone alone has failed as maximal therapy a combination of amiodarone with sotalol may be considered. Similarly, addition of mexiletine or procainamide to sotalol or amiodarone is also worth a cautious trial.
5. Combinations of drugs and devices are becoming common. There is an increasing realization that ICDs outperform even amiodarone, a powerful antiarrhythmic drug, in the secondary prevention of sudden cardiac death, yet with an antiarrhythmic d cautiously added to the ICD,[37,79] especially when there is frequ recurrent VT.

PROARRHYTHMIA, QT-PROLONGATION, AND TORSADES DE POINTES

Proarrhythmic Effects of Antiarrhythmics

Proarrhythmia can offset the benefits of an antiarrhythmic agent.[1] There are two basic mechanisms for proarrhythmia: prolongation of the action potential duration and QT-interval (Fig. 8-4), and, second, incessant wide-complex tachycardia often terminating in VF (Fig. 8-6). The former typically occurs with class IA and class III agents, the latter with class IC agents. In addition, incessant VT can complicate therapy with any class I agent when conduction is sufficiently severely depressed. A third type of proarrhythmia is when the patient's own tachycardia, previously paroxysmal, becomes incessant—the result of either class IA or IC agents. Not only is early vigilance required with the institution of therapy with antiarrhythmics of the class IA, IC, and III types, but continuous vigilance is required throughout therapy. Furthermore, the CAST study shows that proarrhythmic sudden death can occur even when ventricular premature complexes are apparently eliminated. Solutions to this problem include (1) avoiding the use of class I, and especially class IC agents, in patients with structural heart disease; (2) not treating unless the overall effect will clearly be beneficial; and (3) ultimately defining better those subjects at high risk for

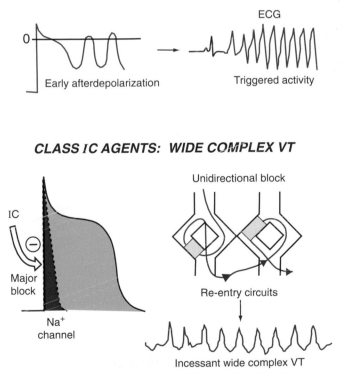

Figure 8-6 Major proarrhythmic mechanisms. *Top*: Class IA and class III agents widen the action potential duration and in the presence of an early afterdepolarization can give rise to triggered activity known as torsades de pointes. Note major role of QT prolongation (Fig. 8-4). *Bottom*: Class IC agents have as their major proarrhythmic mechanism a powerful inhibition of the sodium channel, particularly in conduction tissue. Increasing heterogeneity together with unidirectional block sets the stage for re-entry circuits and monomorphic wide complex ventricular tachycardia. (*Figure © LH Opie, 2005.*)

arrhythmia and arrhythmic death. The latter would now often be treated by an ICD.

Long-QT Syndrome and Torsades de Pointes

The long-QT syndrome (LQTS) with delayed repolarization is clinically recognized by a prolonged QT or QTc (corrected for heart rate exceeding 440 milliseconds) or QTU-interval. LQTS may be either an acquired or a congenital abnormality. The realization that quinidine, disopyramide, procainamide, and related class IA agents, class III agents, and others (Fig. 8-4) can all prolong the QT-interval has led to a reassessment of the mode of use of such agents in antiarrhythmic therapy. Of the class III agents, sotalol may be particularly prone to cause torsades de pointes because of its reverse use dependency, so that bradycardia prolongs the action potential duration even more. By contrast, when amiodarone is given to patients not receiving diuretics or other drugs, who are not hypokalemic and without preexisting QT prolongation, torsades de pointes is very rare. Perhaps amiodarone via its mixed class effects such as sodium and calcium channel inhibition and β-blockade overrides the capacity of its class III side effects that produce torsades. Serious problems may arise when QT prolongation by sotalol or class 1A drugs or even amiodarone is combined with any other factor increasing the QT-interval or QTU, such as bradycardia, hypokalemia, hypomagnesemia, hypocalcemia, intense or prolonged use of potassium-wasting diuretic therapy, or combined class IA and class III therapy. A number of noncardiac drugs prolong the QT-interval by blocking the I_{Kr} potassium channels (Fig. 8-4), including tricyclic antidepressants, phenothiazines, erythromycin, and some antihistamines, such as terfenadine and astemizole. Note that a drug concentration that might slightly prolong the action potential plateau in some patients might in others produce excessive prolongation.

Treatment The management of patients with drug-induced torsades includes identifying and withdrawing the offending drug(s), replenishing the potassium level to 4.5 to 5 mmol/l and infusing intravenous magnesium (1 to 2 g). An interesting new approach is by chronic therapy with the potassium-retaining aldosterone blocker, spironolactone.[82] In resistant cases, isoproterenol or temporary cardiac pacing may be needed to increase the heart rate and shorten the QT-interval. Isoproterenol is contraindicated in ischemic heart disease and the congenital long-QT syndrome.

Congenital Long-QT Syndrome These are examples of the channelopathies, which are congenital disorders of the cardiac ion channels predisposing to lethal cardiac arrhythmias. The three major causes are LQT1; LQT2, a defect in the rapid component of the repolarizing potassium current; and LQT3, a defect in the sodium channel that allow excess entry of sodium ions. LQT3 is logically treated by sodium channel inhibitors (class I drugs) of which mexilitine and flecainide have been documented.[28,83] For LQT1, the action potential does not shorten as it should during the tachycardia of exercise, so that a β-blocker is used to avoid the tachycardia.

Section B   WHICH ANTIARRHYTHMIC DRUG OR DEVICE?

PAROXYSMAL SUPRAVENTRICULAR TACHYCARDIA (PSVT)

Acute Therapy Understanding the mechanism responsible for the arrhythmia (Fig. 8-7) is the key to appropriate therapy for paroxysmal supraventricular tachycardia (PSVT).[84] Atrioventricular nodal re

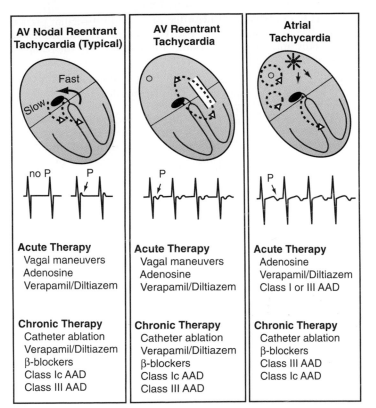

Figure 8-7 Mechanisms and therapy of paroxysmal supraventricular tachycardia. *Left panel* corresponds to Fig. 8-2, left middle panel. *Middle panel* (bypass tract) corresponds to Fig. 8-2, top right. *AAD* = antiarrhythmic drugs. (Modified from Ferguson and DiMarco, Circulation 2003;107:1096.)

trant tachycardia (AVNRT) and atrioventricular reentrant tachycardia (AVRT) are the forms most frequently seen in patients without structural heart disease, and maintenance of both arrhythmias depends on intact 1 : 1 AV nodal conduction. Many patients learn on their own to abort episodes soon after initiation with vagal maneuvers such as gagging, Valsalva, or carotid massage. In infants, facial immersion is effective. If the arrhythmia persists, sympathetic tone increases and these maneuvers then become less effective.

Parenteral Therapy During PSVT, bioavailability of orally administered drugs is delayed, so parenteral drug administration is often required.[85] One report described oral self-administration of crushed diltiazem and propranolol, but this is not frequently recommended.[86] Adenosine and a nondihydropyridine CCB (either verapamil or diltiazem) are the intravenous (IV) drugs of choice.[84,87] After IV administration, adenosine is cleared from the circulation within seconds by cellular uptake and metabolism.[72] Administration of an IV bolus results in transient AV nodal block when the bolus reaches the heart, usually within 15 to 30 seconds. Central administration results in a more rapid onset of effect, and dosage reduction is required. The recommended adult dosage for peripheral IV infusion is 6 mg followed by a second dose of 12 mg, if necessary. Higher doses may be required in selected patients or if venous access is poor. Because adenosine is cleared so rapidly, sequential doses do not result in a cumulative effect. Most patients report transient dyspnea or chest pain after receiving a bolus of adenosine. Sinus bradycardia with or without accompanying AV block is also common after PSVT termination. However, the bradycardia typically resolves within seconds and is

replaced with a mild sinus tachycardia. Atrial and ventricular premature beats may occur and can reinitiate PSVT or atrial fibrillation. (For
further details and Drug Interactions of Adenosine, see this chapter,
p. 248–249).

Verapamil and diltiazem, administered IV, are alternates to adenosine.[72,88] Both of these drugs affect the calcium-dependent AV nodal
action potential and facilitate AV nodal block. The recommended
initial dose of verapamil is 5 mg IV infused over 2 minutes. A second
dose of 5 to 7.5 mg may be given 5 to 10 minutes later, if necessary.
Diltiazem, 20 mg initially, followed by a second dose of 25 to 35 mg,
is equally effective.[89] PSVT termination within 5 minutes of the end
of the first or second infusion is expected in more than 90% of
patients with AVNRT or AVRT (Fig. 8-7). Verapamil and diltiazem are
vasodilators and may produce hypotension if the PSVT does not
terminate. Atrial arrhythmias and bradycardia may also be seen.
CCBs should not be used to treat preexcitation arrhythmias (WPW
syndrome) or wide-complex tachycardias unless the mechanism
of the arrhythmia is known to be AV nodal dependent. Drug-induced
hypotension with persistent arrhythmia may lead to cardiovascular
collapse and ventricular fibrillation (VF) in these settings, as in
neonates.[90]

Adenosine versus CCBs In most patients with PSVT caused by an AV
node-dependent mechanism, either adenosine or a CCB can be
selected.[87,91] Adenosine is preferred in infants and neonates, patients
with severe hypotension, if intravenous β-blockers have been recently
administered, and in those with a history of heart failure and poor
left ventricular function. CCBs are preferred in patients with venous
access unsuitable for delivering a rapid bolus infusion, in patients
with acute bronchospasm, and in the presence of agents that interfere
with adenosine's actions or its metabolism.[84]

Atrial tachycardias may be due to a number of possible mechanisms,
and few data about acute termination of atrial tachycardias (not
involving the AV Node) are available.[87] CCBs or β-blockers may be
effective when there is sinus node reentry or in some automatic atrial
tachycardias. Atrial tachycardias related to reentry around scars are
often drug resistant, and their management should resemble that of
atrial flutter (see below).

Chronic Therapy of PSVT Many patients with recurrent PSVT do not
require chronic therapy. If episodes produce minor symptoms and can
be broken easily by the patient, chronic drug therapy may be avoided.
When recurrent episodes produce significant symptoms or require
outside intervention for termination, either pharmacologic therapy or
catheter ablation is appropriate. In AV node-dependent PSVT, CCBs
and β-blockers are the first-line choices. Flecainide and propafenone
also are effective and are frequently used in combination with a β-
adrenergic blocker.[22,92,93] Sotalol, dofetilide, azimilide, and amiodarone may be effective but are second- or third-line agents. Chronic
drug therapy of atrial tachycardias (as opposed to AV nodal reentry
tachycardias) has not been extensively studied in clinical trials.
Empiric testing of β-blockers, CCB, and either class I or class III antiarrhythmics may be appropriate.[87]

Radiofrequency Catheter Ablation This has dramatically altered the management of symptomatic supraventricular tachycardias. Although
antiarrhythmic drug therapy is usually efficacious in 70% to 90% of
PSVT patients, up to half of these patients will have unwanted side
effects. Catheter ablation is an attractive alternative for AV nodal reentrant tachycardias and AV reentrant tachycardias with or without manifest preexcitation that is highly effective, produces a life-long "cure,"
and in experienced centers, is a low-risk procedure.[94] Many symptomatic patients will prefer to undergo catheter ablation even before

undergoing any trials of drug therapy. Therefore, current guidelines allow catheter ablation to be offered to patients as either a first option before any chronic drug trials or if drug treatment has been unsuccessful.[84,87] In general, if a small volume of cardiac tissue forms a critical part of the arrhythmia mechanism, the tachycardia can be permanently cured by radiofrequency catheter ablation. Hence other tachycardias that are routinely cured by targeted ablation include atrial flutter, atrial tachycardia, right ventricular outflow tract and idiopathic left ventricular (fascicular) tachycardias, bundle branch reentrant tachycardia, and some ventricular tachycardias with a focal origin (Fig. 8-8).

ATRIAL FIBRILLATION

Atrial fibrillation (AF) is the most common sustained arrhythmia encountered by internists and cardiologists treating adult patients.[95] The electrocardiogram in atrial fibrillation is characterized by an undulating baseline without discrete atrial activity. The atrial electrograms show a mostly disorganized pattern with rates averaging over 350 per minute. These rapid atrial rates bombard the AV node during all phases of its refractory period. Some impulses that do not conduct to the ventricle will reset the refractory period of the AV node and thereby delay or prevent conduction of subsequent impulses, a phenomenon called "concealed conduction." Patients with atrial fibrillation may present with a variety of symptoms, including palpitations, exercise intolerance, dyspnea, heart failure, chest pain, syncope, and dizziness. Some patients, however, are asymptomatic during some, or even all, episodes. Symptoms during atrial fibrillation can be caused by the increase in or the irregularity of the ventricular rate and by the loss of organized atrial contraction. Atrial fibrillation is also frequently associated with sinus node dysfunction or AV conduction disease, and patients may experience severe symptoms as a result of bradycardia. Loss of atrial contraction, disturbed atrial endothelial function, and activation of coagulation factors all predispose toward clot formation in the atria. Therapy of atrial fibrillation, therefore, may

SITES AMENABLE TO CATHETER ABLATION
Possible indications

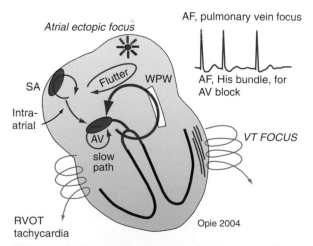

Figure 8-8 Possible sites for intervention by catheter ablation techniques. *AF* = atrial fibrillation; *AV* = atrioventricular node; *flutter* = atrial flutter; *RVOT* = right ventricular outflow tract; *SA* = sinoatrial node; *VT*, ventricular tachycardia; *WPW* = Wolff-Parkinson-White preexcitation syndrome.

involve measures to control ventricular rates, to restore and maintain sinus rhythm, and to prevent thromboembolic complications.

Presentation of AF Atrial fibrillation may present in a number of ways, and a classification based on its temporal pattern is often used.[96,97] At the time of first presentation of an acute episode of atrial fibrillation, the future temporal pattern may be difficult to predict so first episodes are often classified separately. If episodes are self-terminating within <7 days (usually less than 1 day), they are classified as *paroxysmal*. When episodes require drug or electrical therapy for termination, they are classified as *persistent*. Persistent atrial fibrillation that is resistant to cardioversion or in which cardioversion is not attempted is classified as *permanent*. Unfortunately, individual patients may experience both paroxysmal and persistent episodes in an unpredictable pattern, but the terms are helpful in analyzing trials dealing with drug therapy for atrial fibrillation.

Rate Control in Atrial Fibrillation

The two major and sometimes controversial policies are rate control versus rhythm control. Controlling abnormal ventricular rates improves symptoms in most patients. Intravenous therapy is usually employed in patients who present acutely with severe symptoms. In this situation, rapid relief of these symptoms is important. In less symptomatic patients, oral therapy may be initiated. Except in patients with preexcitation, rate control is usually achieved with drugs that act primarily on the AV node (Table 8-7). The adequacy of rate control is assessed by the patient's symptoms and measurement of heart rate both at rest and during moderate activity. The resting heart rate should be between 60 and 100 beats per minute at rest and between 90 and 115 beats per minute with moderate exercise. In general, rate control should not be assessed by a resting electrocardiogram alone and a Holter monitor (aim for average heart rate approximately 80

Table 8-7	Drug Loading and Maintenance Regimens for Control of Ventricular Rate in Atrial Fibrillation		
		Acute Intravenous Therapy	**Chronic Oral Therapy**
β-Blockers	Metoprolol	2.5–5 mg every 5 min up to 15 mg	50–200 mg/day
	Propranolol	0.15 mg/kg (1 mg every 2 min)	40–240 mg/day
	Esmolol	0.5 mg/kg bolus, then 0.05–0.2 mg/kg per min	NA
	Pindolol	NA	7.5–30 mg/day
	Atenolol	5 mg over 5 min, repeat in 10 min	25–100 mg/day
	Nadolol	NA	20–80 mg/day
Calcium-channel blockers	Verapamil	0.075–0.15 mg/kg over 2 min; 0.005 mg/kg per min	120–360 mg/day
	Diltiazem	0.25 mg/kg over 2 min followed by 5–15 mg/h	120–360 mg/day
Cardiac glycoside	Digoxin	0.75 mg–1.5 mg in divided doses over 12–24 h	0.125 mg–0.375 mg/day

Other β-blockers in addition to those listed may also be useful. NA, not available. For doses see ref 96; see Table 8-2 for other indications (verapamil, diltiazem).

beats/minute) or some form of exercise testing is better. More pronounced slowing may lead to syncope or fatigue. Consistently faster rates may result in a tachycardia-induced cardiomyopathy. Rate-induced ventricular dysfunction is fortunately reversible if adequate rate control is achieved.

Choice of Drugs Digoxin has historically been the drug of choice for rate control in atrial fibrillation, but its limitations must be recognized.[98,99] The effects of digoxin are mediated by an enhancement of vagal tone. It is less effective during states of high sympathetic tone such as is commonly seen at the onset of an episode, during exercise, or in critically ill patients. Even if digoxin is given intravenously, there is a delay of about 60 minutes before the onset of any therapeutic effect, and the peak effect is not seen before 6 hours. Digoxin is most effective as oral therapy in stable elderly patients who do not exercise vigorously, or who may have underlying conduction disease or in combination with either a CCB or a β-blocker. *β-Blockers* will all slow ventricular rates in atrial fibrillation, and many are available as intravenous, oral short-action, or oral long-action preparations (see Table 1-3). In patients with moderate slowing of heart rate at rest, a β-blocker with intrinsic sympathomimetic activity (e.g., pindolol) may help to prevent further drug-induced bradycardia. The *nondihydropyridine CCBs*, verapamil and diltiazem, reduce heart rates in atrial fibrillation during both rest and exercise.

Combinations of two AV-nodal blocking agents may be more effective than higher dose therapy with a single drug and are required for optimal rate control in many patients. Concomitant disease also influences the choice of agents for rate control in atrial fibrillation. CCBs should be avoided in patients with congestive heart failure due to systolic dysfunction but may produce added benefit in patients with hypertension and good systolic function. Digoxin is often chosen, either alone or in combination, in patients with heart failure. Here combination with carvedilol is logical and effective in reducing the ventricular rate and increasing the ejection fraction.[100] Adding digoxin may also allow lower doses of other AV nodal inhibitors. In patients with reactive airway disease, β-blockers must be used very cautiously, if at all.

Pacemakers In some patients, it is not possible to achieve effective rate control during atrial fibrillation. In patients with paroxysmal atrial fibrillation, bradycardia during periods when the patient is in sinus rhythm may prevent administration of therapy that would be effective during an episode. In patients with persistent or permanent atrial fibrillation, bradycardia during sleep or rest may limit control of rates during exercise or stress. Implantation of a permanent pacemaker may be required in such patients. Ablation of AV conduction and insertion of an adaptive rate pacemaker constitutes an effective strategy in patients in whom control of inappropriately rapid rates cannot be achieved with pharmacologic therapy alone. A dual-chamber pacemaker with mode switching during periods of atrial fibrillation may be used in patients with paroxysmal atrial fibrillation. A single-chamber pacemaker is used in patients with permanent atrial fibrillation. Thus, *ablate and pace* is one good approach to rate control.

Ventricular Preexcitation with Atrial Fibrillation This combination presents a unique problem (see WPW, Fig. 8-2). Agents acting primarily on the AV node may paradoxically increase ventricular rates either by shortening the effective refractory period of the accessory pathway or by eliminating concealed conduction into the accessory pathway. Agents that prolong the anterograde refractory period of the accessory pathway (e.g., procainamide, flecainide, and amiodarone) should be used both for rate control and to affect conversion, but urgent electrical cardioversion is often necessary.

Restoration and Maintenance of Sinus Rhythm

Restoration and maintenance of sinus rhythm is the alternate management strategy in patients with atrial fibrillation. The agents used for conversion of acute episodes and for long-term prevention of recurrence of atrial fibrillation are listed in Table 8-8.

Pharmacological Conversion of AF Drugs are often used alone or with direct current shocks to restore sinus rhythm. Drug therapy is superior to placebo in patients with atrial fibrillation of recent onset, but many episodes will terminate spontaneously without specific therapy within the initial 24 to 48 hours. Most studies suggest higher pharmacological conversion rates in patients with atrial flutter than in atrial fibrillation. The combined American and European guidelines recommend three intravenous drugs, flecainide, ibutilide, and propafenone, with a class IA recommendation for conversion of atrial fibrillation of ≤7 days duration.[96] Oral administration of dofetilide, flecainide, and propafenone was also considered to be effective. Amiodarone was given a class IIa recommendation because of its delayed onset of action, but amiodarone may be useful in many patients because it also slows ventricular rates and unlike the others, has no risk of post-conversion ventricular arrhythmias. Quinidine was considered to be effective but was given a lower rating because of its potential for toxicity.[7,96,101] All drugs are less effective in atrial fibrillation of more than 7 days in duration when oral dofetilide, requiring hospitalization, was the only agent given a class I recommendation.

Intermittent oral administration of single doses of flecainide (200 to 300 mg) or propafenone (450 to 600 mg) when an episode begins—the "pill-in-the-pocket technique"—may be effective in selected patients with atrial fibrillation and no structural heart disease.[102,103] The major potential complication of this approach is the possibility for organization and slowing of the arrhythmia to atrial flutter, which

Table 8-8	Recommended Antiarrhythmic Drug Doses for Pharmacological Cardioversion and Prevention of Recurrences of Atrial Fibrillation		
		IV or Oral Therapy for Rapid Conversion	Chronic Oral Drug Therapy to Prevent Recurrence*
Class IA	Procainamide	500–1200 mg IV over 30–60 min	2000–4000 mg/day
	Quinidine sulfate	Not recommended	600–1200 mg/day
	Disopyramide	Not recommended	450–600 mg/day
Class IC	Flecainide	1.5–3.0 mg/kg IV over 10 min†; 200–300 mg orally	150–300 mg/day
	Propafenone	1.5–2 mg/kg IV over 10–20 min†	400–600 mg/day
Class III	Ibutilide	1 mg IV over 10 min, repeat once	Not available
	Sotalol	Not recommended	160–320 mg/day
	Amiodarone	5–7 mg/kg IV over 30 min, then 1.2–1.8 mg/day	400–1200 mg/day for 7 days, then taper to 100–300 mg/day
	Dofetilide	Insufficient data	125–500 µg every 12 h

*Initiation of oral therapy without loading may also result in conversion.
†Not available in North America.
IV = intravenous.
For doses, see ref 96.

may then conduct with a 1:1 AV ratio at a very high ventricular rate. Intermittent drug self-administration should be used cautiously and only in patients likely to tolerate this potential proarrhythmic effect. The efficacy of this approach should be monitored before being used on an outpatient basis.

Drug Therapy with Electrical Cardioversion Some antiarrhythmic drugs (e.g., ibutilide or dofetilide) can facilitate cardioversion by lowering the atrial defibrillation threshold. Other drugs may suppress immediate or early recurrence of atrial fibrillation after successful cardioversion. Recurrence of atrial fibrillation is common after cardioversion and is a major limitation to the technique.

Maintenance of Sinus Rhythm After Cardioversion In most patients, atrial fibrillation proves to be a recurrent disorder. Unfortunately, the effectiveness of available antiarrhythmic agents is quite limited.[19,96] In patients with paroxysmal atrial fibrillation, reduction in the frequency and severity of episodes is the usual goal of therapy. In patients with persistent atrial fibrillation, prolongation of the interval between cardioversions is a reasonable target.

Selection of Antiarrhythmic Drug Drugs from classes IA, IC, and III are more effective than placebo for maintaining sinus rhythm in patients with atrial fibrillation.[19,96] Only limited data are available comparing two or more agents in similar populations. In the Canadian Trial of Atrial Fibrillation (CTAF),[104] amiodarone was superior to sotalol or propafenone. In a substudy of the Atrial Fibrillation Follow-up Investigation of Rhythm Management (AFFIRM) trial, amiodarone was superior to both sotalol and a mixture of class I drugs.[20] However, most clinicians select an antiarrhythmic drug based on the desire to minimize toxicity, even at the expense of efficacy. Therefore, *current guidelines follow an algorithm based on the patient's clinical characteristics* (Fig. 8-9). In patients with no or minimal structural heart disease, the first-line agents are flecainide, propafenone, or sotalol. Amiodarone or dofetilide are secondary options. In patients with congestive heart failure, only amiodarone and dofetilide are known to be effective. In patients with coronary artery disease, class Ic agents are associated with increased mortality, so sotalol followed by amiodarone or dofetilide should be selected. In hypertensive patients without left ventricular hypertrophy ($\leq 1.4\,cm$ wall thickness), flecainide or propafenone may be safely used as first-line agents followed by sotalol, amiodarone, or dofetilide. In patients with left ventricular hypertrophy, only amiodarone is recommended.

Proarrhythmia Risk This drug selection algorithm is heavily influenced by the potential for each drug to cause certain types of proarrhythmia in susceptible individuals. All agents, with the possible exception of dofetilide, may cause sinus node dysfunction or AV block. Atrial flutter with 1:1 conduction is a risk with flecainide, propafenone, and quinidine unless other agents to block AV nodal conduction are also used. Flecainide increased mortality in patients with ischemic heart disease and propafenone probably has a similar effect. Agents in classes IA and III prolong the QT-interval and may result in polymorphic ventricular tachycardia (VT). Patients with left ventricular hypertrophy and congestive heart failure are particularly susceptible to proarrhythmia during attempts at therapy for atrial fibrillation.

Renin-Angiotensin Inhibition The development or recurrence of atrial fibrillation may be influenced by drugs that are not usually considered to be antiarrhythmic agents. There is a lower prevalence of atrial fibrillation among patients treated with trandolapril[105] and when irbesartan is added to amiodarone therapy.[106] Studies are underway to determine if anti-inflammatory agents also will decrease the incidence or prevalence of atrial fibrillation.

REPEAT PAROXYSMAL OR PERSISTENT AF

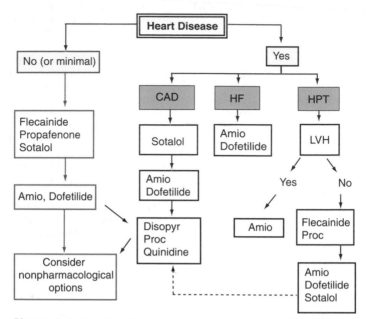

Figure 8-9 Algorithm for drug therapy for paroxysmal or (when rhythm control is selected) for persistent atrial fibrillation. *Amio* = amiodarone; *CAD* = coronary artery disease; *HF* = heart failure; *HPT* = hypertension; *LVH* = left ventricular hypertrophy; *proc* = procainamide. (*Modified from Fuster et al.* J Am Coll Cardiol *2001;38:1231.*)

Postoperative Atrial Fibrillation Atrial fibrillation in the early postoperative period after cardiac surgery is often self-limited and may not require long-term therapy.[107] In untreated patients, the incidence may be 30% to 40% after coronary revascularization and is even higher in patients undergoing valve surgery. Based on data from randomized trials, short-term therapy with β-blockers and/or amiodarone decreases the incidence of atrial fibrillation.[108,109]

Rate Control Versus Rhythm Control The limited efficacy of antiarrhythmic drugs for maintenance of sinus rhythm and the improvement in symptoms and function noted with effective rate control led several groups of investigators to compare the rate control and rhythm control strategies in randomized clinical trials. The largest of these trials, AFFIRM,[110] enrolled 4060 patients having either persistent or paroxysmal atrial fibrillation who, in addition, had one or more risk factors for stroke or death. The average age was 70 years and 71% had a history of hypertension. Patients could be in sinus rhythm at the time of enrollment. Patients were randomized to either rate or rhythm control strategies using any approved therapy. Anticoagulation was to be continued indefinitely in the rate control group and was encouraged, but not mandated, in the rhythm control group if sinus rhythm had been apparently maintained for at least 4 weeks, and preferably 12 weeks, of therapy. The prevalence of sinus rhythm in the rhythm control group was 82%, 73%, and 63% at the 1-, 3-, and 5-year follow-up visits.

Outcomes in AFFIRM Study Total mortality was not statistically different between the two strategies with a trend in favor of rate control. Stroke rates were also not different between the two groups. Most strokes occurred in patients who had either stopped anticoagulation or had a subtherapeutic (i.e., <2.0) international normalized ratios (INR).

Quality of life and functional status measurements also showed no advantage with either strategy. The AFFIRM investigators concluded that either a rate control or a rhythm control strategy was appropriate in atrial fibrillation with risk factors for stroke or death and that anticoagulation should be continued in such patients even if they are apparently maintaining sinus rhythm.

Smaller Studies on Rate versus Rhythm Control These conclusions from AFFIRM are supported by several smaller studies comparing rate control and rhythm control strategies. The Pharmacological Intervention in Atrial Fibrillation (PIAF) Trial[111] randomly assigned 252 patients with persistent atrial fibrillation to rate control with diltiazem or rhythm control with amiodarone with cardioversions as required. After 1 year, symptom relief and quality of life measures for the two groups were similar. The rhythm control group had a slightly better (6 minutes) walk distance but had experienced more hospitalizations. The Rate Control Versus Electrical Cardioversion for Persistent Atrial Fibrillation (RACE) study[112] included 522 patients with persistent atrial fibrillation of less than 1 years' duration and one or two prior electrical cardioversions. Once again, there was no overall difference in the primary end-point, but subgroup results in women and in hypertensive patients favored rate control. In RACE, at the end of follow-up, only 39% of the rhythm control group was still in sinus rhythm. Finally, the Strategies of Treatment of Atrial Fibrillation study[113] randomly assigned 200 "high-risk" patients to either rate control or rhythm control. Again, there was no difference between the groups in major endpoints. As in RACE, most patients eventually developed permanent atrial fibrillation. Another large trial, Atrial Fibrillation in Congestive Heart Failure trial (AF-CHF)[114] is now underway, focusing on patients with symptomatic heart failure, but results are not expected for several years.

Guidelines of the American Academy of Family Physicians and the American College of Physicians These guidelines recommend rate control with chronic anticoagulation as the strategy for the majority of patients with atrial fibrillation.[19,115] However, physicians managing patients with atrial fibrillation should base individual therapy on the patient's symptoms, quality of life, and tolerance for procedures. Importantly, it has not been demonstrated that even an apparently successful rhythm control strategy eliminates a need for anticoagulation in patients with risk factors for stroke, especially because even in those with an apparently well controlled rhythm, there are still frequent episodes of subjectively undetected episodes of atrial fibrillation.[116] It should also be emphasized that the majority of patients in these trials tolerated the arrhythmia sufficiently well to allow randomization. It is likely that severely symptomatic patients and younger patients without structural heart disease were underrepresented.

Nonpharmacologic Approaches to the Maintenance of Sinus Rhythm Given the disappointing results of pharmacologic therapy in the maintenance of sinus rhythm after cardioversion, there is growing interest in nonpharmacologic approaches. The initial surgical experience with the "corridor" and "maze" procedures plus the observation that ectopic beats originating from a muscular sleeve surrounding the pulmonary vein orifices can initiate atrial fibrillation, paved the way for radiofrequency catheter-based ablation of atrial fibrillation.[117–119] Focal pulmonary vein stenosis has been a major complication but newer techniques in which the pulmonary veins are circumferentially isolated in conjunction with the placement of additional left atrial ablation lines, have resulted in a major improvement both in terms of procedural success and complication rates. The ideal candidates are younger patients with paroxysmal atrial fibrillation and without structural heart disease. More recent modifications suggest that radiofrequency ablation may also be effective in older patients and in those with underlying structural heart disease.

Anticoagulation for Atrial Fibrillation Nonvalvular atrial fibrillation is associated with an increased risk for stroke. Loss of atrial systolic function results in sluggish blood flow in the atrium. Atrial distention disturbs the atrial endothelium and activates hemostatic factors leading to a hypercoagulable state.[19,96,120] Several factors increase the risk for stroke in patients with atrial fibrillation. The primary risk factors are increased age, history of stroke or transient ischemic attack, hypertension, left atrial enlargement, diabetes, and congestive heart failure. Separate guidelines for anticoagulation around the time of cardioversion and during chronic therapy have been published.[121] For cardioversion of acute episodes that are of less than 48 hours duration, anticoagulation is not required. For episodes that are of greater than 48 hours duration or when the duration is uncertain, 3 to 4 weeks of anticoagulation with warfarin (INR between 2 and 3) before cardioversion is recommended. Alternatively, a transesophageal echocardiogram during anticoagulation can be used to exclude the presence of a left atrial thrombus. If none is found, cardioversion may be performed while anticoagulation is continued. Even in patients without risk factors for stroke, anticoagulation is maintained for at least 4 weeks after conversion. In the AFFIRM trial, the majority of strokes occurred in patients with either subtherapeutic INRs or those who were not on warfarin.[110] Furthermore, many brief recurrences of atrial fibrillation may be asymptomatic. Hence the current trend is for lifelong anticoagulation unless there is unequivocal proof that recurrences are not occurring. Randomized trials show the benefit of anticoagulation with warfarin in patients with nonvalvular atrial fibrillation, yet it is often difficult to judge when a patient's risk for stroke is high enough to warrant long-term therapy.[96,121] Some guidelines recommend warfarin for all patients older than 65 years of age or with a risk factor, while others define an intermediate risk group between ages 65 and 75 with no or minor heart disease and without hypertension in which either aspirin or warfarin would be acceptable.[96,121] Current trials focus on the oral direct thrombin inhibitor ximelagatran[122] or aspirin and clopidogrel.

ATRIAL FLUTTER

Traditionally, atrial flutter has been defined as a regular atrial rhythm with a rate between 250 and 350 beats per minute in the absence of antiarrhythmic drugs. Several electrophysiologic mechanisms are responsible. The most common form, typical or classical atrial flutter, involves a macroreentrant circuit with a counterclockwise rotation in the right atrium.[123] This circuit passes through the isthmus between the inferior vena cava and the tricuspid valve. Atrial activity is seen on the electrocardiogram as negative flutter waves in the inferior leads II, III, and aVF. Less commonly, a reverse circuit involving a clockwise rotation occurs. These two forms are also called "isthmus-dependent flutters." Other atrial rhythms at similar rates that do not require conduction through the isthmus are referred to as atypical flutters. Most clinical reports on the acute management of atrial flutter have included all types of flutter. Atrial flutter is also commonly associated with atrial fibrillation. There is an extensive literature concerning ablation therapy of atrial flutter and some studies on acute conversion rates, but most studies of long-term pharmacologic therapy have combined atrial flutter patients with those with atrial fibrillation.

Acute Therapy Patients with new-onset atrial flutter commonly are usually highly symptomatic. In the absence of antiarrhythmic drug therapy or disease in the AV conduction system, there is typically 2:1 AV conduction, since alternating atrial impulses either conduct normally or encounter the absolute refractory period of the AV node. There is, therefore, little concealed conduction in the AV node, and it is difficult to achieve stable control of ventricular rates by the modest increases in AV nodal refractory periods produced with AV nodal blocking agents. AV nodal blocking agents are, however, important adjuncts to protect against 1:1 AV conduction should drug therapy slow the atrial rate.[123]

As with all reentrant arrhythmias, patients with severe symptoms or hemodynamic collapse during atrial flutter should be electrically cardioverted as soon as possible. Most patients, however, can tolerate rates of 150 beats per minute or less during 2:1 or higher AV block. In such patients, either electrical or pharmacologic conversion may be chosen. Both synchronized direct current shocks and overdrive atrial pacing are effective techniques for effective electrical conversion. Intravenous *ibutilide* (1 to 2 mg IV) is reported to correct 38% to 78% of episodes of atrial flutter.[19,58,61] Ibutilide should not be administered to patients with long-QT interval or with significant hypokalemia or hypomagnesemia. The major complication of intravenous ibutilide is polymorphic ventricular tachycardia (VT) with a long-QT interval, in about 2% of individual trials. Patients with severe left ventricular dysfunction (ejection fraction less than 0.21), left ventricular hypertrophy, bradycardia, electrolyte imbalance, and prolonged QT intervals at baseline are at increased risk for developing polymorphic VT. Women are more susceptible than men.

Drug Choice Randomized, double-blind studies show that IV ibutilide is more effective than IV procainamide or sotalol.[19,58,61] Conversion to sinus rhythm, when it occurs, is seen within 60 minutes, and most commonly within 30 minutes, of the end of the infusion. Polymorphic VT also is seen principally during this interval, but monitoring for at least 4 hours is recommended. Class IC drugs and amiodarone, either IV or orally, are less effective than ibutilide. Dofetilide is also effective for converting atrial flutter, but an IV preparation is not currently available for clinical use.[124] If long-term antiarrhythmic therapy is not planned and there are no contraindications, IV ibutilide and electrical therapy are appropriate first-line choices. If long-term antiarrhythmic therapy is planned, it may be preferable to begin therapy with amiodarone, sotalol, dofetilide, or a class IC agent, often with an AV nodal blocking agent, with electrical cardioversion after 24 to 48 hours of therapy if a pharmacologic conversion does not occur.

Chronic Therapy There are insufficient data on chronic drug therapy of atrial flutter on which to base firm clinical recommendations. For patients with normal atrial anatomy and no history of atrial fibrillation, ablation to produce conduction block in the cavotricuspid isthmus is often preferable to drug therapy. In patients with a history of atrial fibrillation, flutter ablation may eliminate the flutter but atrial fibrillation is likely to recur in the future.[125] Some patients who present with atrial fibrillation and then develop atrial flutter while on an antiarrhythmic drug, will do well on drug therapy after flutter ablation. In patients with concomitant atrial fibrillation and/or abnormal atrial anatomy, chronic drug therapy as discussed above, either alone or in combination with ablation therapy, is the best approach.

Anticoagulation for Atrial Flutter Patients with atrial flutter are at risk for cardioembolic stroke and systemic embolism. Guidelines for anticoagulation during acute and chronic management are the same as those for patients with atrial fibrillation.[121]

VENTRICULAR ARRHYTHMIAS

Acute Management Ventricular tachycardia (VT) with a stable QRS morphology is often referred to as monomorphic VT. Monomorphic VT can present in a variety of cardiac conditions and may be caused by several distinct electrophysiologic mechanisms. Reentry related to scars (myocardial infarction, surgical incisions, and fibrosis) is the most common mechanism seen clinically. Guidelines for pharmacologic management of sustained monomorphic VT are based almost exclusively on experience treating this type of arrhythmia. Unless there is specific clinical information available to suggest another mechanism, therapy for patients with sustained monomorphic VT should be based on a presumed reentrant mechanism.

Hemodynamic Status The patient's hemodynamic status should determine the initial therapy used to terminate an episode of sustained monomorphic VT.[126] Patients who are unconscious, severely hypotensive, or highly symptomatic should be treated with synchronized direct current shocks. Preadministration of an intravenous anesthetic agent or sedative should be used, if possible. Antiarrhythmic drug therapy, if used at all, in this situation is used to prevent recurrences. In patients with stable hemodynamics during sustained VT, pharmacologic termination may be considered. There are only a few randomized trials published dealing with VT termination. Griffith and colleagues[127] evaluated intravenous lidocaine (1.5 mg/kg), disopyramide (2 mg/kg, ≤ 150 mg), flecainide (2 mg/kg), and sotalol (1 mg/kg) in patients with sustained VT induced during electrophysiologic studies. Of the 24 patients in the trial, 20 had coronary artery disease with a history of myocardial infarction. Flecainide and disopyramide were the most effective agents for terminating VT but especially flecainide was associated with significant side effects. All drugs worked best in patients without prior infarctions. They recommended lidocaine as a first-line and disopyramide as a second-line drug, but did not study procainamide.

Procainamide Benefits versus Toxicity Gorgels and colleagues[9] compared intravenous lidocaine (1.5 mg/kg over 2 minutes) and procainamide (10 mg/kg at 100 mg/minute) in 29 patients, 25 with prior myocardial infarction, who presented with hemodynamically tolerated, spontaneous, sustained VT. Patients who failed the initial randomized drug or who developed recurrent VT were crossed over to the other agents. Procainamide at this dose was effective in 12/15 original attempts and in 38 of 48 total episodes. In contrast, lidocaine was effective in only 3/14 initial trials. When all initial and crossover trials were analyzed, lidocaine had been effective in 6 of 31 trials and procainamide in 38 of 48 trials. The major toxicities seen with intravenous procainamide in patients with sustained VT are QRS widening and hypotension. During the infusion, the physician should carefully monitor the QRS complex to detect any change in morphology. Widening of the QRS complex, so that the width approaches the tachycardia cycle length, is a sign of definite toxicity and must be avoided. Moderate hypotension during intravenous procainamide is often well tolerated, but the infusion must be discontinued if symptoms develop or worsen. Slowing the rate of drug infusion decreases the risk of hypotension but also makes termination less likely. If the VT rate does not continue to slow as additional procainamide is given, it is unlikely that the VT will terminate.

Intravenous Amiodarone Intravenous amiodarone can be useful in patients who present with sustained monomorphic VT.[128] Current guidelines suggest it should be preferred over procainamide in patients with severe left ventricular dysfunction,[127] but published data concerning the efficacy of amiodarone for quickly terminating an episode of VT are limited. The most common use of intravenous amiodarone is in patients with either incessant VT or frequent VT episodes.[129-131] In these patients, an initial intravenous bolus of 150 mg over 10 minutes is followed by an infusion of 360 mg (1 mg/minute) over the next 6 hours and 540 mg (0.5 mg/minute) over the remaining 18 hours. If given during incessant VT, the expected response will be gradual slowing of the VT cycle length with eventual termination. Transition to oral therapy can be made at any time.

Cardiac Arrest and Amiodarone In patients with cardiac arrest due to VF, amiodarone can be an *adjunct to defibrillation* (see Fig. 11-7). Two randomized trials have addressed this issue. In the ARREST study,[46] intravenous amiodarone (300 mg) was given to patients not resuscitated after three or more precordial shocks, rather late in the resuscitation attempts (mean time, over 40 min). Patients who received amiodarone were more likely to survive to hospital admission (44% versus 34% with placebo, $P = 0.03$), but survival to hospital discharge was not significantly improved (13.4% versus 13.2%). The ALIVE study compared amiodarone (5 mg/kg estimated body weight) and lidocaine (1.5 mg/kg) in patients with out-of-hospital VF.[43] The mean interval from paramedic dispatch to drug administration was 25 ± 8 minutes. Amiodarone gave better survival-to-hospital admission (22.8% amiodarone versus 12% lidocaine). Survival to hospital discharge (5% amiodarone, 3% lidocaine) was not significantly improved. These two studies indicate that amiodarone may be useful for resuscitating some cardiac arrest victims. Antiarrhythmic therapy in this setting is an adjunct to defibrillation. Prevention of recurrent episodes of VT or VF after electrical termination is the primary reason for drug administration during resuscitation.

Chronic Therapy of VT Antiarrhythmic drugs are used in patients with a history of sustained VT and cardiac arrest to decrease the probability of recurrence or to improve symptoms during a recurrence. In several randomized trials, antiarrhythmic drug therapy has produced less benefits than implantable cardioverter-defibrillators (ICDs) when either approach is selected as initial therapy.[132-136] In patients with life-threatening arrhythmias, antiarrhythmic drugs are often used in conjunction with ICDs. In these patients, an additional role for antiarrhythmic drug therapy is to modify the arrhythmia so that it can be painlessly terminated by antitachycardia pacing.

Drug Selection and Electrophysiological Testing The best method for selecting an antiarrhythmic drug for patients with prior sustained VT or VF remains uncertain. One approach is based on suppression of spontaneous nonsustained ventricular tachycardia and premature beats during electrocardiographic (ECG) monitoring. Unfortunately, in many individuals, the frequency and type of spontaneous ventricular ectopic activity is not reproducible, and suppression during drug therapy may not correlate with outcome. In the Cardiac Arrhythmia Suppression Trial (CAST),[29,137] patients who initially "responded" to drug therapy had a higher mortality if they were continued on an antiarrhythmic drug than if they were randomized to placebo. The alternative approach for selecting chronic therapy is the use of serial electrophysiologic studies with programmed ventricular stimulation.[138] After a baseline electrophysiologic study is performed, and ventricular arrhythmia is induced, drug therapy is then initiated, and ventricular stimulation is repeated. Suppression of the ability to induce a sustained VT or VF is used as a predictor of an effective drug as suggested by numerous observational reports. This impression has not been supported by several randomized trials.[139-141]

Is antiarrhythmic therapy selected by electrophysiologic studies better than empirically chosen amiodarone? In the CASCADE study, amiodarone was superior to the class I drugs tested, but a high arrhythmia recurrence rate was noted, and many patients received an ICD.[139] Should drug selection be based on serial ambulatory electrocardiographic monitoring or serial electrophysiologic testing? In patients with a history of a sustained ventricular arrhythmia who were randomly assigned to six class I agents and to sotalol.[140,141] Both techniques for drug selection were associated with a high failure rate overall (58% at 2 years). Of these drugs, sotalol appeared to be superior. In a third trial patients with prior myocardial infarction, a left ventricular ejection fraction of <41%, and spontaneous nonsustained VT were randomly assigned to either no specific antiarrhythmic therapy or to drug therapy selected by serial electrophysiologic testing.[142] Patients who received drug therapy predicted to be effective did slightly worse than the control group who did not receive therapy unless they received an ICD. *These trials have left unresolved the best way to select antiarrhythmic drugs for patients with ventricular arrhythmias.* Both electrophysiologic study and ECG monitoring approaches have not proved to be consistently reliable, and in any event the characteristics of the spontaneously occurring arrhythmia may differ from that induced at the time of the electrophysiologic study.

Antiarrhythmic Drugs in ICD Recipients Antiarrhythmic drugs are used in conjunction with an ICD in many patients. The purpose of such therapy is to decrease the need for shocks by decreasing arrhythmia frequency or by allowing termination by antitachycardia pacing. Class I drugs and amiodarone can increase defibrillation thresholds, and this should be taken into account if there is a narrow safety margin between the defibrillation threshold and programmed energy. Pacifico et al.[38] reported that sotalol increased time-to-therapy delivery in ICD patients. The Antiarrhythmics Versus Implantable Defibrillators (AVID) trial investigators also reported[143] that adding an antiarrhythmic drug decreased the probability of recurrence after a first appropriate ICD therapy, but even with antiarrhythmic drug treatment, most patients had recurrences.

Ventricular Tachycardia in the Absence of Structural Heart Disease In patients without structural heart disease, treatment of VT requires a different approach. The two most common types of monomorphic sustained VT in patients without structural heart disease arise in the right ventricular outflow tract (RVOT) or in the inferior left ventricular septum and have characteristic ECG patterns and mechanisms.[144] When VT starts in the RVOT, the ECG will show a predominant left bundle block pattern with an inferior axis. This arrhythmia presents with both nonsustained bursts and, less commonly, sustained episodes that are often provoked by stress or exercise. The postulated mechanism is cyclic adenosine monophosphate-mediated triggered activity. Acutely, this arrhythmia responds to *intravenous β-blockers or verapamil.* Chronic oral therapy with agents such as verapamil, β-blockers, flecainide, or propafenone, is very effective. In idiopathic left ventricular VT, calcium-channel–dependent reentry occurs in or near the left posterior fascicle. The ECG shows a left-axis deviation and a right bundle branch block pattern. This arrhythmia terminates with verapamil administration, and *verapamil* is also the preferred choice for chronic therapy. Both these forms of VT are susceptible to catheter ablation (Fig. 8-8) and many individuals will prefer to undergo ablation as opposed to lifelong drug therapy, particularly because many of these patients are young.

Channelopathies There is a rapidly expanding fund of knowledge about arrhythmias caused by genetic mutations in ion channels.[145] For patients with an inherited long-QT syndrome, β-blocker therapy is often effective. Genotyping of individual patients is still not commonly available, but mutation-specific therapy for patients with long-QT syndrome and other genetically determined arrhythmias may be possible in the future.

PRIMARY PREVENTION OF SUDDEN CARDIAC DEATH IN HEART FAILURE

Post–Myocardial Infarction

In patients with symptomatic ventricular arrhythmias, trial data have conclusively demonstrated the superiority of the ICD over drugs, primarily amiodarone.[79] In regard to the *primary* prevention of sudden cardiac death in patients without symptomatic arrhythmias, three trials of patients with underlying coronary artery disease, almost all postinfarct, and low ejection fractions have provided guidelines (MADIT I,[146] MUSTT,[142] and MADIT II[147]).

1. In patients with an ejection fraction of ≤30% and a QRS width ≥120 milliseconds, the MADIT II trial demonstrated a mortality benefit from the ICD-irrespective of the presence or absence of nonsustained ventricular tachycardia on the Holter (Fig. 8-10). However, a shorter QRS does not preclude benefit, a situation that needs further exploration.

2. In patients with an ejection fraction of >30% to 40%, current strategies based upon the MUSTT and MADIT I trials recommend Holter monitoring, and for those with documented nonsustained ventricular tachycardia, for this to be followed by invasive electrophysiologic testing. If sustained arrhythmias are inducible, the ICD is a preferred form of therapy.

3. In patients with an ejection fraction of <40%, there is no need for further arrhythmia evaluation unless the patient is experiencing symptomatic palpitations, near syncope, or syncope.

The problem arises in the extrapolation of these trials to predischarge survivors of an acute myocardial infarction, because none of the trials address the issue in patients this early after an acute myocardial infarction. The decision is further complicated by changes in the ejection fraction during the first 4 weeks after infarction, especially in patients receiving reperfusion therapy. Many would advocate that one should wait a month and then reevaluate the patient and treat according to the algorithm developed for patients with chronic coronary artery disease. The role of the ambulatory external defibrillator during the "waiting period" is currently under the subject of an ongoing trial.

ICDs in Dilated Cardiomyopathy

All of the above trials included patients with coronary artery disease, so that the only unresolved issue is the role of the ICD for the primary prevention of sudden cardiac death in congestive heart failure without coronary artery disease (dilated cardiomyopathy). Results of smaller trials have, however, not been conclusive[41,148] and further data are awaited. In the DEFINITE multicenter study on 458 patients with a mean ejection fraction of 21% and almost all on modern medical therapy including β-blockers and ACE inhibitors, the ICD substantially reduced arrhythmic but not all-cause mortality.[149] A large multicenter trial on about 2500 patients with heart failure, the Sudden Cardiac Death-Heart Failure Trial (SCD-HeFT), showed a 23% fall in mortality compared to placebo with ICD therapy but no difference with amiodarone treatment.[150] Results were equally impressive whether or not the origin of the heart failure was ischemic or nonischemic, the first time this has been shown. Thus all patients with significant heart failure and left ventricular systolic dysfunction are potential candidates for ICD therapy in addition to optimal medical therapy.

In the future, more exact risk stratification will probably help guide the decision whether or not to use an ICD. In the meantime, a practical point is that lack of β-blocker use is an important risk predictor of arrhythmia,[151] also in SCD-HeFT.[150] Of note, in those with severe LV dysfunction (mean ejection fraction only 21%) plus an arrhythmia marker, optimal medical therapy including β-blockade and ACE inhibition reduced the annual mortality to only 6% to 7%, and such therapy should be instituted before an ICD is considered.[149,151]

POST-MI ICD POLICY

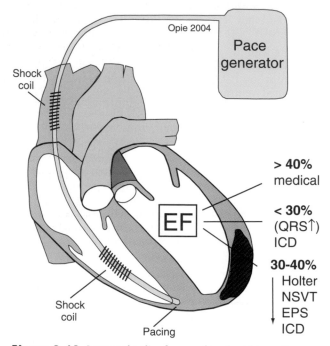

Figure 8-10 Suggested policy for use of implantable cardioverter defibrillator *(ICD)* in patients with post-myocardial infarction *(MI)* heart failure. If the ejection fraction *(EF)* is above 40%, only medical therapy is given. Below 30% and especially in the presence of QRS widening, an ICD is implanted. Biventricular pacing may also be indicated (see text). Between 30% and 40%, nonsustained ventricular tachycardia *(NSVT)* on the Holter leads to electrophysiological stimulation *(EPS)*. If such stimulation produces sustained VT, then an ICD is chosen. For references, see text.

ICD plus Cardiac Resynchronization Therapy

The above arguments for ICD placement in selected patients with severe heart failure lead to a further question: Can added cardiac resynchronization therapy (CRT) by biventricular pacing do even better? This issue arises especially in those with a prolonged QRS interval, who in their own right are candidates for resynchronization. In the large COMPANION study this combination of devices reduced all-cause mortality in those with class III or IV chronic heart failure (QRS interval ≥120 milliseconds) by 36% (Fig. 8-10).[152] Unfortunately the effect of an ICD alone was not assessed, so that the benefits of this combined approach beyond an ICD alone are not yet firmly established. CRT acts in complex ways to achieve some remodeling of the failing LV. Although CRT can give benefit even with "narrow" QRS, a wide QRS means a greater likelihood of mechanical delay and thus a greater potential for success.[153]

SUMMARY

1. *Antiarrhythmic drug classification.* These are grouped into four classes: class I, sodium channel blockers; class II, β-adrenergic blockers; class III, repolarization blockers; and class IV those agents that block the calcium current in the AV node, such as some calcium channel blockers (verapamil and diltiazem) and adeno-

sine. Class I agents are used less and less because of adverse long term effects, except for the acute use of intravenous lidocaine or procainamide, and agents which are safe only in the absence of structural heart disease (flecainide and propafenone). Class II, the β-blockers, are especially effective in hyperadrenergic states such as chronic heart failure, some repetitive tachycardias and ischemic arrhythmias. Among class III agents, amiodarone is a powerful antiarrhythmic agent, acting on both supraventricular and ventricular arrhythmias, but potentially toxic, sometimes even when used in a very low dose, and therefore often not regarded as a first-line agent except when intravenously given as in cardiac arrest. Class IV agents are excellent in arresting acute supraventricular tachycardias (adenosine preferred), and also reduce ventricular rates in chronic atrial fibrillation (verapamil and diltiazem).

2. *Current trends.* The complexity of the numerous agents available and the ever-increasing problems with side effects and proarrhythmic events have promoted a strong trend toward intervention by ablation or devices. For example, an implantable cardioverter-defibrillator (ICD) is now increasingly used in the presence of severe heart failure.

3. *Supraventricular arrhythmias.* In terms of drug effects, the acute therapy of supraventricular arrhythmias is assuming an increasingly rational basis with a prominent role for adenosine, verapamil, or diltiazem in inhibition of supraventricular tachycardias involving conduction through the AV node. Sodium blockers can inhibit the bypass tract or retrograde fast AV nodal conduction, as can class III agents, such as sotalol or amiodarone. Ablation is increasingly used for long-term management of most symptomatic cases of SVT.

4. *Atrial flutter.* Ibutilide, given intravenously, or dofetilide, given orally, are effective for drug-induced reversion of atrial flutter. These should not be given to patients at risk of torsades de pointes (check QT-interval, electrolyte status and other drugs taken). Cardioversion is often the treatment of choice. Ibutilide sensitizes the flutter to the effects of cardioversion. Ablation is often chosen for chronic therapy.

5. *Acute onset atrial fibrillation.* For acute onset atrial fibrillation, control of the ventricular rate can be achieved by AV nodal inhibitors, such as verapamil or diltiazem, or intravenous β-blockade by esmolol, metoprolol, or propranolol, or by combinations. Pharmacological conversion can usually be achieved by intravenous ibutilide or, if there is no structural heart disease, flecainide or propafenone. Note the risk of post-conversion ventricular arrhythmias. Amiodarone has a slower onset of action but also slows the heart rate and has no post-conversion ventricular arrhythmias. If drugs fail to restore sinus rhythm, direct current defibrillation given externally or (even better) transvenously has a very high success rate.

6. *Recurrent atrial fibrillation: rate control.* For patients with recurrent forms of atrial fibrillation, the choice between rate and rhythm control is never easy. With either policy, optimal anticoagulation should be continued indefinitely, since many episodes of atrial fibrillation are asymptomatic and unsuspected. The AFFIRM and smaller European trials have, however, changed practice by showing that rate control has similar outcomes to rhythm control. *One practical policy* is to attempt cardioversion for the first episode of atrial fibrillation. Then if this arrhythmia returns and is asymptomatic, rate control is in order. Although digoxin may suffice for some elderly patients, additional verapamil, diltiazem or β-blocker therapy or combination therapy is necessary for most. Radiofrequency ablation of the AV node (followed by pacing) is

increasingly selected for patients who find drugs difficult or who are refractory to their effects.

7. *Algorithm for rhythm control for recurrent atrial fibrillation.* In patients with no or minimal structural heart disease, the first-line agents are flecainide, propafenone, or sotalol. Amiodarone or dofetilide are only secondary options in view of their potentially serious side effects. In patients with congestive heart failure, only amiodarone and dofetilide are effective. In patients with coronary artery disease, sotalol followed by amiodarone or dofetilide should be selected. In hypertensive patients without left ventricular hypertrophy or other structural heart disease, flecainide or propafenone may be safely used as first-line agents followed by sotalol, amiodarone, or dofetilide. In patients with left ventricular hypertrophy, only amiodarone is recommended. Addition of angiotensin receptor blockers or ACE inhibitors may help to reduce recurrences. Repetitive cardioversion may also be required. There may be a pulmonary vein rapidly firing focus that responds to ablation.

8. *Chronic atrial fibrillation.* Here again the choice is between rate and rhythm control with careful anticoagulation. However, defibrillation is less likely when atrial fibrillation is more than 7 days in duration when dofetilide is chosen.

9. *Ventricular arrhythmias* and their therapy remain controversial and constantly evolving. Antiarrhythmic drug therapy may be only one avenue of overall management, as ICDs are increasingly used in severe ventricular arrhythmias, especially with a low ejection fraction. A distinction must be made between suppression of premature ventricular complexes, which is useless, and the control of VT/VF, which can prolong life. In acute AMI, lidocaine is no longer given prophylactically. In post-infarct patients, β-blockers remain the drugs of choice, while amiodarone has good evidence in its favor.

10. *Implantable cardioverter defibrillators (ICD).* In CHF, optimal management of the hemodynamic and neurohumoral status, including the use of ACE inhibitors and β-blockade, must be instituted before the prophylactic use of antiarrhythmic drugs or an ICD. In severe heart failure ICD therapy is probably the single most important aspect of antiarrhythmic therapy. The combination of ICD and cardiac resynchronization by biventricular pacing is increasingly considered, especially when there is QRS prolongation.

11. *Hybrid pharmacologic drugs and device or ablation therapy* is an option increasingly used for disabling atrial fibrillation or for severe and serious ventricular arrhythmias. Thus, β-blockade or amiodarone may be combined with ICDs to give optimal results.

12. *New antiarrhythmic agents* have been investigated in recent years. Most have been variations of the class IC or class III drugs that are already available. In many instances the assessment of these drugs has revealed a negative benefit-risk ratio. Only ibutilide and dofetilide have so far been approved for clinical use. Ibutilide is given intravenously and dofetilide orally. Both benefit atrial tachyarrhythmias, yet both have prominent warnings regarding torsades. Of the other drugs, dronedarone may eventually have the advantages of amiodarone, without the disadvantages of the extracardiac side effects.

REFERENCES

1. CAST Investigators. Preliminary report: effect of encainide and flecainide on mortality in randomized trial of arrhythmia suppression after myocardial infarction. The Cardiac Arrhythmia Suppression Trial (CAST) Investigators. *N Engl J Med* 1989;321:406–412.

2. Teo KK, Yusuf S, Furberg CD. Effects of prophylactic antiarrhythmic drug therapy in acute myocardial infarction. An overview of results from randomized controlled trials. *JAMA* 1993;270:1589–1595.

3. Connolly SJ. Evidence-based analysis of amiodarone efficacy and safety. *Circulation* 1999;100:2025–2034.

4. Vorperian VR, et al. Adverse effects of low dose amiodarone: a meta-analysis. *J Am Coll Cardiol* 1997;30:791–798.

5. Task Force of the Working Group on Arrhythmias of the European Society of Cardiology. The Sicilian Gambit. A new approach to the classification of antiarrhythmic drugs based on their actions on arrhythmogenic mechanisms. *Circulation* 1991;84:1831–1851.

6. Sheldon R, et al. On behalf of the CIDS Investigators. Identification of patients most likely to benefit from implantable cardioverter-defibrillator therapy. The Canadian Implantable Defibrillator Study. *Circulation* 2000;101:1660–1664.

7. Coplen SE, et al. Efficacy and safety of quinidine therapy for maintenance of sinus rhythm after cardioversion. A meta-analysis of randomized control trials. *Circulation* 1990;82:1106–1116.

8. Morganroth J, et al. Flecainide vs. quinidine for treatment of ventricular arrhythmias: a multicenter study. *Circulation* 1983;67:1117–1123.

9. Gorgels AP, et al. Comparison of procainamide and lidocaine in terminating sustained monomorphic ventricular tachycardia. *Am J Cardiol* 1996;78:43–46.

10. Volgman AS, et al. Conversion efficacy and safety of intravenous ibutilide compared with intravenous procainamide in patients with atrial flutter or fibrillation. *J Am Coll Cardiol* 1998;31:1414–1419.

11. Kosowsky BD, et al. Long-term use of procaine amide following acute myocardial infarction. *Circulation* 1973;47:1204–1210.

12. Singh BN. Routine prophylactic lidocaine administration in acute myocardial infarction. An idea whose time is all but gone? *Circulation* 1992;26:1033–1035.

13. Sadowski ZP, et al. Multicenter randomized trial and systemic overview of lidocaine in acute myocardial infarction. *Am Heart J* 1999;137:792–798.

14. ACC/AHA Guidelines, et al. ACC/AHA guidelines for the management of patients with acute myocardial infarction: executive summary. *Circulation* 1996;94:2341–2350.

15. CASH Study, et al. Preliminary results of the Cardiac Arrest Study Hamburg (CASH). *Am J Cardiol* 1993;72:109F–113F.

16. Reiffel JA, Blitzer M. The actions of ibutilide and class Ic drugs on the slow sodium channel: new insights regarding individual pharmacologic effects elucidated through combination therapies. *J Cardiovasc Pharmacol Ther* 2000;5:177–181.

17. Cahill SA, Gross GJ. Propafenone and its Metabolites Preferentially Inhibit IKr in Rabbit Ventricular Myocytes. *J Pharmacol Exp Ther* 2003.

18. Reiffel JA, Hahn E, Hartz V. Sotalol for ventricular tachyarrhythmias; beta blocking and class III contributions, and relative efficacy versus class 1 drugs after prior drug failure. *Am J Cardiol* 1997;79:1048–1053.

19. McNamara RL, et al. Management of atrial fibrillation: review of the evidence for the role of pharmacologic therapy, electrical cardioversion, and echocardiography. *Ann Intern Med* 2003;139:1018–1033.

20. AFFIRM Investigators. First Antiarrhythmic Drug Substudy. Maintenance of sinus rhythm in pateints with atrial fibrillation. *J Am Coll Cardiol* 2003;42:20–29.

21. Ruffy R. Flecainide. *Electrophysiology Review* 1998;2:191–193.

22. UK Propafenone PSVT Study Group. A randomized, placebo-controlled trial of propafenone in the prophylaxis of paroxysmal supraventricular tachycardia and paroxysmal atrial fibrillation. *Circulation* 1995;92:250–257.

23. Stoobrand R, et al. Propafenone for conversion and prophylaxis of atrial fibrillation. *Am J Cardiol* 1997;79:418–423.

24. Kochiadakis GE, et al. Amiodarone versus propafenone for conversion of chronic atrial fibrillation: results of a randomized, controlled study. *J Am Coll Cardiol* 1999;33:966–971.

25. Natale A, Beheiry S, Leonelli F, et al. Intermittent administration of 1c antiarrythmic drugs for sporadic episodes of atrial fibrillation: safety and long-term efficacy (Abstract). *Circulation* 1999;100(Suppl 1):1–102.

26. Joglar JA, Hamdan MH, Page RL. Propafenone. *Cardiac Electrophysiol Rev* 1998;28:204–206.

27. IMPACT Research Group. International mexiletine and placebo antiarrhythmic coronary trial: 1. Report on arrhythmia and other findings. *J Am Col Cardiol* 1984;4:1148–1163.

28. Priori SG, et al. Molecular biology of the long QT syndrome: impact on management. *Pacing Clin Electrophysiol* 1997;20:2052–2057.

29. CAST-II Study. The Cardiac Arrhythmia Suppression Trial II (CAST-II) Investigators. Effect of the antiarrhythmic drug moricizine on survival after myocardial infarction. *N Engl J Med* 1992;327:227–233.

30. Ellison KE, et al. Effect of beta-blocking therapy on outcome in the Multicenter UnSustained Tachycardia Trial (MUSTT). *Circulation* 2002;106:2694–2699.

31. Dargie HJ. Beta blockers in heart failure. *Lancet* 2003;362:2–3.

32. MERIT-HF Study Group. Effect of metroprolol CR/XL in chronic heart failure: Metoprolol CR/XL Randomized Trial in Congestive Heart Failure (MERIT-HF). *Lancet* 1999;353:2001–2007.

33. CIBIS II Study. The Cardiac Insufficiency Bisoprolol Study II (CIBIS-II): a randomised trial. *Lancet* 1999;353:9–13.

34. Exner DV, et al. Beta-blocker use and survival in patients with ventricular fibrillation or symptomatic ventricular tachycardia: The Antiarrhythmics Versus Implantable Defibrillators (AVID) Trial. *J Am Coll Cardiol* 1999;34:325–333.

35. Boutitie F, et al. Amiodarone interactions with beta-blockers. Analysis of the merged EMIAT (European Myocardial Infarct Trial) and CAMIAT (Canadian Amiodarone Myocardial Infarct Trial) databases. *Circulation* 1999;99:2268–2275.

36. Wiest D. Esmolol: A review of its therapeutic efficacy and pharmacokinetic characteristics. *Clin Pharmacokinet* 1995;28:190–202.

37. Manz M, et al. Interactions between drugs and devices: experimental and clinical studies. *Am Heart J* 1994;127:978–984.

38. Pacifico A, et al. Prevention of implantable-defibrillator shocks by treatment with sotalol. d,l-Sotalol Implantable Cardioverter-Defibrillator Study Group. *N Engl J Med* 1999;340:1855–1862.

39. Gottlieb SS, et al. Effect of beta-blockade on mortality among high-risk and low-risk patients after myocardial infarction. *N Engl J Med* 1998;339:489–497.

40. ESVEM Investigators. Electrophysiologic Study Versus Electrocardiographic Monitoring for selection of antiarrhythmic therapy of ventricular tachycardia. *Circulation* 1989;70:1354–1360.

41. Strickberger SA, et al. Amiodarone versus implantable cardioverter-defibrillator: randomized trial in patients with nonischemic dilated cardiomyopathy and asymptomatic nonsustained ventricular tachycardia–AMIOVIRT. *J Am Coll Cardiol* 2003;41:1707–1712.

42. Nademanee K, et al. Amiodarone and post-MI patients. *Circulation* 1993;88: 764–774.

43. Dorian P, et al. Amiodarone as compared with lidocaine for shock-resistant ventricular fibrillation. *N Engl J Med* 2002;346:884–890.

44. Crystal E, et al. Atrial fibrillation after cardiac surgery: update on the evidence on the available prophylactic interventions. *Card Electrophysiol Rev* 2003;7:189–192.

45. Amiodarone Trials-Meta-Analysis Investigators (ATMAI). Effect of prophylactic amiodarone on mortality after acute myocardial infarction and in congestive heart failure; Meta-analysis of individual data from 6500 patients in randomized trials. *Lancet* 1997;350:1417–1424.

46. Kudenchuk PJ, et al. Amiodarone for resuscitation after out-of-hospital cardiac arrest due to ventricular fibrillation. *N Engl J Med* 1999;341:871–878.

47. Julian DG, et al. Randomized trial of effect of amiodarone on mortality in patients with left ventricular dysfunction after recent myocardial infarction. EMIAT. *Lancet* 1997;347:667–674.

48. Cairns JA, et al. Randomised trial of outcome after myocardial infarction in patients with frequent or repetitive ventricular premature depolarisations: CAMIAT. Canadian Amiodarone Myocardial Infarction Arrhythmia Trial Investigators. *Lancet* 1997;349:675–682.

49. Welch PJ, et al. Management of ventricular arrhythmias. *J Am Coll Cardiol* 1999;34:621–630.

50. Doval HC, et al. Randomized trial of low-dose amiodarone in severe heart failure. *Lancet* 1994;344:493–498.

51. Singh SN, et al. For the Survival trial of Antiarrhythmic Therapy in Congestive Heart Failure. Amiodarone in patients with congestive heart failure and asymptomatic ventricular arrhythmia. *N Engl J Med* 1995;333:77–82.

52. Roy D, et al. Amiodarone to prevent recurrence of atrial fibrillation. Canadian Trial of Atrial Fibrillation Investigators. *N Engl J Med* 2000;342:913–920.

53. Kato R, et al. Electrophysiologic effects of the levo- and dextrorotatory isomers of sotalol in isolated cardiac muscle and their in vivo pharmacokinetics. *JACC* 1986;7:116–125.

54. SWORD Investigators, et al. Prevention of sudden death in patients with LV dysfunction after myocardial infarction. The SWORD trial. *Lancet* 1996;348:7–12.

55. ESVEM Investigators, Mason JW. For the Electrophyisologic Study Versus Electrocardiographic Monitoring Investigators. A comparison of seven antiarrhythmic drugs in patients with ventricular tachyarrhythmias. *N Engl J Med* 1993;329:452-458.

56. Murray KT. Ibutilide. *Circulation* 1998;97:493–497.

57. Bernard EO, et al. Ibutilide versus amiodarone in atrial fibrillation: a double-blinded, randomized study. *Crit Care Med* 2003;31:1031–1034.

58. Stambler BS, et al. Efficacy and safety of repeated doses of ibutilide for rapid conversion of atrial flutter or fibrillation. *Circulation* 1996;94:1613–1621.

59. Guo GB, et al. Conversion of atrial flutter by ibutilide is associated with increased atrial cycle length variability. *J Am Coll Cardiol* 1996;27:1083–1089.

60. VanderLugt J, et al. Efficacy and safety of ibutilide fumarate for the conversion of atrial arrhythmias after cardiac surgery. *Circulation* 1999;100:369–375.

61. Oral H, et al. Facilitating transthoracic cardioversion of atrial fibrillation with ibutilide pretreatment. *N Engl J Med* 1999;340:1849–1854.

62. Kowey PR, VanderLugt JT, Luderer JR. Safety and risk/benefit analysis of ibutilide for acute conversion of atrial fibrillation/flutter. *Am J Cardiol* 1996;78(suppl 8A): 46–52.

63. Boriani G, et al. A multicentre, double-blind randomized crossover comparative study on the efficacy and safety of dofetilide vs sotalol in patients with inducible sustained ventricular tachycardia and ischaemic heart disease. *Eur Heart J* 2001;22: 2180–2191.

64. Torp-Pedersen C, et al. Dofetilide in patients with congestive heart failure and left ventricular dysfunction. *N Engl J Med* 1999;341:857–865.

65. Brendorp B, et al. Survival after withdrawal of dofetilide in patients with congestive heart failure and a short baseline QTc interval; a follow-up on the Diamond-CHF QT substudy. *Eur Heart J* 2003;24:274–279.

66. Fermini B, et al. Use-dependent effects of the class III antiarrhythmic agent NE-10064 (azimilide) on cardiac repolarization: block of delayed rectifier potassium and L-type calcium currents. *J Cardiovasc Pharmacol* 1995;26:259–271.

67. Camm A, et al. Mortality in patients following a recent myocardial infarction: a randomized, placebo-controlled trial of azimilide, using heart rate variability for risk stratification. *Circulation* 2004;109:990–996.
68. Singer I, et al. Azimilide decreases recurrent ventricular tachyarrhythmias in patients with implantable cardioverter defibrillators. *J Am Coll Cardiol* 2004;43:39–43.
69. Sun W, et al. Electrophysiological effects of dronedarone (SR33589), a noniondinated benzofuran derivative, in the rabbit heart. *Circulation* 1999;100:2276–2281.
70. Touboul P, et al. Dronedarone for prevention of atrial fibrillation: a dose-ranging study. *Eur Heart J* 2003;24:1481–1487.
71. Tzivoni D, et al. Treatment of torsade de pointes with magnesium sulfate. *Circulation* 1988;77:392–397.
72. DiMarco JP. Adenosine and digoxin, in *Cardiac Electrophysiology: from Cell to Bedside*, 3rd edit, Zipes DP, Jalife J, eds. Philadelphia: WB Saunders; 2000:933–938.
73. Markowitz SM, et al. Adenosine-sensitive ventricular tachycardia. Right ventricular abnormalities delineated by magnetic resonance imaging. *Circulation* 1997;96:1192–1200.
74. Garratt CJ, et al. Use of intravenous adenosine in sinus rhythm as a diagnostic test for latent pre-excitation. *Am J Cardiol* 1990;65:868–873.
75. Jaeggi E, et al. Adenosine-induced atrial pro-arrhythmia in children. *Can J Cardiol* 1999;15:169–172.
76. Marcus FI. Drug combination and interactions with class III agents. *J Cardiovasc Pharmacol* 1992;20:S70–S74.
77. Channer KS. The drug treatment of atrial fibrillation. *Br J Clin Pharmacol* 1991;32:267–273.
78. Okishige K, et al. Experimental study on the electrophysiological effects of the combination of the antiarrhythmic drugs aprindine and verapamil. *Arch Int Pharmacodyn* 1991;314:44–56.
79. Bokhari F, et al. Long-term comparison of the implantable cardioverter defibrillator versus amiodarone: eleven-year follow-up of a subset of patients in the Canadian Implantable Defibrillator Study (CIDS). *Circulation* 2004;110:112–116.
80. Luderitz B, Manz M. Pharmacologic treatment of supraventricular tachycardia: the German experience. *Am J Cardiol* 1992;70:66A–74A.
81. Yeung L, et al. Propafenone-mexiletine combination for the treatment of sustained ventricular tachycardia. *J Am Coll Cardiol* 1992;20:547–551.
82. Etheridge SP, et al. A new oral therapy for long QT syndrome: long-term oral potassium improves repolarization in patients with HERG mutations. *J Am Coll Cardiol* 2003;42:1777–1782.
83. Windle JR, et al. Normalization of ventricular repolarization with flecainide in long QT syndrome patients with SCN5A: deltaKPQ mutation. *Ann Noninvasive Electrocardiol* 2001;6:153–158.
84. Ferguson JD, DiMarco JP. Contemporary management of paroxysmal supraventricular tachycardia. *Circulation* 2003;107:1096–1099.
85. Hamer AW, et al. Failure of episodic high-dose oral verapamil therapy to convert supraventricular tachycardia: a study of plasma verapamil levels and gastric motility. *Am Heart J* 1987;114:334–342.
86. Alboni P, et al. Efficacy and safety of out-of-hospital self-administered single-dose oral drug treatment in the management of infrequent, well-tolerated paroxysmal supraventricular tachycardia. *J Am Coll Cardiol* 2001;37:548–553.
87. Blomstrom-Lundqvist C, et al. ACC/AHA/ESC guidelines for the management of patients with supraventricular arrhythmias—executive summary: a report of the American College of Cardiology/American Heart Association Task Force on Practice Guidelines and the European Society of Cardiology Committee for Practice Guidelines (Writing Committee to Develop Guidelines for the Management of Patients With Supraventricular Arrhythmias). *Circulation* 2003;108:1871–1909.
88. Mangrum J, DiMarco J. Acute and chronic pharmacologic management of supraventricular arrhythmias, in *Cardiovascular Therapeutics: A Companion to Braunwald's Heart Disease*, 2nd ed, Antman E, et al, eds. Philadelphia: WB Saunders; 2002:423–444.
89. Dougherty AH, et al. Acute conversion of paroxysmal supraventricular tachycardia with intravenous diltiazem. IV Diltiazem Study Group. *Am J Cardiol* 1992;70:587–592.
90. Epstein ML, et al. Cardiac decompensation following verapamil therapy in infants with supraventricular tachycardia. *Pediatrics* 1985;75:737–740.
91. DiMarco JP, et al. Adenosine for paroxysmal supraventricular tachycardia: dose ranging and comparison with verapamil. Assessment in placebo-controlled, multicenter trials. The Adenosine for PSVT Study Group. *Ann Intern Med* 1990;113:104–110.
92. Dorian P, et al. A randomized comparison of flecainide versus verapamil in paroxysmal supraventricular tachycardia. The Flecainide Multicenter Investigators Group. *Am J Cardiol* 1996;77:89A–95A.
93. Akhtar M, et al. Role of adrenergic stimulation by isoproterenol in reversal of effects of encainide in supraventricular tachycardia. *Am J Cardiol* 1988;62:45L–49L.
94. Scheinman M, Huang S. The 1998 NASPE prospective catheter ablation reg' *Pacing Clin Electrophysiol* 2000;23:1020–1028.
95. Lip G, et al. Atrial fibrillation, in *Cardiology*, 2nd edit., Crawford M, DiMarco J, ' W, eds. London: Elsevier; 2004:699–716.
96. Fuster V, et al. ACC/AHA/ESC Guidelines for the management of patie atrial fibrillation: executive summary a report of the American C Cardiology/American Heart Association Task Force on Practice Guidelines Conferences (Committee to Develop Guidelines for the Managment of P Atrial Fibrillation) Developed in collaboration with the North Americ Pacing and Electrophysiology. *Circulation* 2001;104:2118–2150.

97. Gallagher MM, Camm J. Classification of atrial fibrillation. *Am J Cardiol* 1998;82: 18N–28N.

98. The Digitalis in Acute Atrial Fibrillation (DAAF) Trial Group. Intravenous digoxin in acute atrial fibrillation. Results in a randomized, placebo-controlled multicentre trial in 239 patients. *Eur Heart J* 1997;18:649–654.

99. Sarter BH, Marchlinski FE. Redefining the role of digoxin in the treatment of atrial fibrillation. *Am J Cardiol* 1992;69:71G–78G; discussion 78G–81G.

100. Khand AU, et al. Carvedilol alone or in combination with digoxin for the management of atrial fibrillation in patients with heart failure? *J Am Coll Cardiol* 2003;42:1944–1951.

101. Reimold SC, et al. Assessment of the efficacy and safety of antiarrhythmic therapy for chronic atrial fibrillation: observations on the role of trial design and implications of drug-related mortality. *Am Heart J* 1992;124:924–932.

102. Boriani G, et al. Oral propafenone to convert recent-onset atrial fibrillation in patients with and without underlying heart disease. A randomized, controlled trial. *Ann Intern Med* 1997;126:621–625.

103. Capucci A, et al. Effectiveness of loading oral flecainide for converting recent-onset atrial fibrillation to sinus rhythm in patients without organic heart disease or with only systemic hypertension. *Am J Cardiol* 1992;70:69–72.

104. Roy D, et al. Amiodarone to prevent recurrence of atrial fibrillation. Canadian Trial of Atrial Fibrillation Investigators. *N Engl J Med* 2003;342:913–920.

105. Pedersen OD, et al. Trandolapril reduces the incidence of atrial fibrillation after acute myocardial infarction in patients with left ventricular dysfunction. *Circulation* 1999;100:376–380.

106. Madrid A, et al. Use of irbesartan to maintain sinus rhythm in patients with long-lasting persistent atrial fibrillation: a prospective and randomized study. *Circulation* 2002;106:331–336.

107. Crystal E, et al. Interventions on prevention of postoperative atrial fibrillation in patients undergoing heart surgery. A meta-analysis. *Circulation* 2002;106:75–80.

108. Mahoney EM, et al. Cost-effectiveness of targeting patients undergoing cardiac surgery for therapy with intravenous amiodarone to prevent atrial fibrillation. *J Am Coll Cardiol* 2002;40:737–745.

109. Barucha D, Kowey P. Management and prevention of atrial fibrillation after cardiovascular surgery. *Am J Cardiol* 2000;85:20D–24D.

110. AFFIRM Investigators. The Atrial Fibrillation Follow-up Investigation of Rhythm Management. A comparison of rate control and rhythm control in patients with atrial fibrillation. *N Engl J Med* 2002;347:1825–1833.

111. Hohnloser S, et al. Rhythm of rate control in atrial fibrillation—Pharmacological Intervention in Atrial Fibrillation (PIAF): a randomised trial. *Lancet* 2000;356: 1789–1794.

112. van Gelder IC, et al. For the Rate Control versus Electrical Cardioversion for Persistent Atrial Fibrillation Study Group. A comparison of rate control and rhythm control in patients with recurrent persistent atrial fibrillation. *N Engl J Med* 2002;347:1834–1840.

113. Carlsson J, et al. Randomized trial of rate-control versus rhythm-control in persistent atrial fibrillation: the Strategies of Treatment of Atrial Fibrillation (STAF) study. *J Am Coll Cardiol* 2003;41:1690–1696.

114. The AF-CHF Trial Investigators. Rationale and design of a study assessing treatment strategies of atrial fibrillation in patients with heart failure: The Atrial Fibrillation and Congestive Heart Failure (AF-CHF) trial. *Am Heart J* 2002;144:597–607.

115. Snow V, et al. Management of newly detected atrial fibrillation: a clinical practice guideline from the American Academy of Family Physicians and the American College of Physicians. *Ann Intern Med* 2003;139:1009–1017.

116. Israel CW, et al. Long-term risk of recurrent atrial fibrillation as documented by an implantable monitoring device: implications for optimal patient care. *J Am Coll Cardiol* 2004;43:47–52.

117. Hissaguerre M, et al. Spontaneous initiation of atrial fibrillation by ectopic beats originating in the pulmonary veins. *N Engl J Med* 1999;339:659–665.

118. Pappone C, et al. Mortality, morbidity, and quality of life after circumferential pulmonary vein ablation for atrial fibrillation: outcomes from a controlled nonrandomized long-term study. *J Am Coll Cardiol* 2003;42:185–197.

119. Oral H, et al. Catheter ablation for paroxysmal atrial fibrillation: segmental pulmonary vein ostial ablation versus left atrial ablation. *Circulation* 2003;108: 2355–2360.

120. Wang TJ, et al. A risk score for predicting stroke or death in individuals with new-onset atrial fibrillation in the community. The Framingham Heart Study. *JAMA* 2003;290:1049–1056.

1. Albers GW, et al. Antithrombotic therapy in atrial fibrillation. *Chest* 2001;119: 194S–206S.

Olsson S, Executive Steering Committee, on behalf of the SPORTIF III Investigators. Stroke prevention with the oral direct thrombin inhibitor ximelagatran compared with warfarin in patients with non-valvular atrial fibrillation (SPORTIF III)l: ranmised controlled trial. *Lancet* 2003;362:1691–1698.

rgatroyd F. Atrial tachycardias and atrial flutter, in *Cardiology*, 2nd edit., ford M, DiMarco J, Paulus W, eds. London: Elsevier; 2004:717–728.

RH, et al. Intravenous dofetilide, a class III antiarrhythmic agent, for the terion of sustained atrial fibrillation or flutter. Intravenous Dofetilide Investigam Coll Cardiol 1997;29:385–390.

DM, et al. Long-term outcome of patients after successful radiofrequency or typical atrial flutter. *Pacing Clin Electrophysiol* 2003;26:53–58.

126. AHA Guidelines. For cardiopulmonary resuscitation and emergency cardiovascular care. *Circulation* 2000;102:1–384.
127. Griffith MJ, et al. Relative efficacy and safety of intravenous drugs for termination of sustained ventricular tachycardia. *Lancet* 1990;336:670-673.
128. Kowey PR, et al. Intravenous amiodarone. *J Am Coll Cardiol* 1997;29:1190–1198.
129. Levine JH, et al. Intravenous amiodarone for recurrent sustained hypotensive ventricular tachyarrhythmias. Intravenous Amiodarone Multicenter Trial Group. *J Am Coll Cardiol* 1996;27:67–75.
130. Scheinman MM, et al. Dose-ranging study of intravenous amiodarone in patients with life-threatening ventricular tachyarrhythmias. The Intravenous Amiodarone Multicenter Investigators Group. *Circulation* 1995;92:3264–3272.
131. Kowey PR, et al. Randomized double-blind comparison of intravenous amiodarone and bretylium in the treatment of patients with recurrent, hemodynamically destabilizing ventricular tachycardia or fibrillation. The Intravenous Amiodarone Multicenter Investigators Group. *Circulation* 1995;92:3255–3263.
132. DiMarco JP. Implantable cardioverter-defibrillators. *N Engl J Med* 2003;349:1836–1847.
133. AVID Investigators. A comparison of antiarrhythmic-drug therapy with implantable defibrillators in patients resuscitated from near-fatal ventricular arrhythmias. *N Engl J Med* 1997;337:1576–1583.
134. Connolly SJ, et al. Canadian implantable defibrillator study (CIDS): a randomized trial of the implantable cardioverter defibrillator against amiodarone. *Circulation* 2000;101:1297–1302.
135. Kuck KH, et al. Randomized comparison of antiarrhythmic drug therapy with implantable defibrillators in patients resuscitated from cardiac arrest: the Cardiac Arrest Study Hamburg (CASH). *Circulation* 2000;102:748–754.
136. Connolly SJ, et al. Meta-analysis of the implantable cardioverter defibrillator secondary prevention trials. AVID, CASH and CIDS studies. Antiarrhythmics vs Implantable Defibrillator study. Cardiac Arrest Study Hamburg . Canadian Implantable Defibrillator Study. *Eur Heart J* 2000;21:2071–2078.
137. Echt DS, et al. Mortality and morbidity in patients receiving encainide, flecainide, or placebo. The Cardiac Arrhythmia Suppression Trial. *N Engl J Med* 1991;324:781–788.
138. Steinbeck G, Greene HL. Management of patients with life-threatening sustained ventricular tachyarrhythmias—the role of guided antiarrhythmic drug therapy. *Prog Cardiovasc Dis* 1996;38:419–428.
139. CASCADE Investigators. Randomised antiarrhythmic drug therapy in survivors of cardiac arrest (The CASCADE Study). *Am J Cardiol* 1993;72:280–287.
140. Mason JW. A comparison of electrophysiologic testing with Holter monitoring to predict antiarrhythmic-drug efficacy for ventricular tachyarrhythmias. Electrophysiologic Study versus Electrocardiographic Monitoring Investigators. *N Engl J Med* 1993;329:445–451.
141. Mason JW. A comparison of seven antiarrhythmic drugs in patients with ventricular tachyarrhythmias. Electrophysiologic Study versus Electrocardiographic Monitoring Investigators. *N Engl J Med* 1993;329:452–458.
142. Buxton AE, et al. For the Multicenter Unsustained Tachycardia Trial Investigators. A randomized study of the prevention of sudden death in patients with coronary artery disease. *N Engl J Med* 1999;341:1820–1890.
143. Steinberg JS, et al. Antiarrhythmic drug use in the implantable defibrillator arm of the Antiarrhythmics Versus Implantable Defibrillators (AVID) Study. *Am Heart J* 2001;142:520–529.
144. Borggrefe M, et al. Ventricular tachycardia, in *Cardiology*, 2nd edit., Crawford M, DiMarco J, Paulus W, eds. London: Elsevier; 2004:753–764.
145. Priori SG, et al. Task Force on Sudden Cardiac Death of the European Society of Cardiology. *Eur Heart J* 2001;22:1374–1450.
146. Moss AJ, et al. For the Multicenter Automatic Defibrillator Implantation Trial (MADITT) Investigators. Improved survival with an implanted defibrillator in patients with coronary artery disease at high risk for ventricular arrhythmia. *N Engl J Med* 1996;335:1933–1940.
147. Moss AJ, et al. Prophylactic implantation of a defibrillator in patients with myocardial infarction and reduced ejection fraction. *N Engl J Med* 2002;346:877–883.
148. Bänsch D, et al. Primary prevention of sudden cardiac death in idiopathic dilated cardiomyopathy: the Cardiomyopathy Trial (CAT). *Circulation* 2002;105:1453–1458.
149. Kadish AH. For the DEFINITE Investigators. Prophylactic ICD implantation in patients with non-ischemic dilated cardiomyopathy. The DEFibrillators In Non-Ischemic Cardiomyopathy Treatment Evaluation trial. *N Engl J Med* 2004;350:2151–2158.
150. Bardy, G. Sudden cardiac death in heart failure trial (SCD-HeFT). www.theheart.org. March 8, 2004.
151. Grimm W, et al. Noninvasive arrhythmia risk stratification in idiopathic dilated cardiomyopathy: results of the Marburg Cardiomyopathy Study. *Circulation* 2003;108:2883–2891.
152. Bristow MR, et al. Cardiac resynchronization therapy with or without an implantable defibrillator in advanced chronic heart failure. *N Engl J Med* 2004;350:2140–2150.
153. Kass DA. Predicting cardiac resynchronization response by QRS duration: the long and short of it. *J Am Coll Cardiol* 2003;42:2125–2127.
154. Steinbeck G, et al. A comparison of electrophysiologically guided antiarrhythmic drug therapy with beta-blocker therapy in patients with symptomatic, sustained ventricular tachyarrhythmias. *N Engl J Med* 1992;327:987–992.
155. MUSTT Investigators. For the Multicenter Unsustained Tachycardia Trial (MUSTT) Investigators. A randomized study of the prevention of sudden death in patients with coronary artery disease. *N Engl J Med* 1999;341:1882–1890.

Antithrombotic Agents: Platelet Inhibitors, Anticoagulants, and Fibrinolytics

Harvey D. White • Bernard J. Gersh • Lionel H. Opie

The Emperor said:	"I wonder whether breathlessness results in death or life?"
Chi'i P answered:	"When there are blockages in the circulation between the viscera, then death follows."
The Emperor said:	"What can be done with regard to treatment?"
Chi'i P replied:	"The method of curing is to establish communication between the viscera and the vascular system."

THE YELLOW EMPEROR'S CLASSIC OF
INTERNAL MEDICINE (CIRCA 2000 BC)

MECHANISMS OF THROMBOSIS

Pro- and Antiaggregatory Factors

The proaggregatory and antiaggregatory factors of the hemostatic system are normally finely balanced, opposing mechanisms. To protect against vascular damage and the risk of bleeding to death, the proaggregatory system is poised to rapidly form a thrombus to limit any potential hemorrhage. As long as the vascular endothelium is intact, at least four different mechanisms keep the blood flowing (Fig. 9-1). As coronary endothelial damage appears to be a prominent feature of ischemic heart disease, there is a constant threat that anti-aggregatory forces will be overcome by the proaggregatory forces, with the risk of further vascular damage and, potentially, thrombosis (Fig. 9-2).

The *formation of thrombus* occurs in three steps: (1) exposure of the circulating blood to a thrombogenic surface, such as damaged vascular endothelium resulting from a ruptured atherosclerotic plaque; (2) a sequence of platelet-related events involving platelet adhesion, platelet activation, and platelet aggregation (Fig. 9-3), with release of substances that further promote aggregation and cause vasoconstriction; and (3) triggering of the clotting mechanism. Thrombin plays an important role in the formation of fibrin, which crosslinks to form the backbone of the thrombus. Thrombin itself is a very powerful stimulator of platelet adhesion and aggregation. Once formed, the thrombus may be broken down by plasmin-stimulated fibrinolysis. The typical arterial thrombus at the site of a coronary stenosis has a white head due to platelet aggregation, and a red tail due to stasis beyond the lesion.

The three main types of agent discussed in this chapter act at different stages of the thrombotic process. First, platelet inhibitors act on arterial thrombi and help prevent consequences such as myocardial infarction and transient ischemic attacks (TIAs). Second, anticoagulants given acutely (e.g., heparin) limit the further formation of fibrin,

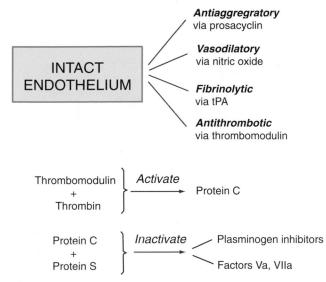

Figure 9-1 Factors protecting against coagulation directly or indirectly depend on an intact endothelium. *tPA* = tissue plasminogen activator. (*Figure © LH Opie, 2005.*)

REGULATION OF PLATELET AGGREGATION

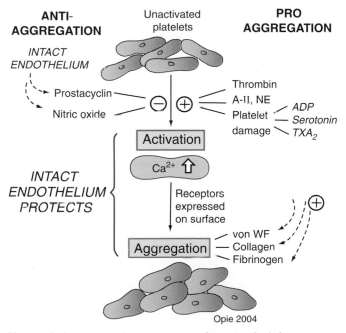

Figure 9-2 Balance of antiaggregatory forces on the left and proaggregatory forces on the right. These promote or inhibit platelet activation, dependent on an increased platelet calcium level (Fig. 9-3), which results in platelet aggregation and thrombosis. The proaggregatory forces are set in motion by endothelial and platelet injury. *A-II* = angiotensin II; Ca^{2+} = calcium, *NE* = norepinephrine, TXA_2 = thromboxane A_2, *VWF* = von Willebrand factor. (*Figure © LH Opie, 2005.*)

PLATELET INHIBITORS

Opie 2004

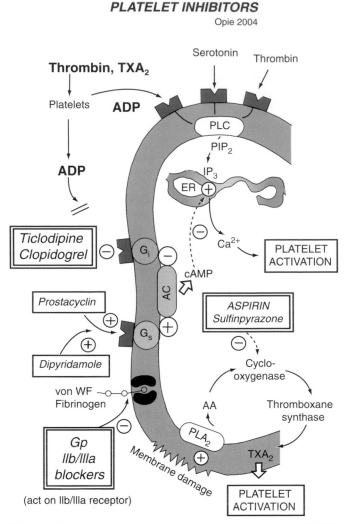

Figure 9-3 Mechanism of action of aspirin including Gp IIb/IIIb inhibitors and other antiplatelet agents in the light of the platelet activation cycle, that leads to activation of the Gp IIb/IIIa receptor. The self-augmenting platelet activation cycle alters membrane configuration, "exposing" the receptors with further activation of the Gp IIb/IIIa receptor. Note that formation of IP_3 is crucial in mobilizing calcium from the endoplasmic reticulum. This cycle also depends on formation of thromboxane A_2. All these agents, acting via different mechanisms, to inhibit the calcium-dependent pathways of platelet activation. AC = adenyl cyclase; ADP = adenosine diphosphate; Ca^{2+} = calcium; $cAMP$ = cyclic adenosine monophosphate; ER = endoplasmic reticulum, G_i = G-protein, inhibitory form; Gp = glycoprotein; G_s = G-protein, stimulatory form; IP_3 = inositol trisphosphate; PIP_2 = phosphatidylinositol diphosphate; PLA_2 = phospholipase A_2; TXA_2 = thromboxane A_2. (*Figure © LH Opie, 2005.*)

and, when given chronically (e.g., warfarin), help prevent thromboembolism from a dilated left atrium or from veins. Third, fibrinolytic agents are most useful in the clinical syndromes of acute arterial thrombosis and occlusion, such as myocardial infarction and peripheral arterial thrombosis. The different sites of action of these three types of agent mean that combination therapy can be beneficial. For example, fibrinolytic agents are used together with antiplatelet agents and anticoagulants in the management of acute myocardial infarction but the greater efficacy of combinations is offset by the increased incidence of bleeding.

Platelet Function In addition to acting against arterial thrombosis, platelet inhibitors protect against other proposed consequences of platelet malfunction, such as excessive vasoconstriction. Possibly by releasing platelet derived growth factor (PDGF), platelets may also promote the development of atheroma by stimulating smooth muscle cell proliferation and migration into the subintimal layer, with subsequent synthesis of connective tissue and intimal hyperplasia.

Platelet Adhesion to the Injured Vessel Wall This is the first of the three steps involving platelets in the development of an arterial thrombus (Fig. 9-2). Endothelial injury promotes platelet adhesion in two ways. First, the damaged endothelium releases *von Willebrand factor*, a multimeric glycoprotein synthesized in the endothelial cells to which activated platelets adhere at their glycoprotein receptor sites.[1] Second, microfibrils of collagen from the deeper layers of the vessel become exposed as a result of endothelial injury, thereby promoting platelet adhesion.

Platelet Receptors and Activation Superficial platelet injury activates platelet receptors, which are membrane glycoproteins. Activated receptors bind more readily to von Willebrand factor (receptors glycoprotein Ib and GP IIb/IIIa),[1] subendothelial collagen (receptor glycoprotein Ia), or fibrinogen (receptor glycoprotein IIb/IIIa). These receptors have two functions. They help to activate platelets by releasing calcium from the endoplasmic reticulum (Fig. 9-3) and they allow macromolecules, such as circulating von Willebrand factor, to "chain" receptors together, thereby promoting platelet adhesion. Although it is an end-product of the coagulation process, thrombin also acts as a classic ligand, activating one of the two platelet ADP receptors.[2] The activated receptor then raises platelet calcium by stimulating phospholipase-C (Fig. 9-3).

Platelet Aggregation The critical event is a rise in the intracellular platelet calcium level. Several mediators (including collagen from endothelial injury, thrombin, ADP released from injured platelets, and serotonin released from hemolyzed red cells) act by stimulating the formation of inositol triphosphate (IP_3). The thromboxane A_2 synthesized in the damaged vessel wall inhibits the formation of cyclic adenosine monophosphate (cAMP), thereby removing a brake on the production of IP_3 (Fig. 9-3). IP_3 mobilizes calcium from the endoplasmic reticulum. Enhanced platelet calcium has several consequences, including: (1) stimulation of the pathways breaking down the platelet phospholipids to eventually form thromboxane A_2 (Fig. 9-3) and (2) activation of platelet actin and myosin to cause contraction. Contraction of the platelets or mechanical shear stress[3] exposes the glycoprotein receptors IIb/IIIa and Ib, which mediate the final common pathway of platelet aggregation by allowing a greater rate of interaction with various macromolecules such as von Willebrand factor, fibrinogen, thrombin, and thrombospondin.[3] These macromolecules bind the platelets to each other and to the platelets already adhering to the vessel wall.

Tissue Factor and Activation of Clotting Mechanisms The conversion of prothrombin to thrombin is a crucial step in the coagulation process. Traditionally, the intrinsic and extrinsic pathways are distinguished. The intrinsic coagulation pathway involves a series of interactions that lead to activation of factor IX (forming IXa), that in turn activates factor X to Xa, which acts on prothrombin to form thrombin (Fig. 9-4). In reality, it is the extrinsic coagulation pathway that is predominant in vivo. The immediate trigger to this path is tissue injury that exposes or expresses *tissue factor*, a cell surface glycoprotein that is abundantly expressed in damaged endothelial cells and macrophages,

INTRINSIC AND EXTRINSIC COAGULATION PATHS

Opie 2004

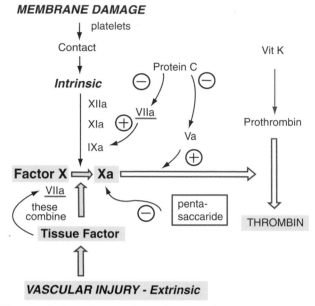

Figure 9-4 Intrinsic and extrinsic coagulation pathways. Note inhibitory role of protein C, and roles of factor Xa and vitamin K in promoting formation of prothrombin. For further role of prothrombin see Fig. 9-7. (*Figure © LH Opie, 2005.*)

as in the atherosclerotic plaque. Tissue factor then forms a complex with and activates factor VII. Factor VIIa in turn promotes the activation of factor X to Xa, both directly and indirectly by activating factor IX (Fig. 9-4). Factor Xa converts prothrombin to thrombin. Tissue factor and tissue factor inhibitor appear to be involved in acute coronary syndromes when the inhibitor levels are lower in coronary sinus blood.[4] In nonvalvular atrial fibrillation, atrial thrombosis may be provoked by local inflammation associated with overexpression of tissue factor.[5] When urgent activation of the clotting mechanism is essential (e.g., a wounded soldier bleeding to death or unstoppable hemorrhage in a patient), then powerful activation of thrombosis at two sites (Fig. 7-4) is achieved by recombinant factor VIIa, licensed in the United States as *Novoseven* only for hemophiliacs with inhibitors to factors VIII and IX.

Prothrombin and Thrombin Prothrombin is one of several vitamin K-dependent clotting factors, and oral anticoagulants such as warfarin are vitamin K antagonists. Thrombin from either source further enhances platelet membrane activation, promoting platelet aggregation and converting fibrinogen to fibrin, which adheres to platelet surfaces to stabilize and fix the arterial thrombus. Thrombin is one of the most powerful activators of platelets. The end result is a platelet- and fibrin-rich thrombus, adherent to the vessel wall. This whole process may be dynamic and repetitive.[6] Fibrinolytic mechanisms involving the conversion of plasminogen to plasmin act by limiting the size of the clot and eventually dissolving part or all of it.

Platelets and Vascular Contraction During and after platelet aggregation, platelets release 5-hydroxytryptamine (serotonin) and other potentially important products, such as platelet factor 4 and β-thromboglobulin, which may help to promote platelet aggregation. Serotonin normally causes vasodilation in the presence of an intact vascular endothelium. In contrast, when the endothelium is damaged, serotonin causes vasoconstriction, which may promote vascular stasis and thrombosis. Hence it is suspected that platelets play a role in vasoconstrictive diseases such as coronary spasm or Raynaud's disease.

ASPIRIN AND CARDIOVASCULAR PROTECTION

Platelet Inhibition Aspirin (acetylsalicylic acid) irreversibly acetylates cyclo-oxygenase (Fig. 9-3), and activity is not restored until new platelets are formed. The cyclo-oxygenase isoform is COX-1, the inhibition of which gives both the therapeutic benefit and the toxic gastric side effects.[7] Aspirin does not strongly inhibit COX-2, which produces the prostaglandins that contribute to the inflammatory response. By inhibiting COX-1, aspirin interferes with the synthesis of prothrombotic TXA_2, important in the platelet activation cycle (Fig. 9-3). This benefit outweighs the possible adverse effects of inhibiting the synthesis of antithrombotic prostacyclin.[7] Being very primitive cells, platelets cannot synthesize new proteins, meaning that aspirin prevents all platelet COX-1 activity for the lifespan of the platelet. Therefore, aspirin stops the production of the proaggregatory thromboxane A_2, and eventually acts as an indirect antithrombotic agent. On the other hand, it also has important nonplatelet effects. In the vascular endothelium it inactivates cyclo-oxygenase, which may diminish the formation of antiaggregatory prostacyclin. The difference is that vascular cyclo-oxygenase can be resynthesized within hours. Despite the potentially conflicting effects of aspirin in reducing the synthesis of both thromboxane A_2 and prostacyclin, the overwhelming clinical message is that the antithrombotic effects predominate.[6] On the negative side, aspirin can cause gastric irritation, and gastrointestinal bleeding requiring hospitalization occurs in 2 per 1000 patients treated per year,[8] with a small increase in risk of hemorrhagic stroke.[9,10] Furthermore, aspirin resistance may limit the response (see later).

Anti-inflammatory Effects Aspirin is a relatively weak antiplatelet agent, and only blocks aggregation in response to stimulation by thromboxane. Its effects can be overcome by other stimuli, particularly thrombin, which is the most powerful stimulus of platelet aggregation.[11] However, it may have important additional effects on platelet-neutrophil interactions,[12] and on inflammation.[13] The beneficial effect of aspirin in preventing myocardial infarction in the US Physicians' Study occurred almost exclusively in individuals with elevated levels of C-reactive protein, suggesting that the clinical benefits of aspirin may be at least partly due to its anti-inflammatory properties, rather than its antiplatelet properties.[13]

Aspirin Resistance This is common, occurring in 5% to 20% (or more) of patients with arterial thrombosis as shown by a recurrent vascular event during long-term follow-up despite an adequate therapeutic dose.[14] When defined as failure of suppression of thromboxane generation with high urinary concentrations of a metabolite of thromboxane A_2, then the risk of myocardial infarction is doubled.[14] When defined by platelet function tests and presumed clinical unresponsiveness to aspirin, there is a long-term trebling of the risk of death, myocardial infarct or stroke.[15] The diverse mechanisms of aspirin resistance include platelet glycoprotein polymorphisms, activation of platelets by pathways other than the cyclo-oxygenase pathway, and enhanced inflammatory activity with increased expression of COX-2 that is not strongly inhibited by aspirin.[14] Ibuprofen but not diclofenac interferes with aspirin protection and increases mortality in those with cardiovascular disease.[16] Laboratory diagnosis is not easy, although a new bedside test should help to confirm clinical suspicions.[17] Clopidogrel, as an add-on or replacement, is a logical although not formally tested, because of its different mode of action and several major studies showing superiority of dual platelet inhibition to aspirin alone.[17]

Clinical Use of Aspirin

Because platelets play such an important role in vascular disease of all kinds, the clinical indications for aspirin are many. A meta-analysis of 135,000 patients in 287 studies confirmed its prophylactic effects after a previous myocardial infarction, in angina, after stroke, and after bypass surgery, and established its efficacy in women as well as in men.[18] Aspirin works in diabetics and in well-treated hypertensive patients.[19,20] The major problem is balancing the benefits of aspirin versus the risks, the chief being major gastrointestinal bleeding and hemorrhagic stroke. When aspirin is used for secondary prevention, the balance strongly favors benefit, when used for primary prevention the best approach is risk factor stratification.

Secondary Prevention by Aspirin All patients with a prior cardiovascular event should be considered for aspirin therapy, which on average reduces the risk of any further vascular event by about one quarter. *In stable angina* in β-blocked patients, aspirin 75 mg daily reduced acute myocardial infarction or sudden death by 34% compared with placebo.[21] The risk reductions extend to those with unstable angina (46%), coronary angioplasty (53%), prior MI (25%), prior stroke or transient ischemic attack (22%), atrial fibrillation (24%), and peripheral arterial disease (23%).[18] *In acute coronary syndromes*, including acute myocardial infarction, aspirin should be given in both the acute and follow-up phases. Theoretically, an initial dose of about 325 mg is preferable. When a Gp IIb/IIIa blocker is used then aspirin is part of the standard background therapy that includes dose-adjusted heparin (this chapter, p. 290). Aspirin is an integral part of postinfarction preventative care.

Primary Prevention by Aspirin: Only for Those at High Risk Our recommendation, supported by a meta-analysis on more than 30,000 subjects, is that aspirin is indicated only in high-risk populations.[18] The protective benefit must exceed that of unwanted side effects. The American Heart Association guidelines propose aspirin for those with a 10-year cardiovascular risk ≥10%.[22] However, even this is controversial. The FDA recently turned down a proposed indication for aspirin in primary prevention of myocardial infarction in those with a 10-year risk of >10%, who were regarded as being at moderate risk. Overall, the data from five trials showed that for every 1000 patients treated for 5 years, five nonfatal MIs would be avoided at a risk of one excess disabling stroke, and two to four serious gastrointestinal bleeds requiring transfusions.[23] Other calculations are also discouraging.[10,24] Clearly, aspirin should not be used prophylactically by the general apparently healthy population, especially by the elderly, in whom decreased renal function is a possible side effect.[25] If used, systolic blood pressure must be well controlled, ideally below 130 mmHg.[20]

Aspirin as an Anti-inflammatory Drug While the above risk factor calculation is an excellent guide, it does not factor in the role of the inflammatory response in the genesis of vascular disease. In the Physicians' Health Study, the benefit of aspirin in primary prevention was largely localized to males with high blood levels of C-reactive protein.[13] Logically, but without prospective trial support, aspirin by its anti-inflammatory effect should be more effective than expected from current risk factor calculations, and might be considered for primary prevention in those with a high C-reactive protein.

Other Indications for Aspirin (1) *Post-coronary bypass surgery*, aspirin should be started within 48 hours of surgery, which reduces total mortality by about two thirds[26] and probably continued indefinitely. (2) *For coronary angioplasty*, pretreatment with aspirin plus acute unfractionated heparin, low-molecular-weight heparin,[27] or bivalirudin[28] are strongly recommended to help prevent acute thrombotic closure. (3) *Prevention of stroke in atrial fibrillation*, when warfarin is contraindicated or the patient is not at high risk of stroke, aspirin should be used. It reduces events by about 25%.[18] (4) For *artificial heart valves*, to prevent emboli; the combination of warfarin and low-dose aspirin has been validated.[29] (5) For *arteriovenous shunts*, aspirin decreases thrombosis; and (6) For *renovascular hypertension*, aspirin may reduce the blood pressure, presumably by inhibiting formation of the prostaglandins involved in renin release.[30]

Low-Dose Aspirin Low doses theoretically retain efficacy yet limit gastrointestinal side effects. Meta-analysis suggests that the dose range should be 75 to 150 mg daily for a wide range of indications.[18] In a follow-up study of patients with non-ST-elevation acute coronary syndromes the optimal dose of aspirin was 75 to 100 mg.[31] How low to go? Aspirin 80 mg/day completely blocks platelet aggregation induced by cyclo-oxygenase.[6] Doses of only 30 mg daily were as effective as higher doses in preventing TIAs,[32] but other end-points were not tested. The problem with these relatively low doses is that the full antithrombotic effect takes up to 2 days to manifest, explaining why higher dose aspirin (about 320 mg) should be given urgently at the onset of symptoms of acute myocardial infarction or unstable angina. Higher dose aspirin, formerly used to prevent recurrences of stroke or transient ischemic attacks, is no longer appropriate.[8,32,33]

Gastric and Other Side Effects of Aspirin High-dose aspirin causes gastrointestinal side effects in many patients, but the standard dose (150 to 300 mg daily) reduces the incidence to about 40% (compared with about 30% for placebo).[34] Gastrointestinal side effects, such as dyspepsia, nausea, or vomiting, may be dose-limiting in about 10% to 20% of patients. Such side effects may be reduced by buffered or enteric-coated aspirin, or by taking aspirin with food. Dose-related gastrointestinal bleeding may occur in about 4% to 5% of patients,[31] with frank malena in about 1% per year and hematemesis in about 0.1% per year. When the aspirin dose is only 30 mg daily, bleeding is substantially reduced but other gastric side effects remain virtually unchanged.[32] Less commonly emphasized side effects but frequent in the elderly even with low-dose aspirin, are impaired renal function and decreased excretion of uric acid.[25]

Contraindications to Aspirin The major contraindications are aspirin intolerance; hemophilia; and history of gastrointestinal bleeding, peptic ulcer, or other potential sources of gastrointestinal or genitourinary bleeding. Congestive heart failure is a contraindication against Alka-Seltzer use (to reduce gastric discomfort) because of its sodium content, as are renal failure, renal stones, or hepatic cirrhosis. Because it retards the urinary excretion of uric acid and creatinine, blood uric acid and creatinine should be monitored, especially in the elderly.[35] Relative contraindications include dyspepsia, iron deficiency anemia, and the possibility of increased perioperative bleeding.

Drug Interactions with Aspirin Concurrent warfarin and aspirin therapy increases the risk of bleeding, especially if doses are high. Among nonsteroidal anti-inflammatory drugs (NSAIDs), ibuprofen but not diclofenac interferes with the cardioprotective effects of aspirin.[16] Angiotensin-converting enzyme (ACE) inhibitors and aspirin have potentially opposing effects on renal hemodynamics, aspirin inhibiting and ACE inhibitors promoting the formation of vasodilatory prostaglandins. Two meta-analyses have addressed this issue. When ACE inhibitors are chronically used for heart failure or postinfarct protection or for high-risk prevention, they are still beneficial in 22,060 patients even when aspirin is added.[36] Yet aspirin did reduce the ACE inhibitor effect on myocardial infarction ($P < 0.01$) and on mortality ($P < 0.04$).[36] In 96,712 patients with acute myocardial infarction (AMI), there was no interaction over 30 days.[37] A practical policy is to keep the aspirin dose low especially in those with hemodynamic problems such as heart failure.[38] The risk of aspirin-induced gastrointestinal bleeding is increased by alcohol, corticosteroid therapy, and other NSAIDs. The efficacy of enteric-coated preparations may be reduced by antacids, which alter the pH of the stomach. Phenobarbital, phenytoin, and rifampin decrease the efficacy of aspirin through induction of the hepatic enzymes metabolizing aspirin. The effect of oral hypoglycemic agents and insulin may be enhanced by aspirin. Aspirin may reduce the efficacy of uricosuric drugs such as sulfinpyrazone and probenecid. Both thiazides and aspirin retard the urinary excretion of uric acid, increasing the risk of gout.

TICLOPIDINE, CLOPIDOGREL, AND OTHER ANTIPLATELET AGENTS

Ticlopidine

Ticlopidine *(Ticlid)* and clopidogrel are both thienopyridine derivatives that irreversibly inhibit the binding of ADP to its receptor on the platelets, thereby preventing the transformation of the glycoprotein IIb/IIIa receptor into its active form (Fig. 9-3). Ticlopidine can cause neutropenia, liver abnormalities, and thrombotic thrombocytopenia, so that it is less safe than clopidogrel. Both agents when added to aspirin give added antiaggregatory effects and improve clinical outcomes.[18]

Pharmacokinetics The kinetics of ticlopidine tablets are nonlinear, with a markedly decreased clearance on repeated dosing. Thus it takes 4 to 7 days to achieve maximum inhibition of platelet aggregation when given with aspirin.[39] However, a quicker response can be achieved by oral loading. Ticlopidine is largely metabolized by the liver, followed by renal excretion. The plasma half-life on constant dosing is 4 to 5 days.

Indications Ticlopidine has two licensed indications in the United States, to prevent repeat stroke or TIA in those intolerant of or resistant to aspirin, and coronary artery stenting, for up to 30 days after stenting and with aspirin. In practice it is also used in other conditions when aspirin is contraindicated or has failed. A standard dose is 250 mg taken twice daily with food to lessen intolerance and to increase absorption. Ticlopidine reduces the risk of fatal and nonfatal thrombotic stroke in patients who have had TIAs, and in those who have had a completed thrombotic stroke.[40,41] In patients undergoing coronary artery stenting, treatment must be begun 3 days prior to the procedure, or alternatively given as a loading dose of 500 mg at the time of the procedure and continued for 2 to 4 weeks. It is contraindicated in bleeding disorders, or preexisting depression of neutrophils or of platelets.

Side Effects and Essential Precautions The major side effect of ticlopidine is neutropenia, which occurs in 2.4% and is the subject of a boxed warning in the package insert. Thrombotic thrombocytopenia, which is usually life-threatening, occurs in approximately 0.01% of patients. Minor bleeding may also occur in up to 10%, skin rashes in up to 15%, liver toxicity in 4%, and diarrhea in 22%, but all of these are reversible.[42] The neutropenia occurs within the first 3 months of treatment. It is therefore essential that a complete blood count and white cell differential be performed before starting treatment, and every 2 weeks until the end of the third month, according to the manufacturer's information.

Clopidogrel

Structurally similar to ticlopidine, clopidogrel seems substantially safer with a low rate of myelotoxicity (0.8%, package insert) and an incidence of gastrointestinal complications similar to aspirin. It acts on platelets, as ticlopidine does, at a different site from aspirin by irreversibly inhibiting the binding of ADP to its platelet receptor, thereby preventing platelet activation and hence the transformation of the glycoprotein IIb/IIIa receptor into its active form (Fig. 9-3). Thus clopidogrel has assumed considerable importance in the treatment of acute coronary syndromes (Table 9-1; Fig. 9-5). Compared to ticlopidine, meta-analysis suggests a superior reduction of major adverse cardiac events,[43] to which may be added better tolerability (less gastrointestinal and allergic side effects). As with aspirin, clopidogrel resistance also occurs,[44] and one cause may be interaction with statins (see later).

Clinical Trials In *atherosclerotic vascular disease* the CAPRIE Trial,[45] on 19,185 patients given either aspirin 325 mg or clopidogrel 75 mg daily, showed an 8.7% reduction in the composite endpoint of ischemic stroke, myocardial infarction, or vascular death with clopidogrel. There was no excess of neutropenia with clopidogrel, and severe gastrointestinal bleeding was more common with aspirin. In *non-ST-elevation acute coronary syndromes*, regardless of whether they are managed conservatively or invasively, clopidogrel provides benefit (combined with aspirin). In the CURE trial of 12,562 patients, clopidogrel

ACUTE CORONARY SYNDROME

Opie 2004

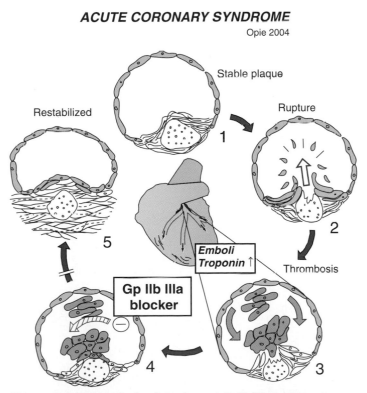

Figure 9-5 Proposed role of platelets and GpIIb/IIIa inhibitors in acute coronary syndromes. The sequence starts with rupture of the plaque, thrombosis, platelet activation, and aggregation (Fig. 9-3), followed by eventual restitution of the vascular endothelium, and a larger plaque. Note that there is no complete coronary occlusion as would be the case in acute myocardial infarction. Hypothetically, microembolization down the coronaries leads to release of troponin, the marker for high risk (Fig. 11-3).

Table 9-1 GP IIB/IIIA Receptor Antagonists: Key Pharmacological Properties

Compound and Indications	Supporting Trials	Pharmacokinetics	Doses (All with Aspirin and Heparin)*	Special Points	Side Effects and Contraindications
Abciximab 1. Percutaneous interventions (PCI) 2. Unstable angina requiring PCI within 24 hrs	CAPTURE EPIC EPILOG EPISTENT GUSTO4-ACS ADMIRAL ACE	Monoclonal antibody. High affinity to platelet receptor (low K_D); 67% bound to receptor; plasma $t\frac{1}{2}$ 10–30 min; remains platelet-bound in circulation up to 15 days with some residual activity	0.25 mg/kg bolus 10–60 before PCI, then 0.125 µg/kg/min up to max of 10 µg/min over 12 hrs, up to 24 hrs if ACS with planned PCI (stop 1 h after PCI)	Keep vials in cold (not frozen); filter bolus injection before use, use in-line filter for infusion; discard vial after use	Bleeding—most contraindications relate to risk of bleeding. Extra care at puncture sites. Thrombocytopenia (<100,000/µL) in 4.5% with standard dose heparin vs. 2.1% in placebo + heparin. Caution: platelet count before starting, 2–4 h after bolus and 24 h before discharge of patient. Hypersensitivity is rare.
Eptifibatide 1. Non-ST elevation acute coronary syndromes (ACS), also if PCI 2. PCI including stents	IMPACT-II PURSUIT ESPIRIT	Cyclic heptapeptide. Lower receptor affinity than others; plasma $t\frac{1}{2}$ 2–3 h; renal clearance 50%	In ACS, 180 µg/kg bolus, then 2 µg/kg/min up to 72 hrs; if PCI, continue until 18–24 h after PCI, max 96 h. For elective PCI, 180 µg/kg bolus just before PCI, infuse as above, repeat bolus after 10 min, continue infusion for 12–24 h	Store vials at 2–8°C but can keep at room temperature up to 2 months.	Bleeding, as above Renal disease: if creatinine clearance <50 ml/min or if serum creatinine >2 mg/dL. 180 µg/kg bolus then reduce dose to 1.0 µg/kg/min. For PCI, repeat bolus after 10 min. Thrombocytopenia risk probably similar to other agents (see text)
Tirofiban 1. Non-ST elevation acute coronary syndromes (ACS)	PRISM PRISM-Plus RESTORE TARGET TACTICS	Peptidomimetic nonpeptide. Intermediate affinity for receptor, closer to abciximab. Hence 35% unbound in circulation, renal (65%) and fecal (25%) clearance.	Two stage infusion: 0.4 µg/kg/min for 30 min, then 0.1 µg/kg/min throughout angiography and for 12–24 h after angioplasty.†	Store vials at room temperature, 25°C or 77°C protected from light (easiest to store)	Bleeding, as above Renal disease: ↓ dose if creatinine clearance <30 ml/min Thrombocytopenia: 1.5% vs. 0.6% heparin alone. Do platelet count before (C/I if count <150,000/µL), 6 h after initial dose, then daily, stop if platelets <90,000/µL

*For heparin doses, see text.
†For high dose bolus and infusion, see Valgimili et al. *J Am Coll Cardiol* 2004;44:14.

reduced the combined incidence of death, nonfatal myocardial infarction and stroke by 20% (*P* < 0.001) over an average 9-month follow-up period.[46] There was an excess of major bleeding with clopidogrel (3.7% versus 2.7%, *P* = 0.003). In the PCI-CURE trial of 2658 patients, pretreatment with clopidogrel for a median of 10 days prior to PCI reduced the combined 30-day incidence of death, nonfatal myocardial infarction, and urgent target vessel revascularization by 30% (*P* = 0.03).[47] Long-term benefit of clopidogrel plus aspirin after PCI was shown in the CREDO trial.[48] At 1 year, the composite end-point of death, myocardial infarction, or stroke was reduced by 27% in the clopidogrel group.

Pharmacokinetics Clopidogrel itself is an inactive prodrug that requires in vivo oxidation by the hepatic and/or intestinal cytochrome CYP3A4 isoenzyme, providing the basis for a possible and controversial *drug interaction* with those statins such as atorvastatin (but not pravastatin or rosuvastatin) also metabolized by this isoenzyme.[44,49,50] The onset of action on platelets occurs within hours of a single oral dose, but steady-state inhibition is only found between 3 and 7 days (package insert). A 600-mg *loading dose* of clopidogrel achieves maximal inhibition of platelets approximately in 2 hours,[51] whereas a 300-mg loading dose does not achieve maximal platelet inhibition until after 24 to 48 hours, both doses being more powerful than ticlopidine.[51] Even the 300-mg loading dose gives better clinical results than no loading and than ticlopidine,[52] which might explain why one study that gave no loading dose found a better clinical outcome with ticlopidine.[53] Kinetics of clopidogrel are nonlinear, with a markedly decreased clearance on repeated dosing. When dosing is stopped, it takes about 5 days for the effect on platelets to wear off.

Indications, Dose, and Use Clopidogrel is indicated for (1) *reduction of atherosclerotic events* (myocardial infarction, stroke, vascular death) in patients with atherosclerosis documented by recent stroke, recent myocardial infarction, or with established peripheral arterial disease; and (2) for *acute coronary syndromes* whether or not percutaneous intervention (PCI) (with or without stent) or coronary artery bypass grafting (CABG) is applied. In practice it is also used for aspirin resistance or intolerance, and for elective PCI.[54] Clopidogrel (300 to 600 mg orally and then 75 mg/day) should be considered in all patients with non-ST-elevation acute coronary syndromes, but because it increases bleeding, it is not given when urgent CABG is likely. A reasonable alternative approach is to withhold clopidogrel until the coronary anatomy is known and if PCI is planned to give a 600-mg loading dose which has a maximal antiplatelet effect within 2 hours.[51] All such patients should have expeditious angiography. An early invasive approach (within 4 to 48 hours) is associated with improved outcomes in patients with ST-segment depression, diabetes, or elevated troponin T levels.[55] No dose adjustment of clopidogrel is needed for the elderly nor with renal impairment (package insert). After PCI, clopidogrel gives benefit at least 1 year when added to low-dose aspirin.[48] Clopidogrel may be used as a loading dose of 600 mg before PCI in low-risk patients with coronary disease.[54] Clopidogrel has *side effects* similar to those of aspirin without evidence of significant neutropenia or thrombocytopenia. However, neutropenia at a very low rate of 0.02% cannot be excluded, versus 2.4% for ticlopidine (package inserts). The real cost of the benefits of clopidogrel lies in increased serious extracranial bleeds.[18] *Contraindication:* active bleeding. In summary, clopidogrel is an effective agent, safer than ticlopidine, and often added to aspirin to obtain better platelet inhibition and clinical results. For elective PCI, it may be able to replace GpIIb/IIIa blockers.

Dipyridamole and Sulfinpyrazone

In general, platelet inhibition by dipyridamole with or without aspirin or sulfinpyrazone with or without aspirin, produces results very similar to those seen with aspirin alone.[18] By contrast, clopidogrel or ticlopidine add to the effects of aspirin, reducing vascular events by about 20%.[18] Therefore *dipyridamole* is no longer the non-aspirin antiplatelet agent of choice. The only licensed indication of dipyridamole is for prosthetic mechanical valves, in combination with anticoagulation by warfarin.[56] It might help to reduce repeat stroke when combined with aspirin,[57] and this is the subject of an ongoing European-Australian trial. Note the dangerous drug interaction of dipyridamole with adenosine (see Chapter 8). *Sulfinpyrazone* inhibits cyclo-oxygenase, with effects similar to those of aspirin yet more expensive than aspirin. It requires multiple daily doses, and has no benefit in patients already on aspirin.[18] However, in contrast to aspirin it is also a uricosuric agent. In the United States, the only licensed indication is chronic or intermittent gouty arthritis.

GLYCOPROTEIN IIb/IIIa RECEPTOR ANTAGONISTS

These agents inhibit the platelet glycoprotein Gp IIb/IIIa receptor, one of the integrin adhesion receptors that is technically known the $\alpha_{IIb}\beta_3$ receptor (Fig. 9-3).[58] There are three IIb/IIIa antagonists: abciximab, tirofiban, and eptifibatide, with somewhat different approved indications in the United States (Table 9-2). They have all been studied on a background of aspirin and antithrombotic therapy (Table 9-1). As a group they involve risk of increased bleeding, rarely even fatal,[59] especially at the arterial access site when there is cardiac catheterization. All may cause rare but serious thrombocytopenia.[60] All are contraindicated in the presence of a bleeding site or bleeding potential, or preexisting thrombocytopenia. All are administered with either enoxaparin or low-dose intravenous unfractionated heparin controlled by activated partial thromboplastin times (aPPT) or by activated clotting times (ACT). All are given intravenously and only for a limited time, to tide the patient through the clinical acute coronary syndrome or to cover the intervention. Unless given to selected higher risk patients, their use in acute coronary syndromes can be disappointing. Thus far, oral IIb/IIIa inhibitors have had neutral or negative results in large trials, emphasizing that these agents must be given intravenously.

Table 9-2	Antiplatelet and Antithrombotic Therapy in Acute Coronary Syndromes (ACS) and in Percutaneous Coronary Intervention (PCI)		
Condition	**Antiplatelet Agents**	**Antithrombotics**	**Fibrinolytics**
ACS	Aspirin, Clopidogrel (if no CABG)	Heparin or LMWH	None
ACS, high risk*	Above, plus Eptifibatide/tirofiban	Heparin or LMWH	None
PCI	Aspirin, Clopidogrel	Heparin or LMWH	None
PCI, high risk[†]	Above, plus Abciximab/ Eptifibatide	Heparin or LMWH[‡]	None

*Elevated troponins, ischemic ST-depression or similar, ongoing ischemia.
[†]ACS, recent MI, bypass-graft stenosis, chronically occluded coronary arteries, angiographic intracoronary stenosis (for definitions and details of doses, see Lange and Hillis, *N Engl J Med*, 2004;350:277–280).
[‡]For advantages and risks of LMWH, see SYNERGY.[100]
CABG = coronary artery bypass graft; LMWH = low-molecular-weight heparin.

Clinical Trials Various clinical trials have shown the consistent beneficial effects of IIb/IIIa antagonists in patients presenting with *acute coronary syndromes (ACS) without ST-elevation,* that is, unstable angina or
non-ST-elevation myocardial infarction (see Fig. 11-3). In a meta-
analysis of 16 randomized trials of IIb/IIIa antagonists, involving
a total of 32,135 patients, mortality was reduced by 30% at 48 to
96 hours ($P < 0.03$). Longer term, at 6 months, the composite end-
point of death/myocardial infarction/revascularization was only
reduced by 10%.[61] It should, moreover, be emphasized that there were
few deaths and that the majority of "myocardial infarcts" were diagnosed only by elevated serum biomarkers.

Mortality Two meta-analyses suggest mortality reduction of about 15%
to 30% when these agents are combined with PCI.[62,63] Abciximab
combined with stenting reduces mortality when compared with stenting alone.[64,65]

ACS Without Planned PCI The IIb/IIIa antagonists have also been tested
on a background of aspirin therapy in approximately 18,000 patients
with unstable angina in whom percutaneous interventions were not
planned. With approximately 2200 end-points and an 11% reduction
in death or myocardial infarction at 30 days, the evidence strongly
supports the use of these agents in most patients presenting at high
or intermediate risk, that is, those presenting within 24 hours of the
latest episode of prolonged pain, rest pain, or increasingly frequent
angina on minimal exertion. Triage according to the degree of risk is
increasingly accepted, although there as yet no prospective studies
base on such triage. Judging from retrospective analysis, the patients
most likely to benefit are those undergoing early percutaneous coronary interventions, those with ST-segment changes on the admission
electrocardiogram, and those with abnormal troponin levels.[66-68]
In the PRISM-Plus Study,[69] patients with intracoronary thrombus
were at high risk. Other high-risk patients, such as diabetics or those
already on aspirin therapy at admission, are also likely to obtain
benefit from treatment.[67] In those at lower risk, there is no evidence
of benefit.

Acute Coronary Syndrome with Planned PCI Three trials show the value of
starting IIb/IIIa antagonists prior to PCI.[67,70,71] There was an overall
34% reduction in death or myocardial infarction (from 3.8% with
placebo to 2.5%) prior to the intervention, and a further incremental
48% reduction during the 48 hours following the procedure.[72]

Stenting Plus IIb/IIIa Blockade The combination of stenting and IIb/IIIa
blockade by abciximab gives better 6-month outcome results than
stenting alone or balloon angioplasty plus abciximab.[73] Especially
impressive were the results in the diabetic subgroup, in whom
other previous data suggests that PCI without IIb/IIIa blockade is
less effective than bypass grafting. Conversely, in nondiabetic
patients there was no benefit, using repeat revascularization as an
end-point.[73]

Combination with Unfractionated or Low-Molecular-Weight Heparin In almost
all the major trials thus far reported, the IIb/IIIa antagonists have been
added to background therapy by aspirin and unfractionated heparin.
This in turn calls for constant monitoring of the heparin dose by aPPT
or ACT testing, with weight-adjusted low dose heparin dosing. In a
pilot study of 746 patients with non-ST-elevation acute coronary syndrome randomized to receive either unfractionated heparin or enoxaparin on a background of aspirin plus eptifibatide, enoxaparin was
associated with lower rates of major bleeding (1.8% versus 4.6%, $P = 0.03$), ischemia on ST-segment monitoring within the first 48 hours
(14.0% versus 25.1%, $P = 0.0002$), and death or myocardial infarc-
tion (5.0% versus 9.0%, $P = 0.03$).[74] In another study, on high-risk

patients with acute coronary syndromes receiving aspirin and tirofiban, enoxaparin was noninferior to unfractionated heparin.[75]

Abciximab

Abciximab *(ReoPro)* is a monoclonal antibody against the IIb/IIIa receptor. It consists of a murine variable portion of the Fab fragment combined with the human constant region. Abciximab also blocks the binding of vitronectin to its receptor ($\alpha_v\beta_3$) on endothelial cells, but it is not known whether this has any therapeutic advantage. Inhibition of platelet aggregation is maximal at 2 hours after a bolus injection, and returns to almost normal at 12 hours. However, the antibody is transmitted to new platelets and can be detected 14 days after administration. Its action can be reversed by repeated platelet transfusions. Abciximab is very effective in patients undergoing percutaneous interventions,[64,65,70,76,77] which is currently its only license in the United States, unless dealing with unstable angina not responding to medical therapy with PCI planned within 24 hours (Table 9-2). If there is no PCI, there is no benefit of abciximab (GUSTO-4-ACS study; see Table 11-1). A controversial use of abciximab is with stenting in ST-elevation MI, the large CADILLAC trial giving no added outcome benefit when given at the time of PCI, and the smaller ACE study giving the benefit to abciximab (see Table 11-3). In the ADMIRAL trial (see Table 11-3), abciximab given in the emergency room or prehospital showed benefit. Also in MI, abciximab with half dose of a lytic agent gave some benefit at the cost of increased bleeding (GUSTO-5 study; see Table 11-3).

Dose, Side Effects, and Contraindications An initial bolus is followed by an infusion to a maximum of 24 hours (Table 9-2). Careful control of heparin is important to lessen bleeding, using a reduced dose as with all GpIIb/IIIa inhibitors. In EPILOG[77] heparin was given as an initial bolus of 70 U/kg, or less according to the initial ACT time (maximum initial bolus, 7000 units), followed by 20 U/kg boluses as needed to keep the ACT at 200 seconds (see package insert). Acute severe *thrombocytopenia* (platelet count of <20,000), a class side effect, occurs in approximately 0.5% to 1.0% of patients.[54] It is therefore very important that platelet counts are performed in the first few hours after beginning the infusion. There have been concerns about antibody formation with readministration of abciximab, which may cause severe thrombocytopenia in about 2.4%.[78] Thus previous thrombocytopenia is a clear *contraindication* to readministration, and, as there are alternative effective IIb/IIIa blockers available, these should be considered if such blockade is needed. If thrombocytopenia occurs, platelet aggregation returns to 50% of baseline within 1 day in most patients.

Tirofiban

Tirofiban *(Aggrastat)* is a highly specific nonpeptide peptidomimetic IIb/IIIa inhibitor, inherently less likely to cause hypersensitivity than a monoclonal antibody. Nonetheless the end result of both methods of blockade is inhibition of fibrinogen and Von Willebrand factor binding to the IIb/IIIa receptor (Fig. 9-3). It has an acute onset and a half-life of about 2 hours. Indications, dosage, side effects, and contraindications are in Table 9-2. In the TACTICS trial on patients with unstable angina, tirofiban with PCI was compared to tirofiban alone, and the combination was better except for the low-risk group of patients, arguing for the value of risk assessment in acute coronary syndromes (see Fig. 11-3). *Heparin* must be carefully controlled. In PRISM-Plus, the initial bolus of unfractionated heparin was 5000 units, followed by 1000 U/hour to keep the aPPT twice the control value.[67] Tirofiban is licensed only for ACS, but is the easiest of the three agents to store (vials at room temperature). Increased bleeding is given in the tirofiban package insert as the most common adverse event. In those who received heparin and tirofiban the incidence of severe thrombocytopenia ($<$50,000/mm^3) was 0.3% versus 0.1% for those who received heparin alone (package insert).

Comparison with Abciximab In patients receiving triple antiplatelet therapy (aspirin, clopidogrel, and a IIb/IIIa inhibitor) plus heparin, tirofiban was compared with abciximab in 4812 patients undergoing PCI for an acute coronary syndrome or for stable angina.[79] The tirofiban dose was 10 µg/kg bolus and 0.15 µg/kg/minute infusion for 18 to 24 hours (more than in the package insert; see Table 9-2) and the abciximab dose was a bolus of 0.25 mg/kg, followed by an infusion of 0.125 µg/kg for 12 hours, as in the package insert. By 30 days, myocardial infarction had occurred in 6.9% of tirofiban patients versus 5.4% of abciximab patients (P = 0.04). Minor bleeding was more frequent with abciximab (5.6% versus 3.3% with tirofiban, P = 0.002), which suggests that abciximab was more effective in inhibiting platelet activity than tirofiban. At 6-month follow-up of the TARGET trial,[79] there was no difference in the composite end-point of death, myocardial infarction, or urgent revascularization. Thus, overall, and at these doses, and long-term, the agents were equal.

Eptifibatide

Eptifibatide *(Integrilin)* is a synthetic cyclic heptapeptide. Structural differences from tirofiban mean that they bind at different sites on the receptor, yet with the same end-result. The affinity for the receptor is, however, lower than with the other IIb/IIIa blockers, which explains the higher dose in absolute terms. Indications, dosage, side effects, and contraindications are in Table 9-2. Unfractionated heparin was given in the PURSUIT trial as a bolus of 5000 units (weight adjusted), and then infused at 1000 U/hour to keep the aPPT at between 50 and 70.[71] As for all IIb/IIIa blockers, the major problem is increased bleeding. Although the package insert claims that thrombocytopenia ($<$100,000/mm^3) is not increased, in PURSUIT[71] profound platelet depression ($<$20,000/mm^3) occurred in 0.3% eptifibatide versus 0.1% in controls, both groups receiving aspirin and heparin. Thus, thrombocytopenia is a risk as with other IIb/IIIa blockers. Eptifibatide is currently the only IIb/IIIa blocker that is licensed for both ACS and for PCI.

Current Status of Gp IIb/IIIa Blockers These agents, combined with aspirin and heparin, benefit patients who have acute coronary syndromes without ST-elevation (Fig. 9-5) yet with high risk of myocardial infarction, such as those with elevated troponin levels, in whom intervention by PCI is also indicated. In low risk patients they do not give added benefit beyond aspirin and heparin. Their use in acute myocardial infarction with stenting is controversial. When correctly used, they do appear to be relatively cost-effective.[65,80]

ACUTE ANTICOAGULATION: HEPARIN

Mechanism of Action and Use

Heparin is a heterogeneous mucopolysaccharide with extremely complex effects on the coagulation mechanism and on blood vessels. It also exerts indirect antiplatelet effects by binding to and inhibiting von Willebrand factor. Furthermore, chronic heparin administration has poorly-understood effects in lessening experimental atheroma and in promoting angiogenesis.[81] The major effect of heparin is on the interaction of antithrombin-III and thrombin, to inhibit the thrombin-induced platelet aggregation that initiates unstable angina and venous thrombosis (Fig. 9-6). Inhibition of thrombin by heparin requires: (1) binding of heparin to antithrombin-III by a unique

THROMBOSIS AND LYSIS

Opie 2004

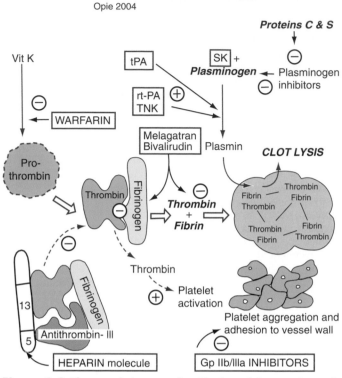

Figure 9-6 The coagulation cascade with sites of therapeutic attack. Crucial to the formation of the clot is the conversion of fibrinogen into fibrin and the binding of fibrin to thrombin, followed by crossbinding of fibrin. Antithrombin-III prevents the binding of fibrinogen to thrombin, and hence is an anticoagulant. **Heparin** promotes the activity of antithrombin-III. Warfarin works by inhibiting the production of prothrombin. Once fibrin is thrombin-bound, heparin has no effect, because antithrombin-III no longer interacts with thrombin. Hirudin acts by inhibiting the interaction of fibrinogen and thrombin. To break down the fibrin-thrombin combination requires fibrinolytics. **Fibrinolytics** act by promoting the conversion of plasminogen to plasmin, which is fibrinolytic. Plasminogen activators include *tPA* (alteplase), reteplase (*rt-PA*), tenecteplase (*TNK*), or the streptokinase (*SK*)-plasminogen complex. They all catalyze the conversion of plasminogen to plasmin. *tPA* = tissue-type plasminogen activator; *Gp* = glycoprotein; *Vit K* = vitamin K. (*Figure © LH Opie, 2005.*)

pentasaccharide segment of the heparin molecule; and (2) simultaneous binding of heparin to thrombin by 13 additional saccharide units.[82] Heparin-antithrombin-III also inhibits factor Xa and a number of other clotting factors. The dose-effect relationship is difficult to predict because heparin is a heterogeneous group of molecules extracted by a variety of procedures, and its strength varies from batch to batch. Heparin also binds variably to plasma proteins, endothelial cells, and macrophages. Such binding inactivates some of the heparin, the remainder leaving the circulation by the renal route. These complexities, added to the difficulty of controlling the dose, mean that heparin is far from ideal as an intravenous anticoagulant.

Intravenous Unfractionated Heparin The standard intravenous regimen for use in acute myocardial infarction or unstable angina is a 5000 IU intravenous bolus, followed by 1000 IU/hour in patients weighing ≥80 kg and 800 IU/hour in those weighing <80 kg,[83] maintained for 48 hours or more,[84] with the dose adjusted according to the aPPT (see next section). The heparin may be diluted in either isotonic saline or dextrose water (which may be better in acute myocardial infarction). Ultra-low-dose intravenous heparin (1 IU/kg/hour for 3 to 5 days, or about 1700 IU/day) seems to be as effective as other methods in preventing postoperative deep vein thrombosis.

Controlling the Dose of Intravenous Heparin When heparin is administered after fibrinolytic therapy to patients with acute myocardial infarction[85] or unstable angina,[86] meticulous laboratory control of the heparin dose is required to maintain the aPPT between 1.5 and 2.0 times normal, or between 50 and 75 seconds, with monitoring at 6, 12, and 24 hours.[85] Higher aPPTs increase the risk of cerebral bleeding without conferring any survival advantage.[85,87] The use of nomograms results in fewer subtherapeutic aPPTs, and there may also be less bleeding. If the aPPT is 3 times the control value, the infusion rate should be decreased by 50%; if 2 to 3 times the control value, the infusion rate should be decreased by 25%; if 1.5 to 2 times the control value, there should be no change. If the aPPT is less than 1.5 times the control value, the infusion should be increased by 25% to a maximum rate of 2500 IU/hour. At the same time, overheparinization should be guarded against to avoid cerebral bleeding. The inherent limitation of the aPPT is that different commercial reagents give different aPPT values.[82] In practice the activated clotting time (ACT) is often used (see later).

Subcutaneous Unfractionated Heparin This route is as good as any other for the treatment of deep vein thrombosis, unless it is proximal.[82] After the initial intravenous loading dose, heparin may be given as a deep subcutaneous injection of 10,000 IU 8-hourly or 15,000 IU 12-hourly, using a different site at each rotation. The required dose is about 10% higher than with the intravenous route. Low-dose subcutaneous heparin is adequate in the prophylaxis of surgical thromboembolism, where the schedule is 5000 IU subcutaneously 2 to 8 hours prior to operation and then every 12 hours for 7 days.[82]

Heparin: Precautions and Side Effects There is an increased risk of heparin-induced hemorrhage in patients with subacute bacterial endocarditis or hematological disorders such as hemophilia, hepatic disease, or gastrointestinal or genitourinary ulcerative lesions. There is a narrow therapeutic window for the use of heparin in conjunction with fibrinolytic therapy.[87,88] To avoid intracerebral hemorrhage, the recommended doses of heparin should not be exceeded. Platelet abnormalities may also, paradoxically, predispose towards heparin thrombosis, characterized by a "white clot."[89] Some patients are *resistant to heparin*, and in these patients administration of high-dose heparin with aPPT monitoring every 4 hours is advised. Heparin is derived from animal tissue, and occasionally causes allergy. *Heparin overdosage* is treated by stopping the drug and, if clinically required, giving protamine sulfate (1% solution) as a very slow infusion of no more than 50 mg in any 10-minute period.

Heparin-Induced Thrombocytopenia and Thrombosis Syndrome (HITS or HITTS) This occurs in about 10% of patients after heparin treatment for 5 days or more, but is usually reversible on heparin withdrawal. The diagnosis is made when the platelet count drops by 50% or more. Usually, the thrombocytopenia is asymptomatic and transient (HIT type 1). Sometimes there is an immune-mediated potentially fatal syndrome in which the immunoglobulins bridge platelets causing both thrombocytopenia and thrombosis (HIT type 2).[90] Heparin or low-molecular-weight heparin (LMWH) must be discontinued on suspicion, and if continued acute anticoagulation is needed, a heparinoid or a direct thrombin inhibitor may be used. In the United States, *lepirudin* is licensed for HIT. Elsewhere, *danaparoid* is a heparinoid commonly used. Other treatment options are bivalirudin (not yet licensed in the

United States for this purpose), r-hirudin, argatroban, dextransulfate, and dermatansulfate.

Indications for Heparin

Acute Myocardial Infarction Heparin is given together with thrombolysis or primary angioplasty. Early high-dose heparin, prior to coronary angioplasty, does not restore coronary patency, contrary to earlier claims from a pilot study.[91] In patients with borderline heart failure, sodium loading can be avoided by the use of calcium heparin (Calciparine, 5000 to 20,000 USP units/ampoule) and by diluting heparin in dextrose water rather than in saline.

Heparin in Acute Coronary Syndromes Unfractionated heparin remains the gold standard in acute coronary syndromes, although under severe challenge by LMWH. In patients with unstable angina, dose-adjusted heparin added to aspirin helps to prevent myocardial infarction.[92] An intravenous bolus of 5000 IU should be given followed by an infusion of 1000 IU/hour,[92] and after 6 hours the dose should be adjusted to an aPPT of 1.5 to 2.0 times baseline, or 50 to 75 seconds, and continued for 2 to 7 days.[86] Reinfarction may occur following the cessation of intravenous heparin as a result of *"heparin rebound"*[92] and the procoagulant state that ensues. Rebound, worse within 24 hours of heparin cessation, also occurs with LMWH and could be lessened by gradual weaning from the heparin preparation used, together with delayed patient discharge after heparin cessation.[93]

Heparin in PCIs Although no placebo-controlled trials have been performed, heparin is indicated because of the risk of acute thrombotic closure. The standard heparin regimen is 100 IU/kg, with additional weight-adjusted boluses to achieve and maintain an activated clotting time (ACT) of 300 seconds. Alternatively, further boluses can be given if the procedure is prolonged beyond 1 hour. In Europe, higher doses (140 IU/kg) are used with no monitoring of the ACT and no additional heparin during the procedure.[54] If a Gp IIb/IIIa antagonist is coadministered, a low-dose, weight-adjusted heparin regimen is recommended. For example, with abciximab an initial bolus of 70 IU/kg is followed by additional boluses of 20 U/kg to maintain an activated clotting time of at least 200 seconds.[77] Heparin should be discontinued immediately after the interventional procedure.

Anticoagulation in Pregnant Women Unfractionated or low-molecular-weight heparin should be used (see Table 11-8), but unfractionated heparin can cause osteoporosis if given in doses of >20,000 IU daily for more than 5 months.[82]

Low-Molecular-Weight Heparins

These agents are about one third of the molecular weight of heparin, and are also heterogeneous in size. LMWHs have greater bioavailability and a longer plasma half-life than standard heparin. Approximately 25% to 30% of the molecules of various preparations contain the crucial 18 or more saccharide units needed to bind to both antithrombin-III and thrombin. In addition, they bind effectively to and inhibit factor Xa (Fig. 9-6). The ratio of LMWHs binding to antithrombin III and inhibition of factor Xa:IIa (where IIa is activated prothrombin) varies with each agent; for example, 2:1 with dalteparin and 3:1 with enoxaprin.[94] The bleeding side effects of LMWHs can be reduced by administration of protamine sulfate, although anti-Xa activity is not completely neutralized. LMWHs can be given subcutaneously in a fixed dose once daily, hence are much easier to use than standard unfractionated heparin. But, are they safer and better?

Dalteparin (Fragmin) This agent comes in a single-dose prefilled syringe or as multidose vials. Each syringe contains 2500 to 10,000 international units of antifactor Xa (see Fig. 9-4) equal to 16 to 64 mg of dalteparin. It is given as a deep subcutaneous injection and NOT (as the manufacturers stress) intramuscularly. In the FRISC study the dose was 120 IU twice daily plus aspirin for 6 days, then 7500 IU for 35 to 45 days, starting on admission for unstable angina. At 6 days the composite end-point of death or myocardial infarction was reduced from 4.8% with aspirin to 1.8% with dalteparin plus aspirin ($P = 0.001$),[95] but by 6 months these differences were no longer apparent. Compared with dose-adjusted heparin given over 1 week, dalteparin was no better (package insert). Dalteparin was also part of early invasive policy, at similar doses and continued for 3 months.[96] In the United States, dalteparin is licensed for prevention of ischemic complications in unstable angina and non-Q wave myocardial infarction, and for prevention of deep vein thrombosis. It is contraindicated by major bleeding or thrombocytopenia or past HIT syndrome. There is a boxed warning against its use with spinal anesthesia. Pregnancy, category B (Table 11-8).

Enoxaparin (Lovenox) This agent, also given by subcutaneous injection, comes in concentrations of 100 or 150 mg/ml, in prefilled single-dose syringes or as ampules. Indications are similar to those for dalteparin, with also treatment of acute deep vein thrombosis. Warnings are similar to those for dalteparin plus warning against use with prosthetic valves especially in pregnant women (pregnancy category B). The dose for unstable angina is 1 mg/kg every 12 hours with aspirin for a minimum of 2 days and continued until the patient is stable. This drug has been well-studied in several major trials (see next section). It is excreted renally. Risks for bleeding are severe renal impairment (creatinine clearance <30 ml/min), increasing age, female gender, and cotherapy with NSAIDs, or aspirin and especially clopidogrel. Dose reduction, to lessen these risks must be individualized, but could be by 50% or even more. Contraindications include prior major bleeding or HIT, thrombocytopenia, and spinal anesthesia (boxed warning).

Acute Coronary Syndromes Several trials show the superiority or equivalence of LMWH to unfractionated heparin. Most trials have used enoxaparin, and because of differences between the agents the results cannot be generalized to class effects. Compared with unfractionated heparin in two trials on non-ST-elevation acute coronary syndromes, ESSENCE and TIMI-11B, enoxaparin reduced the combined end-points of death/MI/urgent revascularization, and the benefit was still apparent at 2 years.[97] A prespecified meta-analysis showed a 23% relative reduction in death or myocardial infarction at day 8 ($P = 0.02$), with a similar reduction at 43 days.[98] In the Aggrastat to Zocor (A to Z) trial on high-risk patients with acute coronary syndromes, patients received either enoxaparin or unfractionated heparin on a background of aspirin and tirofiban.[75] The results fulfilled the prespecified noninferiority criteria. *Heparin rebound* also occurs with LMWH and may be lessened by gradual weaning and/or by delayed patient discharge for observation after LMWH cessation.[93]

PCIs The Superior Yield of the New Strategy of Enoxaparin, Revascularization and Glycoprotein IIb/IIIa Inhibitors (SYNERGY) trial randomized 9978 high-risk patients undergoing a planned early invasive treatment strategy to receive either unfractionated heparin or enoxaparin.[99] The primary composite end-point of death or myocardial infarction at 30 days was similar in the two groups. There was also no difference in the number of abrupt closures or unsuccessful procedures. The trial also showed that crossing over from one antithrombin to another was associated with worse outcomes and increased bleeding. However, the greater convenience of enoxaparin was bought at the cost of increased bleeding. In those undergoing bypass surgery, the modest increase in bleeding with enoxaparin was nonsignificant. Some interventionalists will regard this risk of bleeding as tolerable, and will feel free to give enoxaparin to all high-risk patients with acute coronary syndrome (see Fig. 11-3). Others will continue to prefer unfractionated heparin as the drug of choice.

Choice of Low-Molecular-Weight or Unfractionated Heparin Low-molecular-weight heparin is in general preferred to unfractionated heparin because it is convenient, inexpensive, and eliminates the need for aPPT monitoring, and avoids the problem of intravenous site infections. A systematic review of 21,946 patients showed the superiority of enoxaparin over unfractionated heparin.[100] However, other LMWHs have different properties so that there still is uncertainty about the comparison of LMWHs as a class with unfractionated heparin, yet it is difficult to ignore the evidence favoring enoxaparin. In community hospitals without catheterization facilities, LMWH could be administered prior to transfer of patients for revascularization procedures. In patients undergoing PCI, the role and safety of LMWH has been clarified by the SYNERGY trial. Many interventionalists feel that the inability to monitor the degree of anticoagulation with LMWH in contrast to unfractionated heparin is at present a potential disadvantage when PCI is undertaken.

Thrombolysis with LMWH versus Unfractionated Heparin Can LMWH be used with benefit in acute myocardial infarction? In the AMI-SK study,[101] streptokinase plus enoxaparin gave better early angiographic patency than streptokinase alone with fewer clinical events at 30 days. Major bleeding increased from 2.5% to 4.8% ($P = 0.13$). The ASSENT-3 and ASSENT-3 Plus trials examined the combination of the fibrinolytic agent tenecteplase (TNK) conveniently given as a single bolus, and LMWH enoxaparin, also easy to give. In both studies the enoxaparin reduced the primary end-point defined as death, reinfarction or refractory ischemia at 30 days, significantly ($P < 0.001$) in the larger in-hospital study[102] yet only with a trend ($P = 0.08$) in the out-of-hospital study.[103] Intracranial hemorrhage increased especially in patients older than 75 years of age (6.7% versus 0.8% with unfractionated heparin). In another similar but small comparative trial, the enoxaparin plus TNK group had markedly fewer cardiac events within 30 days (4.4% versus 15.9% in the unfractionated heparin group, $P = 0.005$), without any difference in major bleeding.[104] Thus, on balance, enoxaparin did better than unfractionated heparin. Yet, given the increased bleeding rates seen with enoxaparin in the ASSENT-3 Plus trial, and the need to define the bleeding risks of high-risk subgroups (e.g., the elderly, women, patients with low bodyweight and patients with renal dysfunction), further trials will be needed to evaluate low-molecular-weight heparins in conjunction with new fibrinolytic regimens.

Direct Thrombin Inhibitors

The direct thrombin inhibitors, such as hirudin and bivalirudin (previously known as hirulog), directly inhibit soluble and clot-bound thrombin without depending on antithrombin III for anticoagulant activity. They have high specificity and potency for thrombin inhibition, and do not promote platelet aggregation. At therapeutic concentrations that prolong the aPPT to twice normal, heparin inhibits only 20% to 40% of clot-bound thrombin activity, whereas direct thrombin inhibitors achieve at least 70% inhibition.[105]

Lepirudin (Refludan) This recombinant hirudin is licensed only for HIT and the associated thromboembolic disorder to prevent further thromboembolism. It is contraindicated in pregnancy (category B) and in breast feeding, with a bold-font warning against use with thrombolytic agents or in bleeding disorders. To avoid the occasional development of anaphylactoid shock[105a] that may occur with the recommended initial bolus dose (0.4 mg/kg), the bolus is omitted and replaced by a reduced dose infusion (0.1 mg/kg/h) that is adjusted by the aPPT (1.5 to 2.5). It is almost exclusively cleared in the kidneys, so that renal impairment calls for lower doses (see package insert for table). For *unstable angina* in the OASIS-2 Study, patients were randomized to receive either lepirudin or heparin both groups also given aspirin.[106] Lepirudin reduced the rate of death and reinfarction at 3 days, at the cost of increased major bleeding requiring transfusion.

Bivalirudin (Angiomax) Thus far bivalirudin, previously called hirulog, is the only anticoagulant that reduces both the ischemic and the bleeding complications associated with PCI.[107] It is easy to use, inactivates thrombin and blocks thrombin-mediated platelet activation and aggregation (Fig. 9-6).[107] The fact that bivalirudin binds reversibly to thrombin may explain its safety profile advantage over heparin and hirudin.[108] Nonetheless, its only licensed use in the United States is for unstable angina when it should be given with aspirin and strictly speaking only to patients undergoing balloon angioplasty. Safety and efficacy has not been shown when given together with IIb/IIIa blockers. Despite this limiting label, in a meta-analysis of six trials totalling 5674 patients, 4603 of whom underwent elective PCIs, bivalirudin reduced the risk of death or myocardial infarction by almost 30% at 30 to 50 days, equivalent to 14 fewer events per 1000 patients treated ($P < 0.02$).[109] There was also a 60% reduction in major bleeding, with 58 fewer events per 1000 patients treated ($P < 0.001$).

In patients undergoing elective PCI with a stent, bivalirudin is an effective alternative to unfractionated heparin plus a IIb/IIIa blocker, all the patients receiving aspirin and clopidogrel, as judged by a 30-day follow up.[28] Again, major bleeding was less common with bivalirudin (2.4% versus 4.1%, $P < 0.001$). The 6-month follow-up, presented verbally, found that the survival curves seemed to be separating in favor of bivalirudin, with 1-year results to come. The bivalirudin dose was 0.75 mg/kg prior to the intervention followed by an infusion of 1.75 mg/hour for the duration of the procedure. Overall, for urgent PCI it is a *cost-effective alternative to heparin plus IIb/IIIa blockade*. The question as to whether better outcomes can be achieved by the addition of IIb/IIIa antagonists will be addressed by the ACUITY trial. For evaluation in acute myocardial infarction, more studies are also needed. Bivalirudin added to streptokinase in the HERO-2 trial reduced the rate of reinfarction compared with unfractionated heparin, yet (in contrast to other studies) bleeding increased somewhat.[110]

Novel Long-Term Anticoagulants

Fondaparinux (Arixstra) This synthetic pentasaccharide is an antithrombin-dependent indirect inhibitor of activated factor X (Xa) (Fig. 9-4). It has a longer half life (approximately 15 hours) than unfractionated or low-molecular-weight heparin, and needs no monitoring. In the United States it is licensed only for prevention of deep vein thrombosis. The risk of hemorrhage increases with impaired renal function, when the dose must be reduced. Thrombocytopenia can occur and platelet counts should be monitored. The dose is 2.5 mg daily, subcutaneously. In the PENTALYSE study,[111] 326 patients with ST-elevation MI treated with alteplase were randomized to receive either fondaparinux, first intravenously, and then subcutaneously, in various doses or unfractionated heparin. At 90 minutes there was no difference in coronary patency, judged by TIMI flow grades. At 6 days there were trends toward less reocclusion and more major bleeding with fondaparinux. Bigger trials are needed.

Ximelagatran (Exanta) Not yet available commercially, this is an oral direct thrombin inhibitor (Fig. 9-6) that is rapidly metabolized to its active form, melagatran. Because its metabolism and excretion through the kidneys are independent of the hepatic cytochrome P450 enzyme system, there is little potential for interaction with other drugs. No coagulation monitoring is necessary, hence it is a potential replacement for warfarin. Doses of 24 to 30 mg twice daily are effective for the prevention and treatment of venous thromboembolism.

To prevent repeat coronary events after a recent myocardial infarction, ximelagatran was compared with placebo, both plus aspirin in the ESTEEM trial.[103] At 6 months the combined incidence of death, MI, and recurrent ischemia was reduced in absolute terms by 3.6% and in relative terms by 24% by ximelagatran, with no evidence of a dose response over the range 24 to 60 mg twice daily. Major and minor bleeding increased from 13% to 22%. As seen in other ximelagatran trials, about 5% of patients developed elevated alanine transaminase levels between 2 and 6 months after the start of treatment.

When tested in patients with atrial fibrillation in the SPORTIF-III study, ximelagatran (36 mg twice daily) was associated with similar bleeding and decreased stroke and systemic embolization events rates, when compared to those seen with adjusted-dose warfarin.[112] SPORTIF-V, with nearly 4000 patients with nonvalvular atrial fibrillation and one other stroke risk factor, has now been verbally reported. Taken together with the earlier trial, there is noninferiority of ximelagatran to warfarin for the risk of stroke and systemic embolization with the benefit of less major bleeding, but a sevenfold excess of liver damage.[113] The latter typically resolves spontaneously or on drug withdrawal, but requires monitoring of liver function for the first 6 months and periodically thereafter. Otherwise, this agent is potentially very attractive as a warfarin replacement because it has no apparent interactions with other drugs and needs no monitoring, thus being much more convenient for doctor and patient.

ORAL ANTICOAGULATION: WARFARIN

Warfarin (Coumarin, Coumadin, Panwarfin) is the most commonly used oral anticoagulant because a single dose produces stable anticoagulation as a result of excellent oral absorption and a circulating half-life of about 37 hours. Warfarin also has remarkably few side effects, apart from bleeding. However, it interacts with many other drugs. In general, when comparing warfarin with aspirin, higher intensity warfarin is more effective, but associated with more bleeding. Low intensity warfarin and aspirin are approximately equal in efficacy and safety.[114]

Mechanism of Action As a group, the oral anticoagulants inactivate vitamin K in the hepatic microsomes, thereby interfering with the formation of vitamin K-dependent clotting factors such as prothrombin (Fig. 9-6). In addition factor X may be reduced.[114] Because of the long half-life of prothrombin, there is a delay in the onset of action of 2 to 7 days.

Pharmacokinetics After rapid and complete absorption, oral warfarin is almost totally bound to plasma albumin, with a half-life of 37 hours. It is metabolized in the hepatic microsomes to produce inactive metabolites excreted in the urine and stools.

Dose A standard procedure is to give warfarin 5 mg/day for 5 days, checking the prothrombin time daily until it is in the therapeutic range, and then to check it three times weekly for up to 2 weeks. Lower starting doses should be given in the elderly and in those with increased risk of bleeding. Warfarin should be commenced at least 4 days before heparin is discontinued to allow for the inactivation of circulating vitamin K-dependent coagulation factors; the heparin can be discontinued once the INR has been in the therapeutic range for 2 days.[114] Avoidance of a large primary dose may prevent an excess fall of prothrombin, and may also decrease the risk of skin necrosis. Only when an urgent effect is required, an initial loading dose of warfarin 10 to 15 mg daily should be used. Patients with heart failure or liver disease require lower doses. The usual dose maintenance is 4 to 5 mg daily, but may vary from 1 mg to 20 mg daily. This wide range means that doses must be individualized according to the INR (see next section).

INR Range The effect of warfarin is monitored by reporting the INR, which represents the prothrombin time according to international reference thromboplastin, as approved by the World Health Organization. Prosthetic heart valves require the greatest possible intensity of safe anticoagulation, and the recommended INR range is rather variable, from 2.0 to 4.5, with lower values for those with bioprosthetic valves and mechanical aortic rather than mitral valves.[114] However, a meta-analysis on 23,145 patients recommended higher values with a target of more than 3.0 (see later).[115] Less intense anticoagulation with an INR of 2.0 to 3.0 is appropriate for patients who have deep vein thrombosis with pulmonary embolism, those at risk of thromboembolism, and those who have thromboembolism and are thought to be at high risk of stroke. In patients with atrial fibrillation without valvular heart disease, the lower limit is an INR of 1.5.[116] Once the steady-state warfarin requirement is known, the INR need only be checked once every 4 to 6 weeks.

Self-Monitoring and Computerized Algorithms In selected patients, self-monitoring offers ease and independence of travel, supported by the results of randomized comparative studies.[114] Together with computer-guided dose adjustment, now available, the intelligent patient may outclass the experienced physician.

Dose Reduction The dose should be reduced in the presence of congestive heart failure, liver damage from any source (alcohol, malnutrition), or renal impairment (which increases the fraction of free drug in the plasma). Thyrotoxicosis enhances the catabolism of vitamin K, reducing the dose of warfarin needed, whereas myxedema has the opposite effect. In the elderly, the dose should be reduced because the response to warfarin increases with age. A high intake of dietary vitamin K (green salads) reduces the efficacy of warfarin. Some fad diets alternate high and low salad periods, which causes INR control to vacillate.

Drug Interactions with Warfarin Warfarin is known to interact with approximately 80 other drugs. It is inhibited by drugs such as cholestyramine that reduce the absorption of vitamin K and of warfarin, and drugs such as barbiturates or phenytoin that accelerate warfarin degradation in the liver. Potentiating drugs include the cardiovascular agents allopurinol, quinidine and amiodarone (see p. 242), and cephalosporins that inhibit the generation of vitamin K.[114] Drugs that decrease warfarin degradation and increase the anticoagulant effect include a variety of antibiotics such as metronidazole (*Flagyl*) and co-trimoxazole (*Bactrim*), and the anti-ulcer agent, cimetidine.

Antiplatelet drugs such as aspirin, clopidogrel and NSAIDs may potentiate the risk of bleeding, but this varies considerably between individual patients. High doses of aspirin (>1.5 g per day) impair the synthesis of clotting factors. Sulfinpyrazone powerfully displaces warfarin from blood proteins, reducing the required dose of warfarin down to 1 mg in some patients. The safest rule is to tell patients on oral anticoagulation not to take any over-the-counter drugs without consultation, and for the physician to checklist any new drug used. If in doubt, the INR should be monitored more frequently. This is also necessary when dietary changes are anticipated, as during travel.

Contraindications These include recent stroke, uncontrolled hypertension, hepatic cirrhosis, and potential gastrointestinal and genitourinary bleeding points such as hiatus hernia, peptic ulcer, gastritis, gastro-esophageal reflux disease with overt bleeding, colitis, proctitis, and cystitis. If anticoagulation is deemed essential, the risk-benefit ratio must be evaluated carefully. Old age is not in itself a contraindication against anticoagulation, although the elderly are more likely to bleed.

Pregnancy and Warfarin The latter is contraindicated in the first trimester due to its teratogenicity, and 2 weeks before birth due to the risk of fetal bleeding. The alternative, unfractionated heparin, may be less effective than warfarin and there is a warning against LMWH issued by the FDA. One approach is to use heparin or LMWH in the first trimester, warfarin in the second trimester until about 38 weeks, changing to heparin/LMWH which is discontinued 12 hours before labor induction, restarted postpartum, and overlapped with warfarin for 4 to 5 days. Heparin should be monitored twice weekly by aPPT, and LMWH by anti-Xa levels. Heparin requirements go up in the third trimester because heparin-binding proteins increase.

Complications and Cautions The most common complication is bleeding, while rare but very serious is *warfarin-associated skin necrosis*. The cause is not well understood. It may occur between the third and the eighth day of therapy. Protein-C deficiency (Fig. 9-4) may be a predisposing factor, especially when high-dose warfarin is initiated after cardiopulmonary bypass (which lowers protein-C levels). The best protection is to start with lower doses under the cover of heparin. To carry on with warfarin despite the necrosis, reduce the dose to about 2 mg daily, cover with heparin, and gradually increase warfarin over several weeks.[114]

Warfarin Overdose and Bleeding Excess hypoprothrombinemia without bleeding, or with only minor bleeding, can be remedied by dose reduction or discontinuation. The risk of bleeding can be reduced dramatically by lowering the intended INR from 3.0 to 4.5 down to 2.0 to 3.0, which generally can be achieved by reducing the warfarin dose by only 1 mg daily.[114] Even high INR values up to 9 can (in the absence of bleeding) be managed by dose omission and then reinstating warfarin at a lower dose. If bleeding becomes significant, or if the INR is >9, 3 to 5 mg of oral vitamin K_1 is given to reduce the INR within 24 to 48 hours. The subcutaneous route gives variable results and should be avoided, rather using the slow intravenous route (5 to 10 mg over 30 minutes) for an emergency.[114] In patients with prosthetic valves, vitamin K should be strictly avoided because of the risk of valve thrombosis, unless there is a life-threatening intracranial bleed. In patients unresponsive to vitamin K, the treatment of choice is: (1) a concentrate of the prothrombin group of coagulation factors including II, IX and X; (2) fresh frozen plasma (15 ml/kg); and (3) a transfusion of fresh, whole blood.

Indications for Warfarin

Acute Myocardial Infarction Mural thrombosis and the subsequent incidence of systemic thromboembolism are more common within the first 3 to 6 months in patients with large anterior Q-wave infarctions, apical dyskinetic areas identifiable by echocardiography, severe left ventricular dysfunction, congestive heart failure, or atrial fibrillation.[117]

Furthermore, the likelihood of systemic thromboembolism is greatest in the first 3 months after discharge. Evidence supports the use of oral warfarin for a 3–6-month period in postinfarction patients at high risk of systemic embolism because of atrial fibrillation, congestive heart failure or mobile mural thrombus,[118] aiming at an INR of 2.0 to 3.0.

Low Ejection Fractions These may be an indication for long-term anticoagulation. In the SOLVD study, 80% with a prior myocardial infarction, there was a 24% reduction in mortality in those with ejection fractions of <35%.[119] Of note, there have been no prospective randomized trials of long-term anticoagulation in such patients. Large trials such as the WATCH trial (Warfarin and Antiplatelet Therapy in Chronic Heart Failure) and the WARCEF trial (Warfarin Versus Aspirin in Reduced Ejection Fraction) are currently ongoing.

Chronic Postinfarction Treatment In a meta-analysis that covered 21,319 patients in 30 trials,[120] and four other studies, Hirsh and colleagues[114] concluded: High-intensity oral anticoagulation (INR 3.0 to 4.0) reduces the combined risk of death, MI, and ischemic stroke, but increases the risk of major bleeding. The combination of low-intensity oral anticoagulation (INR < 2.0) with aspirin carries no benefit beyond aspirin alone. The combination of moderate-intensity anticoagulation (INR 2.0 to 3.0) with low-dose aspirin is as effective as high intensity warfarin, but carries a similar increased risk of bleeding. Moderate-intensity without aspirin has not been assessed. Aspirin and oral anticoagulation are associated with almost identical total mortality rates, but they have different side effects. The incidence of bleeding is higher in patients given anticoagulants and the incidence of gastrointestinal problems higher in those given aspirin. For a prolonged antithrombotic effect after infarction, it is much simpler to use aspirin. The recommended dose is 75 to 150 mg daily.[18]

Current Recommendations We do not advise using oral anticoagulants routinely after infarction; rather, there should be a careful evaluation of the needs of each individual patient, with a preference for aspirin started as soon as possible after the onset of myocardial ischemia and continued indefinitely unless there are clear contraindications. Warfarin should be used for patients at high risk of embolization because of atrial fibrillation, congestive heart failure, mobile mural thrombus or prior venous thromboembolism.

Venous Thromboembolism In patients with deep venous thrombosis, warfarin should be initiated concurrently with intravenous heparin or LMWH.[121] Thereafter, oral anticoagulation alone should be continued for longer than 3 months. A less intensive regimen (INR 2.0 to 3.0) is effective and safer than a more intensive regime (INR 3.0 to 4.5).[114] Long-term follow-up by low intensity warfarin (INR 1.5 to 2.0) reduces repeat events.[122] Indefinite treatment should be considered in patients with recurrent venous thrombosis, or with risk factors such as antithrombin-III deficiency, protein-C or protein-S deficiency, persistent antiphospholipid antibodies, or malignancy. For documented *pulmonary embolism*, either LMWH or unfractionated heparin should be given followed by oral warfarin continued for approximately 6 months in the absence of recurrences. However, should there be a recurrence, indefinite therapy should be considered.

Atrial Fibrillation: Indications for Warfarin Atrial fibrillation in the presence of heart disease is strongly associated with thromboembolism. There is no proof that rhythm control is better than rate control to reduce the risk of stroke (see AFFIRM study, Chapter 8), and either policy requires anticoagulation. In general, the benefits of warfarin far exceed the risk of hemorrhage.[114] The only clear indications for withholding warfarin are: (1) lone atrial fibrillation in younger patients; and (2) a bleeding diathesis. Cardioversion increases the risk of an embolus in patients with atrial fibrillation. After 3 days of atrial fibrillation, anti-coagulation for 3 weeks is strongly recommended (if feasible) prior to elective cardioversion, followed by another 2 to 4 weeks of anti-coagulation thereafter.[123] However, the recent AFFIRM trial data[124] and the realization that many recurrences are asymptomatic has certainly suggested that in some patients the duration of anticoagulation even after resumption of sinus rhythm should be lifelong. In *nonvalvular atrial fibrillation*, adjusted-dose warfarin (INR 2.0 to 3.0) is superior to the combination of low-intensity warfarin (INR < 1.0) with aspirin (325 mg).[125] Two other trials have also reported trends suggesting that adjusted-dose warfarin may be superior to fixed minidose warfarin or a combined aspirin regimen.[126,127]

Mitral Stenosis or Regurgitation. In patients with mitral valve disease, the risk of thromboembolism is greatest in those with atrial fibrilla-tion, marked left atrial enlargement or previous embolic episodes; and anticoagulation is strongly indicated in patients with any of these fea-tures. In contrast, anticoagulation is not indicated in patients with mitral stenosis with sinus rhythm. A strong argument can be made for earlier anticoagulation if the left atrium is significantly dilated.

Hypertensive Heart Disease. Anticoagulation is indicated only if there is marked left atrial or left ventricular enlargement, or in the presence of atrial fibrillation, always provided that there is tight control of blood pressure.

Dilated Cardiomyopathy. There is a substantial risk of systemic embolism, particularly if there is atrial fibrillation. Although anti-coagulants are effective in reducing thromboembolism, the risk versus benefit is the subject of ongoing trials.

The Tachycardia/Bradycardia Syndrome. This condition may be com-plicated by atrial fibrillation and thromboembolism. Anticoagula-tion should be considered, especially if there is underlying organic heart disease, such as ischemic heart disease, hypertension or cardiomyopathy.

Atrial Septal Defects. In older patients with atrial septal defects and pul-monary hypertension, anticoagulation is strongly recommended as prophylaxis against *in situ* pulmonary arterial thromboses or, rarely, paradoxical emboli. Anticoagulation is also required for patients with repaired septal defects who subsequently develop atrial fibrillation.

Thyrotoxic Heart Disease. In patients with atrial fibrillation and thyro-toxicosis, the first aim is to render the patient euthyroid, which reverts the atrial fibrillation in the majority.[128] It is generally accepted but without definitive proof that anticoagulants are required in the interim, particularly in the presence of associated heart failure. In the remainder, cardioversion should be performed at about the 16th week after the patient becomes euthyroid. Anticoagulation cover is required, and should be maintained for 4 weeks after conversion.[128]

Intermittent Atrial Fibrillation. When this lasts a few hours, the choices vary from no treatment in lone atrial fibrillation (see next paragraph) to warfarin in those elderly patients who are thought to be at higher risk.

"Lone" Atrial Fibrillation. In the absence of any other cardiac or pre-cipitating condition, such as thyrotoxicosis, embolism is rare. In patients younger than 60 years of age without hypertension, the risk of thromboembolism is no greater than in any age- and sex-matched population, so the morbidity of anticoagulant therapy outweighs the potential advantages.[129] Elderly patients with "lone" atrial fibrillation have an increased risk of TIAs or stroke, and anticoagulant or even aspirin therapy should be considered.[130]

Patients Presenting with Atrial Fibrillation and Acute Embolic Stroke. Although anticoagulation is required, cerebral hemorrhage must first be excluded by computed tomography or MRI, which, in the case of large strokes, must be delayed for about 1 week to allow full evolution to occur.[131]

Atrial Fibrillation: Conclusions There is strong evidence for the use of low-intensity anticoagulation in "high-risk" patients, and warfarin is much more effective than aspirin in preventing stroke in these patients.[132-134] Patients should be risk-stratified, and warfarin should be used in those at high risk and aspirin only in those at low risk. The major risk factors are older than 65 years of age, a history of hypertension, diabetes, congestive heart failure, and a history of stroke or TIA.[132] Increased LA dimension is a risk factor in some but not all studies. Patients with a recent TIA or minor stroke are at particularly high risk of a recurrence.[134]

Warfarin for Prosthetic Heart Valves Warfarin is recommended in patients with mechanical prosthetic heart valves, usually at a level of 2.5 to 3.5,[114] but with a meta-analysis proposing a relatively high target INR of 3.0 to 4.5, with aortic valves at the lower end and mitral valves at the higher end of the INR range.[115] The combination of aspirin (100 mg) and warfarin is also efficacious, with a target INR of close to 3.0.[29] Dipyridamole (400 mg daily) may be chosen if aspirin is contraindicated or if further therapy is required; for example, when there are continued emboli despite treatment with aspirin plus warfarin. In patients with bioprosthetic mitral valves, the risk of thromboembolism is highest in the first 6 to 12 weeks, when warfarin is mandatory. Thereafter, aspirin may be given or antithrombotic therapy may be discontinued if there are no other indications. There is strong evidence supporting the continuation of warfarin when mitral bioprosthetic valves are combined with atrial fibrillation, a large left atrium or left ventricular failure. The risk is particularly low in patients with bioprosthetic aortic valves, so aspirin for 6 to 12 weeks is appropriate.[117]

Possible Indications for Warfarin *Cerebrovascular accidents and TIAs.* There is no evidence to support anticoagulation in patients who have had a completed stroke. When patients present with an acute stroke and atrial fibrillation, warfarin is indicated providing cerebral hemorrhage is excluded by computed tomography. In patients with recent TIAs, aspirin is recommended rather than anticoagulation. In those intolerant of aspirin, clopidogrel is the next best option. Warfarin is recommended only when symptoms persist despite aspirin or clopidogrel therapy, or when there is a major cardiac source of embolism.

Primary Pulmonary Hypertension. This entity includes a variety of histological appearances and probably pathogenic mechanisms. Anticoagulation is widely accepted without randomized trial evidence. Ongoing trials should clarify matters further.

Mitral Valve Prolapse. In patients with definite echocardiographic documentation of mitral valve prolapse and evidence suggestive of thrombotic or thromboembolic events, warfarin or platelet inhibitors may be indicated.

Low-Dose Warfarin: Is It Indicated to Prevent Thrombosis?

Elevated levels of factor VII have been shown to be associated with an increased incidence of primary thrombotic events[135] and occur in patients with acute coronary syndromes.[136] Low-dose warfarin is theoretically attractive yet not supported by trial data.

In *postinfarct patients,*[137] fixed-dose warfarin (1 mg or 3 mg) did not add to the clinical benefits of 160 mg of aspirin. In another postinfarct study, CHAMP, United States veterans who had suffered myocardial infarction were randomized to receive either 162 mg or 81 mg of aspirin plus warfarin and followed up for a median follow-up of 2.7 years. The target INR was 1.5 to 2.5 (measured median, 1.8).[138] There the combination gave on clinical benefit beyond that with aspirin alone. However, major bleeding was almost doubled in the aspirin plus warfarin group. Aspirin alone is therefore preferable to combination therapy with aspirin plus low-dose warfarin.

Prevention of cardiac ischemic events. In the Thrombosis Prevention Trial,[139] 5499 men aged between 45 and 69 years with a high risk score for development of ischemic heart disease were randomized to receive either low-intensity warfarin (to achieve an INR of 1.5), controlled-release aspirin 75 mg, a combination of both drugs, or a placebo. Either warfarin or aspirin reduced ischemic events by about 20%. There was a trend for greater efficacy with the combination of warfarin and aspirin, which reduced ischemic events by 34% (equivalent to 4 fewer events per 1000 patients treated for 1 year). However, the incidence of hemorrhagic strokes and fatal strokes increased (1.5 events per 1000 patients treated per year compared with 0.2 events in the aspirin group). There was also an increase in ruptured aortic aneurysms.

Atrial fibrillation. In the SPAF trial of patients with atrial fibrillation, low-dose warfarin (INR 1.2 to 1.5) was less effective in preventing ischemic stroke and systemic embolism than warfarin adjusted to an INR of 2.0 to 3.0.[140,141]

In *aortocoronary saphenous vein bypass grafts* showed that there was no significant difference in angiographic outcomes between patients given low-dose warfarin (1 mg increasing up to 4 mg unless the INR was >2.0, with a mean INR of 1.4) and those given a placebo.[142]

In *recurrent ischemic stroke* (non-cardioembolic), warfarin with a mean INR 2.1 was no better than aspirin 325 mg per day.[143]

Recurrent venous thromboembolism. Standard preventive therapy includes 3 to 12 months of full-dose warfarin with an INR between 2.0 and 3.0. Thereafter, long-term low intensity warfarin therapy with an INR of 1.5 to 2.0 is much better than placebo with only an increase in minor bleeds.[122]

Based on the above trials, the only real place for a low-dose warfarin regime is in the long-term prevention of repeat venous thromboembolism.

Oral Anticoagulation by Warfarin: Summary A minority of patients with acute myocardial infarction qualify for limited anticoagulation for 3 to 6 months. Very few require prolonged anticoagulation. Oral anticoagulants are indicated in many patients with atrial fibrillation and in those with prosthetic heart valves. They are used in both the treatment and prevention of venous thrombosis and pulmonary embolism. Long-term anticoagulation requires careful consideration of the risk : benefit ratio for the individual patient. For example, while a patient with chronic atrial fibrillation may benefit from meticulous anticoagulation, aspirin may be a safer choice for a relatively non-compliant patient.

FIBRINOLYTIC (THROMBOLYTIC) THERAPY

Goals of Fibrinolysis The goals of reperfusion therapy are early patency, increased myocardial salvage, preservation of left ventricular function and lower mortality.[144,145] Apart from greater salvage, a patent infarct-related artery also improves remodeling, enhances electrical stability, reduces long-term mortality, and has the potential to provide collaterals to another infarct zone in the event of reinfarction.[146] Increased patency of the infarct-related coronary artery at 90 minutes correlates with a mortality reduction at 30 days,[147] and patency of this artery may determine the benefit from late reperfusion.[148] From these facts it follows that the major aim is to achieve early reperfusion with short "symptom-to-needle" and "door-to-needle" times in patients with suspected acute myocardial infarction and ST-segment elevation or new-onset left bundle branch block.[145,149,150] Now that primary PCI is established as providing better reperfusion than lysis except within the first few hours,[151] the symptom-to-balloon time and door-to-balloon times are crucial. Early reperfusion can be achieved by either fibrinolysis or by PCI. The principle of modern fibrinolytic therapy is the use of agents such as alteplase, reteplase, tenecteplase and streptokinase (Table 9-3), which convert plasminogen into active plasmin (Fig. 9-6). Because fibrinolytic agents simultaneously exert clot dissolving and procoagulant actions and have significant serious side effects, they *must not be used in unstable angina* where they have no benefit and may in fact increase the incidence of myocardial infarction.

Early Reperfusion: The Golden Hours Dramatic reductions in mortality can be achieved if treatment is obtained during the "golden" first hour. In the MITI Trial, alteplase and aspirin were started as soon as possible either at home or in hospital.[152] Reperfusion within 70 minutes reduced the early death rate from 8.7% to 1.2%, while infarct size fell from 11.2% to 4.9%, when compared with a longer delay of up to 180 minutes. The CAPTIM trial of prehospital administration of thrombolytics versus primary PCI on admission to hospital convincingly demonstrated the benefits of fibrinolytic treatment within 2 hours.[151]

The Window of Opportunity In the FTT Collaborative Overview of 58,000 randomized patients in fibrinolytic trials,[150] mortality was reduced by 25% in patients randomized between 2 and 3 hours after symptom onset and by 18% in patients randomized between 4 and 6 hours. Patients randomized between 7 and 12 hours still had a 14% reduction in mortality, the later benefit perhaps related more to the

Table 9-3 **Characteristics of Fibrinolytic Agents**

	Streptokinase	Alteplase (tPA)	Reteplase	Tenecteplase
Fibrin selective	No	Yes	Yes	Yes >tPA
Plasminogen binding	Indirect	Direct	Direct	Direct
Duration of infusion (min)	60	90	10 + 10	5–10 sec
Half-life (min)	23	<5	13–16	20
Fibrinogen breakdown	4+	1–2+	Not known	>tPA
Early heparin	Probably yes	Yes	Yes	Yes
Hypotension	Yes	No	No	No
Allergic reactions	Yes	No	No	No
Approximate cost/dose	$562/1.5 MU	$2974/100 mg	$2872 per kit	$2832/50-mg vial
TIMI reflow grade 3, 90 min	32[87]	45*–54[87]	60*	= tPA[†]
TIMI reflow 2–3 at 90 minutes	53[180]–65[181]	81[182]–88[183]	83*	No data
at 2–3 hours	70[184]–73[182]	73[184]–80 (PI)	No data	No data
at 24 hours	81[180]–88[181]	78[185]–89 (PI)	No data	No data

*Bode et al., *Circulation*, 1996;94:891.
†Canon et al., *Circulation*, 1998;98:2805; PI = package insert. For other data sources, see Marder and Sherry.[186]
MU = million units; > = more than; < = less than.

benefits of a patent infarct-related artery than to myocardial salvage.[148,153] An additional 1.6 lives were lost per 1000 patients treated for every hour of delay in treatment. A time window of 12 hours is now widely accepted for the administration of fibrinolytic therapy.[153]

Prehospital Fibrinolysis Pooling of data from five studies has shown a significant difference in 30-day overall mortality.[145] In the CAPTIM study, 840 patients were randomized to receive either prehospital fibrinolysis (using an accelerated infusion of alteplase) or primary PCI.[154] Those treated with prehospital fibrinolysis commenced treatment on average 60 minutes sooner than those randomized to primary PCI. Rescue PCI was subsequently performed in 26% of the prehospital fibrinolysis group. At 30 days the combined incidence of death, MI or disabling stroke was similar in both treatment groups. Comparing those randomized in the first 2 hours versus later, there was less cardiogenic shock and a strong trend to a lower mortality.[151] Follow-up at 2.5 years (unpublished data, CAPTIM Study Group, 2002) showed that the mortality difference between the two treatment strategies had increased over time (6.7% with fibrinolysis versus 8.8% with primary PCI). The advantages of domiciliary fibrinolysis must be balanced against the complications of early reperfusion, such as ventricular fibrillation and symptomatic bradycardia, which might have to be managed at home. The added delay in reaching hospital means that early complications such as shock might also have to be managed at home.

Minimizing Delays The CAPTIM data raise major societal issues. "Most important, how can we most effectively increase the number of patients who present immediately after the onset of symptoms, and how can we provide prehospital fibrinolytic therapy?" ask Giugliano and Braunwald.[148] Every step of the delay should be streamlined: the patient's recognition of symptoms; the arrival of paramedics; initiation of fibrinolytic therapy if possible; the transit time to hospital; and the in-hospital "door-to-needle" or "door-to-balloon" times. When the latter exceeds 60 min, benefit starts to be lost (Fig. 9-7). Thus the "symptom-to-balloon" time is inversely related to mortality.[155]

Recognition of Reperfusion In the absence of early coronary angiography, two simple clinical indicators of reperfusion are rapid relief of chest pain and rapid relief of ST-segment elevation. Rises in the plasma biomarkers such as myoglobin, troponin T, or creatine kinase isoenzymes reflect enzyme washout from the reperfused area. Of these measures, ST resolution is a major determinant of prognosis.

Adjunctive Therapy to Prevent Reinfarction Major contributory factors to restenosis include the presence of a residual luminal stenosis, and the persistence of residual thrombus (the latter is a powerful thrombogenic surface). Successful lysis reexposes the site of the original thrombus, namely the plaque fissure. Three recent trials have tested and established the hypothesis that therapy adjunctive to the fibrinolytic agent could reduce reinfarction. The ASSENT-3 trial[102] tested half-dose tenecteplase plus enoxaparin or abciximab versus full-dose tenecteplase plus unfractionated heparin. The GUSTO-V trial tested abciximab (versus placebo) in conjunction with reteplase.[156] The HERO-2 trial compared bivalirudin with unfractionated heparin both with streptokinase.[110] Although reinfarction was reduced in all three trials, mortality at 30 days did not change. As yet, the adjunctive therapies tested have not been sufficiently convincing to induce major changes in clinical practice.

Which Fibrinolytic? Several large trials randomizing over 100,000 patients have compared the effects of streptokinase and alteplase (Table 9-4). In the GUSTO-I Trial, in which alteplase was infused over 90 minutes, there was a 14% relative and a 1% absolute mortality

TIMING OF PCI VS LYSIS

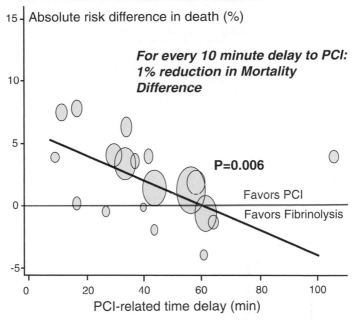

Figure 9-7 PCI-related time delay. Absolute risk reduction in 4- to 6-week mortality with primary PCI as a function of the door-to-PCI time. The sizes of the circles reflect the sample size of the individual studies. Values >0 represent benefit and values <0 represent harm. The solid red line represents the weighted meta-regression. Using only fibrin-specific agents, the equipoise of time-to-treatment is 113 minutes. (*Figure based on personal communication, Dr. Eric Bates, University of Michigan Medical School, Ann Arbor, Michigan, USA.*)

reduction with alteplase compared with streptokinase,[84] at the cost of two extra strokes per 1000 patients randomized. In the GUSTO-III Trial, reteplase was the equivalent to accelerated alteplase. In the ASSENT-2 Trial, tenecteplase was equivalent to alteplase, but there was less major bleeding.[157] Reteplase and tenecteplase have the advantage of bolus administration, tenecteplase being given only once. The bolus agents do not reduce mortality but are certainly more convenient, simpler to use and help to reduce medication errors. Of all the agents, alteplase, streptokinase, tenecteplase and reteplase are licensed in the United States for mortality reduction in AMI. All have similar contraindications (Table 9-5). It appears that we have reached a "reperfusion ceiling" and the scene is set for a major breakthrough using a new generation of thrombolytics but with no obvious contenders on the horizon.

Alteplase (tPA, Tissue Plasminogen Activator)

Tissue plasminogen activator (*Activase in the United States, Actilyse in Europe*) is a naturally occurring enzyme that binds to fibrin with a greater affinity than streptokinase or urokinase; and once bound, it starts to convert plasminogen to plasmin on the fibrin surface. Hence it is relatively "clot-selective," and in clinical doses some systemic effects do occur. The very short half-life of alteplase mandates co-therapy with intravenous heparin to avoid reocclusion.

Dose of Alteplase Standard intravenous regimens administer two thirds of the total dose of 100 mg over the first 30 minutes, starting with an

Table 9-4 Side Effects of Streptokinase, Alteplase, and Tenecteplase in the GUSTO-I and ASSENT-2 Trials

	Streptokinase (GUSTO)[87]	Alteplase (GUSTO)[87]	Alteplase (ASSENT-2)[14]	Tenecteplase (ASSENT-2)[14]
Patient number	10,410	10,396	8461	8488
Mortality at 30 days	7.4%	6.3%*	6.2%	6.2%
Overall stroke	1.40%	1.55%	1.66%	1.78%
Hemorrhagic stroke[†]	0.54%	0.72%*	0.93%	0.94%
Major bleeds	6.3%*	5.4%	5.9%	4.7%*
Allergic reactions	5.8%*	1.6%	0.2% (ana)	0.1% (ana)
Hypotension	12.5%	10.1%	16.1%	15.9%

All three agents were used in conjunction with intravenous heparin.
*Significant difference.
[†]For risk factors, see Simoons et al.[187] In patients with streptokinase and no risk factors, the probability of stroke is 0.3%. In patients with alteplase and 3 risk factors, the probability is >3%. Ana = anaphylaxis.

initial bolus of 15 mg, then 50 mg over 30 minutes, then 35 mg over 1 hour. The dose of the infusion should be reduced for patients weighing less than 68 kg. An initial heparin bolus of 5000 IU is standard, although lower doses should be considered in the elderly and in patients of low bodyweight. Intravenous heparin should be continued for at least 48 hours, adjusted to an aPPT of 50 to 75 seconds.[85] Chewable aspirin should be started as soon as possible.

Contraindications to Alteplase (Table 9-5) These relate chiefly to hemorrhage, for example, any recent hemorrhage or cerebrovascular accident. Menstruation is not a contraindication.[158] Diabetic retinopathy should no longer be considered a contraindication because vitreous hemorrhages are due to vitreous detachment rather than a thrombotic abnormality, and there have been no reports of intraocular hemorrhage in large clinical trials despite the inclusion of patients with diabetic proliferative retinopathy.[159] Gentamicin sensitivity is a specific exclusion for alteplase therapy, because gentamicin is used in the preparation of alteplase.

Cost-Effectiveness of Alteplase An important disadvantage of alteplase is its cost—about five times that of streptokinase. In an analysis of the GUSTO-I Trial, the additional cost of accelerated alteplase compared with streptokinase per extra life-year saved was US$27,382 (in 1992 dollars), being most cost-effective in older patients (>65 years) with anterior infarcts ($13,410) and least cost-effective in younger patients (≤40 years) with inferior infarcts ($203,071).[160]

Tenecteplase

Tenecteplase is a genetically engineered mutant of native tissue plasminogen activator with amino acid substitutions at three sites. These properties result in decreased plasma clearance, a longer half life (Table 9-3), increased fibrin specificity, and resistance to the plasminogen activator inhibitor (PAI-1). In the ASSENT-2 Trial, a single bolus of tenecteplase (in a weight-adjusted dose of 0.5 mg/kg) was compared with accelerated alteplase. At 30 days, mortality was the same with both agents (6.18% with tenecteplase versus 6.15% with alteplase), as was the stroke rate.[157] However, there was less major bleeding with tenecteplase (4.7% versus 5.9%, $P < 0.01$). Thus the same or marginally better clinical results can be found with only one bolus of TNK-tPA versus the infusion required for alteplase, so that tenecteplase is now one of the most popular of the lytic agents.

Reteplase

Reteplase (*Retavase*) is a deletion mutant of alteplase with elimination of the kringle-1, finger and epidermal growth factor domains, as well as some carbohydrate side chains. This results in prolonged plasma clearance, so that a double-bolus regimen (10 U + 10 U intravenously, each over 10 minutes and 30 minutes apart) can be used. Heparin must not be given through the same intravenous line (physical incompatibility). In the INJECT Trial[161] mortality was similar with reteplase and streptokinase, and in the GUSTO-III Trial,[83] mortality was similar with reteplase and alteplase. The stroke rates in GUSTO-III were also similar (1.64% with reteplase versus 1.79% with alteplase). It is licensed for use in AMI to improve postinfarct ventricular function, to lessen the incidence of congestive heart failure, and to reduce mortality.

Streptokinase

Streptokinase has no direct effect on plasminogen (Fig. 9-6). It works by binding with plasminogen to form a 1:1 complex that becomes an active enzyme to convert plasminogen to plasmin.[149] In addition, streptokinase may increase circulating levels of activated protein-C, which enhances clot lysis.[162] The second and third generation of thrombolytics are superior drugs but streptokinase is cheap and still widely used in many parts of the world. The standard rate of infusion is 1.5 million IU of streptokinase in 100 ml of physiological saline over 30 to 60 minutes.[163]

Streptokinase and Heparin Although a meta-analysis does not recommend the use of intravenous heparin with streptokinase,[164] this issue remains controversial. Of note, the optimal aPPT at 12 hours after the administration of fibrinolytic therapy (including streptokinase) is 50 to 70 seconds, as shown by mortality data.[85] To achieve this with streptokinase, adjunctive heparin therapy is required. Intravenous heparin should especially be considered in patients with anterior infarctions (because of the larger size of the infarct and the additional risk of left ventricular thrombus and embolism) and in those with inferior infarctions at high risk of systemic emboli.

We recommend heparin on the basis of the following trials. First, in an analysis of 68,000 patients (all of whom received aspirin, 93% of whom received fibrinolytic therapy and many of whom received streptokinase), the benefits of added heparin translates into a benefit:risk ratio of 5 deaths and 3 infarctions prevented at a cost of 3 transfusions per 1000 patients treated and a nonsignificant increase in stroke.[164] Second, in the 5-year follow-up of United States patients in the GUSTO-I Trial,[165] mortality was similar in the alteplase group and the streptokinase plus intravenous heparin group, but significantly higher in the streptokinase plus subcutaneous heparin group.

Side Effects and Contraindications of Streptokinase In the GUSTO-I Trial,[84] there were two more hemorrhagic strokes per 1000 patients treated with alteplase than with streptokinase ($P < 0.03$; Table 9-5). Allergic reactions and hypotension were more common with streptokinase. The overall incidence of major bleeding was similar with both regimens. Major bleeding requires cessation of the fibrinolytic agent and adjunctive heparin, administration of protamine sulfate to reverse the actions of heparin, and fresh frozen plasma or whole blood. *Contraindications* are similar to those against alteplase, with the exception of gentamicin sensitivity. Additional contraindications are: (1) major recent streptococcal infection, because antistreptococcal antibodies cause resistance to streptokinase; and (2) previous treatment by streptokinase, because the antibodies diminish efficacy and there is an increased risk of allergy.

Table 9-5	**Contraindications to the Use of Fibrinolytic Therapy**

- Suspected aortic dissection
- Any previous history of hemorrhagic stroke
- History of nonhemorrhagic stroke or central nervous system damage within 1 yr
- Head trauma or brain surgery within 6 mo
- Internal bleeding within 6 wk
- Active bleeding or known bleeding disorder (but not menstruation)
- Major surgery, trauma or bleeding within 6 wk
- Traumatic cardiopulmonary resuscitation within 3 wk
- Oral anticoagulant therapy
- Persistent serious hypertension (systolic blood pressure of >180 mmHg or diastolic blood pressure of >110 mmHg)
- Puncture of noncompressible blood vessel within 2 wk
- Peptic ulcer disease documented by endoscopy with symptoms occurring within the previous 3 mo
- Dementia
- Known intracranial neoplasm
- Acute pancreatitis
- Pregnancy or within 1 wk postpartum
- Transient ischemic attack within 6 mo
- Infective endocarditis
- Active cavitating pulmonary tuberculosis
- Advanced liver disease
- Intracardiac thrombi

Agents Undergoing Assessment

Saruplase, or prourokinase, is a recombinant single-chain form of urokinase. Its mechanism of action is not fully elucidated, but it is known that it is not fibrin specific. The 30-day mortality rates are similar with saruplase and streptokinase, with similar rates of intracranial hemorrhage. Saruplase is administered as a 20-mg bolus followed by a 60-mg infusion over 1 hour. Single-bolus regimens are being developed.

Staphylokinase is a 136-amino acid protein, produced by *Staphylococcus aureas*, which forms a 1 : 1 complex with plasminogen. This is then converted to a staphylokinase-plasmin complex, which is rapidly neutralized by α_2-antiplasmin in the absence of fibrin. Staphylokinase is therefore highly fibrin-specific and may be active against platelet-rich thrombi. Staphylokinase causes antigenicity, and antibody titers remain elevated for months. Nonimmunogenic forms may yet be developed. A number of angiographic trials have reported coronary flow rates similar to those achieved with alteplase.

Monteplase (Eisai Co., Ltd., Tokyo, Japan) is a newly developed mt-PA constructed by substituting only one amino acid in the epidermal growth factor domain and is expressed in baby Syrian hamster kidney cells. Monteplase has a prolonged half-life of >20 minutes, compared with 4 minutes for native t-PA, so it can be given intravenously by bolus injection.

Current Status of Fibrinolytics

The lack of any major breakthroughs with the agents currently under evaluation has stimulated renewed interest in combination therapy with reduced dose fibrinolytics and different regimens of antithrombotic agents, e.g., IIb/IIIa inhibitors, direct thrombin inhibitors, LMWH, etc. If the results of recent trials are a portent for the future, the rate of progress is likely to be slow with minor increments in efficacy likely but no striking breakthroughs. Almost half of all patients receiving fibrinolytic therapy fail to achieve normal coronary flow by 90 minutes after the initiation of fibrinolysis, half have intermittent patency or suffer reocclusion,[145] and a quarter of those with angiographic evidence of epicardial blood flow do not have myocyte perfusion according to contrast echocardiography[166] or magnetic resonance imaging.[167,168] Myocyte perfusion may be impaired by platelet, white blood cell, or fibrin plugging; vasospasm; or swelling of endothelial tissue. Newer therapies are therefore required to improve myocyte reperfusion. Bolus administration of some of the newer drugs may enable earlier treatment and prehospital fibrinolysis. Greater efficacy may also be achieved with adjunctive antiplatelet[169] or antithrombin therapies.[170]

Myocardial malperfusion, whether due to microvascular dysfunction, "reperfusion injury," or both, is a major determinant of prognosis and constitutes one of the new frontiers of reperfusion therapy. Many approaches have looked promising in the experimental animal but no trial has yet reached its primary end-point. For the present this is an area of intense interest but perhaps more needs to be understood about the mechanisms in patients with atherosclerotic vessels as opposed to the experimental animal. The best way to optimize myocardial perfusion is to establish patency of the infarct related artery as quickly as possible.

Active Intervention: Fibrinolysis or Angioplasty?

The premise that the best form of reperfusion therapy is mechanical is now firmly established for patients presenting 3 hours or more after symptom onset, but the outcomes are highly dependent on the expertise and logistics present in individual institutions. Primary angioplasty has the distinct advantage of lower bleeding rates than fibrinolytic therapy, and achieves higher TIMI grade 3 flow rates in the infarct-related artery.[171] In patients with cardiogenic shock, the 1-year survival rate was 22% higher with angioplasty or surgery than with medical treatment.[172] A meta-analysis of 23 randomized trials documented a benefit from primary PCI on both short and longer term mortality and morbidity.[173]

Facilitated Intervention A challenging hypothesis is that reduced dose fibrinolytics can be combined with subsequent angioplasty, thereby helping to avoid the adverse effects of long delays to angioplasty. The concept of facilitated PCI is supported by data from the four PAMI trials,[174] in which the presence of TIMI grade 3 flow prior to PCI was associated with higher 6-month survival rates. However, these data are observational. In a trial comparing facilitated PCI (using half-dose alteplase) with primary PCI,[175] facilitated PCI was safe, and there was no difference in left ventricular ejection fraction. At least three trials comparing facilitated PCI with primary PCI are currently underway. Regimens combining fibrinolytic therapy with adjunctive antiplatelet and antithrombotic therapies prior to PCI will also need to be tested in prospective randomized trials.

"Rescue" Angioplasty Some degree of resistance of thrombi to lysis can be expected in perhaps 10% to 15% of patients; the cause may include deep fissuring or rupture of the plaque or platelet-rich thrombus, which is very resistant to lysis. Rescue angioplasty may be beneficial in patients with continuing pain or hemodynamic instability, or as in the CAPTIM study, if very early fibrinolysis appears to have failed.[154] Adjunctive therapy with IIb/IIIa antagonists may enhance the safety and clinical outcome of rescue angioplasty.[176]

Effect of Time Delay PCI and fibrinolysis may be considered to be similarly effective in patients presenting within 3 hours, as shown in PRAGUE-2 study,[177] while within the first 2 hours the CAPTIM data argue for fibrinolysis.[151] Other trials have shown that the advantage of PCI is greater in patients treated late.[178] Fibrinolytic therapy may be the treatment of choice in the first 2 hours, and PCI the treatment of choice both in patients with contraindications against fibrinolytic therapy and in those presenting after 3 hours, provided that the procedure can be performed with less than 60 minutes of PCI-related time delay (Fig. 9-7). Much depends on how soon the patient can reach a center with excellent PCI facilities. Unfortunately, however, fewer than 30% of patients in the United States and <20% in Europe have access to primary PCI, and in many cases, logistical delays in arranging the procedure mean that reperfusion is not achieved within this timeframe.

Adjunctive Antiplatelet Therapy Platelets play a pivotal role in the pathophysiology of acute myocardial infarction. They are involved not only in the initiation of clot formation after plaque fissuring or rupture, but also in the propagation of clot, the secretion of plasminogen activator inhibitor (PAI-1), which causes clots to become resistant to lysis, and the secretion of thromboxane A_2, which causes vasoconstriction. They may also embolize to cause plugging of the microvasculature.[179] Secretion of platelet factor IV lessens the effects of heparin, and α_2-antiplasmin may interfere with fibrinolysis. Specific platelet binding sites for tissue plasminogen activator and plasminogen may also play a role in reducing the efficacy of fibrinolytic therapy. Platelet thrombi are themselves resistant to fibrinolytic therapy. Therefore antiplatelet therapy may benefit intervention.

Gp IIb/IIIa Inhibitors Plus Primary Angioplasty in AMI? On their own, these agents are not very successful in achieving normal coronary flow. As reviewed in Chapter 11 (Table 11-3), and taking into account the results of the ADMIRAL, the CADILLAC, and the ACE trials, it is controversial whether IIb/IIIa antagonists are of benefit when given at the time of stenting, although they may improve coronary flow if given prior to PCI (Van't Hof, 2003, ON-TIME study, unpublished). We take the view that IIb/IIIa antagonists are not recommended unless the patient is in cardiogenic shock or has a large thrombus load at the time of stenting or there is some other compelling indication. Overall, despite their theoretical attraction, the IIb/IIIa inhibitors have shown only a modest benefit in the setting of primary PCI, perhaps because much of the distal embolic material is atherosclerotic debris and not just a mixture of platelets and fibrin.

S U M M A R Y

1. *Antiplatelet agents: Aspirin.* This well tested, widely used, and cheap agent is beneficial in a wide variety of vascular disorders, including the prevention and treatment of coronary heart disease. It inhibits platelet cyclo-oxygenase (COX-1) over a wide dose range. However, because side effects such as gastrointestinal hemorrhage are dose-related, lower doses are preferred. Prophylactic aspirin is indicated for all stages of symptomatic ischemic heart disease, including chronic effort angina, unstable angina, acute myocardial infarction, postinfarction management, coronary artery bypass grafting (CABG), and percutaneous coronary intervention (PCI). Primary prevention by aspirin should be considered only for high-risk patients. For those at moderate risk, there are almost as many disabling strokes and major bleeds as MIs prevented.

2. *Ticlopidine and clopidogrel.* These antiplatelet agents preferred for stroke prevention in aspirin intolerance, and both have a role in the prevention of acute thrombotic closure after coronary artery stenting. Unlike ticlopidine, clopidogrel does not have thrombocytopenia as a possible side effect. Therefore clopidogrel is by far

preferred for use with stenting, when a new trend not fully studied is the use of initial high-dose clopidogrel to replace a GpIIb/IIIb blocker. Clopidogrel should be continued together with aspirin for 12 months following stenting or for non-ST elevation acute coronary syndromes. There may be an adverse interaction with some statins such as atorvastatin and simvastatin that are metabolized by the same liver enzyme, P-450 3A4.

3. *Other antiplatelet agents*, such as sulfinpyrazone and dipyridamole, are used less, although they do have specific indications. For example, dipyridamole is indicated in patients with mechanical prosthetic valves who are intolerant of aspirin or require additional antithrombotic protection.

4. *Glycoprotein IIb/IIIa receptor blockers*, including abciximab, tirofiban, and eptifibatide, act by blocking the final pathway of platelet aggregation. Given intravenously, they are often used in acute coronary syndromes, especially when there is high risk of myocardial infarction or to cover PCIs. They give outcome benefit beyond that obtained by aspirin and heparin, yet at the risk of increased bleeding and rare but serious thrombocytopenia. In patients with ST-elevation myocardial infarction, treated with fibrinolytics, the IIb/IIIa blockers in combination do not reduce mortality yet bleeding is clearly increased. In the setting of primary PCI results are inconsistent. There is a modest benefit in higher risk patients or when given prior to transfer to a facility with a catheter laboratory.

5. *Intravenous unfractionated heparin* has a rapid onset of action, and thus remains the backbone of anticoagulation in acute myocardial infarction with or without thrombolysis. Other indications include the acute coronary syndromes, PCIs, and venous thromboembolism. In all these situations it is combined with aspirin. The drawback of heparin is that its strength and effects cannot be predicted, so that its use must be carefully controlled by repetitive measurements of aPPT (activated partial thromboplastin time).

6. *Low-molecular-weight heparin* is easier to administer than unfractionated heparin, being given in standard doses subcutaneously without the need for aPPT testing. Enoxaparin is superior in patients not undergoing intervention and equal to unfractionated heparin when used prior to intervention, as shown in three trials in acute coronary syndromes. The SYNERGY study argues for the efficacy and safety of combining low-molecular-weight heparin with Gp IIb/IIIa antagonists and with intervention at the cost, however, of increased bleeding.

7. *Direct thrombin inhibitors* are more effective than unfractionated heparin in unstable angina, but carry a higher risk of major bleeding except for bivalirudin. With PCI, bivalirudin is associated with less bleeding and similar outcomes to patients treated with unfractionated heparin and IIb/IIIa antagonists.

8. *Warfarin* has a slow onset of action over several days. Prolonged postinfarction anticoagulation is indicated only for patients at high risk of thromboembolism. Anticoagulation with warfarin is essential for those with prosthetic mechanical heart valves. For patients with atrial fibrillation, there is now substantial evidence showing that warfarin is superior to aspirin in stroke prevention. The oral direct thrombin inhibitor *ximelagatran* is very promising and is currently under evaluation. However, the possible adverse role of mild liver damage must first be clarified.

9. *Fibrinolytic agents* form the basis of therapy in the early stages of acute myocardial infarction, and are usually given in combination with oral aspirin and dose-adjusted heparin. Of practical value are the newer agents with a longer plasma half-life, tenecteplase and

reteplase, that need only one or two (respectively) bolus injections versus the infusion over 90 minutes needed for front-loaded alteplase, still the gold standard. Even the newer agents do not remove the risks of bleeding and intracranial hemorrhage. For those at high risk of intracranial bleeds, such as elderly hypertensive females, streptokinase lessens the risk. If patients present after 3 hours of onset of AMI, and the facilities are available and the expertise and logistics are up to standard, the best approach to opening the occluded infarct-related artery is primary percutaneous coronary intervention (PCI). The admission to balloon time should be 90 minutes or less. The next generation of distal protection devices may improve distal myocardial reperfusion.

10. *Ongoing trials* are testing various combinations of fibrinolytic agents with antiplatelet therapies, including Gp IIb/IIIa antagonists, low-molecular-weight heparins, or direct antithrombin agents, with or without facilitated PCI. It remains to be determined whether these combinations can safely enhance therapeutic efficacy. Yet, more important than the type of reperfusion regiment used, is the urgent need to make the "symptom-to-needle" or the "symptom-to-balloon" time as short as possible.

11. *Future progress.* Overall, the rate of progress has slowed and we are in an era in which the window of opportunity for benefit versus risk is extremely narrow. To place new developments into perspective, it should be emphasized that the major yield from a society perspective is to treat all eligible patients with ST-elevation myocardial infarction as quickly as possible. Unfortunately, many patients, including those at highest risk, receive no reperfusion therapy at all. It is here that the least amount of effort could provide the highest yield.

REFERENCES

1. Lip GY, et al. von Willebrand factor: a marker of endothelial dysfunction in vascular disorders? *Cardiovasc Res* 1997;34:255–265.
2. Nylander S, et al. The relative importance of the ADP receptors, P2Y12 and P2Y1, in thrombin-induced platelet activation. *Thromb Res* 2003;111:65–73.
3. Jurk K, et al. Thrombospondin-1 mediates platelet adhesion at high shear via glycoprotein Ib (GPIb): an alternative/backup mechanism to von Willebrand factor. *FASEB J* 2003;17:1490–1492.
4. Golino P, et al. Involvement of tissue factor pathway inhibitor in the coronary circulation of patients with acute coronary syndromes. *Circulation* 2003;108:2864–2869.
5. Nakamura Y, et al. Tissue factor expression in atrial endothelia associated with nonvalvular atrial fibrillation: possible involvement in intracardiac thrombogenesis. *Thromb Res* 2003;111:137–142.
6. Fuster V, et al. Aspirin as a therapeutic agent in cardiovascular disease. *Circulation* 1993;87:659–675.
7. Awtry EH, et al. Aspirin. *Circulation* 2000;101:1206–1218.
8. UK-TIA Study Group. The United Kingdom Transient Ischaemic Attack (UK-TIA) Aspirin Trial: final results. *J Neurol Neurosurg Psychiatry* 1991;54:1044–1054.
9. Ridker PM, et al. Low-dose aspirin therapy for chronic stable angina. A randomized placebo-controlled clinical trial. *Ann Intern Med* 1991;114:835–839.
10. Hayden M, et al. Aspirin for the primary prevention of cardiovascular events: a summary of the evidence for the U.S. Preventive Services Task Force. *Ann Intern Med* 2002;136:161–172.
11. Heras M, et al. Effects of thrombin inhibition on the development of acute platelet-thromubus deposition during angioplasty in pigs. *Circulation* 1989;79:657–665.
12. López-Farré A, et al. Effects of aspirin on platelet-neutrophil interactions. Role of nitric oxide and endothelin-1. *Circulation* 1995;91:2080–2088.
13. Ridker PM, et al. Inflammation, aspirin and the risk of cardiovascular disease in apparently healthy men. *N Engl J Med* 1997;336:973–979.
14. Eikelboom JW, et al. Aspirin-resistant thromboxane biosynthesis and the risk of myocardial infarction, stroke, or cardiovascular death in patients at high risk for cardiovascular events. *Circulation* 2002;105:1650–1655.
15. Gum PA, et al. A prospective, blinded determination of the natural history of aspirin resistance among stable patients with cardiovascular disease. *J Am Coll Cardiol* 2003;41:961–965.
16. MacDonald TM, et al. Effect of ibuprofen on cardioprotective effect of aspirin. *Lancet* 2003;361:573–574.
17. Bhatt DL. Aspirin resistance: more than just a laboratory curiosity. *J Am Coll Cardiol* 2004;43:1127–1129.

18. Antithrombotic Trialists' Collaboration. Collaborative meta-analysis of randomized trials of antiplatelet therapy for prevention of death, myocardial infarction and stroke in high-risk patients. *Br Med J* 2002;324:71–86.
19. Hansson L, et al. For the HOT Study Group. Effects of intensive blood-pressure lowering and low-dose aspirin in patients with hypertension: principal results of the Hypertension Optimal Treatment (HOT) randomised trial. *Lancet* 1998;351: 1755–1762.
20. Meade TW, et al. On behalf of the MRC General Practice Research Framework. Determination of who may derive most benefit from aspirin in primary prevention: subgroup results from a randomised controlled trial. *Br Med J* 2000;321:13–17.
21. Juul-Möller S, et al. For the Swedish Angina Pectoris Aspirin Trial (SAPAT) Group. Double-blind trial of aspirin in primary prevention of myocardial infarction in patients with stable chronic angina pectoris. *Lancet* 1992;340:1421–1425.
22. Pearson TA, et al. AHA Guidelines for Primary Prevention of Cardiovascular Disease and Stroke: 2002 Update: Consensus Panel Guide to Comprehensive Risk Reduction for Adult Patients Without Coronary or Other Atherosclerotic Vascular Diseases. American Heart Association Science Advisory and Coordinating Committee. *Circulation* 2002;106:388–391.
23. Fleming T, et al. Report from the 100th Cardiovascular and Renal Drugs Advisory Committee meeting: US Food and Drug Administration: December 8–9, 2003 Gaithersburg, Md. *Circulation* 2004;109:e9004–9005.
24. Sanmuganathan PS, et al. Aspirin for primary prevention of coronary heart disease: safety and absolute benefit related to coronary risk derived from meta-analysis of randomised trials. *Heart* 2001;85:265–271.
25. Segal R, et al. Early and late effects of low-dose aspirin on renal function in elderly patients. *Am J Med* 2003;115:462–466.
26. Mangano DT. Aspirin and mortality from coronary bypass surgery. *N Engl J Med* 2002;347:1309–1317.
27. Ferguson JD, et al. Contemporary management of paroxysmal supraventricular tachycardia. *Circulation* 2003;107:1096–1099.
28. Lincoff AM, et al. REPLACE-2 Investigators. Bivalirudin and provisional glycoprotein IIb/IIIa blockade compared with heparin and planned glycoprotein IIb/IIIa blockade during percutaneous coronary intervention: REPLACE-2 randomized trial. (Erratum in: 2003;289:1638). *JAMA* 2003;289:853–863.
29. Turpie A, et al. A comparison of aspirin with placebo in patients treated with warfarin after heart-valve replacement. *N Engl J Med* 1993;329:524–529.
30. Imanishi M, et al. Aspirin lowers blood pressure in patients with renovascular hypertension. *Hypertension* 1989;14:461–468.
31. Peters RJ, et al. Effects of aspirin dose when used alone or in combination with clopidogrel in patients with acute coronary syndromes: observations from the Clopidogrel in Unstable angina to prevent Recurrent Events (CURE) study. *Circulation* 2003;108:1682–1687.
32. Dutch TIA Trial Study Group. A comparison of two doses of aspirin (30 mg vs 283 mg a day) in patients after a transient ischemic attack or minor ischemic stroke. *N Engl J Med* 1991;325:1261–1266.
33. Taylor D, et al. Low-dose and high-dose acetylsalicylic acid for patients undergoing carotid endarterectomy: a randomised controlled trial. *Lancet* 1999;353:2179–2184.
34. Peto R, et al. UK-TIA Study Group. United Kingdom Transient Ischaemic Attack (UK-TIA) Aspirin Trial: interim results. *Br Med J* 1988;296:316–320.
35. Segal R, et al. Early and late effects of low-dose aspirin on renal function in elderly patients. *Am J Med* 2002;115:462–466.
36. Teo KK, et al. Effects of long-term treatment with angiotensin-converting-enzyme inhibitors in the presence or absence of aspirin: a systematic review. *Lancet* 2002;360:1037–1043.
37. Latini R, et al. Clinical effects of early angiotensin-converting enzyme inhibitor treatment for acute myocardial infarction are similar in the presence and absence of aspirin: systematic overview of individual data from 96,712 randomized patients. Angiotensin-converting Enzyme Inhibitor Myocardial Infarction Collaborative Group. *J Am Coll Cardiol* 2000;35:1801–1807.
38. van Wijngaarden, et al. Effects of acetylsalicylic acid on peripheral hemodynamics in patients with chronic heart failure treated with angiotensin-converting enzyme inhibitors. *J Cardiovasc Pharmacol* 1994;23:240–245.
39. Steinhubl SR, et al. Ticlopidine pretreatment before coronary stenting is associated with sustained decrease in adverse cardiac events: data from the Evaluation of Platelet IIb/IIIa Inhibitor for Stenting (EPISTENT) Trial. *Circulation* 2001;103:1403–1409.
40. Gent M, et al. The Canadian American Ticlopidine Study (CATS) in thromboembolic stroke. *Lancet* 1989;1:1215–1220.
41. Hass W, et al. A randomized trial comparing ticlopidine hydrochoride with aspirin for the prevention of stroke in high-risk patients. Ticlopidine Aspirin Stroke Study Group. *N Engl J Med* 1989;321:501–507.
42. Anonymous. Ticlopidine [editorial]. *Lancet* 1991;337:459–460.
43. Bhatt DL, et al. Meta-analysis of randomized and registry comparisons of ticlopidine with clopidogrel after stenting. *J Am Coll Cardiol* 2002;39:9–14.
44. Bates ER, et al. Drug-drug interactions involving antiplatelet agents. *Eur Heart J* 2003;24:1707–1709.
45. CAPRIE Steering Committee. A randomized, blinded trial of clopidogrel versus aspirin in patients at risk of ischemic events (CAPRIE). *Lancet* 1996;348:1329–1339.
46. The Clopidogrel in Unstable Angina to Prevent Recurrent Events Trial Investigators. Effects of clopidogrel in addition to aspirin in patients with acute coronary syndromes without ST-segment elevation. *N Engl J Med* 2001;345:494–502.

47. Mehta SR, et al. Clopidogrel in Unstable angina to prevent Recurrent Events trial (CURE) Investigators: Effects of pretreatment with clopidogrel and aspirin followed by long-term therapy in patients undergoing percutaneous coronary intervention: the PCI-CURE study. *Lancet* 2001;358:527–533.

48. Steinhubl SR, et al. Early and sustained dual oral antiplatelet therapy following percutaneous coronary intervention: a randomized controlled trial. *JAMA* 2002;288: 2411–2420.

49. Saw J, et al. Lack of adverse clopidogrel-atorvastatin clinical interaction from secondary analysis of a randomized, placebo-controlled clopidogrel trial. *Circulation* 2003;108:921–924.

50. Lau WC, et al. Contribution of hepatic cytochrome P450 3A4 metabolic activity to the phenomenon of clopidogrel resistance. *Circulation* 2004;109:166–171.

51. Müller I, et al. Effect of a high loading dose of clopidogrel on platelet function in patients undergoing coronary stent placement. *Heart* 2001;85:92–93.

52. Bertrand ME, et al. Double-blind study of the safety of clopidogrel with and without a loading dose in combination with aspirin compared with ticlopidine in combination with aspirin after coronary stenting: the clopidogrel aspirin stent international cooperative study (CLASSICS). *Circulation* 2000;102:624–629.

53. Mueller C, et al. A randomized comparison of clopidogrel and aspirin versus ticlopidine and aspirin after the placement of coronary artery stents. *J Am Coll Cardiol* 2003;41:969–973.

54. Kastrati A, et al. A clinical trial of abciximab in elective percutaneous coronary intervention after pretreatment with clopidogrel. *N Engl J Med* 2004;350:232–238.

55. Cannon CP, et al. Comparison of early invasive and conservative strategies in patients with unstable coronary syndromes treated with a glycoprotein IIb/IIIa inhibitor tirofiban. *N Engl J Med* 2001;344:1879–1887.

56. Penny W, et al. Antithrombotic therapy for patients with cardiac disease. *Curr Probl Cardiol* 1988;13:433–513.

57. Diener H, et al. European Stroke Prevention Study 2: dipyridamole and acetylsalicylic acid in the secondary prevention of stroke. *J Neurol Sci* 1996;143:1–13.

58. Madan M, et al. Glycoprotein IIb/IIIa integrin blockade. *Circulation* 1998;98:2629–2635.

59. Brown DL. Deaths associated with platelet glycoprotein IIb/IIIa inhibitor treatment. *Heart* 2003;89:535–537.

60. Brown DL, et al. Effect of glycoprotein IIb/IIIa inhibitors on the individual components of composite endpoints used in clinical trials of unstable angina and non-Q-wave myocardial infarction. *Cardiovasc Drugs Ther* 2000;14:301–306.

61. Kong D, et al. Clinical outcomes of therapeutic agents that block the platelet glycoprotein IIb/IIIa integrin in ischemic heart disease. *Circulation* 1998;98:2829–2835.

62. Kong DF, et al. Meta-analysis of survival with platelet glycoprotein IIb/IIIa antagonists for percutaneous coronary interventions. *Am J Cardiol* 2003;92:651–655.

63. Karvouni E, et al. Intravenous glycoprotein IIb/IIIa receptor antagonists reduce mortality after percutaneous coronary intervention. *J Am Coll Cardiol* 2003;41:26–32.

64. EPISTENT Investigators. Randomised placebo-controlled and balloon-angioplasty-controlled trial to assess safety of coronary stenting with use of platelet glycoprotein-IIb/IIIa blockade. *Lancet* 1998;352:87–92.

65. Topol E, et al. For the EPISTENT Investigators. Outcomes at 1 year and economic implications of platelet glycoprotein IIb/IIIa blockade in patients undergoing coronary stenting: results from a multicentre randomised trial. *Lancet* 1999;354: 2019–2024.

66. Heeschen C, et al. For the PRISM Study Investigators. Troponin concentrations for stratification of patients with acute coronary syndromes in relation to therapeutic efficacy of tirofiban. *Lancet* 1999;354:1757–1762.

67. PRISM-Plus Study. The Platelet Receptor Inhibition in Ischemic Syndrome Management in Patients Limited by Unstable Signs and Symptoms (PRISM-Plus) Study Investigators. Inhibition of the platelet glycoprotein IIb/IIIa receptor with tirofiban in unstable angina and non-Q-wave myocardial infarction. *N Engl J Med* 1998;338: 1488–1497.

68. White H. Low-molecular-weight heparin and platelet glycoprotein IIb/IIIa receptor blockade in acute coronary syndromes: complementary or competing therapies. *J Invas Cardiol* 2000;12 (Suppl A):6A–13A.

69. Zhao X-Q, et al. For the PRISM-Plus Investigators. Intracoronary thrombus and platelet glycoprotein IIb/IIIa receptor blockade with tirofiban in unstable angina or non-Q-wave myocardial infarction: angiographic results from the PRISM-PLUS Trial (Platelet Receptor Inhibition for Ischemic Syndrome Management in Patients Limited by Unstable Signs and Symptoms). *Circulation* 1999;100:1609–1615.

70. CAPTURE Investigators. Randomized placebo-controlled trial of abciximab before and during coronary intervention in refractory unstable angina; The CAPTURE Study. *Lancet* 1997;349:1429–1435.

71. PURSUIT Trial Investigators. Inhibition of platelet glycoprotein IIb/IIIa with eptifibatide in patients with acute coronary syndromes. *N Engl J Med* 1998;339:436–433.

72. Boersma E, et al. Platelet glycoprotein IIb/IIa receptor inhibition in non-ST-elevation acute coronary syndromes: early benefit during medical treatment only, with additional protection during percutaneous coronary intervention. *Circulation* 1999;100:2045–2048.

73. Lincoff AM, et al. Complementary clinical benefits of coronary-artery stenting and blockade of platelet glycoprotein IIb/IIIa receptors. *N Engl J Med* 1999;341:319–327.

74. Goodman SG, et al. Randomized evaluation of the safety and efficacy of enoxaparin versus unfractionated heparin in high-risk patients with non-ST-segment elevation acute coronary syndromes receiving the glycoprotein IIb/IIIa inhibitor eptifibatide. *Circulation* 2003;107:238–244.

75. Blazing MA, et al. for the A to Z Investigators. Safety and efficacy of enoxaparin vs unfractionated heparin in patients with non-ST-segment elevation acute coronary syndromes who receive tirofiban and aspirin: a randomized controlled trial. *JAMA* 2004;292:55–64.

76. EPIC Investigators. Use of a monoclonal antibody directed against the platelet glycoprotein IIb-IIIa receptor and high risk angioplasty. *N Engl J Med* 1994;330: 956–961.

77. EPILOG Investigators. Platelet glycoprotein IIb-IIIa receptor blockade and low-dose heparin during percutaneous coronary revascularization. *N Engl J Med* 1997;336: 1689–1696.

78. Tcheng J, et al. Readministration of abciximab is as effective as first time administration with similar risks: results from the ReoPro Readministration Registry (R[3]) [abstract]. *J Am Coll Cardiol* 1999;33 (Suppl A):14A–15A.

79. Moliterno DJ, et al. For the TARGET Investigators. Outcomes at 6 months for the direct comparison of tirofiban and abciximab during percutaneous coronary revascularisation with stent placement: the TARGET follow-up study. *Lancet* 2002; 360:355–360.

80. Szucs T, et al. Economic assessment of tirofiban in the management of acute coronary syndromes in the hospital setting: an analysis based on the PRISM PLUS Trial. *Eur Heart J* 1999;20:1253–1260.

81. Sasayama S. Effect of coronary collateral circulation on myocardial ischemia and ventricular dysfunction. *Cardiovascular Drugs Ther* 1994;8 (Suppl 2):327–334.

82. Hirsh J, et al. Guide to anticoagulant therapy. Part 1: Heparin. *Circulation* 1994;89: 1449–1468.

83. GUSTO-III Investigators. (The Global Use of Strategies to Open Occluded Coronary Arteries). A comparison of reteplase with alteplase for acute myocardial infarction. *N Engl J Med* 1997;337:1118–1123.

84. GUSTO Investigators. An international randomized trial comparing four thrombolytic strategies for acute myocardial infarction. *N Engl J Med* 1993;329:673–682.

85. Granger C, et al. For the GUSTO-I Investigators. Activated partial thromboplastin time and outcome after thrombolytic therapy for acute myocardial infarction: results from the GUSTO-I Trial. *Circulation* 1996;93:870–878.

86. Becker R, et al. Relation between systemic anticoagulation as determined by activated partial thromboplastin time and heparin measurements and in-hospital clinical events in unstable angina and non-Q wave myocardial infarction. Thrombolysis in Myocardial Ischemia IIIB Investigators. *Am Heart J* 1999;131:421–433.

87. GUSTO-IIa Investigators. Randomized trial of intravenous heparin versus recombinant hirudin for acute coronary syndromes. *Circulation* 1994;90:1631–1637.

88. Antman EM. For the TIMI 9A Investigators. Hirudin in acute myocardial infarction: safety report from the Thrombolysis and Thrombin Inhibition in Myocardial Infarction (TIMI) 9A Trial. *Circulation* 1994;90:1624–1630.

89. Hunter J, et al. Heparin induced thrombosis: an important complication of heparin prophylaxis for thromboembolic disease in surgery. *Br Med J* 1993;307:53–55.

90. Harenberg J, et al. Heparin-induced thrombocytopenia: pathophysiology and new treatment options. *Pathophysiol Haemost Thromb* 2002;32:289–294.

91. Liem A, et al. High dose heparin as pretreatment for primary angioplasty in acute myocardial infarction: the Heparin in Early Patency (HEAP) Randomized Trial. *J Am Coll Cardiol* 2000;35:600–604.

92. Théroux P, et al. Reactivation of unstable angina after the discontinuation of heparin. *N Engl J Med* 1992;327:141–145.

93. Bijsterveld NR, et al. Recurrent cardiac ischemic events early after discontinuation of short-term heparin treatment in acute coronary syndromes: results from the Thrombolysis in Myocardial Infarction (TIMI) 11B and Efficacy and Safety of Subcutaneous Enoxaparin in Non-Q-Wave Coronary Events (ESSENCE) studies. *J Am Coll Cardiol* 2003;42:2083–2089.

94. Armstrong P. Heparin in acute coronary disease: requiem for a heavyweight? [editorial]. *N Engl J Med* 1997;337:492–494.

95. FRISC Study Group. Fragmin During Instability in Coronary Artery Disease (FRISC). Low molecular-weight heparin during instability in coronary artery disease. *Lancet* 1996;347:561–568.

96. FRISC II Prospective Randomized Multicenter Study. Long-term low-molecular-mass heparin in unstable coronary artery disease. Fragmin and fast revascularisation during instability in coronary artery disease investigators. FRISC II Prospective Randomized Multi-Center Study. *Lancet* 1999;354:708–715.

97. Antman EM, et al. Enoxaparin is superior to unfractionated heparin for preventing clinical events at 1-year follow-up of TIMI 11B and ESSENCE. *Eur Heart J* 2002;23:308–314.

98. Antman EM, et al. For the TIMI IIB (Thrombolysis in Myocardial Infarction) and ESSENCE (Efficacy and Safety of Subcutaneous Enoxaparin in Non-Q-QWave Coronary Events). Assessment of the treatment effect of enoxaparin or unstable angina; non-Q-wave myocardial infarction TIMI-IIb ESSENCE Meta-Analysis. *Circulation* 1999;100:1602–1608.

99. SYNERGY Trial Investigators. Enoxaparin vs unfractionated heparin in high-risk patients with non-ST-segment elevation acute coronary syndromes managed with an intended early invasive strategy: primary results of the SYNERGY randomized trial. *JAMA* 2004;292:45–54.

100. Petersen JL, et al. Efficacy and bleeding complications among patients randomized to enoxaparin or unfractionated heparin for antithrombin therapy in non-ST-segment elevation acute coronary syndromes: a systematic overview. *JAMA* 2004;292:89–96.

101. Simoons M, et al. Improved reperfusion and clinical outcome with enoxaparin as an adjunct to streptokinase thrombolysis in acute myocardial infarction. The AMI-SK study. *Eur Heart J* 2002;23:1282–1290.

102. ASSENT-3 Investigators. Efficacy and safety of tenecteplase in combination with enoxaparin, abciximab or unfractionated heparin: the ASSENT-3 randomised trial in acute myocardial infarction. *Lancet* 2001;358:605–613.

103. Wallentin L, et al. Oral ximelagatran for secondary prophylaxis after myocardial infarction: the ESTEEM randomised controlled trial. *Lancet* 2003;362:789–797.

104. Antman EM, et al. Enoxaparin as adjunctive antithrombin therapy for ST-elevation myocardial infarction: results of the ENTIRE-Thrombolysis in Myocardial Infarction (TIMI) 23 Trial. *Circulation* 2002;105:1642–1649.

105. Weitz J, et al. Clot-bound thrombin is protected from inhibition by heparin—antithrombin III but is susceptible to inactivation by antithrombin III-independent inhibitors. *J Clin Invest* 1990;86:385–391.

105a. Greinacher A, et al. Lepirudin anaphylaxis and Kounis syndrome (letter). *Circulation* 2004;109:e315.

106. OASIS-2 Investigators. Organisation to Assess Strategies for Ischemic Syndromes. Effects of recombinant hirudin (Lepirudin) compared with heparin on death, myocardial infarction, refractory angina, and revascularisation procedures in patients with acute myocardial ischaemia without ST elevation: a randomised trial. *Lancet* 1999;353:429–438.

107. Reed MD, et al. Clinical pharmacology of bivalirudin. *Pharmacotherapy* 2002;22:105S–111S.

108. Parry M, et al. Kinetic mechanism for the interaction of hirulog with thrombin. *Biochem* 1994;33:14807–14814.

109. Kong D, et al. Clinical outcomes of bivalirudin for ischemic heart disease. *Circulation* 1999;100:2049–2053.

110. HERO-2 Trial Investigators. Thrombin-specific anticoagulation with bivalirudin versus heparin in patients receiving fibrinolytic therapy for acute myocardial infarction: the HERO-2 randomised trial. *Lancet* 2001;358:1855–1863.

111. Coussement PK, et al. A synthetic factor-Xa inhibitor (ORG31540/SR9017A) as an adjunct to fibrinolysis in acute myocardial infarction. The PENTALYSE study. *Eur Heart J* 2001;22:1716–1724.

112. SPORTIF-III Randomized Control Trial. Olsson, SB; Executive Steering Committee. Stroke prevention with the oral direct thrombin inhibitor ximelagatran compared with warfarin in patients with non-valvular atrial fibrillation (SPORTIF II): randomized controlled trial. *Lancet* 2003;362:1691–1698.

113. Eikelboom J, et al. Ximelagatran or warfarin in atrial fibrillation? *Lancet* 2004;363:734; author reply 734, 736.

114. Hirsh J, et al. American Heart Association/American College of Cardiology Foundation guide to warfarin therapy. *J Am Coll Cardiol* 2003;41:1633–1652.

115. Vink R, et al. The optimal intensity of vitamin K antagonists in patients with mechanical heart valves: a meta-analysis. *J Am Coll Cardiol* 2003;42:2042–2048.

116. Singer D. Randomized trials of warfarin for atrial fibrillation. *N Engl J Med* 1992;327:1451–1453.

117. Hirsh J, et al. Guide to anticoagulant therapy. Part 2: Oral anticoagulants (published erratum appears in Circulation 1995;91:A55-A56). *Circulation* 1994;89:1469–1480.

118. Vaitkus P, et al. Embolic potential, prevention and management of mural thrombus complicating anterior myocardial infarction: a meta-analysis. *J Am Coll Cardiol* 1993;22:1004–1009.

119. Al-Khadra A, et al. Warfarin anticoagulation and survival: a cohort analysis from the Studies of Left Ventricular Dysfunction. *J Am Coll Cardiol* 1998;31:749–753.

120. Anand SS, et al. Oral anticoagulant therapy in patients with coronary artery disease: a meta-analysis. *JAMA* 1999;282:2058–2067.

121. Samama M, et al. For the Prophylaxis in Medical Patients with Enoxaparin Study Group. A comparison of enoxaparin with placebo for the prevention of venous thromboembolism in acutely ill medical patients. *N Engl J Med* 1999;341:793–800.

122. Ridker PM, et al. Long-term, low-intensity warfarin therapy for the prevention of recurrent venous thromboembolism. *N Engl J Med* 2003;348:1425–1434.

123. Pritchett E. Management of atrial fibrillation. *N Engl J Med* 1992;326:1264–1271.

124. AFFIRM Investigators. First Antiarrhythmic Drug Substudy. Maintenance of sinus rhythm in pateints with atrial fibrillation. *J Am Coll Cardiol* 2003;42:20–29.

125. Stroke Prevention in Atrial Fibrillation Investigators. Adjusted-dose warfarin versus low-intensity, fixed-dose warfarin plus aspirin for high risk patients with atrial fibrillation: Stroke Prevention in Atrial Fibrillation III Randomised Clinical Trial. *Lancet* 1996;348:633–638.

126. Gullov A, et al. Fixed minidose warfarin and aspirin alone and in combination vs adjusted-dose warfarin for stroke prevention in atrial fibrillation: Second Copenhagen atrial fibrillation, aspirin and anticoagulation study. *Arch Intern Med* 1998;158:1513–1521.

127. Pengo V, et al. Effectiveness of fixed minidose warfarin in the prevention of thromboemolism and vascular death in nonrheumatic atrial fibrillation. *Am J Cardiol* 1998;82:433–437.

128. Dunn M, et al. Antithrombotic therapy in atrial fibrillation. *Chest* 1989;95 (Suppl 2):118S–127S.

129. Kopecky S, et al. The natural history of lone atrial fibrillation: a population-based study over three decades. *N Engl J Med* 1987;317:669–674.

130. Kopecky SL, et al. Lone atrial fibrillation in the elderly (Abstract). *Circulation* 1989;80 (Suppl II):II-409.

131. Cairns JA, et al. Nonrheumatic atrial fibrillation: risk of stroke and role of antithrombotic therapy. *Circulation* 1991;84:469–481.

132. Atrial Fibrillation Investigators. Risk factors for stroke and efficacy of antithrombotic therapy in atrial fibrillation: analysis of pooled data from five randomised controlled trials (published erratum appears in Arch Intern Med 1994; 154: 2254). *Arch Intern Med* 1994;154:1449–1457.

133. Caro J, et al. Atrial fibrillation and anticoagulation: from randomised trials to practice. *Lancet* 1993;341:1381–1384.

134. EAFT Study Group. European Atrial Fibrillation Trial. Secondary prevention in non-rheumatic and atrial fibrillation after transient ischaemic attack or minor stroke. *Lancet* 1993;342:1255–1262.

135. Meade T, et al. Fibrinolytic activity, clotting factors, and long-term incidence of ischaemic heart disease in the Northwick Park Heart Study. *Lancet* 1993;342:1076–1079.

136. Merlini P, et al. Persistent activation of coagulation mechanism in unstable angina and myocardial infarction. *Circulation* 1994;90:61–68.

137. CARS Investigators. Coumadin Aspirin Reinfarction Study. Randomised double-blind trial of fixed low-dose warfarin with aspirin after myocardial infarction. *Lancet* 1997;350:389–386.

138. Fiore LD, et al. Department of Veterans Affairs Cooperative Studies Program Clinical Trial comparing combined warfarin and aspirin with aspirin alone in survivors of acute myocardial infarction: primary results of the CHAMP study. *Circulation* 2002;105:557–563.

139. Medical Research Council's Practice Research Framework. Thrombosis prevention trial: randomised trial of low-intensity oral anticoagulation with warfarin and low-dose aspirin in the primary prevention of ischaemic heart disease in men at increased risk. *Lancet* 1998;351:233–241.

140. Stroke Prevention in Atrial Fibrillation Investigators. Warfarin versus aspirin for prevention of thromboembolism in atrial fibrillation: Stroke Prevention and Atrial Fibrillation II Study. *Lancet* 1994;343:687–691.

141. White HD. Aspirin or warfarin for non-rheumatic atrial fibrillation (Editorial). *Lancet* 1994;343:683–684.

142. Post Coronary Artery Bypass Graft Trial Investigators. The effect of aggressive lowering of low-density lipoprotein cholesterol levels and low-dose anticoagulation on obstructive changes in saphenous-vein coronary-artery bypass grafts. *N Engl J Med* 1997;336:153–162.

143. Mohr JP, et al. A comparison of warfarin and aspirin for the prevention of recurrent ischemic stroke. *N Engl J Med* 2001;345:1444–1451.

144. Gersh BJ, et al. Thrombolysis and myocardial salvage: results of clinical trials and the animal paradigm—paradoxic or predictable? *Circulation* 1993;88:296–306.

145. White H, et al. Clinical cardiology: new frontiers: thrombolysis for acute myocardial infarction. *Circulation* 1998;97:1632–1646.

146. White H. Remodelling of the heart after myocardial infarction. *Aust NZ J Med* 1992;22 (5 Suppl):601–606.

147. Simes R, et al. For the GUSTO-I Investigators. Link between the angiographic substudy and mortality outcomes in a large randomized trial of myocardial reperfusion: importance of early and complete infarct artery repertusion. *Circulation* 1995;91:1923–1928.

148. Giugliano RP, et al. Selecting the best reperfusion strategy in ST-elevation myocardial infarction: it's all a matter of time. *Circulation* 2003;108:2828–2830.

149. Anderson H, et al. Thrombolysis in acute myocardial infarction. *N Engl J Med* 1993;329:703–709.

150. Fibrinolytic Therapy Trial. (FTT) Collaborative Group. Indications for fibrinolytic therapy in suspected acute myocardial infarction; collaborative overview of early mortality and major morbidity results from all randomised trials of more than 1000 patients. *Lancet* 1994;343:311–322.

151. Steg PG, et al. Impact of time to treatment on mortality after prehospital fibrinolysis or primary angioplasty: data from the CAPTIM randomized clinical trial. *Circulation* 2003;108:2851–2856.

152. Weaver WD, et al. For the Myocardial Infarction Triage and Intvervention Trial. Prehospital-initiated vs hospital-initiated thrombolytic therapy. *JAMA* 1993;270:1211–1216.

153. White HD. Optimal treatment of patients with acute coronary syndromes and non-ST-elevation myocardial infarction. *Am Heart J* 1999;138:S105–S114.

154. Bonnefoy E, et al. Primary angioplasty versus prehospital fibrinolysis in acute myocardial infarction: a randomised study. *Lancet* 2002;360:825–829.

155. De Luca G, et al. Symptom-onset-to balloon time and mortality in patients with acute myocardial infarction treated by primary angioplasty. *J Am Col Cardiol* 2003;42:991–997.

156. GUSTO-V Investigators. Reperfusion therapy for acute myocardial infarction with fibrinolytic therapy or combination reduced fibrinolytic therapy and platelet glycoprotein 11b/111a inhibition: GUSTO V randomised trial. *Lancet* 2001;357:1905–1914.

157. ASSENT-2 Investigators. Assessment of the Safety and Efficacy of a New Thrombolytic (ASSENT-2) Investigators. Single-bolus tenecteplase compared with front-loaded alteplase in acute myocardial infarction: the ASSENT-2 double-blinded randomised trial. *Lancet* 1999;354:716–722.

158. Karnash SL, et al. For the GUSTO-I Investigators. Treating menstruating women with thrombolytic therapy: insights from the Global Utilization of Streptokinase and Tissue Plasminogen Activator for Occluded Coronary Arteries (GUSTO-I) Trial. *J Am Coll Cardiol* 1995;26:1651–1656.

159. Mahaffey KW, et al. For the GUSTO- Investigators, 1997. Diabetic retinopathy should not be a contraindication to thrombolytic therapy for acute myocardial infarction: review of ocular hemorrhage incidence and location in the GUSTO-I trial. *J Am Coll Cardiol* 1997;30:1606–1610.

160. Califf RM, et al. Economic and cost-effectiveness in evaluating the value of cardiovascular therapies. The impact of the cost-effectiveness study of GUSTO-1 on decision making with regard to fibrinolytic therapy. *Am Heart J* 1999;137:S90–93.

161. INJECT Trial. International Joint Efficacy Comparison of Thrombolytics. Randomised, double-blind comparison of reteplase double-bolus administration with streptokinase in acute myocardial infarction (INJECT): trial to investigate equivalence (published erratum appears in Lancet 1995; 346: 980). *Lancet* 1995; 346:329–336.

162. Gruber A, et al. Generation of activated protein C during thrombolysis. *Lancet* 1993;342:1275–1276.

163. ISIS-3 Study Group. (Third International Study of Infarct Survival) Collaborative Group. ISIS-3: a randomised comparison of streptokinase vs tissure plasminogen activator vs anistreplase and of aspirin plus heparin vs aspirin alone among 41,299 cases of suspected acute myocardial infarction. *Lancet* 1992;339:753–770.

164. Collins R, et al. Clinical effects of a anticoagulant therapy in suspected acute myocardial infarction: systematic overview of randomised trials. *Br Med J* 1996;313: 652–659.

165. Tardiff BE, et al. Long term results from the Global Utilization of Streptokinase and TPA for Occluded Coronary Arteries (GUSTO-I) Trial: sustained benefit of fibrin-specific therapy (Abstract). *Circulation* 1999;100 (18):I-498–I-499.

166. Ito H, et al. Lack of myocardial perfusion immediately after successful thrombolysis: a predictor of poor recovery of left ventricular function in anterior myocardial infarction. *Circulation* 1992;85:1699–1705.

167. Lauerma K, et al. Multislice MRI in assessment of myocardial perfusion in patients with single-vessel proximal left anterior descending coronary artery disease before and after revascularization. *Circulation* 1997;96:2859–2867.

168. Wu KC, et al. Prognostic significance of microvascular obstruction by magnetic resonance imaging in patients with acute myocardial infarction. *Circulation* 1998;97:765–772.

169. Antman E, et al. For the TIMI IIB Investigators. Enoxaparin prevents death and cardiac ischemic events in unstable angina-non-Q-wave myocardial infarction: results of the Thrombolysis in Myocardial Infarction (TIMI) 11B Trial. *Circulation* 1999;100:1593–1601.

170. White HD, et al. Randomized, double-blind comparison of hirulog versus heparin in patients receiving streptokinase and aspirin for acute myocardial infarction HERO (Hirulog Early Reperfusion/Occlusion) Trial Investigators. *Circulation* 1997;96: 2155–2161.

171. Grines CL, et al. For the Stent Primary Angioplasty in Myocardial Infection Study Group. Coronary angioplasty with or without stent implantation for acute myocardial infarction. *N Engl J Med* 1999;341:1949–1956.

172. Hochman JS, et al. Effects of early revascularization for cardiogenic shock on 1 year mortality: the SHOCK Trial results (abstract). *Circulation* 1999;100 (Suppl I):I-369.

173. Keeley E, et al. Primary angioplasty versus intravenous thrombolytic therapy for acute myocardial infarction: a quantitative review of 23 randomised trials. *Lancet* 2003;361:13–20.

174. Stone GW, et al. Normal flow (TIMI-3) before mechanical reperfusion therapy is an independent determinant of survival in acute myocardial infarction: analysis from the primary angioplasty in myocardial infarction trials. *Circulation* 2001;104: 636–641.

175. Ross AM, et al. A randomized trial comparing primary angioplasty with a strategy of short-acting thrombolysis and immediate planned rescue angioplasty in acute myocardial infarction: the PACT trial. PACT investigators. Plasminogen-activator Angioplasty Compatibility Trial. *J Am Coll Cardiol* 1999;34:1954–1962.

176. Ohman EM, et al. Enhanced early reperfusion at 60 minutes with low-dose reteplase combined with full-dose abciximab in acute myocardial infarction: preliminary results from the GUSTO-4 Pilot (SPED) Dose Ranging Trial. *Circulation* 1998;98 (Suppl I):I-504.

177. Widimsky P, et al. On behalf of the PRAGUE Study Group Investigators. Long distance support for primary angioplasty vs immediate thombolysis in acute myocardial infarction. *Eur Heart J* 2002;2003:94–104.

178. Schomig A, et al. Therapy-dependent influence of time-to-treatment interval on myocardial salvage in patients with acute myocardial infarction treated with coronary artery stenting or thrombolysis. *Circulation* 2003;108:1084–1088.

179. White HD. Future of reperfusion therapy for acute myocardial infarction (Editorial). *Lancet* 1999;354:695–697.

180. Hogg KJ, et al. Angiographic patency study of anistreplase versus streptokinase in acute myocardial infarction. *Lancet* 1990;335:254–258.

181. PRIMI Trial Study Group. Randomised double-blind trial of recombinant prourokinase agaomst streptokinase in acute myocardial infarction. *Lancet* 1989;i: 863–868.

182. GUSTO, et al. The effects of tissue plasminogen activator, streptokinase, or both on coronary artery patency, ventricular function, and survival after acute myocardial infarction (published erratum appears in N Engl J Med 1994;350:516). *N Engl J Med* 1993;329:1615–1622.

183. Purvis JA, et al. Efficacy of 100 mg of double-bolus alteplase in achieving complete perfusion in the treatment of acute myocardial infarction. *J Am Coll Cardiol* 1994;23:6–10.

184. Granger CB, et al. Thrombolytic therapy for acute myocardial infarction: a review (published erratum appears in Drugs, 1993;45:894). *Drugs* 1992;44:293–325.

185. Neuhaus KL, et al. Improved thrombolysis with a modified dose regimen of recombinant tissue-type plasminogen activator. *J Am Coll Cardiol* 1989;14:1566–1569.

186. Marder VJ, et al. Thrombolytic therapy: current status. *N Engl J Med* 1988;318: 1512–1520.

187. Simoons ML, et al. Individual risk assessment for intracranial haemorrhage during thrombolytic therapy. *Lancet* 1993;342:1523–1528.

10

Lipid-Lowering and Antiatherosclerotic Drugs

Antonio M. Gotto, Jr. • Lionel H. Opie

> "In the great majority of cases ordinary atheroma (Greek, meal or porridge) is to blame; this consists of softening, the precursor or arteriosclerosis, with yellowish fatty (cholesterol) areas in the endarterium."
>
> PAUL DUDLEY WHITE, 1944[1]

Blood lipid assessment forms an essential step in the assessment of almost every cardiac patient, whether middle-aged or elderly. Risk factor assessment is integral to the cardiovascular management of all patients: physicians may help guide younger patients towards long-term cardiovascular health by addressing early risk factors, while middle-aged and older patients may need a more intensive approach because of their near-term risk for coronary disease. The widespread availability, persuasive and substantial clinical database, and relative safety of the statins have established pharmacologic control of blood lipids as an increasingly acceptable strategy. Nonetheless, comprehensive lipid management extends beyond drugs to include overall risk factor and lifestyle modification. Regrettably, large numbers of drug-eligible patients who may benefit from statins and other lipid lowering drugs are still not receiving them.[2]

PREVENTION AND RISK FACTORS

Primary prevention in those without evident coronary disease remains a highly desirable aim. Lifestyle interventions (diet, smoking cessation, and physical activity) are the first line of treatment in this population, and may achieve cholesterol reduction in about 50% of those who need primary prevention.[2] In the national American campaign, promoting dietary management and other lifestyle measures has resulted in a reduction of mean blood cholesterol levels and a fall in coronary heart disease (CHD) mortality rate. Primary prevention has two major themes. First, population-wide efforts focus on risk factor modification and education with the goal of staving off the development of coronary disease in the long term (i.e., several decades). Second, within the individual patient, primary prevention intends to identify those patients whose near-term coronary risk (e.g., risk for heart disease within the next 10 years) warrants intensified risk factor modification. The implementation of drug therapy in this latter group has become less controversial in recent years. Clinical trials in the past decade of statins have demonstrated safety and clinical event reduction across the spectrum of cardiovascular risk. Still debated, however, are the fiscal and ethical issues related to the cost-effectiveness of lipid drug therapy in lower risk groups. As less expensive, generic versions of statins become increasingly available, concerns about cost-effectiveness may become moot.

Global Risk Evaluation; ATP III Rather than assign patients to primary or secondary prevention, ATP III argues for three risk categories (Table 10-1): high (CHD or equivalent); medium (2 or more risk factors, 10 year risk of 20% or less) and low (0 to 1 major risk factors, 10 year risk 10% or less). Low-density lipoprotein cholesterol (LDL-C) values

Table 10-1 LDL-C Goals Based on Global Risk in Latest American and European Guidelines

ATP III Risk Categories (Highest to Lowest)	LDL-C Goal

CHD
 CHD Risk Equivalents
   Other cardiovascular disease or
   Diabetes mellitus or
   Aortic aneurysm or
   10 year risk greater than 20%
	<100 mg/dL (2.6 mmol/L)
	 Optional in very high-risk
	   patients: <70 mg/dL
	   (1.8 mmol/L)

Multiple (2+) Risk Factors Moderately high risk (optional)	<130 mg/dL (3.4 mmol/L) <100 mg/dL (2.6 mmol/L)
0–1 Risk Factors	<160 mg/dL (4.1 mmol/L)

European Guidelines Risk Priorities (Highest to Lowest)	

Patients with *established CVD*
 Asymptomatic patients who have
   Multiple risk factors or
   Markedly raised levels of single risk
   factors
 Type 2 diabetes or *type 1 diabetes*
 with Microalbuminuria
	<96 mg/dL (2.5 mmol/L)
	 <115 mg/dL (3.0 mmol/L)

Close Relatives of Patients with early-onset CVD or asymptomatic, high-risk patients	<115 mg/dL (3.0 mmol/L)
Other individuals encountered in routine practice	<115 mg/dL (3.0 mmol/L)

Data from ATP III and joint European Guidelines.[3,3a,4]
CHD = coronary heart disease; CVD = cardiovascular disease; LDL-C = low-density lipoprotein cholesterol.

still play a crucial role in decision making (Table 10-2). Cardiovascular risk management has grown increasingly sophisticated, largely because of the growing acceptance of global risk assessment as the primary mode for determining the intensity of treatment. In the 2001 US Adult Treatment Panel (ATP III) guidelines, the patient's absolute risk for developing CHD in the next 10 years determines the aggressiveness of lipid intervention.[3] This global risk is calculated using an algorithm based on the Framingham Heart Study that considers not only total cholesterol, but also high-density lipoprotein cholesterol (HDL-C), smoking, age, hypertension, and sex. Also featured in ATP III is the concept of the *CHD equivalent*, a risk factor whose presence identifies a patient who should receive treatment as aggressively as someone with a history of heart attack, angina, or revascularization. Included in this category of risk factor are diabetes, noncoronary atherosclerosis (peripheral vascular disease or stroke), and aortic aneurysm.

Other Algorithms Besides the ATP III model, a number of other algorithms are available for estimating absolute risk, including latest guidelines of the Joint Task Force of European and other Societies on Cardiovascular Disease Prevention in Clinical Practice[4] or the PROCAM risk calculators of the International Task Force (http://www.chd-taskforce.com). Differences in the data sets used and the methods for calculation may yield different risk predictions, but these schemas share a common intention: to facilitate the discrimination of higher risk patients from lower risk ones. Such risk estimation should be used to help determine which patients may optimally benefit from drug intervention. Both US and European guidelines prioritize categories of patients and modify the LDL-C goal based on these groups' levels of risk (Table 10-1).

Table 10-2 LDL-C Treatment Thresholds for Diet or Drugs

Risk Category	LDL-C Goal	Diet, Lifestyle Initiation Level	Drug Treatment Initiation Level
0–1 Other risk factors* (Low 10-year risk)	<160 mg/dL (4.14 mmol/L)	≥160 mg/dL	≥190 mg/dL (4.91 mmol/L) (160–189; LDL-C-lowering drug optional)
2+ Other risk factors (10-year risk ≤20%)	<130 mg/dL (3.36 mmol/L) <100 mg/dL (2.6 mmol/L) in higher risk	≥130 mg/dL	10-year risk 10%–20%: ≥130 mg/dL 10-year risk <10%: ≥160 mg/dL
CHD or CHD Risk equivalents (10-year risk >20%)	<100 mg/dL or lower, possibly 70 mg/dL (1.8 mmol/L)†	≥100 mg/dL	≥100 mg/dL†

*Almost all people with 0–1 other risk factors have a 10-year risk <10%: thus, 10-year risk assessment in people with 0–1 risk factor is not necessary.
†Consider such lower levels in the light of PROVE-IT and REVERSAL trials.[3a,6,7] Clinical judgment may call for deferring drug therapy in this subcategory.
CHD = coronary heart disease; LDL-C = low-density lipoprotein cholesterol; TLC = therapeutic lifestyle changes.

Secondary Prevention Since the last edition of this book, there have been major changes in thought in that: (1) any manifestation of vascular disease, whether it be coronary, peripheral or cerebral, or diabetes as a coronary equivalent, is now often regarded as an indication for lipid lowering by a statin,[3,4] irrespective of the baseline cholesterol level because of the high risk for future CHD,[5] and (2) the aim of intensive LDL-cholesterol lowering may now have to be reconsidered, with possibly lower goals in the region of 70 mg/dL (1.8 mmol/L) or even lower in the very high risk patients.[3a,6–8] As most physicians still rely on the blood lipid profile in risk factor management and treat to specific goals, we note that which of the ultra-low values should be the goal is currently under reconsideration by ATP.[3] *Overall, drug-induced LDL-C reduction remains an essential component* of a comprehensive attack on risk factors that also aims to reduce the total risk through BP control, dietary changes, increased exercise, weight loss, and strictly no smoking.

THE ENDOTHELIUM AND INFLAMMATION

A further paradigm shift has been the increasing emphasis on the interactive roles of vascular inflammation and endothelial damage in the genesis of arterial disease.[9,10] Both endothelial dysfunction and the inflammatory process are early events (Fig. 10-1). Links between endothelial damage and atherosclerosis have increasing evidence in their favor, without definite proof of this sequence in humans. The healthy endothelium by producing nitric oxide helps the coronary arteries to dilate when so required by exercise, whereas the damaged endothelium releases endothelin and other vasoconstrictors that also promote vascular smooth muscle growth and thereby contribute to arterial damage. The damaged endothelium also allows neutrophil roll-on, an early event that promotes the adhesion of circulating macrophages, which then penetrate the endothelium to become activated, to participate in the inflammatory process, and to be transformed to foam cells.[10] The presence of oxidized LDL greatly accelerates the whole process. Activity of angiotensin-II contributes by accelerating the formation of oxygen free radicals that in turn promote

ENDOTHELIUM AND VASCULAR DISEASE

Opie 2004

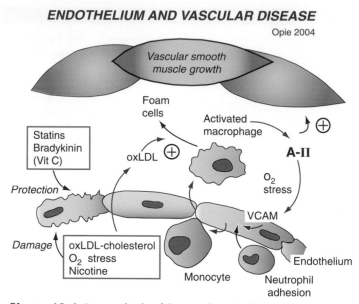

Figure 10-1 Proposed role of the vascular endothelium in atherogenesis. Note: (1) Early endothelial damage, prompted by several factors including oxidized low-density lipoprotein (*ox LDL*), and hypothetically prevented by treatment. Neutrophils roll on and adhere to the damaged endothelium to promote adhesion of macrophages. Vascular cell adhesion molecule (*VCAM*) promotes the binding of macrophages to the endothelium, after which they penetrate the endothelium to become activated and, by uptake of ox LDL, to become foam cells. Activated macrophages also synthesize angiotensin II (*A-II*) that in turn promotes oxidative stress that stimulates the formation of VCAM. A-II also promotes growth of vascular smooth muscle cells, an integral part of atherogenesis. (*Figure © LH Opie, 2005.*)

the formation of oxidized LDL, thereby enhancing the inflammatory process. Increasing evidence shows that there is an important cytokine-mediated inflammatory component to the atherosclerotic process.[10] Statin therapy lowers the blood levels of C-reactive protein, an inflammatory marker and therefore has an anti-inflammatory effect that may contribute to the benefit associated with this drug class.[6,10] Direct measurement of the *coronary atheroma volume* by intravascular ultrasound shows that LDL-C lowering must drop to about 75 mg/dL (about 2.0 mmol/L) or below will prevent plaque progression.[7,8]

BLOOD LIPID PROFILE

Blood Cholesterol and Lipoproteins Although desirable blood cholesterol value may be below 200 mg/dL or 5.2 mmol/L,[3] or even much lower at 150 mg/dL or 3.9 mmol/L (Table 10-3), it needs reemphasizing that the cholesterol level is only part of the patient's absolute global risk. Furthermore, it is the LDL level that is the real goal of therapy, with optimal levels now appearing to be even less than 100 mg/dL.[6-8] Every increment of 25 mg/dL in LDL-C gives about an equal increase in risk.[11] LDL-C values above 130 mg/dL despite diet warrant drug therapy in those at medium risk, while in those at highest risk with CHD or equivalents, the goal is <100 mg/dl or <70 mg/dL in some cases (Table 10-1).

High-density lipoproteins (HDL) are a new focus of interest (Table 10-3). In vitro, HDL aids in clearing cholesterol from foam cells, which develop in the diseased arteries (Fig. 10-2). A low HDL-C is an added risk factor, being strongly and inversely associated with risk for CHD.[3]

Table 10-3	Role of Total Cholesterol, HDL-C, and Triglyceride Values in Management of Lipid Disorders
Values	**Drug Management**
Serum Cholesterol Levels[†]	
~150 mg/dL (3.9 mmol/L)[‡]	? New lower goal for CHD or equivalent
<175 mg/dL (4.5 mmol/L)	Goal for diabetes or CHD or equivalent
<190 mg/dL (5.0 mmol/L)	General goal; desirable; check LDL
>190–239 mg/dL (5.0–6.2 mmol/L)	Only if total risk low; check LDL
≥240 mg/dL (6.2 mmol/L)	Govern by LDL
Serum HDL-C Levels	
>60 mg/dL (1.6 mmol/L)	*High*, protective. Leave.
<40 mg/dL (1.03 mmol/L), in women <46 mg/dL (1.2 mmol/L)[†]	*Low*. Risk factor. Consider drug treatment if other risks.* Otherwise exercise and diet
Triglyceride (Fasting) Levels	
<150 mg/dL (1.69 mmol/L)	Normal
180–199 mg/dL (1.69–2.25 mmol/L)	*Borderline;* nondrug treatment (loss of weight, increased exercise, moderate alcohol intake, dietary therapy)
250–499 mg/dL (2.26–5.63 mmol/L)	*High;* lifestyle treatment; drugs if high LDL-C or low HDL-C
>500 mg/dL (5.65 mmol/L)	*Very high*, urgent treatment needed; risk of pancreatitis.

*Other risk factors for coronary heart disease (CHD), besides cholesterol levels, defined by ATP III as family history of premature CHD, smoking, hypertension, age (men ≥45, women ≥55), and HDLC <40 mg/dL (1.03 mmol/L).
[†]European standards, others from ATP II.
[‡]Extrapolation by one of authors (LHO) from REVERSAL study.[7]

Because this is a continuously variable relation, and because a low HDL-C is often associated with other lipid abnormalities, for example, high triglyceride, an HDL-C below 40 mg/dL (<1.03 mmol/L) is seen in ATP III partially as a marker for other risk factors as in the metabolic syndrome (see later). In the CARE study, every 10 mg/dL decrease in HDL-C led to a similar 10% increase in risk.[11] A value of 60 mg/dL or more (1.6 mmol/L) is a negative (protective) risk factor.[3] Even minor elevations of HDL-C to only 42 mg/dL or 1.1 mmol/L are associated with protection in some large studies.[12] Overall, normalization of HDL-C is desirable, but not as essential as reduction of LDL-C (to below 100 mg/dL). Notable is that ATP III guidelines do not propose a target value for HDL-C, although they do recommend correction when possible by lifestyle modification (exercise, modest alcohol intake, loss of weight, non-smoking may all help). A low HDL-C is often part of a *lipid triad*, or atherogenic dyslipidemia, the other two components being elevated triglycerides and small LDL particles. This can be regarded as a risk factor in its own right, and is commonly found in the metabolic syndrome, in type 2 diabetes, and in others with premature CHD.[3] Nicotinic acid is the agent recommended for this lipid triad,[3] together with lifestyle modification. In the future, a variety of more specific agents including HDL-infusion therapy and *torcetrapib*, a partial inhibitor of the enzyme cholesteryl ester transfer protein inhibitor, will become available with expectations of an increase of HDL, a decrease of the atheroma volume and fewer clinical events.[13]

Blood Triglycerides These are commonly high in patients with coronary artery disease, yet any specific role of hypertriglyceridemia in

ROLE OF LIPOPROTEINS IN ATHEROSCLEROSIS
Opie 2004

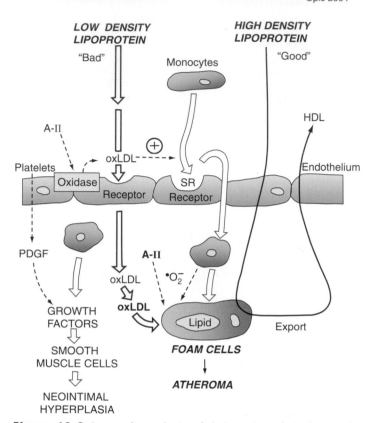

Figure 10-2 Proposed round trip of cholesterol through the vascular endothelium and intima. Low-density lipoprotein (*LDL*) that is oxidized (*ox LDL*) promotes the formation of foam cells. LDL that remains unoxidized can potentially be reexported. High-density lipoprotein (*HDL*) acts hypothetically to help export lipid from the foam cells. *A-II* = angiotensin II; *O^{2-}*, superoxide, representative of free radicals formed either in the endothelium or in foam cells; *Oxidase* = NADPH oxidase; *PDGF* = platelet derived growth factor; *Receptor* = receptor for ox LDL; SR = scavenger receptor. (*Figure © L.H. Opie, 2005.*)

atherogenesis remains controversial, because it is part of the lipid triad. Normal values are below 150 mg/mL (versus the prior cutoff of 200 mg/L).[3] An elevated triglyceride level (>200 mg/dL; 2.3 mmol/L) may be viewed with special concern when combined with high blood LDL-C or low blood HDL-C values (Table 10-3). Hypertriglyceridemia is often part of a *cluster of risk factors* including low HDL-C, obesity, hypertension, and diabetes mellitus.

Metabolic Syndrome The ATP III guidelines recognize as a secondary target of treatment the cluster of risk factors known as the metabolic syndrome. According to ATP III, the metabolic syndrome is present when three or more of the five basic ingredients are present (see Table 7-4). Its presence greatly enhances the risk for coronary morbidity and mortality at any level of LDL-C. The underlying pathology of the metabolic syndrome appears linked to obesity and insulin resistance. After appropriate control of LDL-C, the first lines of therapy are weight control and increased physical activity. A significant increase in HDL-C, though very desirable, may await future therapy.[13]

Non-HDL Cholesterol Increasing emphasis is being placed on the use of non-HDL cholesterol as a secondary target of treatment in patients with triglycerides ≥200 mg/dL (2.26 mmol/L).[14] Measuring non-HDL cholesterol is believed to capture the risk associated with triglyceride-rich particles like very-low-density-lipoprotein (VLDL). The non-HDL-C value is calculated by subtracting the HDL-C value from the total cholesterol value. Treatments that target non-HDL-C include intensified lifestyle measures and possibly drug therapy in high-risk persons. The treatment goals for non-HDL cholesterol are determined by adding 30 mg/dL (0.76 mmol/L) to the LDL-C goals specified in Table 10-2.

Emerging Lipid or Nonlipid Risk Factors Some investigators have put forth *apolipoprotein (apo) B*, a key protein in all major atherogenic lipoprotein fractions, as a more sensitive measure of lipid-based risk than LDL-C.[15] There has not, however, been widespread advocacy for this test, nor has agreement been reached about lipoprotein(a) or homocysteine, two other emerging risk factors. Because of the lack of an overwhelming consensus about the use of novel risk factors, clinicians may derive the most utility from such measurements by using them in patients who appear to be at borderline risk based on traditional risk factors alone. In such cases, an elevated novel risk factor might suggest the intensification of risk factor modification.

C-Reactive Protein This inflammatory marker has gained significant attention because of the increasing attention to the role of inflammation in atherogenesis[10] and especially as a result of a 2003 joint statement from the American Heart Association and the United States Center for Disease Control that endorses its use in assessing those at intermediate risk (10% to 20% 10-year risk) by traditional risk factor assessment.[16] Specifically, a high C-reactive protein (high-sensitivity assay) is an independent risk factor for atherogenesis and adds to the predictive value of other risk factors. The cutoff values are <1.0 mg/L for low risk and >3 mg/L for high risk, the latter tertile indicating an approximate doubling of the relative compared with the low-risk tertile.[16] The presence of an elevated C-reactive protein level may help guide the clinician's decision of whether or not to initiate more aggressive risk reduction.

Treatment Aims: LDL-C Blood lipid normalization remains a cornerstone of the attack on global risk factors. The aims in primary and secondary prevention are shown in Table 10-1. Both European and American guidelines emphasize a low LDL-C (below 100 mg/dL) as the prime aim of therapy in those with established coronary disease or equivalent risks. In other patients, higher values up to 115 mg/dL (3.0 mmol/L) are acceptable according to the European guidelines, with the Americans being somewhat more tolerant, going up to 130 or even 160 mg/dL as the risk level falls (Table 10-1). It has been unclear whether there is a lower limit beyond which no further benefit occurs or whether *"the lower, the better."* This argument is now largely settled in those with a recent acute coronary syndrome because LDL-C values of only 62 mg/dL (1.60 mmol/L) gave convincingly better clinical outcomes than 95 mg/dL (2.46 mmol/L).[6] In a companion study on those with stable coronary disease, high dose atorvastatin reduced atheroma volume at an LDL-C of 79 mg/dl.[7] In a third series, an LDL-C value of about 75 mg/dL (about 2.0 mmol/L) was where progression and regression of the atheroma volume were in balance.[8] Thus a case can be made for an LDL-C goal of <70 mg/dL in selected high risk patients.[3a]

Cholesterol in Special Population Groups

Secondary Hyperlipidemias Diabetes mellitus, hypothyroidism, nephrotic syndrome, and alcoholism should be excluded and remedied if possible. Among drugs causing adverse lipid changes are diuretics, β-blockers, progestogens, and oral retinoids. The latter are supposedly able to retard age-related skin changes at the cost of increasing plasma cholesterol and triglycerides.

Diabetic Patients Patients with diabetes constitute a high-risk group and warrant aggressive risk reduction. Increasingly, type 2 diabetes is regarded as a risk category in its own right and, hence, as a CHD equivalent (Table 10-1). Physicians should evaluate type 2 diabetics not only for LDL-C level, but also for other aspects of the lipid triad (see earlier). There may be a preponderance of smaller, denser atherogenic LDL particles, even although the LDL-C level may be relatively normal. There are few clinical trials that have prospectively evaluated the clinical effect of lipid treatment in diabetic cohorts.[17] The DAIS study reported increased LDL particle size and decreased angiographic coronary lumen size in those who responded to fenofibrate.[18] The CARDS trial is a multicenter, randomized, placebo-controlled primary-prevention study in patients with type 2 diabetes with at least one other risk factor who were treated with atorvastatin, 10 mg/day, compared with placebo.[19] The trial was stopped early because of a statin-induced 37% reduction in the primary endpoint, a composite of serious clinical events. Taken together with a large subgroup analysis from the HPS study,[5] there are strong arguments for considering statin therapy, in addition to lifestyle modification and BP control, in those with type 2 diabetes. Others, however, argue for the primary use of a fibrate, because such therapy also helps increase HDL-C levels.[18]

Elderly Patients Although the relation between cholesterol and coronary disease weakens with age, physicians should continue to consider lipids a modifiable risk factor in the elderly. The absolute risk for clinical coronary disease in the elderly is much higher because age is a powerful risk factor and blood pressure, another risk factor, often increases with age. Furthermore, consider that an elderly patient may have had a lifetime exposure to a coronary risk factor and thus warrants risk factor reduction. The PROSPER study found coronary benefit, but no overall mortality benefit with statin treatment in the elderly (see section on Pravastatin). This trial may have been too short (3 years) to show major benefit on cerebrovascular disease.[12]

Women Women have a lower baseline risk for CHD than men at all ages except perhaps beyond 80 years.[3] Risk lags by about 10 to 15 years, perhaps because of a slower rate of rise of LDL-C, a higher HDL-C, or ill understood genetic protective factors in the heart itself. It is not simply a question of being pre- or postmenopausal. In large statin trials such as the HPS, women experience comparable relative risk reduction to that seen in men.[5]

DIETARY AND OTHER NONDRUG THERAPY

Life Style and Risk Factors Nondrug dietary therapy is basic to the management of all primary hyperlipidemias and frequently suffices as basic therapy when coupled with weight reduction, exercise, ideal (low) alcohol intake, and treatment of other risk factors such as smoking, hypertension or diabetes. Only 1 hour of brisk walking per week increased HDL-C in previously sedentary British women.[20] If lifestyle recommendations, including diet, were rigorously followed, CHD would be largely eliminated in those younger than 70 years of age.[21] However, high-intensity lifestyle modification is required to prevent progression or even to achieve regression of coronary heart disease.

Diet Changes in diet are an absolute cornerstone of lipid-modifying treatment. As a general aim, saturated fats should be less than 7% of the calories, and total fat less than about 30% (Table 10-4). Monoun-

Table 10-4   Suggested Nutrient Composition for Diet

Nutrient	Recommended Intake
Saturated fat	Less than 7% of total calories
Polyunsaturated fat	Up to 10% of total calories
Monounsaturated fat	Up to 20% of total calories
Total fat*	25–35% of total calories
Carbohydrate	50–60% of total calories
Fiber	20–30 grams per day
Protein	Approximately 15% of total calories
Cholesterol	Less than 200 mg/day
Total calories (energy)	Balance energy intake and expenditure to maintain desirable body weight/prevent weight gain

*USA guidelines suggest a range of total fat consumption, provided saturated fats and trans-fatty acids are kept low. A higher intake of unsaturated fats can help reduce triglycerides and raise HDL-C in patients with the metabolic syndrome.

saturates, as in *olive oil*, are relatively beneficial within the framework of total lipid reduction. For information about protective omega-3 fatty acids see later. In addition, patients, especially elderly hypertensive persons, should limit sodium intake (see Chapter 7). In practice, the dietary fatty acid recommendations can be simplified to a reduction of saturated fatty acids, largely of animal origin, and increasing other fatty acids from plants or fish oils. Exceptions: coconut oil and crustacean meat, such as lobsters and prawns, are high in saturated fatty acids.

American Heart Step diets. In 2000, the American Heart Association deemphasized its "Step I/Step II diet" nomenclature in favor of general principles that apply to the collective population (to replace the Step I diet) or more individualized medical nutrition therapy for specific subgroups (to replace the Step II diet). For the general population, a Mediterranean-type diet seems ideal (see later). Higher risk individuals (Table 10-1) may require a stricter diet composed of reduced intake of cholesterol-raising nutrients, saturated fats <7% of total calories, and dietary cholesterol <200 mg per day.

A *Mediterranean-type diet* confers increased postinfarct protection,[22] as discussed under post-myocardial infarction (MI) management (see Chapter 11, p. 371). Patients are told to eat more bread, more fiber, more fresh vegetables, more fish, and less meat, "no day without fruit," and butter and cream are replaced by canola margarine. Olive oil is often used. The more adherence there is to this diet, the better the survival.[23] Note the closely related Indo-Mediterranean diet.[24] Vegetable oils containing the polyunsaturated linoleic acid are not as ideal as once thought. *Omega-3 fatty fish oils* may be protective, at least in the postinfarct period and when the benefit is largely independent of any change of blood lipid levels and may relate to sodium channel blockade. Several good epidemiological studies relate intake of omega-3 fish oils to decreased sudden death or increased life-span. Nonetheless, whatever the merits of the individual nonanimal fatty acid, total lipid intake must be restricted. In brief, the ideal diet is low in total fat, cholesterol, high in fiber, and high in fresh vegetables and fruit, with modest sodium restriction. Much the same diet benefits hypertensives (Chapter 7, p. 184) and is recommended by the American Heart Association, the American Diabetes Association, and the American Cancer Society.[25] The Mediterranean diet seems to confer optimal dietary protection. "Eat Mediterranean, exercise American" is a useful message for patients.

Other dietary options such as consumption of plant stanols/sterols (see Plant Sterol/Stanol Margarines below), increased intake of almonds[26] or walnuts,[27] increased intake of viscous (soluble) fiber (10 to 25 g per day), and decreased intake of *trans* fatty acids may also help manage lipid values.

DRUG-RELATED LIPIDEMIAS

Cardiac Drugs and Blood Lipid Profiles

β-Blockers or diuretics may harmfully influence blood lipid profiles (Table 10-5), especially triglyceride values. Diuretics, in addition, tend to increase total cholesterol unless used in low doses. Nonetheless, cardiac drugs known to be protective, such as β-blockers, should not be withheld on the basis of their lipid effects alone, especially in postinfarct patients when there is clear indication for the expected overall benefit. Statins appear to counter some of the effects of β-blockers on blood lipids.

β-Blockers β-Blockers tend specifically to reduce HDL-C and to increase triglycerides. β-Blockers with high intrinsic sympathomimetic

Table 10-5	Effects of Antihypertensive Agents on Blood Lipid Profiles (Percentage Increase or Decrease)			
Agent	**TC**	**LDL-C**	**HDL-C**	**TG**
Diuretics				
Thiazides[1]	14	10	2	14
Low-dose TZ[2]	0	0	0	0
Indapamide[3]	0	0	0	0
Spironolactone[4]	5	?	?	31
β-Blockers (Grouped >1 Year)[5]	0	0	−8	22
Propranolol[1]	0	−3	−11	16
Atenolol[1]	0	−2	−7	15
Metoprolol[1]	0	−1	−9	14
Acebutolol[2]	−3	−4*	−3	6
Pindolol[1]	−1	−3	−2	7
α-Blockers (Grouped)	−4	−13	5	−8
Doxazosin[2]	−4*	−5*	2	−8
α-β Blocker				
Labetalol[1]	2	2	1	8
Carvedilol[6]	−4	?	7	−20
CCBs (Grouped)[1]	0	0	0	0
Amlodipine[2]	−1	−1	1	−3
ACE Inhibitors (Grouped)	0	0	0	0
Enalapril	−1	−1	3	−7
ARBs (Angiotensin Receptor Blockers)				
Losartan[7]	(0)	(0)	(0)	(0)
Central Agents				
MD + TZ	0	0	0	0

*<0.01 vs. placebo over 4 years.
TC = total cholesterol; LDL = low density lipoprotein; HDL = high-density lipoprotein; TG = triglyceride; MD = methyldopa; TZ = thiazide.
(0) = no long term data.
1 = Frishman, 1992[66]
2 = TOHM Study,[67] chlorthalidone 15 mg/day; acebutolol 400 mg/day; doxazosin 2 mg/day; amlodipine 5 mg/day; enalapril 5 mg/day; data placebo-corrected.
3 = Weidmann et al.[68]
4 = Plouin et al.[69]
5 = Kasiske et al. 1995[70]
6 = Giugliano et al. 1997[71]
7 = Lerch et al. 1998[71a]

activity (ISA) or high cardioselectivity may have less or no effect (as in the case of carvedilol with added α-blockade). The fact that β-blockers also impair glucose metabolism is an added cause for concern when giving these agents to young patients (see Chapter 7, p. 191). Nonetheless, note the strong evidence for protective effects of β-blockers in postinfarct and heart failure patients (Chapter 1, p. 10). In stable effort angina, calcium channel blockers may be preferred to avoid triglyceride elevation and HDL-C decrease with β-blockers. In hypertensives, angiotensin-converting enzyme (ACE) inhibitors, angiotensin receptor blockers (ARBs), and calcium blockers are all lipid-neutral.

Diuretics Doses should be kept low (Chapter 7, p. 194). In ALLHAT, chlorthalidone, 12.5 to 25 mg daily, over 5 years increased total cholesterol by 2 to 3 mg/dL.[28] In the ALPINE study, hydrochlorothiazide, 25 mg, with, in most, added atenolol increased blood triglycerides and apo B, while decreasing HDL-C.[29]

Lipid-Neutral Cardiac Drugs Cardiac drugs that have no harmful effects on blood lipids include the ACE inhibitors, the ARBs, calcium channel blockers, vasodilators such as the nitrates and hydralazine, and the centrally acting agents, such as reserpine, methyldopa, and clonidine. The α-blockers, including prazosin and doxazosin, favorably influence the lipid profiles.

Oral Contraceptives When these are given to patients with ischemic heart disease or those with risk factors such as smoking, possible atherogenic effects of high-estrogen doses merit attention. In postmenopausal women, the cardiovascular benefits of hormone replacement therapy have not been supported by clinical trials. (See *Estrogens* later.)

THE STATINS: HMG CoA REDUCTASE INHIBITORS

The currently available lipid-lowering drugs can be divided into the statins, the bile acid sequestrants, nicotinic acid, the fibrates, and cholesterol absorption inhibitors. These all reduce LDL-C. Of these drugs, statins with their relatively few side effects and predictable benefits for treating LDL-C are now usually the drugs of first choice. They decrease hepatic cholesterol synthesis by inhibiting 3-hydroxy-3-methyl-glutaryl coenzyme A (HMG Co A) reductase (Fig. 10-3). They are highly effective in reducing total cholesterol and LDL-C, they usually increase HDL-C, and long-term safety and efficacy are now established. The landmark Scandinavian Simvastatin Survival study (4S) showed that simvastatin used in secondary prevention achieved a reduction in total mortality and in coronary events.[30] This was soon followed by a successful primary-prevention study with pravastatin in high-risk men.[31] Successful primary prevention of common events has been found in those with LDL-C values near the US national average.[32] An interesting recent concept is that lipid-lowering drugs may act in ways beyond regression of the atheromatous plaque, for example, by improving endothelial function, by stabilizing platelets, or by reduction of fibrinogen (strongly correlated with triglyceride levels), or by inhibiting the inflammatory response associated with atherogenesis.[33] These "nonlipid" benefits are especially invoked as a therapeutic bonus of the statins although their clinical relevance has been notoriously difficult to confirm. The opposing and dominant view is that it is lipid-reduction that matters, especially that of LDL-C (Fig. 10-4).

Class Indications for Statins

In general, depending on the drug chosen (Table 10-6), the patients selected, and whether it is primary or secondary prevention that is the aim, the large statin trials show beyond doubt that cardiovascular endpoints are reduced. In *primary prevention* statins reduce coronary

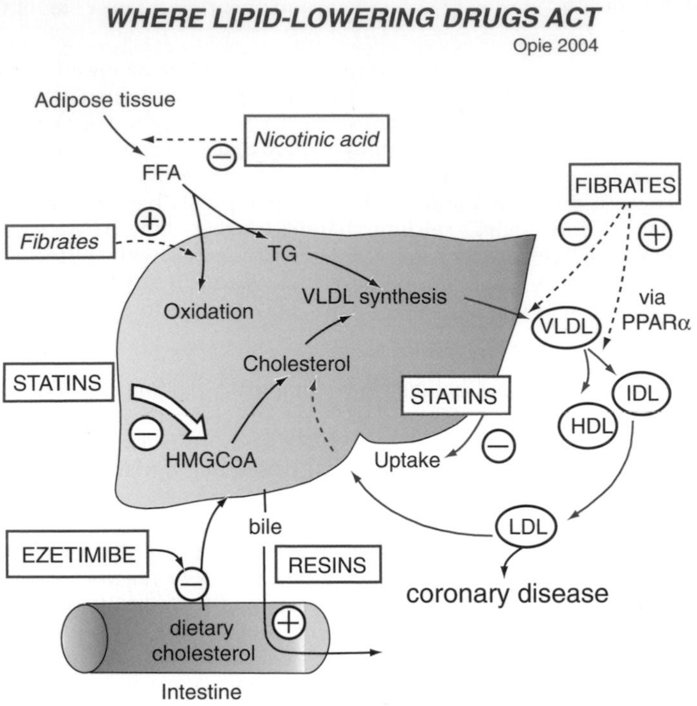

WHERE LIPID-LOWERING DRUGS ACT

Opie 2004

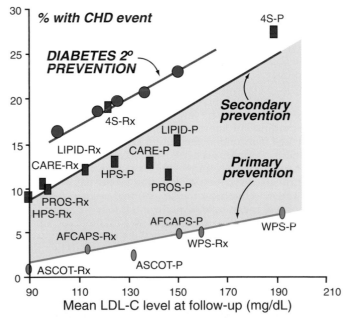

Figure 10-3 Hepatic import and export of lipids is crucial to the sites of action of lipid-lowering drugs. Proposed mechanism of action of statins, fibrates, and nicotinic acid. *FFA* = free fatty acids; *HDL* = high-density lipoproteins; *HMG CoA* = 3-hydroxy-3-methyl-glutaryl-coenzyme A; *IDL* = intermediate density lipoproteins; *LDL* = low-density lipoproteins; *VLDL* = very low density lipoproteins. For *PPAR-α* see text. (*Figure* © *L.H. Opie, 2005.*)

Figure 10-4 The lower the LDL-C, the fewer the events and the greater the benefit. Relation between LDL-C lowering and coronary heart disease (*CHD*) events in major trials for primary and secondary prevention. Note greater effects with secondary than with primary prevention and especially marked effects in diabetics. Modified from Fisher, 2004[74] by addition of new trials. Trials as given in Table 10-7. *P* = placebo arm; *Rx* = treatment arm of the trial indicated. (*Figure* © *LH Opie, 2005.*)

Table 10-6 Pharmacological Properties of Statins

Characteristic	Lovastatin (Mevacor)	Pravastatin (Pravachol)	Simvastatin (Zocor)	Fluvastatin (Lescol)	Atorvastatin (Lipitor)	Rosuvastatin (Crestor)
Usual starting dose (mg/day)	20 mg	40 mg	20–40 mg	20–40 mg	10 mg	10 mg
Expected LDL fall, this dose	24%	34%	38%	25% (40 mg)	39%	52%
Elderly starting dose	Not stated	40 mg start	20 mg or less	→	→	5 mg
Timing of dose	Evening meal	Any time	Evening	Bedtime	Any time	Any time
Maximum daily dose	80 mg	80 mg	80 mg	80 mg	80 mg	40 mg
LDL reduction, max dose	40%	37%	47%	36%	60%	63%
HDL-C increase, max dose	9.5%	13%	8%	5.6%	5%	10%
Mortality reduction in trials	N/D	Yes	Yes	N/D	N/D	N/D
CV endpoint ↓	Yes	Yes	Yes	Probable	Probable	N/D
Stroke reduction	N/D	Yes	Yes	N/D	Probable	N/D
Elimination route, chief	Hepatic and biliary	Hepatic and biliary	Hepatic and biliary	Hepatic and biliary	Hepatic and biliary	Hepatic and biliary
Renal excretion of absorbed dose (%)*	10	20	13	<6	<2	28%
Dose in severe renal failure	20 mg	10 mg	5 mg	→	→	5 mg
Dose with cyclosporine	10 mg	10 mg	5 mg	→	? reduce	5 mg
Digoxin effect	None	None	Small ↑	Small ↑	↑ 20%	None
Mechanism of hepatic metabolism*	Cyto P-450 3A4	Not by P-450, Sulfation Oxidation Isomerization	Cyto P-450 3A4	Cyto P-450 2C9	Cyto P-450 3A4	Cyto P-450 2C9
Hepatic interactions	Erythromycin Ketoconozole	No	Erythromycin Ketoconozole	Clearance↓ cimetidine, ranitidine; ↑ by rifampicin	Erythromycin Ketoconozole	Clearance ↓ cyclosporine, gemfibrozil; ↑ by antacid

*Source: Knopp[42] and package insert for pravastatin; other data from package inserts.
N/D = no data; → = dose unchanged; ↓ = decrease; ↑ = increase; cyto = cytochrome; ? reduce = no clear information in package insert, but warning against myopathy during cotherapy.

morbidity and mortality, and the need for revascularization procedures. Added benefits in *secondary prevention or CHD risk equivalents*, are reduced risks for all-cause mortality and cerebrovascular disease. The number needed to treat to prevent any given major end point makes their use cost-effective, especially in secondary prevention (Table 10-7).

In patients with clinical *congestive heart failure*, statins may be used to slow the progression of coronary atherosclerosis, as part of an overall treatment strategy. In patients with primary *hypercholesterolemia and mixed dyslipidemias*, statins reduce levels of total cholesterol, LDL-C, apo B, and triglycerides. Some are licensed to increase HDL-C. In *homozygous familial hypercholesterolemia* statins are indicated to reduce total cholesterol and LDL-C levels. If at the time of hospital discharge from an *acute coronary event* the LDL-C level equals or exceeds 100 mg/dL (2.6 mmol/L) then statin therapy may be considered. Of note, and as indicated in the package insert for fluvastatin, in hypertriglyceridemic patients the LDL-C may be low or normal despite elevated total cholesterol; statins are not indicated for this situation.

Class Warnings: Liver Damage and Myopathy

The package inserts for statins generally give two warnings in bold: the one regarding liver enzyme elevation and the other, myopathy. Pretreatment *liver function tests* are recommended, repeated after 12 weeks, and then semiannually. In practice, serious liver injury is very rare when compared with placebo.[5] Regarding myopathy and rhabdomyolysis, there is a range of features extending from muscle pains to objective myopathy to severe myocyte breakdown that in turn can cause potentially fatal renal failure by way of myoglobinuria. Myopathy is diagnosed when the creatine kinase blood levels exceeds 10 times normal. The patient is in advance warned that muscle pain, tenderness or weakness must immediately be reported to the physician and the statin, stopped. However, in a very large trial with over 10,000 patients in each group, enzyme-diagnosed myopathy over 5 years occurred only in 0.11% versus 0.06% in controls, and rhabdomyolysis in only 0.05% versus 0.03% in controls. Fatal cases are extremely rare, occurring in only 0 to 0.12 per million prescriptions.[34] Whether regular monitoring of creatine kinase levels will help predict incipient toxicity is controversial. At the very least, a baseline creatine kinase level should be determined before starting a statin. Abnormal enzyme values usually resolve with cessation of treatment. *Predisposing to myopathy* is cotherapy with fibrates, niacin, cyclosporine, erythromycin, or azole antifungal agents. For example, in August 2001, the manufacturer of the drug cerivastatin voluntarily withdrew this statin from the market because of a disproportionate number of reports of rhabdomyolysis-associated deaths, especially when cerivastatin was combined with gemfibrozil. This withdrawal renewed attention to the safety of lipid-modifying drugs. While the relative risk for myopathy may increase when statins or fibrates are administered compared with placebo, the absolute rates of myopathy, much less rhabdomyolysis, are low in reported clinical surveys.[5,34,35] The combination of a statin and fibrate is acknowledged as one that will increase the risk for myopathy, but in general, the incidence of this interaction is about 0.12%.[36] A proposed explanation is that gemfibrozil appears to inhibit the metabolism of statins, especially cerivastatin, thereby increasing active levels of the statin in circulation and enhancing the myopathy risk.[37] The myopathy risk is not an absolute contraindication against combining a statin and a fibrate, yet physicians are cautioned to be mindful of this risk.

Contraindications and Pregnancy Warning Statins are contraindicated in patients with active liver disease or unexplained persistent elevations of serum transaminases. Statins must not be prescribed for women who are pregnant or who are planning to become pregnant (see Table 11-8).

Table 10-7 Key Statin Trials with Major Significant Outcomes

Trial, Statin, 1° or 2° Prevention	Initial Blood Cholesterol (Mean)	Duration and Numbers	Comparator Events per Trial (%)	Statin Events per Trial (%)	Absolute Risk Reduction per Trial	Number Needed to Treat per Trial
4S[32] Simvastatin 40 mg 2° prevention	260 mg/dL; 6.75 mmol/L	5.4yr, median (Pl: 2223 Statin: 2221)	Total deaths 1° end-point 256 (11.5%) 2° end-point 502 (22.6%)	182 (8.2%) 353 (15.9%)	74 (3.3%) 149 (30%)	30 (162/yr) 15 (80/yr)
LIPID[72] Pravastatin 40 mg; 2°	218 mg/dL; 5.63 mmol/L	6.1yr (mean) (Pl: 4502 Statin: 4512)	Deaths: 633 (14.1%) AMI: 463 (10.3%)	498 (11.0%) 336 (7.4%)	135 (3.1%) 127 (2.9%)	33 (201/yr) 36 (220/yr)
WOSCOPS[39] Pravastatin 40 mg; 1°	272 mg/dL; 7.03 mmol/L	4.9yr (mean) (Pl: 3293 Statin: 3302)	Deaths: 135 (4.1%) 1° endpoint: 248 (7.5%)	106 (3.2%) 174 (5.3%)	29 (0.9%) 74 (2.2%)	114 (558/yr) 45 (217/yr)
AFCAPS/ TexCAPS[73] Lovastatin 20 mg 1°	221 mg/dL; 5.71 mmol/L	5.2yr (mean) (Pl: 3301 Statin: 3304)	CAD deaths: 15 (0.5%) AMI* 81 (2.5%) 1° endpoint: 183 (5.5%)	11 (0.3%) 45 (1.4%) 116 (3.5%)	4 (0.2%) 39 (1.3%) 67 (2.0%)	826 (4295/yr) 85 (441/yr) 49 (256/yr)
HPS[5] Simvastatin 40 mg 65% with CHD	228 mg/dL. 5.9 mmol/L	5y (mean) (Placebo: 10267; statin: 10269)	Mortality: 1507 (14.7%) Vascular deaths: 937 (9.1%) Total MI: 1212 (11.8%)	1328 (12.9%) 781 (7.6%) 898 (8.7%)	179 (1.8%) 156 (1.5%) 314 (3.1%)	56 (280/yr) 66 (330/yr) 32 (160/yr)
PROSPER[41] Pravastatin 40 mg High-Risk Elderly	221 mg/dL 5.7 mmol/L	3.2 y (mean) (Placebo: 2913; statin: 2391)	1° endpoint CHD death, nonfatal MI, + stroke: 473 (16.2%)	408 (14.1%)	65 (2.1%)	48 (152/yr)
ASCOT-LLA[47] Atorvastatin 10 mg; 1°; Hypertensive	212 mg/dL 5.48 mmol/L	3.3 y (median) (Placebo: 5137; statin: 5168)	1° endpoint nonfatal MI + CHD death: 154 (3.0%)	100 (1.9%)	54 (1.1%)	90 (297/yr)
PROVE-IT[6] Atorvastatin 80 mg Pravastatin 40 mg Recent ACS, 2°	180 mg/dL; 4.65 mmol/L	2.0y (median) (Pravastatin: 2063; Atorvastatin 2099)	1° composite endpoint: (death plus cardiovascular events): pravastatin, 543 (26.3%)	Atorvastatin, 470 (22.4%)	73 (3.7%)	29 (58/yr)

NB: PROVE-IT compares atorvastatin vs pravastatin, not vs placebo as in others.

*Calculated as primary end-point value minus (unstable angina) minus (fatal CAD).

ACS = acute coronary syndrome; AMI = nonfatal AMI; CAD = coronary artery disease; CHD = coronary heart disease; Pl = placebo.

Cholesterol is an essential component of fetal development, including steroid synthesis and membrane development. Statins are excreted in the mother's milk, so women taking it should not breast-feed.

Lovastatin (Mevacor)

This agent was one of the first available and now is the first generically available (Altocor, Lovastatin tablets). In a landmark study, it reduced cardiac clinical events including heart attacks by 37% in primary prevention in those with initial LDL-C values (221 mg/dL, 5.71 mmol/L) that are "normal" in the general American population, but also with low HDL-C levels (36 mg/dL, 1.03 mmol/L).[32] Besides the class indications (see previously), there is now an important indication for primary prevention.[32]

Dose, Effects, and Side Effects The usual starting dose is 20 mg once daily with the evening meal, going up to 80 mg in one or two doses. In the AFCAPS/TexCAPS primary prevention study, the dose was 20 or 40 mg once daily.[32] Total cholesterol fell by 18%, LDL-C by 25%, and triglycerides by 15%. HDL-C rose by 6%. In the EXCEL study[38] the incidence of liver damage increased from 0.1% to 1.5% in a dose-dependent manner, while myopathy, defined as muscle symptoms plus a CK elevation, occurred in only 0.1%. There are no significant *drug interactions* with the common antihypertensive drugs, or with digoxin. Note the *warnings* about liver enzymes and myopathy, with contraindications including liver disease, pregnancy and lactation (see Class Warnings and Contraindications).

Pravastatin (Pravachol, Lipostat)

The mechanism of action is identical to that of the other statins, so that all are clearly market competitors. Some studies suggest a possible differential beneficial effect on HDL-C compared with other statins (Table 10-6). Pravastatin reduced the risk for coronary morbidity and mortality in high-risk men in the primary-prevention WOSCOPS trial.[39] In the secondary-prevention LIPID trial,[40] pravastatin therapy reduced the risks for death from any cause by 22% (*P* < 0.001) and also decreased the risks for nonfatal MI or CHD death, for stroke, and coronary revascularizations. In another secondary prevention trial, PROVE-IT, moderate LDL-C lowering by pravastatin 40 mg day produced less clinical benefit than aggressive LDL-C lowering by atorvastatin 80 mg daily.[6] The PROSPER trial in the elderly with a mean cholesterol of 5.7 mmol/L (212 mg/dL) and high coronary risk, found that pravastatin, 40 mg/day, reduced the relative risk for CHD death by 24% (*P* = 0.043), chiefly when given for secondary prevention. Results for primary prevention were nonsignificant.[41] There was, however, an increased incidence of gastrointestinal cancer, not seen in other studies with this drug.

Indications Besides indications common to the statins as a class (see previously), pravastatin is licensed for primary prevention in those with hypercholesterolemia to reduce the risk for myocardial infarction (MI), revascularization, and cardiovascular mortality. In patients with previous MI, it is indicated to reduce total mortality by reducing coronary deaths, to reduce recurrent MI, revascularization, and stroke or transient ischemic attacks (TIAs).

Dose and Effects The recommended starting dose is 40 mg at any time of the day, increasing to 80 mg if needed. As with the other statins, liver damage and myopathy are rare, but serious *side effects*. *Cautions and contraindications* are also similar to those for other statins. There is no drug interaction with digoxin. Unlike some other statins, pravastatin is not metabolized by the cytochrome P-450 3A4 pathway (Table 10-6). There may, therefore, be a lower risk for interactions with agents such as erythromycin and ketoconazole that use this pathway.

Simvastatin (Zocor)

This agent was studied in the landmark Scandinavian 4S study that paved the way to widespread acceptance of statins as the cornerstone of lipid-lowering drug therapy.[30] In light of the growing emphasis of global risk assessment as a guide for therapeutic decision making, recent research with simvastatin, as described later, has expanded the types of patients who may be considered for statin treatment.

Major Trials   In the Scandinavian Simvastatin Survival Study (4S) on 4444 patients with increased cholesterol levels, mostly men with past MI, simvastatin reduced LDL-C by 35% over 4 years,[30] total mortality by 30%, cardiac death rate by 42%, and revascularization by 37%. There was no evidence of increased suicide or violent death, previously thought to be a potential hazard of cholesterol reduction. Differences between simvastatin and placebo arms started to emerge after 1 to 2 years of treatment, and most curves were still diverging at 4 years. Longer term follow-up after the trial suggested that benefits were maintained.

Another landmark study, the Heart Protection Study (HPS) of the Medical Research Council/British Heart Foundation, evaluated the role of simvastatin versus placebo in 20,536 high-risk patients for whom guidelines at the time would not have recommended drug intervention.[5] Included patients were 40 to 80 years of age and had total serum cholesterol concentrations of at least 135 mg/dL (3.49 mmol/L). Because only 65% of the patients had a history of CHD at baseline, HPS included many high-risk "primary-prevention" individuals who had never had a coronary event ($n = 7150$). It is important to note, however, that a significant number of these individuals had a CHD-equivalent risk profile: diabetes, peripheral vascular disease, or cerebrovascular disease. Simvastatin reduced the risk for any major vascular event by 24% ($P < 0.0001$) and all-cause mortality by 13% ($P = 0.0003$), with a 17% reduction in deaths attributed to any vascular cause. There were no safety issues with treatment and only an incidence of myopathy of 0.01%. Because there was a similar good response in those with an initial LDL-C below 3.0 mmol/L (116 mg/dL) or total cholesterol below 193 mg/dL (5.0 mmol/L) to those with higher values, *the intriguing interpretation emerges that selection for statin therapy should be by the degree of clinical risk, so that those at high risk should receive a statin irrespective of the initial lipid levels.* This philosophy is reflected in the new labeling (see later).

Indications   These are similar to other statins, plus specific indications in patients with CHD and hypercholesterolemia, for: (1) reduction of coronary and total mortality; (2) reduction of nonfatal MI; (3) reduction of myocardial revascularization procedures; (4) reduction of stroke or transient ischemic attack. Simvastatin also has a license to increase HDL-C in patients with hypercholesterolemia or combined lipidemias, without claiming an effect independent of LDL-C lowering. Based on the results of the HPS, the US Food and Drug Administration approved in 2003 a revised labeling for simvastatin that emphasized high-risk status rather than LDL-C alone as the primary determinant of treatment. Essentially, the new labeling states that simvastatin may be started simultaneously with dietary therapy in patients with coronary disease or with high risk for coronary disease.

Dose   The usual starting dosage is 20 to 40 mg once daily in the evening. In the 4S, the initial dose was 20 mg once daily just before the evening meal, increased to 40 mg if cholesterol lowering was inadequate after 6 weeks.[30] A daily dose of 20 mg has almost exactly the same effect on blood lipids as atorvastatin, 10 mg (manufacturers' information). For patients at high risk, the starting dosage is 40 mg/day as in the HPS. The top dosage is 80 mg daily, giving a mean reduction of LDL-C of 47%.[42] This high dose may be split up, 40 mg in the evening and 20 mg twice during the day (package insert). As in the case of the *side effects* of other statins, liver damage and myopathy are rare but serious. *Cautions and contraindications* are also similar to other statins. There may be a small increase in blood *digoxin* levels. If combined with fibrates or niacin, or with cyclosporine, the dosage should not exceed 10 mg/day. Patients on potent inhibitors of hepatic P-450 3A4, such as ketoconazole, erythromycin, or HIV protease inhibitors, should not be given simvastatin. Note other drug interactions including amiodarone and verapamil (dose no greater than 20 mg daily).

Fluvastatin (Lescol, Lescol XL)

This agent is metabolized mainly by the cytochrome P-450 2C9 isoenzyme, making it less likely to interact with drugs commonly coadministered with those statins that compete for the P-450 3A4 pathway, such as the fibrates. On the other hand, phenytoin and warfarin share metabolism by P-450 2C9, raising the risk for interactions. The same cautions concerning hepatoxicity, myopathy, and rhabdomyolysis that affect other statins also apply to fluvastatin.

Major Trials Although fluvastatin has yet to receive an indication for clinical event reduction, the data are suggestive. The Lescol Intervention Prevention Study (LIPS) compared early initiation of fluvastatin, 80 mg/day, versus placebo in 1677 patients with average cholesterol values, following percutaneous coronary intervention.[43] Survival time free of major adverse cardiac events was longer in the fluvastatin group and there was a 22% relative risk reduction in such events, favoring statin ($P = 0.01$). The Assessment of Lescol in Renal Transplantation (ALERT) trial reported as a secondary end-point a reduced rate of cardiac death or nonfatal heart attack by 35% ($P = 0.005$) with fluvastatin, 40 mg/day, versus placebo in high-risk renal transplant patients.[44]

Indications These are twofold: (1) to lower cholesterol and LDL-C, triglyceride and apo B levels, and to increase HDL-C levels; and (2) to slow the rate of progress of coronary atherosclerosis in those with CHD.

Dose The dosing range of fluvastatin is 20 to 80 mg/day, taken in the evening or at bedtime, and the recommended starting dosage may be determined by the degree of LDL-C reduction needed. For patients needing ≥25% reduction, a starting dosage of 40 mg/day may be used. More aggressive therapy may use the 80 mg dosage, delivered as 40 mg twice daily or as 80 mg once a day in the extended release (Lescol XL) preparation. Patients needing less reduction may be started at 20 mg/day. As with other statins, pregnancy or risk thereof remains a contraindication (category X) as does liver disease.

Atorvastatin (Lipitor)

Atorvastatin, like all statins, interrupts the cholesterol biosynthetic pathway. Atorvastatin has not yet received an indication for reducing clinical cardiovascular events, although an extended license can be anticipated in the light of recent trials.

Major Trials *Secondary prevention.* The Myocardial Ischemia Reduction and Aggressive Cholesterol Lowering (MIRACL) trial[45] and the PROVE-IT[6] trials examined the premise that early treatment with high-dose (80 mg daily) atorvastatin therapy following an acute coronary syndrome would give clinical benefits. Versus placebo, and in a relatively small study, atorvastatin produced modestly significant relative risk reductions for symptomatic ischemia.[45] Versus pravastatin, in a large study on more than 4000 patients, atorvastatin reduced the LDL-C to only 62 mg/dL (1.60 mmol/L) and decreased the composite primary end-point. In those with stable coronary disease, a similar vigorous reduction of LDL-C versus pravastatin decreased the atheroma volume.[7] In the Atorvastatin Versus Revascularization Treatment (AVERT) trial, aggressive lipid lowering by high-dose atorvastatin was marginally better than percutaneous intervention (PCI) in reducing ischemic events in patients with stable effort angina.[46]

Primary prevention. The lipid-lowering arm of the Anglo-Scandinavian Cardiac Outcomes Trial (ASCOT) assessed the clinical effect of atorvastatin, 10 mg/day, versus placebo in 10,305 hypertensive patients with mean total cholesterol 212 mg/dL (5.5 mmol/L), LDL 130 mg/dL (3.4 mmol/L) and a high-risk profile.[47] Originally planned to have a follow-up of 5 years, ASCOT ended early because of clear benefit. Atorvastatin reduced the relative risk for cardiovascular events by 36% (*P* = 0.0005) and for stroke by 27% (*P* = 0.024). There was no effect on the low total mortality rate, and the adverse event rates did not differ between the treatment groups. The Collaborative Atorvastatin Diabetes Study (CARDS) of high-risk diabetics was similarly stopped because of improved clinical endpoints in those treated with atorvastatin, 10 mg daily, versus placebo.

Indications, Doses, and Side Effects Atorvastatin is available as 10-mg, 20-mg, 40-mg and 80-mg tablets. The ASCOT and CARDS Trials suggest that a dosage of only 10 mg daily may help prevent clinical events. The PROVE-IT study shows that high dose atorvastatin, 80 mg/day, reduces LDL-C to very low levels and reduces clinical events in those with a recent acute coronary syndrome. The dose is given once daily at any time of the day, with or without food. A starting dose of atorvastatin, 10 mg, gives good reductions in total cholesterol, LDL-C, apo B, and triglyceride, and a modest increase in HDL-C. Blood lipid levels should be checked 2 to 4 weeks after starting therapy, and the dosage adjusted accordingly. As in the case of the *side effects* of other statins, liver damage and myopathy are rare but serious. *Cautions and contraindications* are also similar to other statins, including the possible adverse drug interactions with fibrates and niacin, drugs that also predispose to myopathy. Other drug interactions include *digoxin* (blood digoxin levels rise about 20%). *Erythromycin* inhibits hepatic cytochrome P-450 to increase blood atorvastatin levels by about 40%. Atorvastatin increases blood levels of some *oral contraceptives*. There is no interaction with warfarin.

Rosuvastatin (Crestor)

Rosuvastatin was approved in the United States in August 2003 for therapy of lipid disorders. The claim is that it is exceptionally potent in reducing cholesterol and LDL-C levels. Rosuvastatin is a hydrophilic compound with a high uptake into, and selectivity for, its site of action in the liver. As with other statins, rosuvastatin produces its lipid-modifying effects by inhibiting the hepatic synthesis of cholesterol, thereby increasing the number of hepatic LDL receptors to enhance uptake and catabolism of LDL. Rosuvastatin's half-life is approximately 19 hours. Like fluvastatin and pravastatin, it is not metabolized by the P-450 3A4 system, thus lessening the risk for certain key drug interactions. There are as yet no major trials with clinical end-points such as cardiovascular morbidity and mortality, or angiographic progression.

Indications Rosuvastatin is indicated as an adjunct to diet to reduce elevated total cholesterol, LDL-C, apo B, non-HDL cholesterol, and triglyceride levels and to increase HDL-C in patients with primary hypercholesterolemia (heterozygous familial and nonfamilial) and mixed dyslipidemia. Rosuvastatin also has a favorable effect on triglycerides in patients with elevated serum triglyceride levels. In patients with homozygous familial hypercholesterolemia, rosuvastatin may be used with other lipid-lowering treatments (e.g., LDL apheresis) or as monotherapy if other treatments are unavailable.

Dose, Effects, and Side Effects Rosuvastatin is supplied in 5-, 10-, 20-, and 40-mg tablets. The recommended starting dosage is 10 mg/day taken with or without food. At this dosage, there is an expected 52% reduction in LDL-C in patients with primary hypercholesterolemia. In these same patients, rosuvastatin produces approximately a 10% increase in HDL-C and a 24% decrease in triglycerides. For patients of advanced age or with renal insufficiency, the recommended starting dose is 5 mg/day. Renal patients may be titrated up to 10 mg/day. Patients receiving concomitant cyclosporine should be limited to rosuvastatin 5 mg/day. In combination with gemfibrozil, rosuvastatin should be limited to 10 mg/day. Its *side effects* and warnings are similar to those of other statins. The access to the maximum 40-mg dose of rosuvastatin is reserved for those patients who do not have adequate response at the 20-mg dose. Uncommon instances of proteinuria with microscopic hematuria have been reported, and the frequency may be greater at the 40 mg (distribution limited in the United States) dose compared with lower doses. However, the interpretation of this finding has proved contentious. In clinical studies of 10,275 patients, 3.7% were discontinued because of adverse experiences attributable to rosuvastatin. The most frequent adverse events (≥2%) included hypertension, myalgia, constipation, asthenia, and abdominal pain. Like fluvastatin, it is metabolized by way of the cytochrome P-450 2C9 isoenzyme and therefore may be less likely to interact with common drugs that use the cytochrome P-450 3A4 pathway, such as ketoconazole or erythromycin. Warfarin interaction becomes an increased risk. Nonetheless, the standard statin warnings against cotherapy with fibrates or niacin remain, although fenofibrate appears safe. Coadministration of cyclosporine or gemfibrozil with rosuvastatin resulted in reduced clearance of this drug from the circulation, so that both are contraindicated. An antacid (aluminium and magnesium hydroxide combination) decreases plasma concentrations of rosuvastatin. and should be taken 2 hours after and not before rosuvastatin.

BILE ACID SEQUESTRANTS: THE RESINS

These agents, cholestyramine (Questran), colesevelam (Welchol) and colestipol (Colestid), bind to bile acids to promote their secretion into the intestine. There is increased loss of hepatic cholesterol into bile acids and hepatic cellular cholesterol depletion, the latter leading to a compensatory increase in the hepatic LDL-receptor population so that the blood LDL is more rapidly removed and total cholesterol falls (Fig. 10-4). There may be a transitory compensatory rise in plasma triglycerides that is usually ignored, but may require cotherapy. The major trial conducted was the Lipid Research Clinics Coronary Primary Prevention Trial,[48] in which cholestyramine modestly reduced CHD in hypercholesterolemic patients, yet without effect on overall mortality. The blood lipid profiles, however, did change in the desired direction. Poor palatability is the major problem. Regarding *drug interactions*, watch for interference with the absorption of digoxin, warfarin, thyroxin, and thiazides, which need to be taken 1 hour before or 4 hours after the sequestrant. Impaired absorption of vitamin K may lead to bleeding and sensitization to warfarin. *Combination therapy* is often undertaken. For example, colestipol has been combined with nicotinic acid and/or lovastatin to achieve angiographic regression of coronary disease. Resins may increase triglycerides such that a second agent such as nicotinic acid or a fibrate may be required to lower triglycerides. Resins should be used with caution in patients with hypertriglyceridemia. Long-term therapy with resins may result in a compensatory increase in HMG CoA reductase activity that tends to increase cholesterol levels. Combination therapy with a statin may exploit the complementary mechanisms of action of these two drug classes.

INHIBITION OF LIPOLYSIS BY NICOTINIC ACID

This was the first hypolipidemic drug to reduce overall mortality.[49] It is the cheapest compound and can be bought over the counter. The basic effect of nicotinic acid may be decreased mobilization of free fatty acids from adipose tissue, so that there is less substrate for hepatic synthesis of lipoprotein lipid (Fig. 10-3). Consequently there is less secretion of lipoproteins so that LDL particles are reduced including the triglyceride-rich component (VLDL). Nicotinic acid is also the drug that best increases HDL-C.[3] This agent is recommended for the *lipid triad* (small LDL, high triglycerides, low HDL-C).[3] The lipid-lowering effects of nicotinic acid are not shared by nicotinamide and have nothing to do with the role of that substance as a vitamin.

Dose, Side Effects, and Contraindications The dosage required for lipid-lowering is up to 4 g daily, achieved gradually with a low starting dose (100 mg twice daily with meals to avoid GI discomfort) that is increased until the lipid target is reached or side effects occur. A lower target dosage (1.5 to 2 g daily) still has a marked effect on blood lipids with better tolerability and the need to be given only in two daily doses. If taken with meals, flushing is lessened. *Niaspan* is an extended release formulation with an initiation starter pack that titrates up the dose to reduce side effects. The recommend maintenance dose is 1 to 2 g once daily at bedtime. On the debit side, this drug has numerous *subjective side effects*, although these can be lessened by carefully building up the dose. Through ill understood mechanisms, nicotinic acid causes prostaglandin-mediated symptoms such as flushing, dizziness, and palpitations. Flushing, very common, lessens with time and with use of the extended release formulation. *Caution* should be used in patients with peptic ulcer, diabetes, liver disease, or a history of gout. Impaired glucose tolerance and increased blood urate are reminiscent of thiazide side effects, also with an unknown basis. Hepatotoxicity may be linked to some *long-acting preparations* (extended-release capsules or tablets), whereas flushing and pruritis are reduced. Myopathy is rare. Use in pregnant women is questionable. Nicotinic acid and statin cotherapy gives a better effect on the lipid levels at the cost of an increased (albeit low) risk of hepatotoxicity and of myopathy, hence the warnings in the statin package inserts.

THE FIBRATES

As a rule, none of the fibrates reduce blood cholesterol as much as do the statins or nicotinic acid. Rather their prime action is to decrease triglyceride, thereby increasing HDL-C, and to increase the particle size of small, dense LDL. Like nicotinic acid, they are therefore suitable for use in atherogenic dyslipidemia.[3] They are first-line therapy to reduce the risk for pancreatitis in patients with very high levels of plasma triglycerides, and may be useful with more modest triglyceride elevations and/or when the prime problem is a low HDL-C.[50] At a molecular level, fibrates are agonists for the nuclear transcription factor peroxisome proliferator-activated receptor-α (PPAR-α) that stimulates the synthesis of the enzymes of fatty acid oxidation, thereby reducing VLDL triglycerides.[3] Although all belong to the same group, structural differences between the compounds seem important because of the very different results of large-scale trials on clofibrate (unfavorable) and gemfibrozil (favorable).

Class Warnings There are five warnings or reservations for this class of drugs, as found in the fenofibrate package insert. First, the early experience with clofibrate suggested that fibrates may increase mortality. This fear has not been borne out by trials of other fibrates, and significant coronary benefits have been reported with gemfibrozil. Second, hepatoxicity may occur, with elevated transaminases in 6% of patients given fenofibrate for 8 to 24 weeks. Third, cholelithiasis is a risk, because fibrates act in part by increasing biliary secretion of cholesterol; however, this was not found in the VA-HIT study.[50] Fourth, there is an important drug interaction with concomitant oral anti-coagulants, so that the warfarin dose needs to be reduced. Fifth, no outcome data exist on combined therapy with statins, with special reference to the potential hazard of myopathy (see section on Combination Therapy).

Gemfibrozil (Lopid)

Major Trials This agent was used in the large Helsinki Heart Study in a primary prevention trial on 2000 apparently healthy men with modest hypercholesterolemia, observed for 5 years.[51] In a dose of 600 mg twice daily there was a major increase in HDL-C (12%), a decrease in total cholesterol and LDL-C (8% to 10%) and a substantial reduction in triglycerides with an overall reduction in coronary events. Although the total death rate was unchanged, the study was not powered to assess mortality. Despite the theoretical risk of gallstone formation, no statistical significant increase was noted.

Benefit in Low HDL-C Men The Veterans Affairs Cooperative Studies Program High-density Lipoprotein Cholesterol Intervention Trial (VA-HIT) was a secondary-intervention trial in men with CHD whose primary abnormality was a low HDL-C, below 40 mg/dL (1.0 mmol/L), with a mean of 32 mg/dL.[50] The LDL-C was 140 mg/dL (3.6 mmol/L) or less, with a mean of 112 mg/dL. Over 5 years, the mean HDL-C was 6% higher, the mean triglyceride 31% lower, the total cholesterol 4% lower, while the mean LDL-C level did not change. There was a 24% reduction in the outcome of death from CHD, non-fatal MI, and stroke. The five-year number needed to treat to prevent one major outcome event was 23, which compared well with the major statin trials. This trial showed that major reduction of total cholesterol or LDL-C was not essential to achieve outcome benefit.

Dose, Side Effects, and Contraindications This agent is currently licensed in the USA for use in the triad of lipid abnormalities, namely low HDL-C levels with high LDL-C, and high triglyceride levels. The dose is 1200 mg given in two divided doses 30 min before the morning and the evening meals. *Contraindications* are hepatic or severe renal dysfunction, and preexisting gallbladder disease (possible risk of increased gallstones, not found in the HIT study). There are *drug interactions* to consider. Because it is highly protein bound, it potentiates warfarin. When combined with statins, there is an increased risk for myopathy with myoglobinuria and further risk for acute renal failure (for perspective, see Combination Therapy).

Bezafibrate (Bezalip in the United Kingdom, Not Available in the United States)

This agent resembles gemfibrozil in its overall effects and side effects and the alterations in blood lipid profile. Whether its added effects on fibrinogen and platelets in patients with hypertriglyceridemia are of clinical relevance is not known. However, these properties are not shared by gemfibrozil. Because plasma glucose tends to fall with bezafibrate, this agent may be useful in diabetic patients or those with abnormal glucose metabolic patterns. As with other fibrates, warfarin potentiation is possible and cotherapy with lovastatin or simvastatin should be avoided. In addition, myositis, renal failure, alopecia and loss of libido may occur. The dose is 200 mg two to three times daily; however, once daily is nearly as good and there is now a slow-release formulation available (*Bezalip-Mono*, 400 mg once daily). Some increase in plasma creatinine is very common and of unknown consequence. The major problem with this agent is that unlike gemfibrozil and simvastatin, there are as yet no major long-term outcome trials with clear results. In the BIP study (Bezafibrate Infarction Prevention) patients with a low HDL-C and modest elevations of LDL-C experienced trends in favor of bezafibrate, but no clear advantage except post hoc in a subgroup of those with initial triglyceride levels >200 mg/dL.[52]

Fenofibrate (Tricor)

This drug, now available in the United States, is a prodrug converted to fenofibric acid in the tissues. The licensed indications are as adjunctive therapy to diet to reduce LDL and total cholesterol, triglycerides, apo B, and to increase HDL-C. The effect on the risk for pancreatitis in those with very high triglyceride levels, typically exceeding 2000 mg/dL, has not been well studied. Tablets are 54 or 160 mg. The dose is 54 to 160 mg once daily (half-life of 20 hours), taken with food to optimize bioavailability. Predisposing diseases such as diabetes and hypothyroidism need to be excluded and treated. Nonetheless, the major outcome trial thus far is in diabetics. The Diabetes Association Intervention Study (DAIS) suggests that treatment with fenofibrate in patients with type 2 diabetes reduces progression of atherosclerosis, with a nonsignficant trend to cardiovascular event reduction.[18]

Weight reduction, increased exercise and elimination of excess alcohol are recognized in the package insert as essential steps in the overall control of the triglyceride levels. In addition, there is a caution that cyclosporine cotherapy may cause renal damage with decreased excretion of fenofibrate and increased blood levels. Note risk of bleeding in those given warfarin (bold warning in package insert). Animal data suggest a deleterious effect in pregnancy. Avoid in nursing mothers (carcinogenic potential in animals). Use caution in elderly or patients with renal dysfunction (renal excretion).

CHOLESTEROL ABSORPTION INHIBITORS: EZETIMIBE

Cholesterol absorption inhibitors selectively interrupt intestinal absorption of cholesterol and other phytosterols. The first of this drug class to reach the market is ezetimibe (Zetia) and has a mechanism of action that differs from those of other classes of cholesterol-reducing compounds. Ezetimibe does not inhibit cholesterol synthesis in the liver, or increase bile acid excretion. Instead, ezetimibe localizes and appears to act at the brush border of the small intestine and inhibits the absorption of cholesterol, leading to a decrease in the delivery of intestinal cholesterol to the liver.[53] This causes a reduction of hepatic cholesterol and an increase in clearance of cholesterol from the blood; this mechanism is complementary to that of the statins. This drug has a half-life of 22 hours and is not metabolized by the cytochrome P-450 system.

Indications As monotherapy in primary hypercholesterolemia, ezetimibe is indicated as adjunctive therapy to diet for the reduction of elevated total cholesterol, LDL-C, and apo B. Ezetimibe may also be used in combination therapy with statins to enhance the lipid reductions associated with that drug class. In homozygous familial hypercholesterolemia, ezetimibe may be combined with atorvastatin or simvastatin, used as an adjunct to other lipid-lowering treatments (e.g., LDL apheresis), or used if such treatments are unavailable. *Ezetimibe* is indicated as adjunctive therapy to diet for the reduction of elevated sitosterol and campesterol levels in patients with homozygous familial sitosterolemia.

Dosage and Effect The recommended dosage of ezetimibe is 10 mg once daily. Ezetimibe can be administered with or without food. The daily dose of ezetimibe may be taken at the same time as the HMG-CoA reductase inhibitor, according to the dosing recommendations for the statin. As fixed dose monotherapy, ezetimibe produces an approximate 12% reduction in total cholesterol; an 18% reduction in LDL-C; and modest beneficial effects on triglycerides and HDL-C. All this happens without any apparent safety concerns. No dosage adjustment is necessary in patients with mild hepatic insufficiency, but the effects of ezetimibe have not been examined in patients with moderate or severe hepatic insufficiency. No dosage adjustment is necessary in patients with renal insufficiency or in geriatric patients. As *cotherapy*, the lipid effects of ezetimibe and a statin appear to be additive. For example, with pravastatin, 10 to 40 mg, LDL-C fell by 34% to 41%, triglyceride by 21% to 23%, and HDL-C rose by 7.8% to 8.4%, with a safety profile similar to pravastatin alone.[54] Coadministration of a resin may dramatically decrease the bioavailability of ezetimibe; therefore its dosing should occur either ≥2 hours before or ≥4 hours after administration of the resin.

COMBINATION THERAPY

Combined Statin plus Fibrate Although the impressive results of the large statin trials have led to an "explosive widening of their use," statins alone are not the answer to all lipid problems.[3] In secondary prevention, the currently ideal lipid levels may be difficult to achieve with only one drug, even if that drug is a statin. In primary prevention, in those with severe hypercholesterolemia, and in familial combined hyperlipidemia with marked triglyceride elevations, combination of a statin with a fibrate is increasingly seen as one answer. Each agent acts by a different mechanism, with more effect on blood lipids than either agent alone. Thus the statin is very effective in the reduction of LDL-C, while the fibrate reduces triglyceride, increases LDL particle size, and increases HDL-C. Two reservations are, first, the absence of any large-scale outcome studies with such combinations (although some are now in planning) and the fear of myopathy. The latter is now increasingly seen as a rather rare event[55] even during combination therapy.[56] A logical combination would be that of a statin plus a fibrate that were metabolized by noncompeting pathways: for example, fluvastatin or rosuvastatin with fenofibrate. Although large trial data support the safety and efficacy of each component of the statin-fibrate combination, it will require a large prospective trial for full reassurance. Vigilance against myopathy must, of course, be maintained until safety is fully assured. Hepatotoxicity seems to be a consistent, but rare side effect of statins, also during combination therapy.[57]

Combined Statin plus Resin or Nicotinic Acid Another choice is between a statin plus a resin, or a statin plus nicotinic acid. In men with coronary disease at high risk for cardiovascular events, colestipol or nicotinic acid was combined with either lovastatin 20 mg twice daily. Both regimens were equally effective on blood lipids.[58] Angiographically measured coronary stenosis was lessened. However, side effects were worse on the nicotinic acid regime. The statin package inserts warn against the combination of a statin with nicotinic acid which is thought to enhance the risk of myopathy. A combination preparation has reached the market that pairs extended release nicotinic acid at doses of 500 mg, 750, and 1000 mg with lovastatin, 20 mg (Advicor). This agent is indicated for treating primary hypercholesterolemia and mixed dyslipidemias where the lipid triad is present.

Sequential Addition of Statin, Nicotinic Acid, Cholestyramine, and Gemfibrozil Coronary patients with mean initial LDL-C levels of 214 mg/dL (5.5 mmol/L, too high), HDL-C levels of 42 mg/dL (1.1 mmol/L, normal), and triglyceride levels of 159 mg/dL (1.8 mmol/L, above ideal) were given sequential therapy, starting with pravastatin that reduced LDL-C by 32% and triglycerides by 15%.[59] Then, addition of 1.5 g of nicotinic acid further reduced LDL-C by 11% and triglycerides by 10%. Cholestyramine addition did little of note, except increase GI symptoms. Gemfibrozil further decreased triglyceride by 37%.

Ezetimibe plus Statins This theoretically sound and easy to manage combination[53] will probably be used more and more in the light of current clinical studies.[54,60] Vycorin is a combination tablet now available.

Other Combinations Because of the enormous popularity of the statins, it is likely that various other combinations will be considered in future, such as a statin with low-dose aspirin and other cardioprotective drugs. Some experts have put forth the concept of a "polypill" that combines several heart-beneficial agents as a potential approach.

SPECIAL PROBLEMS

Pregnancy and Lipid-Lowering Drugs As a group, lipid-lowering drugs are either totally or relatively contraindicated during pregnancy because of the essential role of cholesterol in fetal development. Bile acid sequestrants may be safest, while statins must not be used (see Table 11-8). Women desiring to become pregnant should stop statins for about 6 months before conception. If a patient becomes pregnant when taking such drugs, therapy should be discontinued and the patient apprised of the potential hazard to the fetus (pravastatin package insert).

Lipid Clinic Referrals Cardiologists with the added help of a good dietician should undertake most lipid control in cardiac patients. The major aim in secondary prevention is to reduce LDL-C to below 100 mg/dL (2.6 mmol/L), or even lower (Table 10-1). Advice from a Lipid Clinic should be obtained if there is severe hypercholesterolemia (including the familial homozygous variety) or severe hypertriglyceridemia, or if the lipid profile remains unfavorable despite vigorous diet, exercise, and two-drug treatment.

NATURAL ANTIATHEROSCLEROTIC AGENTS

Estrogens Despite observational studies that noted an association between hormone replacement therapy (HRT) and reduced coronary risk in women, prospective, randomized clinical trials, including the secondary-prevention Heart Estrogen/Progestin Replacement Study (HERS) and the primary-prevention Women's Health Initiative, have reported no clinical cardiovascular benefits with hormone replacement treatment compared with placebo.[61,62] Therefore, it is not possible to recommend HRT as a CHD-prevention strategy in postmenopausal women. Indeed, the evidence of an increased risk for thrombotic complications in the early years of HRT makes such therapy even less attractive for cardiovascular risk management.

Dietary Antioxidants In the light of the negative mega-studies showing no cardiovascular protection by vitamin E, either as primary or secondary prevention (Chapter 11, p. 351), enthusiasm for antioxidant supplements has cooled. A Mediterranean diet is likely to contain adequate amounts of antioxidants mixed in the right proportions.

Plant Sterol/Stanol Margarines Plant sterols can be converted to the corresponding stanol esters that interfere with the intestinal uptake of cholesterol, to cause "cholesterol malabsorption." Daily intakes of 2 to 3 grams per day will reduce LDL by about 6% to 15%.[3] In the United States, *Benecol* margarine is available (dose, between 2 and 2.5 g per day).

Folic Acid The role of homocysteine as a risk factor remains controversial.[3] A level of >14 µmol/L defines hyperhomocysteinemia. In type 2 diabetic patients, homocysteine is an independent risk factor, with increased mortality risk.[63] Overall, there are no good data showing that reducing homocysteine with folic acid lowers the risk for coronary disease.[64]

Alcohol There is a U-shaped relationship between alcohol intake and coronary artery disease, with modest intake rates having a protective effect and higher rates an adverse effect, the latter probably by elevation of triglycerides and blood pressure. Modest quantities of alcohol may promote protection by (1) giving a more favorable blood lipid profile and, in particular, increasing HDL-C; (2) the flavonoids contained in red wine that give experimental coronary vascular protection, perhaps by an antioxidant effect. The potential for abuse makes it difficult to give a whole-hearted endorsement to alcohol consumption as a preventive measure. For teetotallers, a liberal intake of red grape juice or cranberry juice could be equally protective.

Juices, Tea, and Nuts In a variety of studies, red fruit juices such as cranberry juice, purple or red grape juice, black tea, and nuts have shown varying degrees of benefit on lipid profiles or vascular function. Almonds are well studied with a dose-response benefit.[26] Full-dose unblanched almonds (about 75 g/day) reduced LDL-C of hyperlipidemic subjects by 9%, reduced conjugated dienes (evidence of oxidized LDL) by 14%, and raised HDL-C by 4%. Herbal remedies are unsupported by data.

Exercise Besides the protective effects mediated by blood lipid profile changes, as already discussed, regular exercise should help to protect by increasing insulin sensitivity and lessening the risk of maturity onset diabetes.

S U M M A R Y

1. *Major changes.* Advances continue unabated. In primary prevention, there is a new more holistic approach to prevention. In secondary prevention, there are now very strong data favoring intensive statin therapy aimed at very low LDL-levels, called a "sea change in cardiovascular prevention."[65]

2. *In primary prevention* of cardiovascular disease, global risk factor assessment and correction is the favored current approach. The atherogenic components of blood lipids and especially LDL are an important part of an overall risk factor profile that includes factors that cannot be changed, such as age, sex, and family history of premature disease, and those that can, such as blood pressure, diet, smoking, exercise, and weight. The ideal blood cholesterol and LDL-C levels appear to be falling lower and lower, emphasizing the virtues of dietary advice for the population as a whole. The Mediterranean diet and plant stanol ester margarines are among the current dietary approaches.

3. *In secondary prevention,* strict LDL-C-lowering (possibly to even lower values than before) is an essential part of a comprehensive program of risk factor modification. Strict dietary modification is required. Lipidemias secondary to drugs and diseases must be excluded. Among the cardiac drugs tending to cause hyperlipidemias are β-blockers (especially propranolol) and thiazide diuretics. Yet when these drugs are indicated, as, for example, β-blockers are for postinfarct patients, then their protective effect overrides the relatively small changes in blood lipids, especially with statin cotherapy. Careful attention to all other coronary risk factors is essential. The statins (HMG-CoA reductase inhibitors) are extremely impressive, especially in LDL-C reduction, and are widely used.

4. *Increasing use of statins.* The decisive 4S and several other studies have shown substantial total and cardiac mortality reduction when statins are given to postinfarct patients with modest to severe hypercholesterolemia. The Heart Protection Study extends the benefits of statins to all high-risk patients defined by any clinical vascular disease or by diabetes, regardless of baseline total cholesterol or LDL-C. Some statins are now licensed for primary prevention with a lipid-lowering diet. Therefore the strong trend in high-risk patients is to start drug treatment with a statin, concurrently with dietary therapy, especially because statins are easy to use, and have few serious side effects or contraindications. Statins may confer benefits extending

beyond lipid lowering, for example, by protection of the vascular endothelium or by reducing the inflammatory response.

5. *Fibrates* act differently than statins, at a molecular level to modify tissue fatty acid metabolism by stimulation of PPAR-α, and clinically to decrease triglyceride, to increase HDL-C, and to decrease LDL particle size, with only a modest fall in the LDL-C level. Fibrates have received renewed attention and refocused interest with the recognition of low HDL-C and high triglyceride levels as part of the adverse risk profile of the metabolic syndrome.

6. *Combination therapy* is now increasingly used to achieve goal lipid levels. The principle is to combine two different classes of agents with different mechanisms of action, such as a statin and a fibrate or nicotinic acid. Most sources warn against these combinations because of the fear of muscle or renal damage or hepatotoxicity. Nonetheless, there is a growing consensus that judicious use of combination therapy, when required, is likely to confer more benefits than harm. Caution is still required, with regular clinical observation, patient education about side effects and monitoring of creatine kinase and blood liver enzymes. A new and promising combination is that of a statin with a cholesterol absorption inhibitor, ezetimibe.

7. *Hormone replacement therapy* in postmenopausal women can no longer be linked to major cardiovascular benefit. Rather, the decision of whether or not to use HRT must be made on other grounds.

8. *Dietary antioxidants* may be obtained in adequate amounts by following the Mediterranean-type diet, which is ideal for coronary prevention. Vitamin E supplements, in particular, have not given protection either in secondary prevention or as primary prevention in high-risk individuals.

9. *Statins in primary prevention.* Although lifestyle and dietary measures remain the basis of primary prevention, the impressive result of one large statin trial, (AFCAPS/TexCAPS), in individuals with blood cholesterol levels that are within the common range and without known coronary disease, raises important issues for the future prevention of coronary disease.

REFERENCES

1. White PD. *Heart Disease, Third Edition.* 1944, New York: Macmillan Company.
2. Gotto AM, Jr., et al. Eligibility for lipid-lowering drug therapy in primary prevention: how do the Adult Treatment Panel II and Adult Treatment Panel III Guidelines compare? *Circulation* 2002;105:136–139.
3. National Cholesterol Education Program Expert Panel. Detection, evaluation and treatment of high blood cholesterol in adults. (Adult Treatment Panel III). *Circulation* 2002,106:3143–3421.
3a. Grundy SM, et al. Implications of recent clinical trials for the National Cholesterol Education Program Adult Treatment Panel III guidelines. *Circulation* 2004;110:227–239.
4. De Backer G, et al. European guidelines on cardiovascular disease and prevention in clinical practice. *Atherosclerosis* 2003;171:145–155.
5. Heart Protection Study Collaborative Group. MRC/BHF heart protection study of cholesterol lowering with simvastatin in 20536 high-risk individuals: a randomised placebo-controlled trial. *Lancet* 2002;360:7–22.
6. Cannon CP, et al. Intensive versus moderate lipid lowering with statins after acute coronary syndromes. *N Engl J Med* 2004;350:1495–1504.
7. Nissen SE, et al. Effect of intensive compared with moderate lipid-lowering therapy on progression of coronary atherosclerosis: a randomized controlled trial. *JAMA* 2004;291:1071–1080.
8. von Birgelen C, et al. Relation between progression and regression of atherosclerotic left main coronary artery disease and serum cholesterol levels as assessed with serial long-term (>12 months) follow-up intravascular ultrasound. *Circulation* 2003;108:2757–2762.
9. Verma S, et al. Endothelial function testing as a biomarker of vascular disease. *Circulation* 2003;108:2054–2059.
10. Libby P. Inflammation in atherosclerosis. *Nature* 2002;420:868–874.
11. Pfeffer MA, et al. Influence of baseline lipids on effectiveness of pravastatin in the CARE trial. *J Am Coll Cardiol* 1999;33:125–130.
12. Collins R, et al. High-risk elderly patients PROSPER from cholesterol-lowering therapy. *Lancet* 2002;360:1618–1619.

13. Brewer HB, Jr. Increasing HDL Cholesterol Levels. *N Engl J Med* 2004;350:1491–1494.
14. Grundy SM. Low-density lipoprotein, non-high-density lipoprotein, and apolipoprotein B as targets of lipid-lowering therapy. *Circulation* 2002;106:2526–2529.
15. Williams K, et al. Comparison of the associations of apolipoprotein B and low-density lipoprotein cholesterol with other cardiovascular risk factors in the Insulin Resistance Atherosclerosis Study (IRAS). *Circulation* 2003;108:2312–1216.
16. Pearson TA, et al. Markers of inflammation and cardiovascular disease: application to clinical and public health practice: a statement for healthcare professionals from the Centers for Disease Control and Prevention and the American Heart Association. *Circulation* 2003;107:499–511.
17. Lindholm LH. Major benefits from cholesterol-lowering in patients with diabetes. *Lancet* 2003;361:2000.
18. Vakkilainen J, et al. Relationships between low-density lipoprotein particle size, plasma lipoproteins, and progression of coronary artery disease: the Diabetes Atherosclerosis Intervention Study (DAIS). *Circulation* 2003;107:1733–1737.
19. Colhoun HM, et al. Primary prevention of cardiovascular disease with atorvastatin in type 2 diabetes in the Collaborative Atorvastatin Diabetes Study (CARDS): multicentre randomised placebo-controlled trial. *Lancet* 2004;364:685–696.
20. Hardman AE, et al. Brisk walking and plasma high density lipoprotein cholesterol concentration in previously sedentary women. *Br Med J* 1989;299:1204–1205.
21. Kromhout D, et al. Prevention of coronary heart disease by diet and lifestyle: evidence from prospective cross-cultural, cohort, and intervention studies. *Circulation* 2002;105:893–898.
22. de Lorgeril M, et al. Mediterranean diet: traditional risk factors, and the rate of cardiovascular complications after myocardial infarction: final report of the Lyon Diet Heart Study. *Circulation* 1999;99:779–785.
23. Trichopoulou A, et al. Adherence to a Mediterranean diet and survival in a Greek population. *N Engl J Med* 2003;348:2599–2608.
24. Remondino A, et al. β-adrenergic receptor-stimulated apoptosis in cardiac myocytes is mediated by reactive oxygen species/c-Jun NH_2-terminal kinase-dependent activation of the mitochondrial pathway. *Circ Res* 2003;92:136–138.
25. Deckelbaum RJ, et al. Summary of a scientific conference on preventive nutrition: pediatrics to geriatrics. *Circulation* 1999;100:450–456.
26. Jenkins DJ, et al. Dose response of almonds on coronary heart disease risk factors: blood lipids, oxidized low-density lipoproteins, lipoprotein(a), homocysteine, and pulmonary nitric oxide: a randomized, controlled, crossover trial. *Circulation* 2002;106:1327–1332.
27. Morgan JM, et al. Effects of walnut consumption as part of a low-fat, low-cholesterol diet on serum cardiovascular risk factors. *Int J Vitam Nutr Res* 2002;72:341–347.
28. ALLHAT Collaborative Research Group. Major outcomes in high-risk hypertensive patients randomized to angiotensin-converting enzyme inhibitor or calcium channel blocker vs diuretic. The Antihypertensive and Lipid-Lowering Treatment to Prevent Heart Attack Trial (ALLHAT). *JAMA* 2002;288:2981–2997.
29. Lindholm LH, et al. Metabolic outcome during 1 year in newly detected hypertensives: results of the Antihypertensive Treatment and Lipid Profile in a North of Sweden Efficacy Evaluation (ALPINE study). *J Hypertens* 2003;21:1563–1574.
30. Scandinavian Simvastatin Survival Study Group. Randomised trial of cholesterol lowering in 4444 patients with coronary heart disease: the Scandinavian Simvastatin Survival Study (4S). *Lancet* 1994;344:1383–1389.
31. WOSCOPS Study. For the West of Scotland Coronary Prevention Study Group. Prevention of coronary heart disease with pravastatin in men with hypercholesterolaemia. *N Engl J Med* 1995;333:1301–1307.
32. Downs JR, et al. Primary prevention of acute coronary events with lovastatin in men and women with average cholesterol levels: results of AFCAPS/TexCAPS. Air Force/Texas Coronary Atherosclerosis Prevention Study. *JAMA* 1998;279:1615–1622.
33. Ridker P, et al. Long-term effects of pravastatin on plasma concentration of C-reactive protein. *Circulation* 1999;100:230–235.
34. Staffa JA, et al. Cerivastatin and reports of fatal rhabdomyolysis. *N Engl J Med* 2002;539–540.
35. Gaist D, et al. Lipid-lowering drugs and risk of myopathy: a population-based follow-up study. *Epidemiology* 2001;1:565–569.
36. Shek A, et al. Statin-fibrate combination therapy. *Ann Pharmacother* 2001;35:908–917.
37. Prueksaritanount T, et al. Mechanistic studies on metabolic interactions between gemfibrozil and statins. *J Pharmacol Exp Ther* 2002;301:1042–1051.
38. EXCEL Study. Expanded Clinical Evaluation of Lovastatin (EXCEL) Study Results. I. Efficacy in modifying plasma lipoproteins and adverse event profile in 8245 patients with moderate hypercholesterolemia. *Arch Intern Med* 1991;151:43–49.
39. Fibrinolytic Therapy Trial. (FTT) Collaborative Group. Indications for fibrinolytic therapy in suspectred acute myocardial infarction; collaborative overview of early mortality and major morbidity results from all randomised trials of more than 1000 patients. *Lancet* 1994;343:311–322.
40. LIPID Study Group. Prevention of cardiovascular events and death with pravastatin in patients with coronary heart disease and a broad range of initial cholesterol levels. *N Engl J Med* 1998;339:1349–1357.
41. Shepherd J, et al. Pravastatin in elderly individuals at risk of vascular disease (PROSPER): a randomised controlled trial. *Lancet* 2002;360:1623.
42. Knopp RH. Drug treatment of lipid disorders. *N Engl J Med* 1999;341:498–511.
43. Serruys PW, et al. For the Lescol Intervention Prevention Study (LIPS) Investigators. Fluvastatin for prevention of cardiac events following successful percutaneous coronary intervention: a randomized controlled trial. *JAMA* 2002;287:3215–3222.

44. Holdaas H, et al. Effect of fluvastatin on cardiac outcomes in renal transplant recipients: a multicentre, randomised, placebo-controlled trial. *Lancet* 2003;361: 2024–2031.
45. Schwartz GG, et al. Effects of atorvastatin on early recurrent ischemic events in acute coronary syndromes. The MIRACL study: a randomized controlled trial. *JAMA* 2001;285:1711.
46. AVERT Trial. For the Atorvastatin Versus Revascularisation Treatment Investigators. Aggressive lipid-lowering therapy compared with angioplasty in stable coronary artery disease. *N Engl J Med* 1999;341:70–76.
47. Sever PS, et al. Prevention of coronary and stroke events with atorvastatin in hypertensive patients who have average or lower-than-average cholesterol concentrations, in the Anglo-Scandinavian Cardiac Outcomes Trial-Lipid Lowering Arm (ASCOT-LLA): a multicentre randomised controlled trial. *Lancet* 2003;361:1149.
48. The Lipid Research Clinics Coronary Primary Prevention Trial Results 1. Reduction in incidence of coronary heart disease. *JAMA* 1984;251:351–364.
49. Canner PL, et al. Fifteen year mortality in Coronary Drug Project patients: long-term benefit with niacin. *J Am Coll Cardiol* 1986;8:1245–1255.
50. Rubins HB, et al. for the Veterans Affairs Cooperative Studies Program High-Density Lipoprotein Cholesterol Intervention Trial Study Group. Gemfibrozil for the secondary prevention of coronary heart disease in men with low levels of high-density lipoprotein cholesterol. *N Engl J Med* 1999;341:410–418.
51. Frick MH, et al. Helsinki Heart Study: primary prevention trial with gemfibrozil in middle-aged men with dyslipidemia. *N Engl J Med* 1987;317:1237–1245.
52. Boden WE, et al. Raising low levels of high-density lipoprotein cholesterol is an important target of therapy. *Am J Cardiol* 2000;85:645–650.
53. Shepherd J. Combined lipid lowering drug therapy for the effective treatment of hypercholesterolaemia. *Eur Heart J* 2003;24:685–689.
54. Melani L, et al. Efficacy and safety of ezetimibe coadministered with pravastatin in patients with primary hypercholesterolemia: a prospective, randomized, double-blind trial. *Eur Heart J* 2003;24:717–728.
55. Staffa JA, et al. Cerivastatin and reports of fatal rhabdomyolysis. *N Engl J Med* 2002;346:539–540.
56. Tikkanen M. Statins: within-group comparisons, statin escape and comination therapy. *Curr Opin Lipidol* 1996;7:12–20.
57. Athyros VG, et al. Safety and efficacy of long-term statin-fibrate combinations in patients with refractory familial combined hyperlipidemia. *Am J Cardiol* 1997;80:608–613.
58. Brown G, et al. Regression of coronary artery disease as a result of intensive lipid-lowering therapy in men with high levels of apolipoprotein B. *N Engl J Med* 1990;323:1289–1298.
59. Pasternak RC, et al. For the Harvard Atherosclerosis Reversibility Project (HARP) Study Group. Effect of combination therapy with lipid-reducing drugs in patients with coronary heart disease and "normal" cholesterol levels. *Ann Intern Med* 1996;125:529–540.
60. Kerzner B, et al. Efficacy and safety of ezetimibe coadministered with lovastatin in primary hypercholesterolemia. *Am J Cardiol* 2003;91:418–424.
61. Grady D, et al. For the HERS Research Group. Cardiovascular disease outcomes during 6.8 years of hormone therapy: Heart and Estrogen/progestin Replacement follow-up (HERS II). *JAMA* 2002;288:49–57.
62. Writing Group for the Women's Health Initiative Investigators. Risks and benefits of estrogen plus progesterone in healthy postmenopausal women: principal results from the Women's Health Initiative randomized controlled trial. *JAMA* 2000;288:321–333.
63. Hoogeven EK, et al. Hyperhomocysteinemia increases risk of death, especially in type 2 diabetes. 5-year follow-up of the Hoorn Study. *Circulation* 2000;101:1506–1511.
64. Liem A, et al. Secondary prevention with folic acid: effects on clinical outcomes. *J Am Coll Cardiol* 2003;41:2105–2113.
65. Topol EJ. Intensive statin therapy—a sea change in cardiovascular prevention. *N Engl J Med* 2004;350:1562–1564.
66. Frishman WH. *Medical Management of Lipid Disorders. Focus on Prevention of Coronary Artery Disease*, Frishman WH, ed. New York: Futura; 1992.
67. TOMH Study. Treatment of Mild Hypertension study (TOMH). Final results. *JAMA* 1993;270:713–724.
68. Weidmann P, et al. Antihypertensive treatment and serum lipoproteins. *J Hypertens* 1985;3:297–306.
69. Plouin P-F, et al. Are angiotensin enzyme inhibition and aldosterone antagonism equivalent in hypertensive patients over fifty? *Am J Hypertens* 1991;4:356–362.
70. Kasiske BL, et al. Effects of antihypertensive therapy on serum lipids. *Ann Intern Med* 1995;122:133–141.
71. Giugliano D, et al. Metabolic and cardiovascular effects of carvedilol and atenolol in non-insulin-dependent diabetes mellitus and hypertension. A randomized, controlled trial. *Ann Intern Med* 1997;126:955–959.
71a. Lerch M, et al. Effects of angiotensin II-receptor blockade with losartan on insulin sensitivity, lipid profile, and endothelin in normotensive offspring of hypertensive parents. *J Cardiovasc Pharmacol* 1998;31:576–580.
72. Collins R, et al. Clinical effects of anticoagulant therapy in suspected acute myocardial infarction: systematic overview of randomised trials. *Br Med J* 1996;313:652–659.
73. Armstrong P. Heparin in acute coronary disease: requiem for a heavyweight? [editorial]. *N Engl J Med* 1997;337:492–494.
74. Fisher M. Diabetes and atherogenesis. *Heart* 2004;90:336–340.

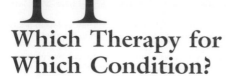

11
Which Therapy for
Which Condition?

Bernard J. Gersh • Lionel H. Opie

**Classification System Modified from that of the American
College of Cardiology and the American Heart Association**

1. **GRADE A:** Data derived from multiple randomized clinical trials involving large numbers of patients

2. **GRADE B:** Data from a limited number of randomized trials involving small numbers of patients or from careful analyses of nonrandomized studies or from large observational registries

3. **GRADE C:** When expert consensus is the primary basis for the recommendation

---

ANGINA PECTORIS

The general approach to angina or any other manifestation of coronary disease has become both more interventional (with increasing use of stents) and more preventative, in that lifestyle modification and aggressive risk factor reduction are now regarded as crucial. Every patient with coronary artery disease requires an assessment of predisposing factors such as diet, smoking, obesity, and lack of exercise, with a search for the metabolic syndrome and diabetes. In exertional angina pectoris, the long-term objectives of treatment are first to improve survival primarily by the prevention of myocardial infarction and death, and second to improve the quality of life by relief of symptoms.[1] Initial examination requires attention to any precipitating factors [hypertension, anemia, congestive heart failure (CHF), tachyarrhythmias, and valve disease]. *The direct attack on coronary disease has two key components, namely lipid lowering and antiplatelet agents.* To these, an angiotensin-converting enzyme (ACE) inhibitor is now increasingly added. The low-density lipoprotein (LDL) target is 100 mg/dl (2.6 mmol/L) or even lower at 70 mg/dL (1.8 mmol/L), often best achieved by a combination of diet and aggressive statin therapy (see Chapter 10), while the optimal aspirin dose range is wide (75 to 325 mg per day). GRADE A Aspirin is strongly indicated in patients without contraindications, and its efficacy in reducing cardiovascular events in stable angina has been confirmed by a meta-analysis of 287 randomized trials.[2] Clopidogrel is the recommended alternative in patients intolerant to aspirin, although never tested in patients with chronic stable angina. Low-intensity anticoagulation with warfarin may give benefit similar to that obtained with aspirin,[3] but this approach is rarely employed. Despite the established links between inflammatory markers and coronary artery disease, there is as yet no role for antibiotic therapy.[4] Of note, both statins and aspirin have anti-inflammatory properties.

Sublingual Nitroglycerin Of the various agents that give pain relief (Fig. 11-1), nitrates are among the most effective although there is no evidence that nitrates reduce mortality in patients with chronic coronary artery disease. Nonetheless, their efficacy in relieving symptoms and

ACTION OF ANTI-ANGINALS

Opie 2005

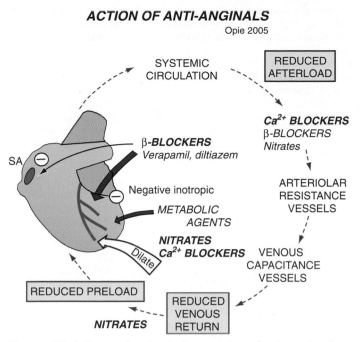

Figure 11-1 Proposed antianginal mechanisms for the major three classes of antianginal agents: nitrates, β-blockers, and calcium channel blockers. (*Figure © L. H. Opie, 2004.*)

improving exercise tolerance justifies their use as standard therapy in conjunction with a β-blocker or calcium channel-blocker (CCB). Thereafter, the addition of long-acting nitrates is indicated. GRADE B Nitrate tolerance remains a major problem, although the precise mechanisms remain unclear. Eccentric dosage schedules with 8- to 12-hour nitrate-free intervals are the most practical method of avoiding tolerance (see Table 2-3). Alternatively, a long-acting mononitrate may be given once a day in the morning; its duration of action is supposedly long enough to see the patient through the day yet short enough to provide a nitrate-free interval at night.

β-Blockers versus Calcium Channel Blockers (CCBs) Which to choose for first-line treatment of angina pectoris is not always easy. Each is combined with nitrates. The meta-analysis of 90 randomized or crossover studies comparing β-blockers, CCBs, and long-acting nitrates demonstrated no significant difference in the rates of cardiac death and myocardial infarction between β-blockers and CCBs.[5] GRADE B Nevertheless, there are groups of patients for whom, on the whole, one of these agents might be preferable. First, in the presence of LV dysfunction, β-blockers are much preferred, because of their capacity to confer postinfarct protection even in the presence of heart failure. GRADE A Specifically, there are strong data favoring carvedilol, metoprolol (Toprol XL), and bisoprolol in heart failure. Of these three agents, metoprolol is the only one licensed for angina in the United States. On the other hand, late heart failure is more prevalent with CCBs as a group, at least in hypertensive patients.[6] Second, in those at risk of acute myocardial infarction, β-blockers protect in the acute and chronic phases. Third, in patients with angina associated with a relatively high heart rate (anxiety), β-blockade is more logical, or if CCBs are used they should be of the non-dihydropyridine variety (heart rate lowering agents). β-Blocker downsides include quality of life problems such as impaired exercise capacity, impotence, and weight gain, besides risk of glucose intolerance, the latter being less likely with carvedilol and CCBs.

The only *absolute contraindications to β-blockers* are severe bradycardia, preexisting high-grade or second-degree atrioventricular block, sick sinus syndrome, asthma, or class IV decompensated congestive heart failure. β-Blockers should be used with caution in patients with chronic obstructive pulmonary disease without frank bronchospasm and in patients with psychological depression or active peripheral vascular disease. Most diabetic patients will tolerate β-blockers, but particular care is needed in patients with insulin-dependent diabetes mellitus with symptomatic hypoglycemia. CCBs may be more effective in directly influencing vascular disease, with evidence that amlodipine both lessens carotid intimal changes in those with coronary disease (see Chapter 3) and reduces the need for repeat percutaneous transluminal coronary angioplasty (PTCA).[7] When coronary spasm is the established cause of the angina, as in Prinzmetal's variant angina, β-blockers are ineffective and probably contraindicated, whereas CCBs work well.

Despite such guidelines, the choice between these two types of agents can often not readily be resolved. β-Blockers are logical initial therapy in the absence of contraindications in those with prior myocardial infarction or left ventricular (LV) dysfunction. Then, if needed, CCBs should be combined with β-blockers and long-acting nitrates. The combination is safest in the case of dihydropyridines, such as long-acting nifedipine and amlodipine, and is pharmacokinetically simplest with those β-blockers, such as atenolol, that are not metabolized by the liver. If side effects from β-blockers are substantial, CCBs in combination with nitrates are the recommended substitute. In this setting long-acting non-dihydropyridine CCBs should be used preferentially. "Triple therapy" with nitrates, calcium antagonists, and β-blockers should not be automatically equated with maximal therapy because patients' reactions vary. In particular, excess hypotension should be avoided.

Other Antianginal Agents Nicorandil, a combined nitrate and ATP-dependent potassium-channel activator, reduced major coronary events in patients with stable angina in the IONA Trial, but there has been no application for its use in the United States.[8] *Ranolazine*, a metabolic agent that inhibits fatty acid oxidation, improves exercise tolerance and, is currently under consideration for approval in the United States.[9] *Trimetazidine* is a similar metabolic agent, widely used as an antianginal in Europe. *Perhexilene*, another metabolic antianginal, is only used when blood levels can be measured. *Ivabradine* is an investigational agent that acts specifically on the current I_f in the sinoatrial node to cause bradycardia. It gives a dose-dependent improvement in exercise tolerance with a lower side effect profile than atenolol.[10,11] Bepridil was withdrawn from the market in the United States in 1998.

Prophylaxis by ACE Inhibitors The role of ACE inhibitors in the routine management of coronary artery disease has been radically expanded by the results and substudies of the HOPE Trial in diabetic and non-diabetic patients,[12,13] and more recently by the EUROPA trial of perindopril in lower risk patients with stable coronary artery disease and no apparent heart failure.[14] The PEACE trial of trandolapril to be presented in 2004, will provide additional data on low-risk patients. Note that each drug should be given exactly as in the trial, that is ramipril 10 mg at night, and perindopril 8 mg in the morning.

No Vitamin E Supplements GRADE A We do not recommend supplemental vitamin E or other antioxidants. The trial data in regard to vitamin E are largely neutral or even negative in two large studies in high-risk or postinfarct patients.[1] Long-term follow-up in HOPE showed an increased risk of heart failure with vitamin E. Rather, we recommend the Mediterranean diet, rich in omega-3 fatty acids (see this chapter, p. 371).[15]

Role of Education in Risk Factor Modification This is a critical component of the integrated management of chronic stable angina and is emphasized by the following mnemonic modified from the ACC/AHA Guidelines (A = Aspirin and ACE inhibitor; B = β-Blocker and Blood pressure; C = Cigarette smoking and Cholesterol; D = Diet and Diabetes; E = Education and Exercise).

Refractory Angina Revascularization is the key when the effort angina is more than mild, especially if symptoms are escalating. The patient population with refractory angina not amenable to revascularization is growing and constitutes a difficult clinical problem. Alternative therapies such as chelation and acupuncture, ineffective in controlled trials, should be avoided. A variety of more promising therapies is available: enhanced external counter pulsation (EECP), spinal cord stimulation (SCS), transcutaneous electrical nerve stimulation (TENS), transmyocardial laser revascularization (TMLR), and gene and stem cell therapy. All of these require the rigorous scrutiny of large, placebo-controlled, randomized trials.[16-22]

Revascularization for Effort Angina

Despite multiple studies over the last 20 years, the issue of timing and type of revascularization, and the long-term consequences thereof, remain to be fully clarified.[23] This is because the techniques for surgical and nonsurgical intervention as well as optimal medical therapy are all constantly improving, with off-pump surgery, drug-eluting stents, statins and tighter blood pressure and glycemic control all giving tangible improvements.[24] For the high-risk patients, surgery remains a very good option, with better results than (old) medical therapy.[23] High risk includes unstable angina, recalcitrant effort angina, left mainstem disease whether symptomatic or not, triple vessel disease, diabetes, and LV dysfunction. In a somewhat lower risk group that excluded left main-stem lesions and poor LV function, stenting was more cost-effective than off-pump surgery with equal improvement in angina and a better quality of life after one year.[25] Off-pump bypass surgery is an attractive option, particularly in elderly patients, in those with peripheral vascular disease, and in the presence of impaired renal function but it is technically more difficult and randomized trials have not demonstrated its superiority over standard "on-pump" surgery. This is an area of continued investigation and evaluation.[26] In an elderly group, mean age 80 years, with severe angina, immediate revascularization gave better symptom relief than did aggressive modern medical therapy, but after 1 year hard endpoints were similar.[23] Thus decisions about the timing and type of intervention must be tailored to the individual and need to take into account all these complex cardiac factors and, in addition, the patient's lifestyle, occupation, other medical conditions, and tolerance of optimal medical therapy.

Percutaneous Coronary Intervention (PCI) The major advances have been in the use of drug-eluting stents and the new antiplatelet agents, namely the intravenous IIb/IIIa inhibitors and clopidogrel. GRADE A The latter agents have substantially decreased peri-procedural complications, particularly in patients with high-risk anatomy. Stents have markedly reduced the need for emergency coronary bypass surgery and the incidence of late stenosis requiring reintervention to the target artery. Yet the hardest end-points of MI and death are unchanged by older model stents in comparison with PTCA alone.[27,28] Nonetheless, the introduction of drug-eluting stents (Fig. 11-2) has had a major impact on restenosis and results at 9 months are very encouraging,[29] but long-term (5-year) follow-up data on drug-eluting stents are needed, especially in high-risk patients with complex lesions such as bifurcation lesions.

Randomized Trials of PCI versus Bypass Surgery The key to selecting the appropriate revascularization strategy whether bypass surgery or PCI, is based on a careful assessment of the coronary anatomy and the

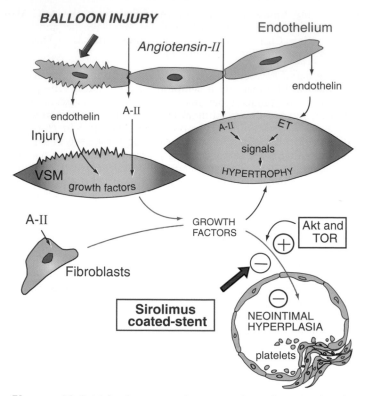

Figure 11-2 Molecular events in restenosis and prevention by sirolimus-coated stent. The balloon-induced injury damages both endothelium and vascular smooth muscle (*VSM*) with release of endothelin (*ET*) and penetration of angiotensin-II (*A-II*). These act to promote growth both of VSM cells and fibroblasts. Growth signals include Akt (protein kinase B) and TOR (= target of rapamycin). The result is neointimal hyperplasia that predisposes to restenosis. With a sirolimus (rapamycin)-coated stent, the growth pathways are inhibited at the site of TOR, and restenosis is much diminished. (*Figure © L. H. Opie, 2004.*)

extent of myocardial jeopardy, the need for "complete" revascularization, left ventricular function, the technical suitability of the lesions for a transcatheter technique, and realistic expectations from the patient of what can be achieved by each procedure. Worldwide, the trend is towards percutaneous coronary intervention for revascularization.[30] In an older patient population it is particularly important to screen for comorbid conditions which can have a crucial impact on procedural success and complications but also upon the long-term outcome. An important trial (AWESOME), employing contemporary PCI techniques but prior to drug-eluting stents, demonstrated similar outcomes in regard to death and myocardial infarction for PCI versus coronary bypass surgery in high-risk patients with medically refractory myocardial ischemia and one or more risk factors for adverse outcomes with coronary bypass surgery.[31] Likewise there were similar results in both diabetic and nondiabetic patients.[32]

ACUTE CORONARY SYNDROMES

Classification has undergone a major change in terminology, based on the presence or absence of electrocardiographic ST-segment elevation at presentation, giving two clear divisions. ST-elevation ACS is treated as acute myocardial infarction (AMI) with the need for urgent revascularization by early fibrinolysis or PCI. The sooner revascularization takes place, the better (Fig. 11-3). In non-ST elevation ACS, including unstable angina, the emphasis is on prevention of throm-

PERIPHERAL HOSPITAL: ACUTE MI
Gersh 2005

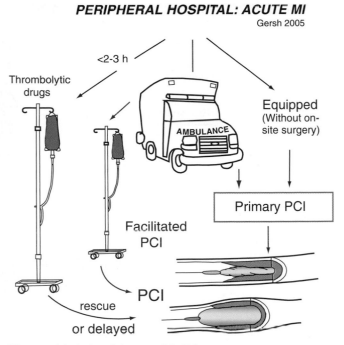

Figure 11-3 Speed is essential. Primary percutaneous coronary intervention (PCI), using a balloon (*bottom right*) and then a stent is the ideal mechanism to achieve reperfusion in acute myocardial infarction, yet is often not available at a peripheral hospital that the patient is rushed to. The subsequent choices are several (*left to right*): (1) thrombolysis is as good as PCI within the first 2 to 3 hours (Table 11-3), especially if followed by transfer to a nearby PCI center; (2) rapid transfer by ambulance to a PCI center, facilitated by thrombolytic therapy; (3) rapid transport to a PCI center; and (4) development of PCI facilities at the peripheral hospital even if no on-site surgery. (*Figure © B. Gersh and L. H. Opie, 2004.*)

bosis by antiplatelet and antithrombotic agents, followed in medium and higher risk groups by rapid PCI (Fig. 11-4). GRADE A General measures include bed rest, immediate relief of ischemia by nitroglycerin (sublingual, spray, or intravenous) with added β-blockers to reduce the myocardial oxygen demand. Morphine sulfate is given intravenously if the pain persists or if the patient is agitated or pulmonary congestion is present. Oxygen is probably best reserved for patients with documented hypoxemia or poor respiratory status.

Antiplatelet and Antithrombotic Therapy for ACS

Aspirin and Clopidogrel Evidence for the efficacy of combined aspirin and heparin is strong.[33] Aspirin should be started immediately and continued indefinitely. The key to effective therapy is to institute all other components in the emergency room as rapidly as possible. GRADE A The role of early clopidogrel given upon admission is still not fully settled. In patients who are unable to take aspirin, the case for clopidogrel as an alternate anti-platelet agent is self-evident. In addition, there is now growing evidence for combining clopidogrel and aspirin on admission, irrespective of whether or not catheterization and PCI is planned.[34,35] In centers in which bypass surgery is performed soon after angiography, it is reasonable to withhold clopidogrel until the coronary anatomy and the revascularization strategy has been determined. Whether the loading dose of clopidogrel should be 300 mg or 600 mg is under evaluation, with early evidence favoring the higher dose, and with the suggestion that added abciximab might become unnecessary.[36,37]

ACUTE CORONARY SYNDROMES: TRIAGE
Gersh 2005

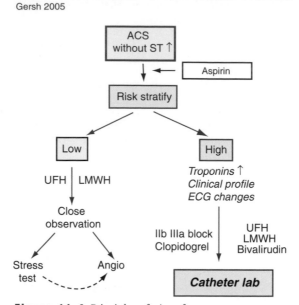

Figure 11-4 Principles of triage for acute coronary syndromes (*ACS*). Those with acute severe prolonged chest pain of cardiac origin and with ST-elevation on the ECG are regarded as acute myocardial infarction and subject to early reperfusion preferably by percutaneous coronary intervention (PCI, Fig. 11-4). The others are stratified according to the risk. With elevated serum troponin levels, and guided by the clinical picture and ECG changes, high and medium risk patients are given Gp IIa/IIIb inhibitors, clopidogrel and unfractionated heparin (*UH*) or low molecular weight heparin (LMWH). *Angio* = coronary angiogram. (*Figure © B. Gersh, 2004.*)

Heparin and Low-Molecular-Weight Heparin The optimum dose of unfractionated heparin is not established, but a weight-adjusted regimen with frequent monitoring to maintain the activated partial thromboplastin time (aPTT) between 1.5 and 2 times controlled is probably the most reasonable.[38] The introduction of low-molecular-weight heparin (LMWH) has been a significant advance in the management of unstable angina. GRADE A The ability to give the drug subcutaneously and without need for aPTT monitoring allows for a longer period of treatment, and consequently offers some protection against the "rebound" phenomenon seen after heparin withdrawal. LMWH offers other potential benefits by acting on both thrombin generation and thrombin activity.

Which LMWH should be used? Since no direct head-to-head comparative trials have been performed, definitive conclusions cannot be drawn. Two trials with enoxaparin, ESSENCE and TIMI IIB have demonstrated a moderate benefit over unfractionated heparin[39,40]; one trial with dalteparin[41] was neutral, and the FRAXIS Trial with nadroparin showed an unfavorable trend.[42] Hence enoxaparin is often preferred. GRADE B

LMWH and PCI Because the level of anticoagulant activity cannot easily be measured in patients receiving LMWH, concern has been expressed concerning its use in patients undergoing coronary angiography. Three studies have shown, however, that PCI can be performed safely in this setting,[43-45] as now confirmed in the large SYNERGY study, though at the cost of a modest increase in bleeding.[46]

Direct Thrombin Inhibitors A meta-analysis of four trials of *hirudin*, the prototype direct antithrombin, demonstrated a modest benefit at best, in comparison with unfractionated heparin, in patients with non-ST-elevation acute coronary syndromes.[47] The downside was increased bleeding. *Bivalirudin*, a direct thrombin inhibitor approved in the United States for clinical use in patients undergoing PCI, seems to be superior to unfractionated heparin with respect to ischemia relief and without increased bleeding.[48] Bivalirudin with the provisional use of IIb/IIIa platelet inhibitors has similar efficacy to unfractionated heparin and routine IIb/IIIa administration but with less bleeding.[49] This remains an area of controversy. The direct thrombin inhibitors are clearly indicated for the treatment of heparin-induced thrombocytopenia (HIT) (see p. 272).

Platelet GP IIb/IIIa Receptor Antagonists These agents have been the subject of intense study and some controversy over the last decade. They constitute an advance in the management of the acute non-ST-elevation acute coronary syndrome and should be used in conjunction with standard antithrombotic agents. However, in those at lower risk, these inhibitors do not give added benefit beyond aspirin and heparin. Thus, a meta-analysis of 31,402 patients with unstable angina/NSTEMI who were not routinely scheduled to undergo coronary revascularization, did not demonstrate any reduction in the endpoints of death or nonfatal myocardial infarction.[50] Rather, benefit is greatest in those with ongoing ischemia or other high-risk features.[1,51-55] Thus when PCI is contemplated, a IIb/IIIa inhibitor should be administered GRADE A either immediately prior to catheterization, when abciximab is often chosen, or "upstream" of the procedure when it is appropriate to use the "small molecule" agents eptifibatide or tirofiban (approved in the United States for this purpose whereas abciximab is not). In lower risk patients without unstable angina, pretreatment with 600 mg of clopidogrel appeared to nullify any additional benefit from abciximab.[37]

Other Antiplatelet Agents Drugs such as sulfinpyrazone, dipyridamole, prostacyclin, prostacyclin analogs, and the thromboxane synthase blockers are not superior to aspirin and have no current role to play in the management of unstable angina/non-Q-wave myocardial infarction. The same applies to the oral IIb/IIIa receptor blockers which are actually harmful.

Thrombolytic Therapy to Be Avoided Despite its beneficial role in patients with acute myocardial infarction presenting with ST-segment elevation, routine thrombolytic therapy cannot be recommended for all, and is absolutely contraindicated in patients with unstable angina or non-ST-segment elevation infarctions. GRADE A Not only is the complication rate increased, but in some studies, overall mortality was higher with thrombolytic treatment.

Anti-ischemic Drugs for Acute Coronary Syndromes (ACS)

Intravenous nitroglycerin is part of the standard therapy, although sometimes it is held in reserve for patients with recurrent pain despite oral nitrates. *β-Blockers*, even in the absence of good trial data, have become a cornerstone of therapy, and should be started early in the absence of contraindications. GRADE B The often-quoted HINT[56] compared the β-blocker metoprolol with placebo in unstable angina with inconclusive results, although the addition of nifedipine to prior β-blocker therapy was clearly beneficial. Thus the arguments for β-blockade largely rest on first principles (reduced myocardial demand) in addition to extrapolation from results in patients with ST-segment elevation and myocardial infarction. It is best to give β-blockers intravenously followed by oral administration in those patients who are at higher risk as well as in patients with ongoing rest pain, whereas oral β-blockers will suffice for patients in lower categories of risk. In patients who are hemodynamically unstable, the choice falls on the ultrashort-acting β-blocker esmolol, known to reduce ischemia in unstable angina.[57] Otherwise the choice of a β-blocker for the individual patient is based upon the pharmacokinetic profile and the experience of the individual physician.

Of the calcium channel blockers, *diltiazem* acts hemodynamically differently from nifedipine, and may be used instead of a β-blocker. Diltiazem compared well with nitrates during the acute phase of unstable angina, with better event-free survival at 1 year.[58] In the absence of coronary spasm the case for nifedipine or any other dihydropyridine CCB is very weak; two randomized trials in unstable angina, including the HINT study,[56] have shown that nifedipine causes harm, presumably by excess hypotension or tachycardia, unless it is combined with a β-blocker. In patients with recurrent ischemia despite β-blockers and nitrates, the addition of a nondihydropyridine CCB is indicated, as it is in the case of patients with contraindications to β-blockers. In patients with refractory angina on maximal medical therapy, intra-aortic balloon counterpulsation may be very effective pending angiography in those patients who are candidates for coronary revascularization in presence of suitable coronary anatomy.

Invasive versus Conservative Strategy in ACS

Although there is general agreement that the first step is to stabilize the patient, there has been considerable debate as to whether the subsequent strategy should be invasive or conservative. The former involves coronary angiography with a view towards coronary revascularization based on the anatomy, whereas the more conservative approach advocates angiography only for patients with recurrent ischemia, either spontaneous or induced by stress testing. Most recent trials strongly favor an invasive approach (Table 11-1), particularly in patients at higher risk and in centers in which facilities for early angiography and PCI are available.[45,59-61] Drug-eluting stents are now state-of-the-art (Fig. 11-4) with zero restenosis after 6 months.[62]

Risk stratification. This is the key to balancing both approaches. GRADE A Subgroups at higher risk who will probably benefit from an early aggressive strategy include patients with elevated serum levels of creatine phosphokinase-MB (CPK-MB) isoenzymes, and/or the troponins, the presence of ST-segment depression or steep symmetrical anterior precordial T-wave inversion on the electrocardiogram, older patients, patients with a history of long-standing angina or prior myocardial infarction, and diabetic patients.[51,63,64] According to the new definition of MI using elevated blood levels of troponins, all patients with non-ST-elevation-MI are considered at high risk and candidates for early angiography. The new biomarkers such as the admission blood sugar,[65] natriuretic peptides, C-reactive protein, and leukocyte myeloperoxidase are currently under investigation, and may help in risk stratification.[66,67] To what extent these markers will provide incremental information is an important, as yet unanswered question. Obviously recurrent pain is a strong indication for early angiography. On the other hand, for patients who initially stabilize and are otherwise considered at low risk, the trend is transfer to a Chest Pain Unit in the Emergency Room for early stress testing, thus avoiding hospitalization.[68]

Long-Term Prophylaxis of Coronary Disease

Overall management of both stable and unstable angina includes a vigorous attack on coronary artery disease. "Antiplatelet agents for all"

Table 11-1 Important Trials in Non-ST Elevation Acute Coronary Syndrome (ACS)

Acronym	Trial Aim/Design	Entry Point	Chief End-Points	Number of Subjects	Chief Results	Reference
ISAR-COOL	Benefit of antithrombotic therapy pre-PCI	Angina at rest with ST↓ or troponin↑	30-day death or large MI; bleeding	410; 207 "cooled off"	No benefit to cooling off	ISAR-cool *JAMA* 2003;290: 1593–1599
GUSTO IV-ACS	Does abciximab benefit ACS if no PCI?	ACS, non-ST↑, including non-ST↑ MI and unstable angina	30-day death or MI; 1-yr data obtained by follow-up	Placebo, 2598 24-h abcx, 2590 48-h abcx, 2612	No 30-day or one year benefit for abcx in absence of early PCI; in subgroups, excess bleeding, mortality	GUSTO IV-ACS *Circulation* 2003;107:437–442
TACTICS-TIMI 18	PCI + tirofiban vs. conservative policy for ACS	ACS, non-ST↑, Pain > 20 min, Enzyme markers	Composite death, MI, rehospitalization at 6 mo	PCI, 1114 Conservative, 1106	Tirofiban + PCI best except for low risk group	TACTICS-TIMI 18 *N Engl J Med* 2001;344:1879–1887
RITA-3	PCI vs. conservative policy for ACS with enoxaparin	Cardiac chest pain at rest, documented CAD, no MI	Death, MI, angina at 4 mo; death or MI at 1yr	PCI, 895 Conservative, 915	Intervention better than conservative therapy	RITA-3 *Lancet*, 2002; 360:743–751
PCI-CURE	Does clopidogrel before and after PCI improve outcome?	Rest angina within 24 h, non-ST↑, enzyme↑	Death, MI, angina at 4 mo; death or MI at 1yr	Clopidogrel, 1313 Placebo. 1345	Clopidogrel added to aspirin before PCI gave better results	PCI-CURE *Lancet* 2001; 358:527–533
SYNERGY	Enoxaparin vs UFH	ACS, non-ST↑ high risk, for early PCI	Death, MI at 30 days; four endpoints at 30 days, death at 1yr	Enoxaparin, 4993 UFH, 4985	Efficacy similar, more bleeding with enoxaparin	SYNERGY *JAMA* 2004;292: 45–54

Abcx = abciximab; CAD = coronary artery disease; GUSTO IV-ACS = global use strategies to open occluded coronary arteries IV-acute coronary syndrome; ISAR = intracoronary stenting with antithrombotic regime cooling off; MI = myocardial infarction; PCI-CURE = percutaneous coronary intervention-Clopidogrel in Unstable angina to prevent Recurrent Events; RITA-3 = Randomised Intervention Trial of unstable Angina-3; TACTICS-TIMI 18 = Treat Angina with Aggrastat and Determine Cost of Therapy with an Invasive or Conservative Strategy-Thrombolysis in Myocardial Infarction; SYNERGY = Superior Yield of the New strategy of Enoxaparin, Revascularization and GlYcoprotein IIb/IIIa inhibitiors; UFH = unfractionated heparin.

(provided that the blood pressure is well-controlled) is now joined by "statins for all," irrespective of cholesterol level according to the Heart Protection Study.[69] GRADE A Clopidogrel is chosen in those who are intolerant to aspirin, and in some patients, warfarin monotherapy is selected. In addition, we recommend an ACE inhibitor for all post-coronary syndrome patients with LV dysfunction or diabetes.[1] GRADE A Long-term ACE-inhibitor prophylaxis by ramipril or perindopril (with other ACE inhibitors not yet tested) is increasingly given for all those with established coronary artery disease.[12,14] GRADE B The *Mediterranean diet* has strong support, especially since it reduced total mortality (this chapter, p. 371). Combined laboratory, epidemiological and clinical trial data strongly suggest that increased dietary omega-3-rich fish oils help to protect from sudden cardiac death.[70] Tight blood pressure and glycemia control is logical though not evidence-based. Other risk factors also need optimizing, including weight loss, increased exercise, and no smoking. Long-term β-blockade is generally recommended although without firm supporting trial data and the side effects of fatigue and weight gain mitigate against an optimal lifestyle.

Prinzmetal's Angina at Rest

This relatively rare condition, much more common in Japan, is often manifest as acute ischemic pain with ST-elevation without myocardial infarction. It requires relief of coronary spasm rather than thrombolytic therapy. β-Blockers are inferior to calcium channel blockers and may aggravate the spasm. GRADE B Short-acting nifedipine, diltiazem, and verapamil all completely abolish the recurrence of angina in approximately 70% of patients with a substantial improvement in another 20%. Starting doses of CCBs are high (e.g., 240 to 480 mg per day of verapamil, 120 to 360 mg per day of diltiazem, and 60 to 120 mg per day of nifedipine). The relatively vasoselective long-acting dihydropyridine amlodipine is also effective. The next step is to add a CCB from another class or a long-acting nitrate.[71] Smoking cessation is imperative. In refractory cases of Prinzmetal's angina associated with coronary artery disease, bypass grafting may be combined with cardiac sympathetic denervation (plexectomy).

EARLY PHASE ACUTE MYOCARDIAL INFARCTION

The management of myocardial infarction (MI) encompasses two different strategies (Fig. 11-5). The early phase of evolving MI is dominated by the need for prompt reperfusion therapy whereas the chronic phase is a dual attack on coronary disease and remodeling. In early phase MI, the earlier reperfusion is achieved the better GRADE A so that time is of the essence, particularly in the first 2 to 3 hours after the onset of symptoms (Table 11-2). Nonetheless, general care is also crucial. Aspirin needs to be given as early as possible, and pain relieved. *Morphine* (4 to 8 mg IV by slow IV push with 2 to 8 mg at 5- to 15-minute intervals) combines a potent analgesic effect with hemodynamic actions that are particularly beneficial in reducing myocardial oxygen demand (MVO_2), namely a marked venodilator action reducing ventricular preload, a decreased heart rate, a mild arterial vasodilator action that may reduce afterload, and a decrease in sympathetic outflow. A "hidden" benefit of morphine may be its capacity, shown experimentally, to precondition the heart, thereby protecting against further ischemia. In the presence of hypovolemia, morphine may cause profound hypotension. The administration of *oxygen* by nasal prongs is almost universal practice in acute myocardial infarction, although whether it does any good is not established. Oxygen, however, should be administered to all patients with overt pulmonary congestion or arterial oxygen desaturation ($SaO_2 < 90\%$). GRADE A

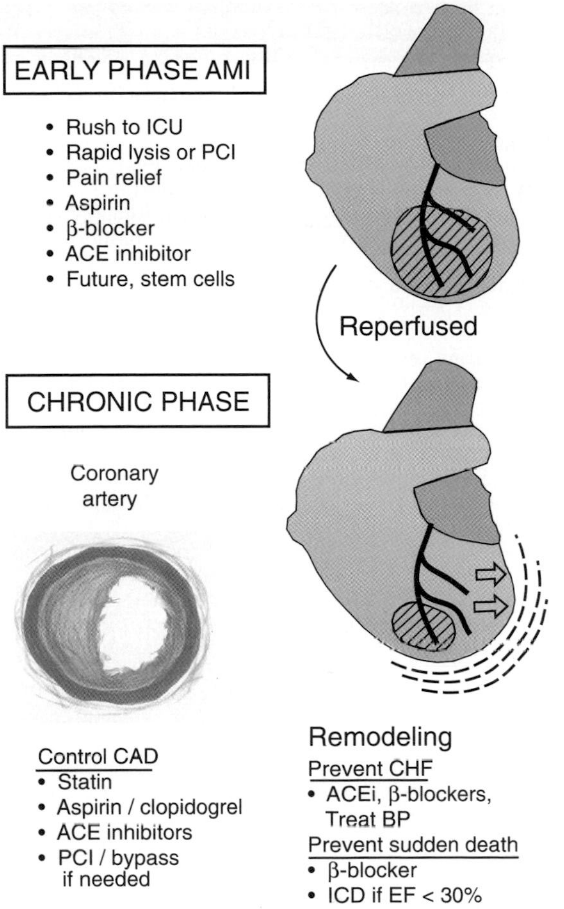

EARLY PHASE AMI

- Rush to ICU
- Rapid lysis or PCI
- Pain relief
- Aspirin
- β-blocker
- ACE inhibitor
- Future, stem cells

Reperfused

CHRONIC PHASE

Coronary
artery

Control CAD
- Statin
- Aspirin / clopidogrel
- ACE inhibitors
- PCI / bypass
  if needed

Remodeling
Prevent CHF
- ACEi, β-blockers,
  Treat BP
Prevent sudden death
- β-blocker
- ICD if EF < 30%

Figure 11-5 Contrasting management of early and chronic phases of MI. In the early phase, the major aim is to achieve reperfusion either by rapid thrombolysis or by percutaneous coronary intervention (PCI), while protecting from pain and starting off cardioprotective drugs such as aspirin, β-blockers and ACE inhibitors (*ACEi*). In the chronic phase, the two major aims are to control coronary artery disease (*CAD*) and to inhibit remodeling, thereby helping to prevent heart failure and sudden death.

Bradyarrhythmias Atropine (0.5 mg IV aliquots to maximum of 2.0 mg) has a vagolytic effect that is useful for the management of bradyarrhythmias with atrioventricular (AV) block (particularly with inferior infarction), sinus or nodal bradycardia with hypotension, or bradycardia-related ventricular ectopy. Small doses and careful monitoring are essential since the elimination of vagal inhibition may unmask latent sympathetic overactivity, thereby producing sinus tachycardia and rarely even ventricular tachycardia (VT) or fibrillation (VF). The role of prophylactic atropine for uncomplicated bradycardia remains questionable.

Sinus Tachycardia This is a common manifestation of early phase sympathetic overactivity, which increases MVO_2 and predisposes to tachyarrhythmias. The first step is to treat the underlying cause—for example, pain, anxiety, hypovolemia, or pump failure—and then to use a β-blocker, which is safe and effective provided that the patient is carefully observed. If the hemodynamic status is borderline, the very short acting esmolol (see next section) may be selected.

Acute Hypertension A high blood pressure must be reduced in all patients in whom thrombolytic therapy is under consideration, to

Table 11-2 **Early Phase Acute Myocardial Infarction: Principles of Management**

1. Minimize pain-to-needle time, urgent hospitalization. Relieve pain by morphine.
2. Aspirin upon suspicion.
3. Duration of pain: if > 3 h, rapid transfer for primary percutaneous coronary intervention (PPCI); consider facilitated PCI. If < 2–3 h, or if excess delay to balloon inflation, give urgent thrombolysis with heparin or low-molecular-weight heparin (bivalirudin considered with streptokinase)
4. Acute angioplasty and stenting in selected patients at centers with documented expertise and good results. (See above about delay times.)
5. Continuing pain. Intravenous nitrates and/or β-blockers. Consider urgent angiography and IABP if the patient is a potential candidate for PCI.
6. Consider indications for early β-blockade, ACE inhibition. Diabetes argues for ACE inhibition or ARB.
7. Management of complications:
   - LVF (after Swan-Ganz catheterization)—ACE inhibitors or ARBs, diuretics, nitrates
   - Symptomatic ventricular arrhythmias: lidocaine; if refractory procainamide, amiodarone
   - Supraventricular arrhythmias (vagal procedures; adenosine or verapamil or diltiazem or esmolol)
   - Cardiogenic shock—acute angioplasty, intra-aortic balloon, bypass surgery.
   - RV infarction—fluids, inotropic support. Avoid nitrates.
   - Rupture of free wall, mitral valve, ventricular septum—cardiac surgery.
   - If patient non-insulin-dependent diabetic: stop oral hypoglycemic, replace by insulin (modified GIK regimen). Strongly consider ACE-inhibition or ARB for all diabetics.

lessen the risk of bleeding. A smooth and careful reduction by intravenous nitroglycerin seems best; other tested drugs include intravenous atenolol or metoprolol or intravenous esmolol (see Chapter 1, p. 29). The latter is especially suitable, because of its very short half-life, when there are possible contraindications including hemodynamic instability. The mean blood pressure should not fall below 80 mmHg.

Acute Reperfusion Therapy for AMI

Removing the thrombotic obstruction to the blood supply remains the most effective mode of preserving the ischemic myocardium and reducing infarct size. Nonetheless, the decision to embark on an approach of "routine" mechanical reperfusion must be driven by the expected outcome, which is, in turn, both operator and institution-dependent. Among the relatively few patients seen within 60 to 70 minutes of symptoms, the extraordinary success of thrombolytics cannot be improved upon. As this time extends to beyond an ill-defined limit of about 2 to 3 hours (Table 11-3) the efficacy of lysis decreases as clots become increasingly resistant, whereas the ability of stents to open arteries probably remains unimpaired.[72] This relative constancy of the benefit of stenting explains why the extra time taken to transfer patients from a peripheral hospital to a PCI center (Fig. 11-3) is justified by better results.

Mechanical Revascularization in AMI Despite the undisputed success of early fibrinolysis, especially in the first 2 to 3 hours, there are considerable limitations to the ability of currently available thrombolytics in achieving "optimal" reperfusion. This provides a strong rationale for the mechanical approaches using primary angioplasty and stents.

Table 11-3 Important Trials in ST-Elevation Acute Coronary Syndromes

Trial Acronym	Trial Aim/Design	Entry Point	Chief End-Points	Numbers	Chief Result	Reference
DANAMI-2	Is primary PCI better than lysis despite transport to PCI center?	Symptoms 30 min to 12 h, ST↑ in two adjacent leads	Reinfarction, death, disabling stroke; composite end-point, all at 30 days	Fibrinolysis, 782 PCI, 790	Primary PCI better if transport ≤ 2 h; composite end-point↓ Mortality →	Danami-2 N Engl J Med 2003; 349:733–742
CAPTIM	Is prehospital lysis better than transport within 1 hr to PCI center?	Symptoms 30 min to 6 h, ST↑ in two adjacent leads or LBBB.	Reinfarction, death, disabling stroke; composite end-point, all at 30 days	Randomized <2 hrs, 460; ≥2 h, 374	Prehospital lysis better if randomized within 2 h	CAPTIM Circulation 2003; 108:2851–2856
PRAGUE-2	Should all patients with AMI be transported to PCI center?	Within 8 h of symptoms, ST-elevation in two leads, new LBBB	30 day mortality; combined end-point of death, reinfarction, stroke	Lysis in local hospital, 421; PCI, 429	Lysis equals PCI if <3 h, PCI superior if <3–12 h	PRAGUE-2 Eur Heart J 2003; 24:94–104
ADMIRAL	Stent ± abciximab for AMI	Pain <12 h, ST↑	Composite 30-day death, reinfarction, revascularization	Abciximab 149; Stent only, 151	Abcx better at 30 days and 6 months	ADMIRAL N Engl J Med 2001; 344:1895–1903

CADILLAC	Is stenting better than PTCA for primary PCI, with or without abciximab (abcx)?	Within 12h of onset of suspected AMI	Reinfarction, death, disabling stroke, ischemia-driven revascularization	2082, 4 groups; PTCA, PTCA + abcx, Stent; Stent + abcx.	Stent best with or without abcx; PTCA improved by abcx; 1 year rehospitalization with stent↓, abcx↑	1. CADILLAC 2002 *N Engl J Med* 2002;346:957–966 2. CADILLAC 2003 *Circulation* 2003;108:2857–2863
ACE	Does abcx add benefit to stent for AMI	Pain 30 min–6 h, ST↑, ongoing ischemia 6–24h	Composite 30-day death, reinfarction, revascularization	Stent alone 200; Stent plus abcx 200	Abcx better at one and 6mo (death, reinfarct)	ACE *JACC* 2003;42:1879–1885
GUSTO-5	Is combined lysis by 1/2 dose reteplase (rTP) with abcx better than full dose rTP?	Within 6h of evolving ST-elevation AMI; no planned PCI	30-day mortality; complications of AMI	Full dose rTP, 8260; Half dose rTP with abcx, 8328	Mortality equal. In abcx group, less reinfarction, ischemia; bleeding↑ (elderly)	GUSTO-5 *Lancet* 2001;357: 1905–1914
ASSENT-3 PLUS	Prehospital TNK + enoxaparin (encx) or unfractionated heparin (UFH)	Symptoms ≤6h, ST↑ in two leads or LBBB	Composite 30-day mortality, reinfarction or refractory ischemia	Enox, 818; UFH, 821	Equal endpoint; with enox, less reinfarction, stroke↑ bleeding↑ (elderly)	ASSENT-3 PLUS *Circulation* 2003;108:135–142

abcx = abciximab; ADMIRAL = Abciximab before Direct angioplasty and stenting in Myocardial Infarction Regarding Acute and Long-term follow-up; AMI = acute myocardial infarction; ASSENT = ASsessment of the Safety and Efficacy of a New Thrombolytic regimen; CADILLAC = Controlled Abciximab and Device Investigation to Lower Late Angioplastic Complications; CAPTIM = Comparison of Angioplasty and Prehospital Thrombolysis in acute Myocardial infarction; LBBB = left bundle branch block; Danami-2 = Danish Multicenter Randomized Study on fibrinolytic therapy versus Acute Coronary Angioplasty in Acute Myocardial Infarction; Lysis = fibrinolysis; PCI = percutaneous coronary intervention; PTCA = percutaneous coronary angiography.

A meta-analysis of 23 trials involving 7739 patients, compared primary PCI (PPCI) with thrombolytic therapy to demonstrate early and one-year benefits for PPCI in terms of death and particularly rein-farction and stroke.[73] Thus there is now consensus that PPCI is the preferred form of reperfusion therapy providing the time delay between balloon inflation versus drug administration is less than 90 minutes. GRADE A Stents lessen the high rates of restenosis and reoc-clusion after balloon angioplasty but without any overall difference in mortality.[74] Drug-eluting stents should give excellent results, but their role in PPCI is still under evaluation. Further improvement in results can be expected from intracoronary thrombectomy as an adjunct to stents, with the future possibility of added benefit from distal protection devices that lessen or prevent the microem-bolization associated with balloon dilation.[75] Intracoronary β-blockade may be a simple procedure to protect the distal myocardium during PCI.[76]

How to do it faster. The quicker the better, whether the reperfusion is by fibrinolysis or by PCI. A delay of only 30 minutes increases 1-year mortality by 7.5%.[77] Three major time delays are (1) onset of patient's pain to arrival of the paramedics, (2) home-to-hospital time, and (3) door-to-needle or to-balloon time in the hospital. The greatest delay is from symptom onset to Emergency Room, and this has changed little over the last decade, being in the range of 85 minutes.[78,79] The next delay is the door-to-balloon time. As little as 60 to 90 minutes was achieved in several randomized trials, yet reality is closer to 2 to 2½ hours in many community and registry studies. To achieve early reperfusion, a logical plan is *prehospital thrombolytic therapy*, which, however, requires intense community organization to get the para-medical team trained and there on time. Fast track assessment and nurse-initiated thrombolysis can cut this patient-to-needle time to below 30 minutes.[80] The evidence regarding prehospital fibrinolysis is very encouraging. Logically, prehospital thrombolysis can be followed by rapid or rescue PCI.[81] A closely related policy is to follow early in-hospital thrombolysis by early PCI.[82]

Thrombolysis Three trials (Table 11-3) have shown the benefit of early fibrinolysis for ST-elevation AMI within 2 to 3 hours of onset of symp-toms. GRADE A In two trials an additional criterion was new onset left bundle branch block. Although fibrinolytic therapy is contraindi-cated in patients with myocardial infarction presenting with ST segment depression, an exception should be made for patients with acute posterior infarction (ST depression ≥2 mm in leads V1+V2 with an R/S ratio ≥ 0.8 or ST segment elevation ≥2 mm in the posterior leads V7, V8, or V9).[83]

Which Thrombolytic Agent? By and large, the debate over which throm-bolytic agent is the most effective was resolved by the first GUSTO trial[84] that demonstrated the superiority of the accelerated regimen of tissue plasminogen activator (tPA, Alteplase) over streptokinase (see Table 9-4). Nonetheless, this came at the price of a slightly but significantly greater risk of intracranial hemorrhage, especially in female patients over the age of 75 years.[85] Single bolus Tenecteplase or TNK, is now the most widely used thrombolytic agent in the United States because of its efficacy and ease of administration. GRADE B TNK and alteplase are equivalent in regard to 30-day mortality, but noncerebral bleeding and blood transfusions were less with TNK.[86] The dose of TNK is weight-adjusted and administered as a single bolus over 5 seconds (versus 90 minutes of variable rate infusion with tPA). *Reteplase (rPA)* is a more fibrin-specific agent administered as two 10-unit bolus given 30 minutes apart. Alteplase and reteplase are equivalent in both mortality and hemorrhage.[87] Overall, we appear to have reached a plateau in that the new fibrinolytics do not result in increased reperfusion rates or reduced mortality. The major strength of the bolus agents (TNK, rPA), lies in their ease of administration resulting in fewer dosing errors.

Limited Benefit of GP IIb/IIIa Inhibitors plus Reperfusion Therapy Glycoprotein IIb/IIIa inhibitors, strongly recommended in those acute coronary syndromes already discussed, provide very limited benefits when added to fibrinolytic agents for acute ST segment elevation myocardial infarction (Table 11-3). Admittedly they improve reperfusion with increased rates of TIMI 3 flow.[88] However, this initial promise has not been translated into a major long-term clinical benefit. In the trials totaling over 22,000 patients, there was a modest benefit on rates of reinfarction, no mortality benefit, and a significant increase in bleeding which is especially marked in the case of abciximab.[48,49,88,89] In the setting of primary PCI, four clinical trials involving over 3000 patients demonstrated that added GP IIb/IIIa inhibition reduced the need for urgent target-vessel revascularization but neither death nor recurrent myocardial infarction.[88,90-93] The largest study, CADILLAC, showed that stents were better than balloons, and that abciximab did not much improve the excellent results with stents. Accordingly the cost-effectiveness of adding abciximab is questioned.[94] Three smaller studies, RAPPORT, ADMIRAL and ACE, argue for added abciximab.[90,92,95]

Facilitated Reperfusion Intense interest currently revolves around strategies for achieving reperfusion prior to balloon inflation, including the use of high-dose heparin, low-molecular-weight heparin,[96] abciximab, clopidogrel, and low-dose tPA. For the community hospital, the optimal reperfusion strategy is not fully clarified and the possibilities are complex[97]—thrombolytics, thrombolytics plus transfer to a referral center, transfer without pretreatment, facilitated PCI, or PPCI without on-site cardiac surgery (Fig. 11-5). These choices are the subject of ongoing trials and particularly in the area of facilitated PCI, there is widespread discussion. At present "one size does not fit all."

Reperfusion Injury and Microvascular Dysfunction Considerable experimental evidence points to a spectrum of reperfusion events, including ventricular arrhythmias, mechanical stunning, and microvascular injury. Reperfusion-induced apoptosis has now been added to this list. Reperfusion injury occurs on reperfusion, not later. Microvascular dysfunction, however, may precede or follow arterial reperfusion. There is now increasing realization that despite restoration of flow to the epicardial infarct-related artery, there remains a persistent impairment of myocardial reperfusion and microvascular dysfunction,[75] which has stimulated multiple trials of widely diverse agents aimed at modifying these pathophysiological consequences of coronary occlusion and reperfusion. To date, the clinical results have been disappointing, in contrast to the experimental data, although some promise has been demonstrated for agents such as adenosine, nicorandil, glucose-insulin-potassium, myocardial cooling, and aqueous oxygen. Early data on mechanical distal protection devices are encouraging and more trials are proceeding. All of these remain investigational at the present time, but it should be emphasized that none of the trials to date have achieved their primary end-point. The problem is that even if these approaches were effective, they are often given too late to make a difference. On the other hand, if utilized very early in the course of MI, the preexisting low mortality rates and high rates of salvage would make it difficult to "demonstrate" a difference.

Reocclusion and Heparin Prophylaxis Reocclusion, which occurs both early and late (weeks or months) after thrombolysis, remains an "Achilles heel" of reperfusion therapy. In a meta-analysis of more than 20,000 patients entered into randomized trials of thrombolytic therapy, the frequency of symptomatic recurrent myocardial infarction during the index hospitalization was 4.2%, together with a 2- to 3-fold increase in 30-day mortality.[98] Irrespective of the timing, reocclusion has markedly deleterious effects of left ventricular function and long-term outcomes. There are many contributory factors, including the severity of the underlying residual stenosis, the persistence of the initial thrombogenic substrate (plaque fissure), and activation of platelets and of the clotting cascade. *Intravenous heparin* has an established place in patients receiving tPA, TNK, or reteplase and should be utilized in the initial 24 to 42 hours to prevent further thrombin generation and reduce the risk of reocclusion. The dose should be adjusted to keep the aPTT between 60 and 80 seconds, taking care to avoid wide swings in the aPTT values. The aPTT should be evaluated 4 to 6 hours following heparin bolus and then checked every 6 to 8 hours thereafter.

The appropriate *duration of heparin therapy* is uncertain, but a reasonable approach is to use intravenous heparin for 48 hours and then to continue for 5 to 7 days in subsets of patients with large anterior infarctions or in those with atrial fibrillation who are considered at high risk for embolism. If chronic anticoagulation is contemplated, warfarin can then be substituted. In patients presenting with acute myocardial infarction and already on chronic warfarin therapy, the use of intravenous heparin should be similar to those not on warfarin. There is a lesser role or no role for routine intravenous heparin in patients receiving streptokinase, unless they are considered at high risk for systemic emboli (large or anterior MI, atrial fibrillation, previous embolus, or known LV thrombus). (For heparin with streptokinase, see Chapter 9, p. 308).

Low-Molecular-Weight Heparins (LMWH) These are increasingly used because of the known deficiencies of heparin as an antithrombotic agent. Trials based upon angiographic patency have suggested that LMWHs lessen reocclusion of the infarct artery, reinfarction, and recurrent ischemic events when compared to unfractionated heparin or placebo. Based upon the ASSENT-3 and ASSENT-3 PLUS trials, in which patients received TNK and either unfractionated heparin or enoxaparin, it is reasonable to consider LMWH as an acceptable alternative to unfractionated heparin. GRADE A There are two contraindications: in patients older than 75 years of age who are receiving fibrinolytic therapy because of increased intracranial bleeding, and renal dysfunction with a creatinine greater than 2.0 to 2.5 mg/dL.[99,100]

Direct Thrombin and Factor Xa Inhibitors These are only licensed for use in patients with heparin-induced thrombocytopenia, but have promise in ST-elevation myocardial infarction. A meta-analysis of 11 trials totaling over 35,000 patients, demonstrated a 20% reduction in recurrent myocardial infarction with bivalirudin or hirudin and with less bleeding following the use of bivalirudin.[101] However, only four of the trials were limited to AMI, with the others being mostly unstable angina. In patients with AMI treated with streptokinase, bivalirudin, in comparison with unfractionated heparin, reduced recurrent infarction but increased bleeding.[102] Thus, in patients with given streptokinase for fibrinolysis, bivalirudin is probably superior to unfractionated heparin. Preliminary studies with *pentasaccharide*, a highly selective inhibitor of Factor Xa[103] warrant further evaluation.

Protecting the Ischemic Myocardium

Prophylactic Early β-Blockade Pooled data on trials of β-blockers given early to about 29,000 patients with myocardial infarction showed a 13% reduction in acute phase mortality.[104] Yet almost all of these studies were gathered in the prethrombolytic era. With thrombolysis, there is no hard evidence on the benefits of β-blockers on early mortality in patients receiving reperfusion therapy. Yet their use is logical, based on their effects on myocardial oxygen demands, their impact on cardiac rupture in the prethrombolytic era, and their theoretical potential to augment coronary perfusion by reducing heart rate and prolonging diastole. β-Blockers are particularly useful in patients with sinus tachycardia, tachyarrhythmia such as atrial fibrillation, hypertension, and recurrent ischemia. Furthermore there are indirect indicators of the benefits of β-blockade. In the three PAMI trials, pre-PCI β-blockers reduced procedural complications, in-hospital death, and 1-year mortality.[105] Furthermore, in a retrospective analysis of five large trials using abciximab during PCI, prior β-blockade reduced mortality.[106] Consequently, the prompt administration of intravenous followed by oral β-blockers in all patients without contraindications, irrespective of the administration of early reperfusion therapy, is recommended. $\boxed{\text{GRADE B}}$ Of note, such prompt β-blockade reduces intracranial hemorrhage in thrombolysed patients.[107] Alternatively, β-blockade can be introduced later, when there is hemodynamic stabilization (late intervention, 25 studies, 24,000 patients) to bring about a 23% reduction in late-phase mortality.[104] The best-tested drugs are metoprolol and atenolol, whereas the short-acting esmolol is preferred when the hemodynamic situation is potentially unstable. In the acute infarct setting, it is essential to pay attention to relative contraindications, particularly when β-blockers are given intravenously.[108]

Early Use of Angiotensin-Converting Enzyme (ACE) Inhibitors or Angiotensin-II Receptor Blockers (ARBs) in AMI This is now common practice based on the logic of improved remodeling and the results of several large well-designed trials, of which the first was the SAVE study with captopril, closely followed by AIRE with ramipril (see Chapter 5). Hence the early use of oral ACE inhibitors in those at high risk (anterior infarcts, clinical LV failure, ejection fraction below 35%, diabetics) is advisable, with long-term use to follow. $\boxed{\text{GRADE A}}$ A logical policy would be to start the ACE inhibitor as soon as the patient is hemodynamically stable and to watch for hypotension or renal impairment. An ARB such as valsartan is a good alternative, giving equal mortality benefit,[109] besides being the therapy of choice if there is intolerance to the ACE inhibitor.

Limitation of Infarct Size Since myocardial infarction is ultimately the consequence of a serious imbalance between myocardial oxygen supply and demand, it is logical and prudent to employ measures aimed at redressing this imbalance. These measures include the treatment of arrhythmias, hypoxia, heart failure, hypertension, and tachycardia. Hypokalemia should be sought and treated. Despite much laboratory evidence that numerous pharmacologic agents such as β-blockers, nitrates, metabolic agents, or free radical scavengers will reduce infarct size, clinical evidence of benefit has been difficult to prove.

Metabolic Support *Glucose-insulin-potassium (GIK)*, a concept that is more than 40 years old, may be particularly effective in those patients who are being reperfused. In the placebo-controlled randomized trial (ECLA) of 407 patients including 62% treated with reperfusion therapy, GIK was associated with significant reduction in the composite end-point of death, nonfatal severe congestive heart failure, and nonfatal ventricular fibrillation.[110] In a recent Netherlands trial of 940 patients undergoing primary PCI, GIK did not result in a significant mortality reduction in all patients, but in a subgroup of patients without signs of heart failure, a significant reduction was seen.[111] The adverse trend in patients with signs of heart failure may be related to the volume load. The attraction of glucose-insulin-potassium is its simplicity and its cost. Further large international trials will soon guide the use or otherwise of GIK. In the meantime, modified GIK infusions can be considered as part of the routine care of diabetics with acute myocardial infarction.[112] *Intravenous magnesium*, otherwise discredited, remains indicated for patients with torsades de pointes-type of ventricular tachycardia and in patients who have low serum magnesium and/or potassium levels frequently associated with chronic diuretic therapy.

Acute Statins If statins have prominent protective "nonlipid" effects, then perhaps they should be started as soon as possible as now being tested. Thus, statins started on admission or within 24 hours thereof, may reduce hospital mortality.[113] In LIPS (Lescol Intervention Prevention Study) patients were randomized to fluvastatin on hospital discharge after PCI by balloon or stenting.[114] Six months later cardiac complications were reduced. Perhaps the strongest case for the early administration of statins is to increase the proportion of patients who are on statins at follow-up. Since statins are safe, we recommend that they be initiated prior to discharge—together with other essentials such as aspirin, an ACE inhibitor (ramipril or perindopril referred), and a β-blocker, as described in the next section.

Arrhythmias in AMI

Therapy of Ventricular Arrhythmias in AMI *Lidocaine* (lignocaine) has been widely used in the prophylaxis and therapy of early postinfarct arrhythmias. Lidocaine is often chosen as the initial when treatment is indicated for premature ventricular extrasystoles (only if therapy is essential), ventricular tachycardia, ventricular fibrillation, or occasionally for wide-complex tachycardias of uncertain origin. Prophylactic lidocaine therapy confers no long term benefits. A meta-analysis of 14 trials shows that lidocaine reduces VF by about one third, but may increase mortality by about the same percentage.[115] *Amiodarone* is now the preferred intravenous antiarrhythmic agent for life-threatening ventricular tachycardias when lidocaine fails. *Interventional techniques* such as atrial or ventricular pacing, stellate ganglion blockade, or radiofrequency catheter ablation may occasionally be life-saving. Treatment of LV failure is an essential adjunct to antiarrhythmic therapy. The possibility of drug-induced ventricular tachycardia or of hypokalemia should always be borne in mind.

Supraventricular Arrhythmias in AMI Atrial fibrillation, flutter, or paroxysmal supraventricular tachycardia are usually transient yet may be recurrent and troublesome. Precipitating factors requiring treatment include hypoxia, acidosis, heart failure with atrial distention, pericarditis, and sinus node ischemia. In the case of supraventricular tachycardia, initial therapy should be carotid sinus massage or other vagal maneuvers. In the absence of LV failure, intravenous diltiazem or verapamil or the ultrashort-acting β-blocker esmolol are all effective in controlling the ventricular rate. Although intravenous diltiazem is licensed in the United States for acute conversion of supraventricular tachycardia, experience in AMI is limited and concurrent use of intravenous β-blockade is a contraindication. In the presence of LV failure, intravenous adenosine (Adenocard) or the careful use of esmolol may be tried. Adenosine cannot be used for atrial fibrillation or flutter because of its ultrashort action. *Cardioversion* may be required in the face of compromised hemodynamics or severe ischemia, starting with a low threshold. To avoid systemic embolization after cardioversion for atrial fibrillation, heparin should be restarted or continued.

LV Failure and Shock in AMI

Swan-Ganz catheterization to measure LV filling pressure and cardiac output allows a rational choice between various intravenous agents that reduce both preload and afterload or chiefly the preload. For several reasons the use of the Swan-Ganz catheterization has declined. For the patient with AMI and pulmonary edema, excess diuresis with preload reduction and relative volume depletion must be avoided.

Reduced ventricular compliance requires higher filling pressures to maintain cardiac output.

Load-Reducing Agents In the intensive care unit setting, intravenous nitroglycerin is the most appropriate preload-reducing agent, particularly in the early hours of acute infarction when ischemia may contribute to LV dysfunction. Where there are no intensive care facilities, intravenous unloading agents such as nitroprusside and nitrates are best avoided. Sublingual agents that reduce the preload (short-acting nitrates) or the pre- and afterload (captopril) should be useful here. The diuretic furosemide, although standard therapy and acting by rapid vasodilation as well as by diuresis, may sometimes paradoxically induce vasoconstriction. Nesiritide, a synthetic natriuretic peptide, is theoretically sound but still under evaluation for acute infarction.

Nitrates in AMI Current indications for nitrate therapy in AMI include recurrent or ongoing angina or ischemia, hypertension, and load reduction in patients with congestive heart failure and mitral regurgitation. Nitrates should not be administered to patients with a systolic blood pressure of less than 90 mmHg, patients with right ventricular infarction or those who received sildenafil (or its equivalent) in the last 24 hours.

Low Cardiac Output in AMI When cardiac output is low in the absence of an elevated wedge pressure or clinical and radiographic evidence of LV failure, it is crucial to exclude hypovolemia (possibly drug-induced), or right ventricular infarction. In the absence of these conditions, the best strategy is to employ ACE inhibitors alone or in combination with a positively inotropic agent such as norepinephrine, dopamine, or dobutamine to bring the systolic blood pressure up to 80 mmHg. However, it is often forgotten that dobutamine by stimulating peripheral β_2-receptors can drop the diastolic blood pressure. Monitoring the hemodynamic response invasively is indispensable. Nitrates are usually contraindicated because their main effect is reduction of the preload. Intra-aortic balloon counterpulsation is useful in some patients. Inotropic support by digitalis in AMI remains controversial (see Chapter 6). The benefits of digoxin in AMI are probably small, so that its use is restricted to patients with frank LV failure not responding to furosemide, nitrates, or ACE inhibitors, or patients with atrial tachyarrhythmias in whom diltiazem or verapamil or esmolol fail or are contraindicated.

Cardiogenic Shock Cardiogenic shock is the leading cause of death in AMI. In severely ill patients with Killip class III or IV features, thrombolytic therapy is not of proven benefit and primary PCI must be considered to treat cardiogenic shock. In the SHOCK Trial,[116] a strategy of emergency angiography with a view to revascularization was associated with a 50.3% mortality at 6 months versus 63.1% among patients who were initially treated with medical therapy ($P = 0.027$). Intra-aortic balloon counterpulsation was utilized in both groups. Coronary bypass surgery is indicated in patients in whom PCI has failed, in the presence of a severe left main coronary artery or three-vessel disease and in patients undergoing concomitant cardiac surgery for mechanical complications. A crucial aspect of the management of cardiogenic shock is the diagnosis and prompt treatment of potentially reversible mechanical complications, for example, rupture (free wall, septum, or papillary muscle), tamponade, and mitral regurgitation. Underlying hypovolemia or dominant right ventricular infarction also needs to be excluded.[117] Such patients need vasopressors such as phenylephrine, vasopressin and dopamine (see Fig. 6-10). A *new paradigm for cardiogenic shock* postulates that activation of inflammatory cytokines leads to increased activity of inducible nitric oxide synthase (iNOS) with increased production of NO and peroxynitrite, all of which have multiple deleterious effects including systemic vasodilation and a low peripheral vascular resistance, thereby simulating gram-negative septic shock.[118] Thus, a new and promising treatment of shock is inhibition of nitric oxide synthase by L-NMMA,[119] currently the subject of a large, multicenter, randomized trial (SHOCK-2).

LONG-TERM THERAPY AFTER AMI

General Management (Table 11-4) Long-term prognosis depends chiefly on the postinfarct LV function, the LV volume, the absence of ischemia, coronary anatomy, and electrical stability.[1] Upon this background, control of risk factors including lipids and blood pressure remains essential. GRADE A Careful choice of long-term protective drugs, giving full reasons, also reassures; those receiving statins feel (and do) better.[120] *Psychosocial factors help to determine prognosis.* Postinfarct patients who are single, isolated or stressed or are depressed may all be suffering from serious psychological depression that is an independent predictor of post myocardial infarction mortality.[121] If tricyclic antidepressants have to be used, they may interfere with treatment of hypertension or cause tachycardia. Pet ownership may provide social support with favorable effects upon outcomes, particularly in the case of dogs.[122] *Lifestyle changes* are often needed. A rehabilitation exercise program combines social support with the

Table 11-4	Postinfarct Follow-up: Principles of Management

1. Risk Factor Modification

No smoking, full lipogram, control of hypertension, aerobic exercise, psychological support. Diabetics: limit HbA1c. For all: strongly consider lipid-lowering drugs (statins), LDL <100 mg/dL (2.6 mmol/L).

2. Assess Extent of Coronary Disease

Residual ischemia? (symptoms, exercise test). Revascularize depending on extent and estimated viability of ischemic tissue.

3. Assess LV Function and Size. Avoid LV Dilation.

If LV dysfunction (low ejection fraction) or anterior MI or diabetes: ACE inhibitor or ARB. Consider aldosterone antagonists (watch serum K^+).

4. Prevention of Reinfarction

- Aspirin; if contraindicated give clopidogrel
- β-Blockade if not contraindicated (severe respiratory disease)
- If contraindicated, verapamil (or diltiazem) if no clinical LV failure
- ACE inhibition or ARB (consider for all)
- Statin therapy, aggressive, to LDL 100 mg/dL, 2.6 mmol/L
- Oral anticoagulation for selected patients

5. Complications Other than Arrhythmias

Postinfarct angina: nitrates, add CCB to β-blocker, consider revascularization
Overt LVF: diuretics, ACE inhibitors or ARBs, β-blocker, aldosterone antagonists, consider digoxin.
Hibernating myocardium: consider revascularization after dobutamine echocardiography or stress scintigraphy or positron emission tomography

6. Complex Ventricular Arrhythmias (VA)

(under evaluation: roles of Holter monitor, EPS, ICD)
Exclude significant coronary disease; assess LV function
LV preserved: effort stress test, exercise rehabilitation
LV 30–40%: Holter, EPS, consider ICD. If no NSVT: β-blockers
If ejection fraction <30%, consider ICD (QRS prolongation >120 msec a possible added risk factor) Role of T-wave alternans under evaluation.
Complex symptomatic VA: consider ICD and amiodarone.

EPS = electrophysiologic stimulation; ICD = implantable cardioverter defibrillator; LDL = low-density lipoprotein; LVF = left ventricular failure; NSVT = nonsustained ventricular tachycardia.

specific benefits of exercise. To stop smoking, patients need enough education and encouragement to become determined in their efforts. Then, if needed, the antidepressant drug bupropion (Wellbutrin) helps them to stop.[123]

Mediterranean Type Diet Epidemiologically, Mediterranean countries have a low incidence of coronary heart disease. In the Lyon Diet Heart Study of Infarct Survivors, a Mediterranean-type diet with a high intake of β-linolenic acid (the precursor of omega-3 long chain fatty acids), vegetables, fruits, and oils (olive and canola) but with reduced butter and red meat, gave striking protection. Total mortality, cardiac death and nonfatal MI fell for up to 4 years of follow-up.[124] In a population-based study in Greece, the closer the adherence to the traditional Mediterranean diet, the greater the longevity.[125] In postinfarct survivors, 1 g daily of fish oil gave cardiovascular protection over 3.5 years.[126,127] In line with the evidence for omega-3 fatty acids, the Nutrition Committee of the American Heart Association now recommends two fatty fish meals per week or dietary fish oil capsules.[128] Closely allied is the beneficial Indo-Mediterranean diet, with much less olive oil and fish, but with more nuts and other plant-based oils (mustard or soy bean).[129] The benefits of red wine have probably been overdramatized, but modest intake of wine with meals is part of the Mediterranean culture. Vitamin E has sadly failed expectations. After 7 years of follow-up in the HOPE study, there was no cardiovascular benefit, but rather increased heart failure.[130]

Hormone Replacement Therapy: Harmful Large landmark clinical trials have provided firm evidence that combination estrogen and progestin replacement therapy should not be used as either the primary or secondary prevention of cardiovascular disease in women. In postmenopausal women who are already taking hormone replacement therapy at the time of myocardial infarction should not continue taking the drugs; neither should HRT be given de novo.

Postinfarct Statins There no longer is any doubt that statins reduce hard end-points in those with coronary disease (see Chapter 10). The only remaining issue is how far to reduce LDL-cholesterol. An elegant study with intravascular ultrasound suggests that 75 mg/dL (1.95 mmol/L) is the equilibrium level at which progression and regression of the plaque is, on average, similar.[131]

Postinfarct β-Blockade Solid evidence shows that postinfarct β-blockade provides benefit. In a very large survey on more than 200,000 patients, late mortality fell by about 40%.[132] GRADE A The present trend is to continue β-blockers indefinitely, together with aspirin, a statin, and, whenever there is LV dysfunction or diabetes, ACE inhibition. β-Blockers protect from the adverse effects of surges of catecholamines, which may explain their effects on sudden cardiac death. In a large Finnish study of infarct survivors, (97% of whom were on β-blockers), the rate of sudden cardiac death after an average of 3.5 years of follow-up was only 3.3% with few arrhythmic events.[133] In the presence of severe respiratory problems but in the absence of heart failure, verapamil is a viable alternative to β-blockade (see next section).

Which subsets of patients are most likely to benefit? Paradoxically, those patients who appear to be at higher risk also benefit most. For example, β-blockade may have its best effects in the presence of heart failure, with all cause mortality reduced by 23%.[134] The mortality reduction also extends to cotherapy with ACE inhibitors, aspirin, and CCBs.[132] Obvious contraindications to β-blockade remain untreated heart failure, severe bradycardia, hypotension, overt asthma, and heart block greater than first degree.

When to Use Calcium Channel Blockers As a group, these agents do not give postinfarct protection.[135] Yet there are good arguments for verapamil or diltiazem in the absence of LV failure, especially when β-blockade is contraindicated by respiratory disease. In the large Danish postinfarct trial (DAVIT II) in which overt LV failure was prospectively excluded, verapamil 120 mg three times daily decreased reinfarction and cardiac mortality.[135] In patients with angina or hypertension not controlled by other agents, verapamil or diltiazem may be helpful.

Aspirin and Clopidogrel Aspirin, the simplest and safest agent, is now established therapy, starting with an oral dose as soon as possible after the onset of symptoms of AMI and continuing indefinitely thereafter (provided that the blood pressure is adequately controlled). GRADE A It prevents reinfarction, stroke, and vascular mortality as shown in numerous trials. The updated meta-analysis suggests a loading dose of at least 150 mg and maintenance dose of 75 to 150 mg daily.[2] The lower doses have fewer side effects. Aspirin may also be selected for postinfarct follow-up of (1) those patients thought to be at risk of thromboembolism in whom oral anticoagulation is not advisable, and (2) those not likely to comply with the stringent requirements for prolonged oral anticoagulation therapy. When aspirin is contraindicated or not tolerated, *clopidogrel* is an excellent alternative that is approved in the United States for the reduction of thrombotic events such as MI, and for use in acute coronary syndromes. In these conditions, clopidogrel given in addition to aspirin extends the benefit. Other antiplatelet drugs such as sulfinpyrazone and dipyridamole have been used in the postinfarct patient, but there is no evidence to suggest that they are any better than aspirin alone.[2]

Warfarin or Ximelagatran Anticoagulation This is usually given for 3 to 6 months after an infarct to patients with prior emboli, in those with LV thrombus (echocardiographically proven), or large anterior infarcts (threatened thrombus), or with established atrial fibrillation, and in patients with contraindications or hypersensitivity to aspirin. Several trials have examined the combined use of warfarin and aspirin in secondary prevention. Patients older than 75 years of age have not been adequately studied. Medium-intensity anticoagulation with a INR of about 2.5 seemed effective, albeit in two relatively small studies,[136,137] whereas low-intensity with an INR of 1.8 in the largest study was not.[138] In another large study mean INR values of about 2.2 to 2.8 reduced nonfatal MI and nonfatal embolic stroke.[139] These modest returns need to be balanced against increased bleeding, greater cost, and added inconvenience to the patient. The role of the oral direct thrombin inhibitor ximelagatran in post-MI patients remains to be determined but a benefit over placebo was established in the ESTEEM trial at the cost of increased leakage of liver enzymes.[96]

ACE Inhibitors for All with Coronary Disease? ACE inhibitors reduce left ventricular remodeling, late mortality, and congestive heart failure, as has been repetitively demonstrated. Since a substantial proportion of the benefit occurs within the first 24 hours, oral ACE inhibitors should be used as soon as the patient is clinically stable. Reduction in ischemic events is achieved by ACE inhibitors. A fascinating aspect of the SAVE and SOLVD Trials (see Chapter 5) was the reduction in recurrent ischemic events in patients treated with ACE inhibitors compared to placebo. This led to three additional large trials of ACE inhibitors in the primary prevention of cardiovascular events in patients with overt coronary disease or at high risk of cardiovascular disease but without significant left ventricular dysfunction[12,14,140,141] Two trials have already demonstrated striking benefits of the ACE inhibitors used (ramipril and perindopril) on cardiovascular events. The results of the ongoing PEACE Trial[140] which includes a high proportion of patients with prior revascularization and on statin therapy, will be crucial in defining whether or not the cardioprotection is a generalized property of ACE inhibitors as a class. Nonetheless, the evidence to date would suggest that it is certainly reasonable to consider prescription of an

ACE inhibitor (preferably ramipril or perindopril in the doses used in the trials) for all post-MI patients irrespective of ejection fraction.

Aspirin Plus ACE Inhibitors Several retrospective studies have demonstrated an interaction between aspirin and ACE inhibitors suggesting that aspirin attenuates the hemodynamic and mortality benefits of ACE-inhibition. However, in one small prospective randomized trial, low-dose aspirin (75 to 160 mg) did not interfere with the efficacy of the ACE inhibitor.[142]

Postinfarct Antiarrhythmic Agents Complex ventricular ectopy and VT in the late-hospital phase of myocardial infarction are predictors of subsequent sudden death after discharge, independently of their frequent association with LV dysfunction. Nonetheless, the hoped for benefit of antiarrhythmic therapy on postinfarct mortality is still elusive. The overall approach is still evolving with β-blockers and amiodarone the only agents showing clear-cut mortality reduction.[104] Amiodarone given to patients with either prior myocardial infarction or congestive heart failure reduced total mortality by 13% and arrhythmic/sudden death by 29%.[143] The major disadvantages of amiodarone remain the side effects and the excessively long duration of action.

Implantable Cardioverter Defibrillators (ICDs) are increasingly used to avoid post-MI arrhythmic death in those with poor LV function. GRADE A Those with an ejection fraction greater than 40% to 45% have too low a risk of arrhythmic death to benefit from an ICD. As shown in the MADIT-2 trial, and now confirmed in SCD-HeFT, those below 30% require an ICD (see Fig. 8-10). Note the somewhat greater benefit in SCD-HeFT found in those with QRS widening ≥120 milliseconds and in those already receiving a beta-blocker.[144] If the ejection fraction is in the 30% to 40% range, most would extrapolate from the MUSTT[145] and MADIT-1[146] trials which support Holter monitoring followed by invasive electrophysiologic testing before deciding on the ICD. Since the ejection fraction may change and improve or deteriorate during the first few weeks post-MI, we suggest a waiting period of approximately 4 weeks before making a definite decision. The role of the ambulatory external defibrillator (AED) during this waiting period is currently the subject of an ongoing randomized trial.

There is an urgent need for new methods of arrhythmia risk stratification. Whether modalities such as T-wave alternans and measurements of autonomic function fulfill their early promise remains to be determined.

ATRIAL FIBRILLATION

The general approach to the therapy of arrhythmias has swung from the widespread use of antiarrhythmic drugs to increasing intervention (Fig. 11-6). As our population ages, the incidence and prevalence of atrial fibrillation is rapidly increasing, giving rise to a "growing epidemic" that has been seriously underestimated.[147] Therapeutic approaches to atrial fibrillation emphasize three main aspects: (1) anticoagulation; (2) cardioversion with maintenance of sinus rhythm by antiarrhythmic agents all having potentially serious side effects or by evolving ablative approaches, primarily catheter-based; or (3) accepting chronic atrial fibrillation with the emphasis on rate control and long-term anticoagulation (Table 11-5). Because cardioversion is associated with temporary atrial "stunning," there is definite risk of thrombus formation even if the atrium is not enlarged. Thus, whenever possible, anticoagulation is required for either cardioversion or rate control. GRADE A Newer techniques such as atrioventricular nodal ablation followed by permanent pacemaker implantation, the implantable atrial defibrillator, the maze cardiac surgical procedure, and, in particular, investigative catheter-based techniques of atrial

ARRHYTHMIA THERAPY

Opie 2004

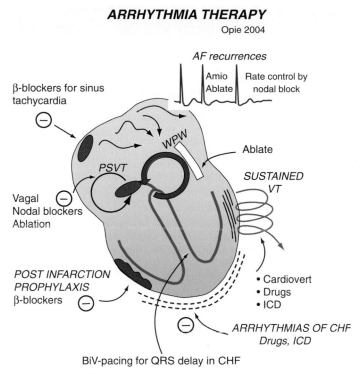

Figure 11-6 Principles of antiarrhythmic therapy, starting from the sinus node (*top left*) and proceeding toward the ventricles: (1) Sinus tachycardia, as in myocardial infarction or anxiety; treated by β-blockade (after excluding causes such as hypovolemia or fever in MI). (2) Atrial fibrillation (*AF*) recurrences prevented by amiodarone (*amio*) or ablation, or choosing rate control by nodal blocking agents. (3) Paroxysmal supraventricular tachycardia (*PSVT*) with nodal reentry paths susceptible to atrioventricular (*AV*) inhibition by nodal blockers such as vagal maneuvers, calcium channel or β-blockers, or AV ablation. (4) Supraventricular tachycardias of the Wolff-Parkinson-White (*WPW*) bypass tract are treated either by AV nodal inhibitors or by catheter ablation of the bypass tract. (5) Sustained ventricular tachycardia (*VT*), especially in the presence of an infarcted or ischemic zone, is based on reentry circuits that require cardioversion if persistent, drug therapy as by amiodarone and in selected patients, an implantable cardioverter defibrillator (*ICD*). (6) Arrhythmias of congestive heart failure (*CHF*) may require either drugs or in selected patients, an ICD. (7) For prevention of sudden cardiac death in CHF with QRS prolongation, biventricular pacing gives excellent results. (8) Postinfarction prophylaxis is best given by β-blockade. (*Figure © L. H. Opie, 2004.*)

fibrillation ablation, are likely to change traditional approaches to management in the next 5 years. Nonetheless, the management of atrial fibrillation, the most common of all arrhythmias, is often not easy (Table 11-5).

Acute Onset Atrial Fibrillation

Urgent control of the ventricular rate, if needed, is achieved by AV nodal inhibitors, such as (1) verapamil or diltiazem, or (2) intravenous beta-blockade by esmolol, or (3) digoxin, or (4) combinations. Other agents that can also be given intravenously include flecainide, propafenone, sotalol, ibutilide, and high-dose amiodarone.[148] Of these, only ibutilide is registered for use in acute atrial fibrillation and only amiodarone is safe for patients with ischemic heart disease or heart failure.[148] With ibutilide there is the risk of torsades especially in those with heart failure.[149] In selected patients

Table 11-5 | Acute Onset Atrial Fibrillation (AF): Principles of Management

Acute Onset

- Correct precipitating factors (dehydration, alcohol, pyrexia, etc.).
- Use intravenous AV nodal inhibitors to control ventricular rate (diltiazem,* verapamil or esmolol; sometimes digoxin or combinations)
- If duration of AF <48 h, first observe for 8 h. Spontaneous reversion is common. If not, consider chemical cardioversion or procainamide infusion 15–20 mg/min up to 1000 mg or ibutilide (care torsades) or high-dose amiodarone infusion (125 mg/h, up to 3 g/24 h).[148]
- Thereafter, electrical cardioversion often required.
- Depending on the local situation, electrical cardioversion may be chosen first

Preparation for Elective Cardioversion

- Control ventricular rate (digoxin if CHF; otherwise start with verapamil or diltiazem or β-blockade). Exclude thyrotoxicosis.
- Oral anticoagulation for 3–4 consecutive weeks with INR of 2–3, or use TEE-guided approach.
  During fourth week, consider amiodarone as 800–1600 mg/day for 1 wk followed by 200–400 mg/day.
- Hospital admission; becoming outpatient procedure
- If patient not receiving amiodarone, start agents that might *chemically cardiovert:* procainamide, sotalol, ibutilide, or dofetilide (ibutilide better than procainamide,[271] risk of torsades with all but most with ibutilide or dofetilide). Flecainide or propafenone only when no structural heart disease, with a β-blocker or verapamil to avoid a fast ventricular rate.
- Electrical cardioversion. If failed, repeat after infused ibutilide and magnesium.[272]

Postcardioversion

Search for underlying causes. Congestive heart failure or hypertension, if present, must be vigorously treated. One of three arrhythmia policies.

1. *Rhythm control. Aim to maintain sinus rhythm* by chronic therapy. Use sotalol or low-dose amiodarone; or if no structural heart disease, flecainide or propafenone (both approved in USA). Procainamide may be used for periods less than 6 mo. Anticoagulation continued for at least 3–6 mo, but usually indefinitely since many episodes are asymptomatic.
2. *Alternate policy:* Leave *drug-free* and if recurrence, control ventricular rate (digoxin if CHF, otherwise β-blocker or verapamil or diltiazem). Oral anticoagulation essential.
3. *Third policy:* Cardiovert, observe on anticoagulation, start antiarrhythmics for second episode.

Repetitive serious AF: focal pulmonary vein ablation or left atrial isolation; surgical Maze procedure. *Under investigation:* dual site atrial pacing; implantable atrial cardioverter defibrillator.

*Diltiazem preferred because of clearly defined dose guidelines in package insert, including rate for prolonged infusion.
INR = international normalized ratio; TEE = transesophageal echocardiography.

without structural heart disease, single loading doses of propafenone[150] or flecainide may also be used, despite their proarrhythmic effects. If still needed, cardioversion is then undertaken either at the end of the drug infusion, which is logical and effective,[148,149] or electively once the patient has been anticoagulated. Factors precipitating atrial fibrillation must also be treated (Table 11-5).

Transvenous low energy cardioversion may be used to obviate the need for general anesthesia. Standard practice has been not to anticoagulate for short duration (<48 hours) atrial fibrillation, which however often spontaneously reverts to sinus rhythm.[151] The use of low-molecular-weight heparins instead of unfractionated heparin in patients with atrial fibrillation is theoretically attractive from a number of standpoints, but recommendations have been largely based on extrapolation from venous thromboembolic disease states.[151] Following cardioversion, self-administration of low-molecular-weight heparins out of hospital prior to full-dose anticoagulation with warfarin may be cost-effective and requires further study.

Atrial Stunning Following cardioversion there may be "temporary stunning" of the atrium, probably a function of the duration of atrial fibrillation. In this situation it is important to emphasize that there is a risk of thrombus formation, even if the atrium is not enlarged or if echocardiography did not show any atrial appendage thrombus. Consequently, whenever possible, anticoagulation should be started prior to elective cardioversion and continued for at least 3 to 4 weeks thereafter. For urgent cardioversion, logic but no trial data would dictate intravenous heparin to cover the procedure. To reduce the risk of atrial stunning, oral verapamil may be given before and just after the cardioversion.[152]

Role of Transesophageal Echocardiography (TEE) The advantage is direct visualization of thrombus in the left atrium or left atrial appendage which if found, contraindicates urgent cardioversion without prior prolonged anticoagulation.[153,154] The TEE-guided early approach utilizes heparin for 24 hours precardioversion and chronic anticoagulation for at least 4 weeks postcardioversion, with the aim of protecting against new left atrial thrombosis during postcardioversion stunning. The advantage of the TEE-guided approach is one of convenience, and theoretically, it should be safer by reducing the overall time during which a patient is exposed to anticoagulation and the risk of bleeding. Technical expertise and experience are crucial for this approach, since the anatomy of the left atrial appendage is complex and small thrombi can easily be overlooked.

Chronic Atrial Fibrillation

Rate Control Versus Sinus Rhythm Rather than aiming to maintain sinus rhythm by antiarrhythmic drugs, another major policy is to accept the existence of atrial fibrillation yet controlling the ventricular response by AV nodal inhibitors, and to provide oral anticoagulation. The logic for this line of therapy is that all the drugs that can be used to maintain sinus rhythm (quinidine, flecainide, propafenone, sotalol, amiodarone, dofetilide) have some potentially serious side effects. Rhythm control offered no advantage over rate control in the AFFIRM Trial that enrolled a total of 4060 patients at high risk for stroke on the basis of either risk factors for stroke or age greater than 65 or both.[155] There was a trend toward more stroke with rhythm control and certainly more hospitalizations. In two other smaller European trials, rate-control was again similar in outcome to rhythm control.[156,157]

The choice between rate and rhythm control is not always easy. The AFFIRM and the European trials have, however, changed practice. A practical policy is to attempt cardioversion for the first episode of atrial fibrillation.[158] Then if this arrhythmia returns and is asymptomatic, rate control is in order. If markedly symptomatic, the preference is for cardioversion covered by anti-arrhythmic drugs. With either policy, optimal anticoagulation should be continued indefinitely, since many episodes of atrial fibrillation are asymptomatic.[155,157] The majority of thromboembolic strokes occurred in patients either not taking warfarin or when INR levels were subtherapeutic.

Rate Control The drugs inhibiting the AV node are digoxin and β-blockers, especially when there is heart failure, with the calcium blockers verapamil and diltiazem for the others. Often several of these must be given in combination. Amiodarone is occasionally used for rate control in patients with heart failure. The heart rate at rest should be 80 beats or less per minute and 110 or less during a 6-minute walk. These are arbitrary limits. When rate control is unsatisfactory, tachy-cardia-induced ventricular dysfunction is a concern. In this setting, radiofrequency ablation of the AV node causing complete heart block with implantation of a permanent pacemaker, may result in a marked improvement in symptoms and, in some patients, ventricular function.[159,160]

Rhythm Control by Elective Cardioversion In chronic atrial fibrillation, having achieved control of the ventricular rate by AV nodal inhibitors, the patient is anticoagulated by warfarin while being maintained on drug therapy which is often amiodarone (Table 11-5). Factors favor-ing drug conversion include a small left atrial size and atrial fibrilla-tion less than 6 months in duration. The risk of embolization at the time of rhythm conversion is about 1% to 2%, so that *prophylactic anti-coagulation* with an INR >2 for at least 3 consecutive weeks is required. Since the recurrence rate of atrial fibrillation is quite high during the first 3 to 6 months following cardioversion, many cardiologists advo-cate a much longer period of post-cardioversion anticoagulation so as to ensure that patients are "covered" by warfarin in the event that they relapse back to atrial fibrillation. Prior to electrical cardioversion, it is reasonable in patients not receiving amiodarone, to attempt a pharmacologic cardioversion using intravenous procainamide or ibutilide[161,162] or less frequently, oral propafenone, flecainide, or disopyramide. GRADE B The latter three drugs should be avoided in the presence of structural heart disease, particularly if significant left ventricular dysfunction is present. Some still use quinidine, when concurrent digoxin is essential to avoid a very fast ventricular rate. This risk may result if the fibrillation is converted to flutter and there is enhanced conduction through the AV node resulting from the vagolytic action of quinidine. For cardioversion failures, repeat under ibutilide cover before considering internal cardioversion. Ibutilide should not, according to the package insert, be given to those already receiving amiodarone, but in practice the added risk is very low.[161]

Recurrent Atrial Fibrillation After two attempts at cardioversion or when atrial fibrillation is known to be recurrent, the drug choice has been between low-dose sotalol or low-dose amiodarone. In the AFFIRM Trial, at 1 year, 62% of patients treated with amiodarone were alive, in sinus rhythm without any additional cardioversion.[155] The corre-sponding figure for sotalol was 23%, no better than the class I agents. Nonetheless, it still makes sense to attempt to maintain sinus rhythm with the less effective but more easily tolerated drug. There is always the option to switch to amiodarone at a later stage. In patients with left ventricular dysfunction, amiodarone and dofetilide are probably the antiarrhythmic drugs of choice (see Fig. 8-9). Sotalol, the class III β-blocker, should benefit those with atrial fibrillation and heart failure but there are no formal studies and torsades is a risk. The ARB irbe-sartan when added to amiodarone gives added protection from recur-rences,[163] and should also help to treat heart failure. In patients with poor LV function in the SOLVD trials, enalapril reduced the subse-quent development of atrial fibrillation.[164]

New Pharmacologic Options for the Maintenance of Sinus Rhythm Drugs for paroxysmal or persistent atrial fibrillation include *dofetilide* (a class III antiarrhythmic drug, I_{Kr} blocker) and *azimilide*, which blocks both rapid (I_{Kr}) and slow components (I_{Ks}) of the potassium channel. Dofetilide is well tested in congestive heart failure to help cardiover-sion and to prevent hospitalization,[165] but there is increased torsades and the dose must be tailored to renal function. Dofetilide must be given under monitoring conditions in hospital and drug interactions are frequent. Azimilide for atrial flutter and fibrillation is still under study.

Chronic Atrial Fibrillation: Anticoagulation Long-term anticoagulation is indicated in most patients with chronic atrial fibrillation, but the key to optimal therapy is risk stratification. In patients younger than 65 years of age without the risk factors of prior transient ischemic attack (TIA) or stroke, congestive heart failure, left ventricular systolic dysfunction, diabetes, or a history of hypertension, the risk of stroke is approximately 1% per year, which is similar to the risk of bleeding on warfarin. On the other hand, warfarin is generally indicated for all patients with clinical risk factors and in those aged 65 years or older. GRADE A Depending upon the perceived risk of bleeding with warfarin, aspirin may be a reasonable substitute even in the elderly at lower risk (e.g., no hypertension, diabetes, prior stroke or TIA, and good LV function).[166] Thus the crucial aspect of the treatment strategy is balancing the risks of bleeding compared with those of stroke. Ongoing trials are comparing the combination of aspirin and clopidogrel with aspirin alone and with warfarin. The oral direct thrombin inhibitor *ximelagatran* (not yet licensed in the United States), that unlike warfarin needs no constant monitoring, was as effective as well-controlled warfarin in preventing stroke and systemic embolic events.[167,168] Ximelagatran caused less bleeding than warfarin. Liver enzyme elevations, characteristically transient or responding to drug withdrawal, were noted in 6%. Thus liver function should be tested monthly for the first 6 months and at intervals thereafter.

Rhythm Control by Maze Operation or Focal Ablation These are important advances. Chronic atrial fibrillation, the most common of all sustained cardiac arrhythmias, increases morbidity and mortality, yet is often therapy-resistant. Hence, Cox and colleagues[169] decided to create an electrical maze. Numerous sutures in a labyrinthine pattern are made to stop potential macro-reentry circuits. Appropriate surgical incisions guide the impulse from the SA to the AV node with exiting blind alleys to allow normal atrial excitation. Sinus rhythm is maintained in a high proportion of patients, although a number will require permanent pacemaker implantation. The procedure continues to undergo modification. The invasive nature of the Maze surgical procedure has prompted investigative studies into catheter-based ablative procedures in the right and left atrium. The finding of a *focal source of atrial fibrillation* in the pulmonary veins by Haissaguerre and colleagues[170] is extraordinarily exciting. The initial procedure has undergone modification so as to encircle the pulmonary veins[171] in addition to other ablative lines in the left atrium and appears to be superior in terms of freedom from recurrences and a low incidence of pulmonary vein stenosis. Long-term follow up is needed.

OTHER SUPRAVENTRICULAR ARRHYTHMIAS

Atrial Flutter Satisfactory control of the ventricular rate may be extremely difficult to achieve, but flutter is easily converted by a low-energy countershock. GRADE A In the prevention of recurrent atrial flutter, sotalol or low-dose amiodarone or dofetilide may be tried. Azimilide is under evaluation. Because the left atrium still contracts, anticoagulation is omitted. For resistant or recurrent cases, catheter ablation of the AV node with pacemaker implantation is increasingly used. Patients with "typical atrial flutter" enjoy a very high success rate with radiofrequency ablation of the flutter circuit (see Fig. 8-8). The combination of atrial fibrillation and atrial flutter can either be treated by drugs, or if refractory, often responds to catheter-induced dissection of the pulmonary vein from the left atrial junction.[172]

Chaotic multifocal atrial tachycardia may respond to verapamil or β-blockade, but there appear to be no formal drug trials and the clinical impression is that this is a very difficult arrhythmia to control. Exclude underlying theophylline toxicity. Intravenous magnesium is effective for rate control and helps to restoration of sinus rhythm.[173]

Supraventricular Tachycardia (Table 11-6) In the standard paroxysmal type (PSVT) with nodal reentry, vagotonic procedures (Valsalva maneuver, facial immersion in cold water, or carotid sinus massage) may terminate the tachycardia. Always auscultate the carotid arteries before performing carotid sinus massage. If these measures fail, the next step is to use intravenous adenosine followed by intravenous diltiazem, or verapamil, or esmolol (see Chapter 8). Adenosine with its ultrashort duration of action is safest, especially if there is a diagnostic problem between PSVT with aberrant conduction and wide complex VT. If these steps fail, vagotonic maneuvers are worth repeating. Thereafter the choice lies between intravenous digitalization or intravenous amiodarone or direct-current cardioversion, and the decision needs to be tempered by the clinical condition of the patient. (Also, in

---

Table 11-6 | Paroxysmal Supraventricular Tachycardia (PSVT): Principles of Management

Entry Point

■ Narrow QRS complex tachycardia; either AV nodal reentry or WPW (Fig. 8-2). If *atrial flutter*, proceed straight to DC cardioversion (may consider ibutilide, torsades risk)

Acute Therapy: Hemodynamically Stable

■ Vagal maneuvers
■ Intravenous AV nodal blockers (adenosine*, verapamil, diltiazem, esmolol; high success rate)
■ Occasionally IV propafenone
■ Synchronized DC cardioversion
■ Burst pacing in selected cases, e.g., post-bypass surgery

Acute Therapy: Hemodynamically Unstable

■ Intravenous adenosine (not other AV nodal blockers)
■ Must cardiovert if adenosine unsuccessful

Follow-up: PSVT with AV Nodal Reentry

■ Self-therapy by vagal procedures
■ Prevention by long-acting AV-nodal blockers (verapamil, diltiazem, standard β-blockers, digoxin)
■ If repetitive attacks, perinodal ablation to inhibit reentry through reentry pathways. Small risk of AV nodal damage requiring permanent pacemaker

Follow-Up: WPW (Delta Wave During Sinus Rhythm)

■ Radiofrequency (RF) catheter ablation of bypass tract
■ Rarely, surgery is performed for associated conditions (young children with associated anomalies; multiple paths)
■ Occasionally drug therapy: class IC or class III agents. Digoxin contraindicated, avoid other AV nodal blockers

Follow-Up: Atrial Flutter

■ Prevent by sotalol, amiodarone, dofetilide or RF ablation of flutter circuits
■ Rate control by AV nodal inhibitors (verapamil, diltiazem, β-blocker, digoxin or combinations)
■ Consider RF AV nodal ablation and permanent pacemaker

Catheter Ablation

■ Treatment of choice for recurrent PVST

*Adenosine preferred, it is ultra short-acting; esmolol action wears off more slowly but fast enough to allow subsequent safer use of verapamil or diltiazem if needed.
AV = atrioventricular; WPW = Wolff-Parkinson-White syndrome.

countries outside the United States, IV flecainide is approved and may be a choice in the absence of structural heart disease.)

Refractory PSVT Patients with supraventricular arrhythmias that are very rapid or refractory to standard drugs, or associated with a wide QRS complex on the standard electrocardiogram (implying either aberration, antegrade preexcitation, or VT) warrant an invasive electrophysiologic study. In the majority of other patients, drug management is successful. Nonetheless, the ease of radiofrequency ablation coupled to the very high success rates and low rates of complications have increasingly led to its use as "first-line therapy," particularly in younger patients who are reluctant to commit to life-long drug therapy, even if the latter is effective.

Prevention of PSVT The best measure is often catheter ablation. Otherwise initiating ectopic beats may be inhibited by β-blockade, verapamil, diltiazem, or by amiodarone. The latter is highly effective for supraventricular arrhythmias including paroxysmal atrial fibrillation and arrhythmias involving accessory pathways; potentially severe side effects may be limited by a low dose (see Chapter 8). The class IC drugs (propafenone or flecainide) are viable alternatives, but should not be used in the presence of structural heart disease.

Wolff-Parkinson-White Syndrome The acute treatment of choice is cardioversion if the patient is hemodynamically compromised. If presenting with narrow complex PSVT, the same intravenous therapy as for standard PVST may be followed (Table 11-6). For follow-up, because of the risk of antegrade preexcitation via the bypass tract, *digoxin is absolutely contraindicated* (because it shortens the refractory period of the tract). Verapamil, diltiazem, and β-blockade may also be dangerous by blocking the AV node and redirecting impulses down the bypass tract. In the prevention of paroxysmal supraventricular tachycardia including atrial fibrillation, radiofrequency catheter ablation of the accessory pathway is usually highly successful and is now standard treatment. Otherwise, low-dose amiodarone is probably best followed by sotalol or propafenone. Prophylactic ablation in asymptomatic patients at high risk may be the best approach, for example, in those 35 years or younger, or with electrophysiologic inducible arrhythmias at an invasive study, or on the basis of occupation or other lifestyle circumstances.[174]

BRADYARRHYTHMIAS

Asymptomatic sinus bradycardia does not require therapy and may be normal, especially in athletes. For symptomatic sinus bradycardia, sick sinus syndrome, and sinoatrial disease, probanthine and chronic atropine are unsatisfactory in the long run so that pacing is usually required. First, however, the adverse effects of drugs such as beta-blockers, digitalis, verapamil, diltiazem, quinidine, procainamide, amiodarone, lidocaine, methyldopa, clonidine, and lithium carbonate should be excluded. In the *tachycardia/bradycardia syndrome*, intrinsic sinus node dysfunction is difficult to treat and once again may require permanent pacing. Standard β-blockers aggravate the bradycardiac component of the syndrome, while pindolol with marked agonist activity (ISA) may be useful. Patients usually end up with a combination of a permanent pacemaker and antiarrhythmic agents. But in some patients the combination of radiofrequency ablation of the AV node followed by permanent pacemaker implantation is a highly effective method of controlling refractory tachycardia. For *AV block with syncope* or with excessively slow rates, atropine or isoproterenol or transthoracic pacing is used as an emergency measure, pending pacemaker implantation. In asymptomatic patients with congenital heart block, the role of permanent pacing is debatable with current trends favoring a more aggressive approach at an earlier age.

VENTRICULAR ARRHYTHMIAS AND PROARRHYTHMIC PROBLEMS

The criteria for instituting drug therapy for ventricular arrhythmias are not clear-cut, although patients with sustained VT (Table 11-7), survivors of previous arrhythmia-related cardiac arrest, and those with severely symptomatic arrhythmias, all require treatment. A full cardiologic assessment is required. An essential adjunct to antiarrhythmic therapy lies in the management of underlying disease such as LVF, ischemia, anemia, thyrotoxicosis, or electrolyte imbalance. The potential hazards of antiarrhythmic therapy were emphasized by the CAST study, which warned that the proarrhythmic effects of some class I agents can actually increase mortality in patients with ischemic heart disease. The only evidence that therapy for asymptomatic nonsustained ventricular tachycardia prolongs life or prevents arrhythmic death comes from the two trials of amiodarone and a subsequent meta-analysis of 13 trials of prophylactic amiodarone (ATMA).[143] The most effective way to prevent sudden cardiac death in patients with coronary disease is to eliminate ischemia and to improve left ventricular function, often by coronary revascularization. GRADE B In the patient who has already survived an episode of cardiac arrest or hemodynamically unstable ventricular tachycardia, coronary revascularization alone will usually not suffice, and an ICD is indicated.

Table 11-7 | Acute Sustained Ventricular Tachycardia

Entry Point: Wide QRS Complex Tachycardia

About 90% will be wide-complex ventricular tachycardia; the others will include PSVT with aberration or WPW with anterograde conduction.

- DC cardioversion—procedure of choice, usually effective
- If DC cardioversion fails or if patient hemodynamically stable:
  —IV amiodarone now often used
  —IV lidocaine (safe but will only revert a minority)
  —IV procainamide (more effective but less safe)
  —Or, where available, IV disopyramide (not in USA)
- If torsades de pointes, IV magnesium sulfate; consider atrial pacing; isoproterenol in an emergency
- If VT recurs soon after cardioversion, repeat the latter under cover of lidocaine or other IV drug
- (Only if PSVT presents as suspected VT, use IV adenosine for diagnosis but *never* verapamil nor diltiazem)

Follow-Up of Acute Attack

- (If PSVT, see Table 11-4)
- If VT (majority), requires thorough cardiological evaluation. Need accurate diagnosis of rhythm, structural heart disease, and LV function, long QT syndrome; arrhythmogenic RV dysplasia
- Empirical drug approach (amiodarone) if patient not candidate for ICD
- EPS-guided choice: current strong trend towards ICD, away from EPS
- Sometimes surgery (LV aneurysm)
- If idiopathic refractory VT, especially RVOT in origin, radiofrequency catheter ablation but verapamil may be effective in RVOT VT and exercise-induced VT in patients without structural heart disease.
- ICD as first line therapy if high risk of sudden death: in survivors of cardiac arrest, in symptomatic VT, or in asymptomatic VT with a low ejection fraction.

EPS = electrophysiological stimulation; ICD = implantable cardioverter defibrillator; PSVT = paroxysmal supraventricular tachycardia; RVOT = right ventricular outflow tract; VT = ventricular tachycardia; WPW = Wolff-Parkinson-White syndrome.

Drug Choice The choice of drug for chronic use is ideally based on prior demonstration during acute and chronic Holter or electrophysiologic testing that the drug actually works and on its potential for toxicity in the patient under study. Unfortunately, neither the Holter nor the electrophysiologic study are reliable guides to long-term efficacy of therapy. Class I agents including quinidine, disopyramide and mexilitine are used less and less. Propafenone is possibly the most effective and least harmful of the class IC agents, although not as good as β-blockade or amiodarone in the CASH study[175] in which the propafenone arm was discontinued. In patients without structural heart disease, the risk of proarrhythmia with both propafenone and flecainide is low. The antiarrhythmic effect of *empiric β-blockade monotherapy* for VT is impressive and reportedly as good as electrophysiologic-guided drug choice. In comparison with other drugs, amiodarone appears to be the most effective antiarrhythmic agent, despite its considerable side effects.

β-Blockers are among the few antiarrhythmic agents with positive long-term beneficial effects in postinfarct patients.[104] GRADE A In those not responding to beta-blockade, or in whom beta-blockade is contraindicated, *low-dose amiodarone* is increasingly used, despite potentially serious side-effects. Like β-blockade, amiodarone appears to give postinfarct protection. Deciding between these agents is somewhat of a personal choice and not entirely evidence based. Yet, in comparison with others, amiodarone is the most effective antiarrhythmic agent despite its considerable side effects that are, however, lower at reduced doses.

Implantable Cardioverter Defibrillators The treatment of recurrent sustained ventricular tachycardia and ventricular fibrillation is difficult and pharmacologic therapy has, in the main, been very disappointing. This failure has stimulated alternative approaches such as surgical or catheter ablation of the ventricular tachycardia-foci and the implantable cardioverter defibrillator (ICD). ICDs give a clear though modest mortality reduction In patients with underlying coronary artery disease, the MUST, MADIT-1, and MADIT-2 trials all show the superiority of the ICD in primary prevention in certain patient subsets (see Table 8-6), as now confirmed in the large Sudden Death in Heart Failure Trial (SCD-HeFT).[144] The advent of the ICD has virtually eliminated surgical procedures such as endocardial resection. Radiofrequency catheter ablation may be very successful in idiopathic or right ventricular outflow tract ventricular tachycardias. By contrast, for the vast majority of patients who have ventricular tachycardia secondary to coronary artery disease and left ventricular dysfunction, catheter ablation remains investigational, although newer mapping techniques are improving success rates.

In patients with ICDs, recurrent discharges are a major source of morbidity, depression, and anxiety. With the back-up of an ICD in place, there is a new role for the use of antiarrhythmic drugs, despite left ventricular dysfunction, whereas these might be contraindicated in patients without devices.[176]

CONGESTIVE HEART FAILURE

General Policy Despite powerful protective agents (ACE inhibitors, ARBs, beta-blockers, spironolactone, eplerenone), the long-term prognosis of CHF remains poor, unless a reversible cause is found. The initial steps in a patient with heart failure include investigation and specific treatment for a cause including ischemic heart disease, hypertension, valvular heart disease, thyrotoxicosis, excess alcohol, and anemia. It is important to obtain a careful family history as familial dilated cardiomyopathy is being increasingly recognized. The past policy was to initiate treatment with diuretics, salt restriction, then digoxin before proceeding to conventional vasodilators. ACE inhibitors and β-blockers are now the cornerstone of therapy, GRADE A increasingly given from the start of symptoms (with diuretics), or even before, in asymptomatic LV dysfunction (without diuretics). The role of *digoxin* in patients with atrial fibrillation cannot be contested. In others, it improves symptoms but not mortality, so that the current trend is to emphasize the agents that improve mortality (ACE inhibitors, ARBs, β-blockers, spironolactone) and then to add digoxin for patients remaining symptomatic. Today there is less emphasis on reaching the therapeutic level of digoxin, with increasing suggestions that previously "normal" levels are less desirable than lower values (see Fig. 6-4). Previous combination "triple therapy" by diuretics, ACE inhibition, and digoxin is now replaced by *"modern quadruple therapy"* (ACE inhibitors or ARBs, β-blockade, diuretics, spironolactone, or eplerenone) or even "quintuple therapy" by including digoxin. How can clinical judgment be aided? Plasma BNP (brain natriuretic peptide) is a rapid and sensitive guide that reflects cardiovascular events and complements clinical decisions.[177,178]

ACE Inhibitors versus ARBs The vast experience gained with ACE inhibitors makes them the gold-standard for renin-angiotensin inhibition (see Chapter 5). When ACE inhibitors cannot be tolerated (cough) then ARBs become a logical replacement but the combination of these is also being advocated for heart failure.[179]

β-Blockers When cautiously added to ACE inhibitors and diuretics in hemodynamically stable patients, beta-blockers consistently decrease mortality by about 30% or even more. GRADE A The patient should be closely supervised during this initial titration because there is the risk of transient deterioration. Trial data favor the use of carvedilol, metoprolol and bisoprolol (see Chapter 1). Of these, only carvedilol and long-acting metoprolol XL are licensed for use in the United States, and only carvedilol is approved for class IV heart failure.[180] Metoprolol XL is licensed only for class II and III heart failure but has an angina license which carvedilol does not in the United States.

Diuretic Therapy Doses and drugs should not be fixed. Diuretics may need to be reduced when the ACE inhibitor is introduced or the dose increased, or diuretic therapy may have to be stepped up in cases of refractory edema. Especially in severe right ventricular failure, the absorption of drugs given orally is impaired and a short course of intravenous furosemide can be very helpful. *Posture* can influence diuretic efficacy. To improve renal perfusion and to increase diuresis, the patient may have to return to bed for 1 to 2 hours of supine rest after taking a diuretic. The principle of *sequential nephron blockade* (see Fig. 4-2) states that different types of diuretics can synergistically be added, such as a thiazide to a loop diuretic. GRADE B

Aldosterone Antagonists The adverse neurohumoral qualities of diuretic therapy, often forgotten, need to be balanced by an ACE inhibitor or ARB, often with spironolactone. Yet especially in patients with poor renal function, these combinations can precipitate hyperkalemia. Nonetheless, the RALES study[181] showed that the addition of spironolactone at an average dose of 25 mg daily while watching K^+ can give substantial clinical improvement and save lives in those with class III or IV heart failure. RALES is complemented by the EPHESUS study that used eplerenone, a selective aldosterone blocker, in post-MI patients with transient heart failure or in the case of diabetics, an ejection fraction of less than 40%.[182] This too was strongly positive. It is highly likely that aldosterone antagonists will be used more frequently and in milder degrees of heart failure, but it remains essential to monitor the serum potassium carefully, particularly when ACE inhibitors or ARBs are also part of the therapeutic attack.

Vasodilators High-dose nitrates (on-off patches) improve exercise tolerance and LV size and function when added to ACE inhibitors, diuretics, and digoxin.[183] In patients with pulmonary congestion, nitrates given at night can decisively improve sleep. For long-term use, the old combination of nitrates plus hydralazine is logical because the hydralazine appears to counteract nitrate tolerance (see Chapter 2), although it is still prudent to maintain a nitrate-free window of 8 to 10 hours depending upon whether symptoms occur primarily at night or with exertion during the day.

Atrial Fibrillation In CHF Atrial fibrillation (AF) both contributes to mortality,[160] and is a marker for severe disease.[184] Both the AF and the heart failure must be treated as vigorously as possible. In selected patients cardioversion under anticoagulation or new atrial pacing techniques or internal cardioversion may be appropriate, but for most strict rate control over 24 hours and anticoagulation with warfarin "remain the mainstays of therapy."[184] Failing rate control, the next option is conversion and maintenance of sinus rhythm with amiodarone, which is well tested in CHF though not approved for atrial fibrillation in the United States. Dofetilide, approved for highly symptomatic atrial fibrillation, converts to sinus rhythm in CHF but only in about 12%.[165] Once sinus rhythm was restored, dofetilide reduced recurrences by 65%. Careful dose adjustment is needed in renal failure. Another major downside is the risk of early torsades de pointes (3.3%).

Ventricular Arrhythmias in CHF The incidence of sudden death seems to be falling since the widespread introduction of ACE inhibitors and now β-blockers. For those who still have severe *significantly symptomatic ventricular arrhythmias*, it is first essential to pinpoint precipitating factors such as hypokalemia, hypomagnesemia, or use of sympathomimetics, phosphodiesterase inhibitors or digoxin. The hemodynamic status of the myocardium must be made optimal because increased LV wall stress is arrhythmogenic. Thereafter, amiodarone remains the drug of choice. Increasingly ICDs are considered for selected high-risk patients with life-threatening arrhythmias, and especially those with an ejection fraction below 30% (see Fig. 8-9). Prophylactic class I antiarrhythmic drug therapy is contraindicated. In contrast, prophylactic β-blockade can be very helpful, especially in those with coronary-related CHF. The role of the ICD versus amiodarone in patients with moderate CHF and low ejection fractions is the subject of two current trials. The preliminary results of one of them, DEFINITE, favor the ICD (see Chapter 8, p. 267).

Severe Intractable CHF Here there are several approaches, including short term "rescue" by intravenous phosphodiesterase inhibitors monitored invasively by Swan-Ganz catheterization. The hope is that tailored intravenous therapy will act as a bridge to oral agents. GRADE C Dobutamine, often used, has three potential hazards: further β-receptor downgrading, increased arrhythmias,[185] and hypotension. In an era when most patients are on β-blockers, milrinone may be a better choice for intravenous therapy in those patients with decompensation. Dopamine remains the agent of choice, though the idea of the renal dose is now discredited (see Chapter 6). Intermittent intravenous nitroglycerin tides some patients over, and is the logical choice for ischemic cardiomyopathy. Recombinant human BNP, nesiritide, is safer than dobutamine[185] with a lower 6-month mortality.[186] In the VMAC Trial, nesiritide caused less hypotension than nitroglycerin.[187] A criticism is that at least some of the studies have been based largely on surrogate endpoints.[178] An LV assist device may "bridge" the gap to transplantation,[188] or may even initiate "reverse remodeling" by myocyte unloading.[189]

Diastolic Dysfunction Traditional concepts emphasize the primary role of systolic ventricular dysfunction. Yet in about 40% to 60% of patients with a clinical diagnosis of heart failure, there is relatively preserved LV systolic function thereby emphasizing the concept of "primary diastolic dysfunction." This usually results from increasing age and/or left ventricular hypertrophy. Although the mortality risk is lower than for systolic failure, there is still a threefold increase.[190] There are few outcome trials. Logically, the fundamental therapy is to aim for regression of LVH, often the underlying cause of diastolic dysfunction. Exclusion of aortic stenosis is essential. In hypertensive hearts, when 24-hour blood pressure control is required. Other measures are: reduction in central blood volume by diuretics, avoiding tachycardia, and the theoretical potential of enhancing LV relaxation by CCBs or ACE inhibitors or ARBs, and of lessening of myocardial collagen by aldosterone antagonists. In one arm of the CHARM studies, in which there was relatively preserved LV function, the ARB candesartan gave only modest benefit.[191] β-Blockers help to prevent ischemia and bradycardia, to improve diastolic filling. In the elderly with increased myocardial stiffness, therapy is still attempted even though LV regression may not be achieved.

New Agents for CHF Atrial natriuretic peptide with diuretic and vasodilator properties can be increased by *atriopeptidase inhibition*.[192] Similarly *nesiritide* has the actions of brain natriuretic peptide. Omapatrilat, a new combined ACE and *neutral endopeptidase inhibitor*, is no more effective than ACE inhibition alone, with, however, a greater incidence of angioedema than standard ACE inhibitors. Of the other new agents, promising are the calcium sensitizers such as *levosimendan* (the subject of a successful trial in acute pulmonary edema; see Chapter 6), and endothelin antagonists. Inhibitors of *tumor necrosis factor-α* (TNF-α) have not lived up to their promise in several well-designed trials.

General Management of CHF Sodium restriction and, in severe cases, water limitation are important ancillary measures. It is often forgotten that in severe CHF there is delayed water diuresis. Weight loss and exercise rehabilitation, as well as psychological support, are all positive procedures. Home nursing helps those with severe limitation of exercise. A short-term high carbohydrate diet by allowing muscle glycogen to breakdown more slowly can increase endurance exercise—of potential interest to CHF patients who need extra energy for that special occasion. A major advance in the management of congestive heart failure is an extensive, nurse-based outpatient program which relies on patient education and regular communication between patient and health care provider. This gives a substantial reduction in hospital admissions.[193]

Summary In asymptomatic LV dysfunction, initial therapy is by ACE inhibition or sometimes by an ARB. Added β-blockade started in very low doses and titrated upward adds decisive benefit. In those with symptomatic CHF, a diuretic is required. Spironolactone or eplerenone is being added earlier than before. Of these agents, ACE inhibitors, ARBs, β-blockers, and spironolactone all improve longevity. GRADE A Digoxin is added for atrial fibrillation or to control symptoms, without expecting any effect on mortality. The "quintuplet combination" of ACE inhibitors or ARBs, β-blockers, diuretics, spironolactone, and digoxin is now increasingly common, followed by addition of vasodilators such as hydralazine and nitrates. The lot of the individual patient with severe CHF can be improved by searching out underlying causes, by diuretic synergism, by adjustment of the dose of the ACE inhibitor and digoxin, by checking on serum potassium and magnesium, and by general management including salt restriction, exercise rehabilitation, psychological support ("keep going, you are doing better than you think") and intensive nurse-based outpatient care of CHF.

ACUTE PULMONARY EDEMA

In acute pulmonary edema of cardiac origin, the initial management requires positioning the patient in an upright posture and oxygen administration. The standard triple drug regime is: morphine, furosemide, and nitrates, to which ACE inhibitors must now be added. If the underlying cause is a tachyarrhythmia, restoration of sinus rhythm takes priority. Morphine sulfate, with both venodilator and central sedative actions, is highly effective in relieving symptoms. Intravenous furosemide, both diuretic and vasodilator, is the other basic therapy. *Acute digoxin* is now used much less, and may be undesirable in view of the prevailing arrhythmogenic environment, unless there is uncontrolled atrial fibrillation.

Nitrates are excellent for unloading of the left heart and relief of pulmonary congestion. Which is better—repetitive furosemide or repetitive intravenous nitrates? Repeated intravenous boluses of high-dose isosorbide (3 mg every 5 minutes) after a single low-dose (40 mg) furosemide were better than repeated high-dose furosemide with low-dose isosorbide,[194] the former treatment reducing the need for mechanical ventilation and the frequency of myocardial infarction.

ACE inhibitors, sublingual captopril or intravenous enalaprilat (1 mg over 2 hours) are logical and achieve load reduction when added to the standard regimen of oxygen, nitrates, morphine, and furosemide.[195,196] In practice, these agents (or ARBs) are often started orally as soon as the hyperacute phase is over.

Other Vasodilators In patients with pulmonary edema secondary to severe acute or chronic mitral or aortic regurgitation, intravenous nitroprusside is probably the agent of choice. Whenever vasodilators are contemplated, particular caution is necessary in the patient with a systolic blood pressure of less than 90 mmHg. In AMI, compounds such as aminophylline and milrinone are best avoided because of their proarrhythmic potential. *Nesiritide* offers the desirable combination of vasodilation and natriuresis (see p. 384).

Severe Hypertension Use carefully titrated intravenous nicardipine or sodium nitroprusside or nitrates or enalaprilat, together with careful pressure monitoring. Oral ACE inhibitors are started as soon as feasible, taking care to prevent hypotension. *Bronchospasm* will usually respond to diuresis or load reduction.

In refractory cases, use rotating tourniquets or intubate with mechanical ventilation. "When in doubt, intubate." A modest amount of evidence supports the use of continuous positive airway pressure (CPAP) given via a face mask to patients with cardiogenic pulmonary edema.[197] Although bilevel positive airway pressure (inspiratory and expiratory pressures respectively 15 and 5 cm H_2O) improves ventilation and vital signs more rapidly than CPAP, the unexpected cost is increased myocardial infarction.[198] Further studies are needed before general use of increased airways pressures can be recommended.

CARDIOMYOPATHY

Hypertrophic Cardiomyopathy

Among patients with symptomatic hypertrophic cardiomyopathy with documented obstruction, there are several treatment options. The principles are threefold. First, lessen the hypercontractile state by a negative inotrope such as a β-blocker or a nondihydropyridine CCB; second, relieve any outflow tract obstruction; and third, prevent potentially fatal arrhythmias. The role of ACE inhibitors and aldosterone antagonists is unproven and currently under evaluation. The finding that a statin regresses cardiac hypertrophy and fibrosis in an animal model is fascinating and unexpected, but far from translation into clinical practice.[199] Likewise are the impressive data with the CCB diltiazem in another animal model.[200]

Negative Inotropes These are β-blockers, nondihydropyridine calcium blockers, and disopyramide. The postulated mechanism of benefit from the negative inotropic action is via a reduction in left ventricular ejection acceleration, which reduces the hydrodynamic force on the protruding mitral leaflet, delaying mitral-septal contact and reducing the outflow tract gradient. Furthermore, the reduction in ventricular afterload and outflow tract gradient may result in a secondary improvement in diastolic function.[201] *High-dose β-blockers*, such as 200 to 400 mg of propranolol per day or its equivalent, are effective in relieving symptoms such as dyspnea, fatigue, or angina in about 50% to 70% of patients. The high doses required may in turn result in dose-limiting side effects. *Calcium channel blockade*, usually verapamil at a dose of 240 to 320 mg per day, is advocated particularly in patients with asthma and other contraindications to β-blockers or else in combination with β-blockers in patients with continued symptoms. Although they are usually well tolerated, caution needs to be exercised since the peripheral vasodilatory effects can lead to increased hemodynamic obstruction and clinical deterioration. This effect is unpredictable, and the consequences may be rapid and serious. In general, maximum symptomatic benefits are obtained by using β-blockers in combination with verapamil. Nifedipine and other dihydropyridines are contraindicated in patients with resting obstruction. Logically, verapamil and diltiazem may be helpful in relieving the diastolic relaxation problems found in the nonobstructive variety, but clinical evidence is sparse.[202] *Disopyramide*, a class I antiarrhythmic with negative inotropic properties, can be used in those with significant outflow tract obstruction. Anticholinergic side effects, especially urinary retention, glaucoma, and dry mouth, are frequent.[203]

Relief of Outflow Tract Obstruction Drug efficacy may decline over the long term, or side effects become a major problem, and in such patients the remaining treatment options are invasive, such as surgical myectomy, dual-chamber pacing, or alcohol septal ablation. *Dual chamber pacing*, programmed with a short AV delay, initially gave encouraging results but the perceived functional improvement is largely a placebo effect apart from a small subset who might benefit. Nonetheless, a logical application of dual chamber pacing is with atrioventricular nodal ablation for refractory atrial fibrillation. *Alcohol septal ablation* is a very promising technique which needs to stand the test of time. The indications are the same as those for surgery, namely, severe symptoms unresponsive to medical therapy. Alcohol is injected into the first septal perforator branch of the left anterior descending coronary artery producing a "controlled infarction." Acute and intermediate-term hemodynamic studies show a marked reduction in outflow tract gradients and excellent improvement in symptoms. Short-term results are very similar to surgical myectomy.[204] The most frequent complication is complete heart block requiring a permanent pacemaker. Caution is advocated until the long-term results are available and the consequences of creating a myocardial infarction are better understood.

Surgery for Obstructive Cardiomyopathy When standard therapy fails, surgical myotomy/myectomy remains the "gold standard." Surgery is associated with relief of symptoms and a substantial decrease in gradient and in the degree of mitral regurgitation, but should be reserved for significant obstruction and symptoms. No randomized trials have been performed to confirm that surgery prolongs life though hemodynamic results are excellent. *Systolic anterior motion of the mitral valve* is an important component of dynamic LV outflow tract obstruction and mitral regurgitation is common. Thus mitral valve repair and rarely replacement may be combined with surgery.[205] A novel repair procedure is by grafting a pericardial patch over the center of the anterior leaflet.[206] A subset of patients with markedly hypertrophied and displaced papillary muscles that contribute to the obstruction may require papillary muscle relocation as part of the surgical procedure.

Management of Arrhythmias in Hypertrophic Cardiomyopathy Patients at high risk for *sudden cardiac death*, usually from ventricular tachycardia or fibrillation,[207] include those with documented ventricular arrhythmias, young patients with a history of syncope, a strong family history of sudden cardiac death, or, highly controversially, certain specific genotypes. The most effective procedure for patients with documented ventricular tachycardia or out-of-hospital cardiac arrest is the implantable cardioverter defibrillator (ICD). Its indications have expanded to asymptomatic patients with a strong family history of sudden cardiac death.[207] Coexisting coronary artery disease seriously impairs the prognosis.[208] *Atrial fibrillation* can be a devastating complication in patients with hypertrophic cardiomyopathy. Treatment options include amiodarone, disopyramide, β- and calcium-channel blockers for rate control, and AV nodal ablation plus permanent pacemaker implantation. Anticoagulation with warfarin is essential.

Dilated Cardiomyopathy

The standard therapy for CHF in this condition consists of diuretics, ACE inhibitors, and β-blockers starting with an ultra low dose. GRADE A Aldosterone antagonists are being utilized increasingly early in the course of the disease. β-Blockers may be particularly useful in the presence of sinus tachycardia or ventricular arrhythmias. Other antiarrhythmic therapy is not as logical as previously thought because most antiarrhythmic drugs can depress LV function. For atrial fibrillation, anticoagulation is mandatory. Inotropic support is reserved for acute deterioration.

Inflammatory and Immunological Factors Specific therapies for these types of myocarditis and dilated cardiomyopathy have met with little clinical success. In recent onset dilated cardiomyopathy and an ejection fraction of less than or equal to 40%, intravenous immunoglobulin was no better than placebo in enhancing spontaneous recovery.[209] Cytokine inhibitors such as TNF-α have been very disappointing. Immunosuppressive therapy for giant cell myocarditis is still under evaluation, but does appear to offer some benefit.[210]

Resynchronization and ICD Therapy In patients with idiopathic dilated cardiomyopathy and heart failure of other etiologies, biventricular pacing is currently an important option in patients with class III to IV symptoms and QRS prolongation of ≥120 milliseconds. GRADE A The potential mechanisms of benefit include shortening of the QRS duration to improve AV synchrony. Other effects may include reduced mitral regurgitation and improved diastolic filling. Benefits consistently shown in randomized trials include better quality of life, functional status, exercise capacity, ventricular function, and lowered mortality from heart failure.[211] The early and consistent improvement in functional capacity far exceeds that found when ACE inhibition or β-blockade therapy is initiated and severely ill patients may be saved from transplantation.[212] In the COMPANION trial designed to assess mortality,[212a] patients were randomly assigned to optimal modern medical therapy, biventricular pacing, or biventricular pacing plus an implantable cardioverter-defibrillator (ICD). All-cause mortality in the pacing group fell by 24% and by about 36% ($P = 0.003$) in the pacing-ICD arm of the trial. Thus in seriously ill heart failure patients with QRS widening already receiving optimal medical treatment, added biventricular pacing with an ICD now offers substantial improvement to their otherwise dismal prognosis. What remains a problem is an inability to predict ahead of time, which patients will or will not benefit from biventricular pacing. The SCD-HeFT trial (Sudden Cardiac Death in Heart Failure Trial), verbally presented, shows that sudden cardiac death can be averted by ICDs in advanced cardiomyopathy.[144]

Cardiac Transplantation and LV Assist Devices These are last resorts. The decision to transplant must not lightly be made until completing the "full house" of modern anti-CHF therapy, adding optimal vasodilator treatment to standard maximal therapy that includes ACE inhibition (and/or ARB), β-blockade, aldosterone blockade, and digoxin. To this long list should be added biventricular pacing and an ICD (see preceding paragraph). Select an experienced transplant center, expert in all phases of care, and don't wait until there is deterioration in the patient's general health. Shortage of donors and of money may limit this advice. Implantable left ventricular assist devices (LVAD) have been used primarily as bridges to transplantation, but some patients have been maintained long term and few have recovered to be weaned. In the REMATCH Trial, the use of an LVAD in patients with advanced heart failure who were ineligible for cardiac transplantation demonstrated a 52% 1-year survival in the device group versus 25% in the medical therapy group ($P = 0.002$).[213] The absolute survival benefit of at 1 year was excellent. Two-year survival was more dismal at only 23% but still compared well with the medical group at 8%. Serious adverse events in the device group such as infection, bleeding, and malfunction of the device were frequent. A major criticism of this study is that medical therapy given in 1998 at the start of the trial was unavoidably incomplete when compared with the current "full house"—then only 51% received ACE inhibitors, 20% β-blockers, 39% spironolactone, and none, it seems, had biventricular pacing. Thus LVAD is still chiefly a bridge to transplantation that has not yet been tested against totally aggressive medical therapy.

Chagas' Heart Disease

The World Health Organization suggests that 15 to 20 million people, primarily in Latin America, are affected by Chagas' disease (a *Trypanosoma cruzi* infection). In the acute phase, antitrypanosomal agents (nifurtimox and benznidazole) are helpful in controlling symptoms, in addition to supportive therapy for congestive heart failure, arrhythmias, and conduction disturbances. Does acute therapy prevent chronic organ damage? One small trial of benznidazole suggests that specific therapy may have a favorable impact on the chronic phase of Chagas' disease.[214] Thus the management of Chagas' disease remains supportive. GRADE C

Restrictive Cardiomyopathy

Restrictive heart disease is not well understood. It may be idiopathic or associated with other diseases such as amyloidosis or endomyocardial disease with or without hypereosinophilia. First exclude constrictive pericarditis, the treatment of which may be curative, whereas the therapy of the restrictive cardiomyopathy is both difficult and highly unsatisfactory. In the elderly, restriction may reflect increased myocardial fibrosis, and the latter can perhaps be countered by ACE inhibitors, ARBs, or aldosterone blockers (see Chapter 5). Once fibrosis has developed, the most important aspect of treatment is to avoid dehydration and overdiuresis, which impairs the left atrial filling pressure, and to control the heart rate in atrial fibrillation. Pharmacologic therapy of restrictive heart disease is extremely difficult. Conduction disease may require a permanent pacemaker. Cardiac transplantation with and without bone marrow transplantation is currently under investigation, as is the role of chemotherapy for some patients with cardiac involvement due to primary amyloidosis. Despite the many treatment strategies, none are based on randomized control data, nor are randomized trials likely.

VALVULAR HEART DISEASE

Rheumatic Fever Prophylaxis Treatment should start as soon as a definitive diagnosis of streptococcal infection has been made; the treatment is either a single dose of benzathine penicillin—1,200,000 units for adults and half dose for children—or a full 10-day course of oral penicillin-V (for children, 250 mg two or three times daily;[215] empirically double this for adults). Thereafter, in selected patients in whom recurrences are feared, the penicillin injection is repeated monthly, or pencillin-V is given as 125 to 250 mg twice daily continuously. The best route is by injection, which is used for 5 years followed by oral prophylaxis possibly for life. For *penicillin allergy*, use sulfadiazine,[215] erythromycin,[216] or the cephalosporins.

General Approach to Valvular Heart Disease As surgical techniques for valve repair and the performance of prosthetic valves have improved, so have the surgical indications become less stringent. Now most patients with LV dysfunction are operated on even if asymptomatic. Thus the tendency is to become more aggressive, particularly in the case of mitral regurgitation, where a strong case can be made for surgical repair in asymptomatic patients with severe mitral regurgitation, even in the face of well preserved LV function. GRADE B An essential component of this strategy lies in the local results in regard to mitral valve repair versus mitral valve replacement. Concomitant therapy in patients with valvular heart disease is not based on trial data but may include diuretics, ACE inhibitors, especially for certain nonstenotic lesions, and vasodilators. Attention to arrhythmias, particularly atrial fibrillation, is essential and rate control with anticoagulation must be considered.

Aortic Stenosis In valvular stenosis, the basic problem is obstructive and requires surgical relief. GRADE A Four advances in understanding are: (1) the knowledge that increased LV pressure sets in motion a series of signaling pathways that lead not only to myocyte hypertrophy but to fibrosis and progressive myocyte death, the latter promoting deterioration from compensated hypertrophy to failure, and arguing for valve replacement while LV function is still relatively preserved[217]; (2) improved surgical techniques allow valve replacement even in those with heart failure so severe that the aortic valve gradient is low[218]; (3) peripheral vasoconstriction can contribute to critically severe heart failure, when careful vasodilator therapy improves the hemodynamic status,[219] so that aortic valve replacement becomes feasible; and (4) the potential but unproven role of medical therapy by statins and other drugs based on the hypothesis that aortic stenosis in the elderly has similar risk factors to coronary artery disease.[220]

Afterload reduction remains generally contraindicated, except in the highly selected,[219] because it increases the pressure gradient across the stenosed valve. Thus, CCBs should not be used to treat any accompanying hypertension except in mild degrees of stenosis. In patients with decompensated heart failure due to systolic dysfunction and severe aortic stenosis, intravenous nitroprusside may play a role as a bridge to valve replacement, but meticulous monitoring is mandatory.[219]

Asymptomatic Patients with Aortic Stenosis In truly asymptomatic aortic stenosis, which is nonetheless hemodynamically significant, the key to the management is careful and regular supervision, with intervention as soon as symptoms appear. Nonetheless, a strong case can be made for surgery for asymptomatic patients with severe aortic stenosis who have left ventricular systolic dysfunction without any evidence of symptomatic cardiac failure and in patients who manifest an abnormal response to exercise, for example, hypotension. A case, albeit a weaker one, can be made for surgery in asymptomatic patients with documented ventricular tachycardia, a valve area of 0.6 cm, or patients with very marked or excessive left ventricular hypertrophy of 15 mm or greater.[221]

Aortic Valve Replacement Surgical therapy is required for those with angina, exertional syncope, or symptoms of LV failure (even if early). Surgery can relieve the hypertrophy, improve the coronary perfusion pressure, and often also correct any accompanying coronary artery disease. The combination of aortic stenosis and gastrointestinal bleeding suggests type 2A Von Willebrand syndrome, which improves with aortic valve replacement.[222] For the future, percutaneous valve replacement is an exciting possibility.[223]

Valvuloplasty for Aortic Stenosis The initial enthusiasm for percutaneous aortic balloon valvuloplasty has been tempered by the long-term results which are disappointing, but it does offer an alternative for patients in whom surgery is contraindicated and in some patients as a bridge to aortic valve replacement, if for one reason or another immediate surgery is inadvisable. There are also subsets of patients with low gradients and poor ventricular function in whom the symptomatic response to balloon valvuloplasty may provide a guide to the success of surgery in the future.[224] The discouraging results of balloon valvuloplasty in the elderly contrast with more positive outcomes in young patients with congenital aortic stenosis.[225]

Mitral Stenosis In mitral stenosis with sinus rhythm, β-blockade improves exercise capacity to lessen possible pulmonary symptoms. This may be particularly helpful in patients with symptomatic mitral stenosis during pregnancy. Prophylactic digitalization is still sometimes used supposedly to avoid a high ventricular rate during intermittent atrial fibrillation; this practice is not supported by the available data. Balloon valvuloplasty is now established for relief of stenosis with selection of patients depending on the echocardiographic characteristics of the valve. Paroxysmal atrial fibrillation precipitating left-sided failure may require carefully titrated intravenous diltiazem, verapamil, or esmolol, provided that the left ventricle itself is not depressed in function (associated mitral regurgitation). In established atrial fibrillation, digitalization is usually not enough to prevent an excessive ventricular rate during exercise, so that digoxin should be augmented by diltiazem, verapamil, or β-blockade. Anticoagulation is essential for those with atrial fibrillation and merits consideration for those in sinus rhythm thought to be at high risk for atrial fibrillation (marked left atrial enlargement or frequent atrial extrasystoles).

Balloon mitral valvuloplasty gives excellent early and late results in rheumatic mitral stenosis. All patients with symptomatic mitral stenosis should be considered for this procedure. GRADE A Contraindications include the presence of left atrial thrombus, severe subvalvular fibrosis or valve calcification, and a significant mitral regurgitation, but this can be determined ahead of time by transesophageal echocardiography. The surgical alternatives are open mitral commissurotomy or mitral valve replacement. The percutaneous technique is comparable to the more invasive surgical approach.[226]

In aortic regurgitation, indications for operation are the development of symptoms, or in the absence of symptoms, evidence of progressive or impending LV dysfunction based upon impaired indices of contractility, a LV ejection fraction of below 55%, or increased left ventricular end diastolic dimensions.[227] GRADE B However, "agreement is greatest where data are fewest"[227] because there are no rigorous trials to support any improved survival using such indicators. In those with systolic hypertension, chronic afterload reduction by long-acting nifedipine is logical.[228] and benefits those with asymptomatic aortic regurgitation. Experimental data show that afterload reduction by ACE inhibitors or ARBs, despite increasing the LV ejection fraction, may adversely influence myocardial contractility so that there is no mandate for their use.[227]

In mitral regurgitation, the disease is more serious because it impacts three primary organs: the LV, the left atrium, and the right ventricle.[227] Hence the criteria for operation are more stringent, with a LV ejection fraction below 60% the best validated predictor of prognosis.[227] Other criteria are persistent atrial fibrillation, a subnormal RV ejection fraction, and an increased LV internal diameter. The current trend is to operate even earlier both to prevent ventricular dilatation and to "preserve the atrium," hopefully avoiding atrial fibrillation. GRADE B Thus the approach to operation has become increasingly aggressive, especially if the likelihood of a repair versus valve replacement is high. The ability to perform a mitral valve repair is based upon the skill and the experience of the surgeon and on the location and type of mitral valve disease that caused mitral regurgitation. Repair is more likely with degenerative as opposed to rheumatic or ischemic involvement of the mitral valves, and transesophageal echocardiography is a critical aspect of pre- and intraoperative strategies.

COR PULMONALE

Therapy of right heart failure is similar to that of left heart failure, except that digoxin appears to be less effective because of a combination of hypoxemia, electrolyte disturbances, and enhanced adrenergic discharge. Thus when atrial fibrillation develops, cautious verapamil or diltiazem is preferred to reduce the ventricular rate. Multifocal atrial tachycardia is associated with chronic lung disease and is a difficult arrhythmia to treat, although success with verapamil has been reported. In general, all beta-blockers should be avoided because of the risk of bronchospasm. Bronchodilators should be β_2-selective. For example, albuterol (salbutamol) has relatively little effect on the heart rate, while unloading the left heart by peripheral vasodilation.

PULMONARY HYPERTENSION

Primary pulmonary hypertension (PPH; both sporadic and familial) includes a variety of pathogenic mechanisms, while excluding pulmonary hypertension secondary to chronic pulmonary disease, congenital heart disease, or secondary to left heart disease. Some identified causes include HIV infection, appetite suppressants (fenfluramine, dexfenfluramine, amphetamines), and probably L-tryptophan, portal hypertension, toxic adulterated rape seed oil previously illegally sold as cooking oil in Spain, and collagen vascular disorders.[229] The hallmark of pulmonary hypertension is the histopathologic similarity shared by the different clinical types, and even on lung biopsy the exact pathogenesis may not be apparent. Long-term anticoagulants are frequently used on the assumption that there is thromboembolism or thrombosis in situ. A number of studies, but no randomized trials, suggest a better survival in patients treated with warfarin.[230] Oxygen supplementation should be used as necessary to maintain saturations of ≈90% at all times, with diuretics for fluid retention, and digoxin if the right ventricle begins to fail.

Calcium Channel Blockers Long-term therapy may give sustained hemodynamic improvement and increased survival in a minority of patients who responded to an acute vasodilator challenge. Currently a trial of long-acting CCBs is appropriate for those patients who have responded to acute testing with short-acting agents such as nifedipine or with inhaled nitric oxide, intravenous adenosine, or intravenous epoprostenol. The problem with CCBs is systemic hypotension, so that other agents more selective for the pulmonary arteries are now preferentially used.

Prostacyclin Analogs A continuous infusion of prostacyclin (epoprostenol sodium) is the only agent demonstrated to decrease mortality in PPH.[229] Currently several analogs with fewer side effects are available with demonstrated benefits on symptoms, exercise capacity, and on hemodynamics. Beraprost is an oral analogue, while iloprost is given by inhalation. Both have shown efficacy over 12 weeks.[231,232] Incomplete evidence suggests long-term survival benefit for beraprost.[229] Beraprost is used in Japan, but not licensed in the United States. Another prostacyclin analogue, treprostinil, is given as a subcutaneous infusion with benefits maintained for up to 18 months.[229] This is also not available in the United States. However, strict evidence favoring a survival benefit for these analogues is still lacking.[229]

Endothelin Receptor Antagonists Bosentan is a nonselective endothelin-1 receptor A and B antagonist, licensed for primary pulmonary hypertension in the United States. It improves exercise capacity in patients with severe symptoms. Problems are potential liver toxicity requiring monthly liver function tests and expense.[229,233]

Phosphodiesterase Inhibitors Logically, an agent that increases vascular levels of cGMP should vasodilate in primary pulmonary hypertension. Sildenafil, a selective inhibitor of cGMP-specific phosphodiesterase-type 5, given as 50 mg every 8 hours, attenuates pulmonary hypertension in animals and improves clinical status over 3 months.[234] Sildenafil is much cheaper than iloprost or bosentan. GRADE B Large comparative multicenter trials are now underway. Other agents undergoing evaluation include L-arginine, specific antagonists of endothelin-1 receptor A, and sildenafil alone or in combination with prostacyclin analogs and endothelin-1 receptor antagonists.

Transplantation and Other Surgical Interventions The most definitive therapy for primary pulmonary hypertension is transplantation but this may be associated with more morbidity and a higher incidence of obliterative bronchiolitis (chronic rejection) in patients with primary pulmonary hypertension than for other disorders. One year mortality is approximately 30%, rising to 80% at 5 years. The limited donor supply and uncertain long-term outcomes remain significant issues.

HEART DISEASE IN DIABETICS

Two major changes have propelled diabetes into the lap of cardiologists. First, diabetes is now recognized as a "coronary heart disease equivalent" by the Adult Treatment Panel (ATP III) of the National Cholesterol Education Program.[235] Second, diabetes is basically a vascular rather than a carbohydrate disorder.[236] For both these reasons, tight control of blood pressure, blood lipids, and all other risk factors is essential. GRADE A For glycemic control, the ideal agents apart from insulin are those that activate the peroxisome proliferator-activated receptors-gamma (PPAR-γ), such as metformin and the thiazolidinediones.[236] These agents help to attenuate insulin resistance, with the further hope, still under test,[237] that they will also retard the progress of diabetic vascular disease.

Blood Pressure The new BP goal is 130/80 mmHg (see Chapter 7). Tight control of BP lessens macrovascular complications,[238] whereas tighter diabetic control lessens only microvascular end-points. In Chapter 5 we argue that ACE inhibitors or ARBs are first choice in all diabetic hypertensives, especially those with underlying nephropathy, as they may also be vascular protective. Nonetheless a variety of agents, including low-dose diuretics, CCBs and β-blockers, will probably all be required to reach adequate control of blood pressure.

Lipids in Diabetes Although elevated LDL levels are common in diabetics, a normal level does not exclude a lipid abnormality because there are smaller denser LDL particles. Apolipoprotein B levels are a better reflection of total atherogenic particle number.[239] Trial data argue that all diabetics should receive a statin, irrespective of lipid levels.[69]

Heart Failure in Diabetics Because of rampant coronary disease and increased hypertension, heart failure is more common, requiring standard therapy but with focused attention on these two precipitating factors. Of note, the antidiabetic thiazolidinediones can cause leg edema and in about 2% overt failure.[240]

AMI in Diabetic Patients The arguments for acute ACE inhibition have been made in Chapter 5 (p. 126). In insulin-requiring diabetics, careful regulation of blood sugar and potassium during a maintained insulin infusion is required. In non-insulin-requiring diabetics, continued use of oral antidiabetic agents might increase mortality because these agents are potassium channel closers with coronary constriction as a side effect. Based on the Swedish DIGAMI study, the therapy of the diabetes should be shifted from an oral agent to a modified GIK regime during the early phase of AMI, followed by insulin for 3 months thereafter.[112]

Interventions in Diabetic Patients The long-term benefits of coronary artery bypass grafting in diabetic patients with angina are well established.[241] However, percutaneous coronary intervention (PCI) with stenting has its strong advocates,[32] especially using a drug-eluting stent combined with a Gp IIa/IIIb inhibitor such as abciximab.[49] The role of revascularization versus medical therapy in diabetic patients with stable angina or in asymptomatic patients with a positive stress test is currently the object of the large multinational trial, BARI 2.[237]

Should all diabetic patients receive an ACE inhibitor or ARB? This possibility is strongly raised by the MICRO-HOPE study in which high risk type 2 diabetics responded to ramipril therapy by reducing nephropathy and total mortality by 24%.[242] In those with type 2 diabetic renal lesions, including microalbuminuria and frank proteinuria, the evidence for renoprotection by an ARB is even better than for an ACE inhibitor.[24,243]

Metabolic Syndrome

This prediabetic state has rapidly increased in incidence and importance to reach alarming proportions (see p. 191). The metabolic syndrome probably constitutes one of the three current epidemics of cardiovascular disease, the others being congestive heart failure and atrial fibrillation. Diagnostic criteria are any three or more of: triglycerides ≥150 mg/dL (1.73 mmol/L); HDL <40 mg/dL (1.1 mmol/L); fasting glucose ≥110 mg/dL; blood pressure ≥130/85 mmHg; and abdominal obesity or a body mass index of >28.8 kg/m^2.[235,239] Any three features constitute the metabolic syndrome. With four or five features in hypercholesterolemic men, but reducing the blood sugar threshold to 99 mg/L (5.5 mmol/L), the risk for coronary disease increases 3.7-fold, and that for diabetes an astounding 24.5-fold compared with no such features.[244] Even only two features, namely an enlarged waist and elevated triglyceride levels, increase the risk of diabetes 3.2-fold.[245] To lessen the development of diabetes requires lifestyle modification by weight loss, less intake of fat and saturated fats, more fiber in the diet, and exercise more than 4 hours per week.[246]

INFECTIVE ENDOCARDITIS

Infective endocarditis remains potentially fatal if not aggressively treated by antibiotics, with or without surgery.[247] New risk factors have replaced the old. Rheumatic valve disease, for long the major predisposing cause, has given way to more modern risk factors such as intravenous drug use, degenerative valve diseases of the elderly, prosthetic valves, and nosocomial disease.[247] In addition, there are increasingly many immunologically compromised patients with HIV/AIDS or undergoing therapeutic immune suppression. Drug-resistant endocarditis is increasing, whether caused by "old pathogens" outwitting the standard antibiotics or by the more new "exotic organisms" that include fungi. To diagnose, echocardiography and transesophageal echos are very helpful but a negative does not rule out the diagnosis. Blood cultures remain the key investigation. Optimal therapy requires identification of the causative organism, which may delay initiation of therapy in subacute endocarditis for a short period. Definitive antibiotic therapy is based on susceptibility testing and requires the advice of an expert in infectious diseases. In culture-negative endocarditis therapy is empiric.

Streptococcus viridans, sensitive to penicillin, is still usually the causative organism in community acquired endocarditis in nonaddicts. Gentamicin may be added to shorten the duration of therapy. If a highly penicillin-resistant streptococcus is suspected, even if not proven, a combination of ampicillin or ceftriaxone with gentamicin is suggested. For highly resistant streptococci[247] or for penicillin allergy, vancomycin is used.

Staphylococcus is the second most common cause of endocarditis, moving up to first place in intravenous drug abusers, who are also at increased risk of gram-negative bacilli and fungal infections, all of which carry a high mortality. *Staphylococcus aureus* is usually penicillin-resistant; use vancomycin or other agents. If vancomycin-resistant, there are several options including cotherapy with cotrimoxazole.[247]

Enterococci, even when fully susceptible to penicillin, respond best to penicillin or vancomycin with an added aminoglycoside such as gentamicin, to achieve a cure rate more rapidly than with penicillin alone. By contrast are the single-drug options of streptococci and staphylococci on native valves.

Indications for Surgery An increasing aggressive approach to early cardiac surgery has favorably influenced the outcome of infective endocarditis. In patients with native valve endocarditis, the indications for surgery are congestive heart failure resulting from valve dysfunction, new valve regurgitation, systemic embolization to vital organs, refractory infection, and a vegetation on echocardiography.[248] This policy reduces 6-month mortality versus medical therapy alone.[248] The approach to prosthetic valve endocarditis, particularly within 3 months of the initial operation, is even more aggressive, with surgery for any signs of prosthetic valve dysfunction or any of the indications for surgery in native valves. Infection of a prosthetic valve by *Staphylococcus aureus*, gram-negative bacilli or fungi provide additional indications for early surgery. In the face of hemodynamic decompensation, surgery should not be delayed pending completion of antibiotic therapy. Relative indications for early surgical intervention include apparent failure of medical therapy as evidenced by persistent bacteremia or fever or an increase in the size of vegetation during treatment. Transesophageal echocardiography is extremely helpful in the detection of intracardiac vegetations and other complications such as perivalvular extension.

Anticoagulant Therapy The decision to initiate or continue anticoagulant therapy in patients with infective endocarditis is often difficult. In those patients already on anticoagulants (e.g., patients with mechanical prostheses or those in whom there are other indications for anticoagulation, such as thrombophlebitis) anticoagulant therapy should be continued or initiated. In the event of a cerebral thromboembolic complication, the risk of anticoagulant-induced hemorrhage must be balanced against the alternate risk of recurrent embolism. Aspirin has no effect on vegetation resolution and valvular dysfunction and is not indicated in the early management of patients with infective endocarditis.

Antibiotic Prophylaxis Against Infective Endocarditis Both American and European practice are based on amoxicillin prophylaxis (Tables 11-8 and 11-9). In 1997, the American Heart Association updated

Table 11-8	American Recommended Antibiotic Regimens for Dental or Respiratory Tract or Esophageal Procedures
Standard general prophylaxis for those at risk	Amoxicillin 2.0 g orally 1 h before procedure For patients unable to take oral medication, ampicillin 2.0 g IV or IM within 30 min before procedure
Oral regimen for amoxicillin or penicillin-allergic patients	Orally 1 h before procedure: Clindamycin 600 mg; or cephalexin or cefadroxil 2.0 g; or azithromycin or clarithromycin 500 mg
Parenteral regimen for ampicillin or penicillin-allergic patients	Within 30 min before procedure: Clindamycin IV 600 mg, or cefazolin 1.0 g IM or IV
Genitourinary or Gastrointestinal procedures High-risk patients (e.g., prosthetic valves)	Ampicillin 2.0 g *plus* gentamicin 1.5 mg/kg, both IM or IV within 30 min before procedure, followed 6 h later by ampicillin 1.0 g IM/IV or oral amoxicillin 1.0 g
GU/GI, high risk, but allergic to ampicillin/amoxicillin	Vancomycin 1.0 g IV slowly over 1–2 h, plus gentamycin 1.5 mg/kg (no more than 120 mg) IM or IV; complete administration within 30 min before procedure
GU/GI, moderate risk	Amoxicillin 2.0 g orally 1 h before procedure or ampicillin 2.0 g IV or IM within 30 min before
GU/GI, moderate risk, allergy to ampicillin/amoxicillin	Vancomycin, 1.0 g IV over 1–2 h, complete 30 min before procedure

Note: follow-up doses no longer recommended. For children's doses and other details see *Circulation* 1997;96:358–366.

Table 11-9	European Recommendations: Antibiotic Prophylaxis of Infective Endocarditis for Adults During Dental Procedures		
Not Allergic to Penicillin		**Allergic to Penicillin**	
Oral Amoxicillin	**IV Amoxicillin or Ampillicin**	**Oral Clindamycin**	**High Risk GU/GI**
2 g 1 h before	2 g before ($\frac{1}{2}$ to 1 h)	600 mg 1 h before (or 500 mg azithromycin-clarithromycin)	Vancomycin 1.0 g IV slowly over 1–2 h, plus gentamycin 1.5 mg/kg (no more than 120 mg) IM or IV; complete administration within 30 min before procedure

For details, see *Eur Heart J* 2004;25:267.

recommendations for the prevention of bacterial endocarditis in individuals at risk. Major changes include: (1) emphasis that most cases of endocarditis are not attributable to an invasive procedure; (2) cardiac conditions are stratified into high, moderate, and negligible risk categories based on the potential outcome of endocarditis when it develops; (3) procedures that may cause bacteremia and for which prophylaxis is recommended are more clearly specified, with an algorithm to more clearly define when prophylaxis is recommended in patients with mitral valve prolapse. Prolapse of mitral valves without any evidence of leak as defined by one or more systolic clicks but with no murmur and no Doppler-demonstrated mitral regurgitation probably does not increase the risk of endocarditis above that of the normal population and does not require prophylaxis.[249]

The updated recommendations suggest that for oral or dental procedures, the initial amoxicillin dose is reduced to 2 g given orally 1 hour before the procedure, and a follow-up dose is not recommended. Among patients unable to take oral medications, intramuscular or intravenous ampicillin 30 minutes before the procedure is recommended. For patients who are allergic to penicillin, erythromycin is no longer recommended but rather clindamycin, cephalexin, or aziothromycin/clarithromycin. The new guidelines have also simplified antibiotic prophylaxis for patients undergoing gastrointestinal or genitourinary procedures. Even in high-risk patients (prosthetic valves, a history of endocarditis, or surgical shunts or conduits), oral prophylaxis can be used although intravenous agents give maximal protection.

Primary Prevention Despite these guidelines, most infectious endocarditis is not preceded by medicosurgical or dental interventions, so the real answer lies in primary prevention.[247] Thus, conditions predisposing the patient to infective endocarditis, such as poor dental hygiene or genitourinary tract pathology, must be eliminated.

PERIPHERAL VASCULAR DISEASE

"Peripheral vascular disease is a marker for systemic atherosclerosis; the risk to limb is low, but the risk to life is high."[250] The basis of therapy is interventional whenever possible, coupled with active medical therapy, the latter previously disappointing but now much more encouraging in the light of several large studies.[250] Large-vessel atheroma is best dealt with by surgery, where the big advance has been the use of catheter-based therapies including stents.

Prophylaxis of Cardiovascular Complications The basis of medical therapy lies in risk factor modification, exercise training, and aspirin.[250] A supervised exercise program can result in a major improvement in motivated patients but the benefits are lost if the patient stops exercising. Control of smoking, hypertension, and hyperlipidemia are logical given the data that almost 70% of peripheral vascular disease is attributable to these known cardiovascular risk factors.[251] In addition, ACE inhibition, clopidogrel and a statin can all be given with large trial justification. In the HOPE study, 4051 patients with peripheral vascular disease were among those given prophylactic ACE inhibition by ramipril (aimed at 10 mg once daily), and they obtained the same striking decrease in cardiovascular events as did others at high risk due to coronary artery disease.[12] In the CAPRIE Study among 5787 patients with peripheral arterial disease, the risk of MI, ischemic stroke, or vascular death was about 24% less in the clopidogrel versus aspirin-treated groups ($P = 0.0028$).[252] In the Heart Protection Study (HPS) the relative risk reduction in the 6758 subjects with peripheral arterial disease was 19% ($P < 0.001$) in those given simvastatin 40 mg daily for about 5 years.[69] Though without formal proof that clopidogrel, aspirin, statin, and ACE inhibitor give additive protection and not adversely interfere, each agent acts by a different mechanism so that we recommend this combination. GRADE B However, of these, only clopidogrel has in its USA license an indication for peripheral vascular disease. Coronary artery disease is often associated and requires therapy in its own right. Ongoing major trials of statins, antiplatelet agents, recombinant growth factors, and immune modulators may result in clinically relevant new advances in the medical management of peripheral vascular disease in the future.

Cilostazol Cilostazol was approved in 2000 in the United States for intermittent claudication. It is a phosphodiesterase-III inhibitor, and therefore contraindicated when there is fear of ventricular arrhythmias, as in heart failure. The usual dose is 100 mg twice daily. It is metabolized by the cytochrome P-450 3A4 system, and hence open to interaction with ketoconazole, erythromycin, and diltiazem, as well as grapefruit juice. All these should be avoided.

Pentoxifylline This agent (*Trental*) decreases blood viscosity and maintains red cell flexibility of the erythrocytes as they are squeezed through the capillary bed. It is licensed for use in intermittent claudication in the United States (600 to 1200 mg daily in three divided doses with meals; side-effect nausea). Yet in a randomized trial of pentoxifylline and cilostazol, pentoxifylline had no effect on maximal walking distance or quality of life. In contrast, cilostazol improved both functional status and the walking impairment questionnaire.[253]

Other Agents Levocarnitine and L-propionyl-carnitine favorably improve the metabolic status of skeletal muscle to lengthen the walking distance. Neither preparation is licensed in the United States. Gingko biloba gives modest success but the mechanisms are unclear.[254] Ineffective therapies that should be discouraged include estrogen replacement, chelation therapy, and vitamin E supplementation.

Claudication plus Hypertension or Angina β-Blockers are still generally held to be relatively contraindicated in the presence of active peripheral vascular disease, although a meta-analysis of 11 pooled trials showed no adverse effects on the walking distance in mild to moderate disease.[255] Verapamil increases pain-free walking time.[256] CCBs may, therefore, be preferred to β-blockers, although there are no comparative studies.

RAYNAUD'S PHENOMENON

Once a secondary cause has been excluded (for example vasculitis, scleroderma, or lupus erythematosus), then calcium channel antagonists are logical. Nifedipine is best tested and one 10-mg capsule may be taken intermittently at the start of an attack. β-Blockers are traditionally contraindicated, although the evidence is not good. Sustained-release glycerol trinitrate patches may be effective in Raynaud's phenomenon, but are limited by the frequency of headaches. Several reports attest to the efficacy of topical glycerol trinitrate in this condition.[257]

BERI-BERI HEART DISEASE

This condition is characterized by high output CHF due to thiamine deficiency. Common in Africa and Asia, in Western countries it is under-diagnosed especially in alcoholics. The basis of treatment is thiamine 100 mg parenterally followed by 50 to 100 mg daily with vitamin supplements, a balanced diet, and abstinence from alcohol. Even in Shoshin beri-beri with peripheral circulatory shock and severe metabolic acidosis, thiamine remains the mainstay of treatment because the acidosis responds poorly to treatment. Diuretics are needed when diuresis is delayed beyond 48 hours of thiamine therapy (Comment by courtesy of Prof. D. P. Naidoo, University of Natal, South Africa).

CARDIOVASCULAR DRUGS IN PREGNANCY

Most cardiovascular drugs are not well studied for safety in pregnancy. ACE inhibitors, ARBs, warfarin and the statins are all clearly contraindicated (Table 11-10). For pregnancy hypertension, methyldopa is best validated, while the diuretics are not as bad as often thought.

CARDIOPULMONARY RESUSCITATION

The clear command remains: "Defibrillate as early and as often as possible." The first essential is actually to shout for help, then to intubate, and to start cardiopulmonary resuscitation (CPR) as soon as possible. The best ratio of chest compressions to ventilation is still not clear. If there is no intubation, clearing the airway is essential. Mouth-to-mouth breathing is unpleasant and probably unnecessary. A recent innovation, still under evaluation, is "reverse" CPR with intermittent back pressure on the prone patient.[258] Out of hospital, when bystanders are involved, well-performed chest compression alone is simple and as effective as combined compression and mouth-to-mouth ventilation. GRADE B Bystander CPR gives a good quality of life to the survivors, but implies a high level of community education.[259] CPR programs focusing on early defibrillation have certainly improved the rate of survival to discharge, and a recent study from Mayo Clinic and Olmsted County, Minnesota, demonstrated that in patients with out-of-hospital cardiac arrest treated by early defibrillation, 40% were discharged neurologically intact. Long-term survival was similar to that among age-, sex-, and disease-matched patients who did not have an out-of-hospital cardiac arrest. These data serve as a benchmark for what can be achieved, particularly in smaller communities with rapid and easy access to trained life support personnel.[260]

American and European recommendations are basically similar,[261] but have become dated because they do not allow for recent studies that have changed practice such as the success of amiodarone versus placebo[262] or lidocaine[263] for out-of-hospital cardiac arrest, and the superiority of vasopressin over epinephrine for asystole.[264] In the algorithm for ventricular fibrillation (Fig. 11-7), there are three rapid successive defibrillations followed by a "loop" of activity. Each loop includes three full dose (360-J) defibrillatory shocks of the traditional monophasic type or 150-J of the biphasic type.[265] Each loop of activity is separated by 10 sequences of 5:1 compression-ventilation sequences preceded by injection of vasoconstrictive doses of epinephrine (1 mg). A single dose (40 units) of vasopressin can be used in place of the initial dose of epinephrine. Note that the use of either epinephrine or vasopressin has been challenged, there apparently being scant data from prospective randomized human trials.[266] The ALIVE study[263] is not clear about the use of epinephrine before randomization into amiodarone or lidocaine groups whereas the earlier amiodarone study[262] first gave 1 mg of epinephrine before randomization into amiodarone or placebo. Therefore we have followed the later protocol and modified the guidelines. Sodium bicarbonate is not recommended except in prolonged resuscitation when respiration is controlled. In the absence of adequate respiration, the CO_2 formed from the bicarbonate permeates into the cell to increase intracellular acidosis.

Apparent asystole (Fig. 11-8) accounts for 20% to 40% of all cardiac arrests and has a dreadful prognosis.[267] Although epinephrine has been recommended in prior guidelines, vasopressin is superior and

Table 11-10 Cardiovascular Drugs in Pregnancy

Drug Category	Potential Adverse Effect on Fetus	Safety in Pregnancy Classification	Trimester Risk(1,2,3)
β-Blockers	Intrauterine growth retardation; neonatal hypoglycemia, bradycardia	C or D	1, 3
Nitrates	None; may benefit by delaying premature labor	C	None
CCBs	None; may delay labor; experimentally embryopathic	C	None
Diuretics			
Thiazides	May impair uterine blood flow; usually regarded as C/I yet meta-analysis suggests safety*	B or C	3
Furosemide	Experimentally embryopathic	C	(1)
Torsemide	None	B	None
Indapamide	None	B	None
ACEi; ARBs	Embryopathic; may be lethal	D or X	(1), 2, 3
Digoxin	None	C	None
Antihypertensives			
Methyldopa	Well tested in pregnancy	B	None
Others as shown	Generally no adverse effects	C	None
Antiarrhythmics			
Amiodarone	Altered thyroid function	D	2, 3
Sotalol	None	B	None
Antithrombotics			
Warfarin	Embryopathic; crosses placenta with risk of fetal hemorrhage	X	1, 3
Heparin	None. Does not cross placental barrier	C	None
Enoxaparin GpIIa/IIIb blockers	No trials in humans	B	Not known
Abciximab	No data in humans	C	?none
Eptifibatide	No data in humans	B	?none
Tirofiban	No data in humans	B	?none
Aspirin	High dose risk of premature close of patent ductus	None	3
Lipid-Lowering Agents			
Nicotinic acid	None	B	None
Gemfibrozil	None	C	None
Statins	Congenital anomalies	X	1, 2, 3

For trimester risk, see *British National Formulary*, Sept 1999, p 620. X-rated, positive evidence of fetal abnormalities or risk that clearly outweighs any possible benefit to the patient; (1) = risk in first trimester not established.
*Collins et al. *Br Med J* 1985;290:17.
ACEi = angiotensin converting enzyme inhibitor; ARB = angiotensin AT-1 receptor blocker; C/I, contraindicated.

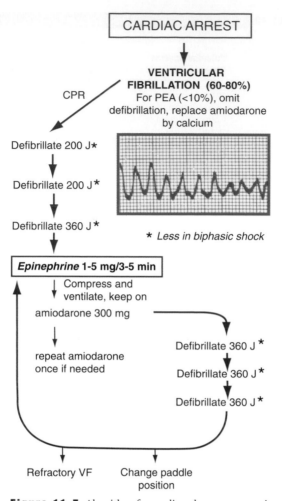

Figure 11-7 Algorithm for cardiopulmonary resuscitation (CPR) when there is ventricular fibrillation or pulseless electrical activity, taking into account the guidelines of the American Heart Association with the International Liaison Committee on Resuscitation,[261] and the amiodarone ARREST and ALIVE studies on out-of-hospital cardiac arrest.[262,263] CPR = cardiopulmonary resuscitation; Epinephrine = adrenaline; PEA = pulseless electrical activity = electromechanical dissociation; VF = ventricular fibrillation.

therefore incorporated into our algorithm. Again, new guidelines are needed.

Electromechanical dissociation is also called *pulseless electrical activity (PEA)*, occurring in up to 10% of cardiac arrests.[267] Now the "loop" omits defibrillation and considers pressor agents and calcium. Epinephrine is again given early and in a randomized American study a high dose (0.2 mg/kg) was better than a standard dose.[268] Calcium chloride is thought to have specific value in the presence of hyperkalemia, hypocalcemia, or excess of calcium antagonists.

When to Call It Off The ethics of when to stop the "loops" and when not to resuscitate are becoming increasingly complex.

Self-Help by Coughing For those many who are alone when having a heart attack and beginning to feel faint, repeated and very vigorous coughing might save them from fatal ventricular fibrillation.[269]

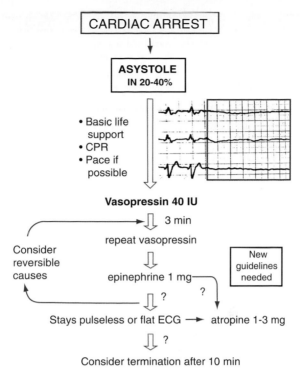

Figure 11-8 Algorithm for asystole, taking into account the new study on superiority of vasopressin over epinephrine.[264] Note that this study upsets previous algorithms, and must still be incorporated into revised guidelines. Asystole accounts for 20% to 40% of cardiac arrests, with a terrible prognosis.[267] *Epinephrine = adrenaline.*

Care of Cardiac Arrest Survivors The patient will have been urgently hospitalized and cardiogenic shock is now the major risk. Prophylactic antiarrhythmic therapy by lidocaine or procainamide for 36 to 48 hours is common practice. Some use intravenous amiodarone. In unconscious patients with spontaneous circulation after recovery from cardiac arrest due to ventricular fibrillation, mild therapeutic hypothermia to 32 to 34°C improves the neurological outcome and long-term survival.[270] Once stabilized, a full cardiac evaluation is required, including echocardiography and coronary angiography.

Long-Term Care The substrate for sustained monomorphic VT is seldom abolished by bypass grafting, so that the indications for cardiac surgery must be decided in their own right. Nevertheless, it makes sense to consider an ischemic etiology in such patients, and aggressively to treat coronary heart disease and LV failure both medically and, where indicated, surgically. Empiric β-blockade is the prime long-term antiarrhythmic treatment unless contraindicated, whereupon empiric amiodarone is the next choice. The implantable cardioverter-defibrillator (ICD) is often regarded as the ultimate treatment and it undoubtedly reduces sudden cardiac death. The ICD has irrevocably altered the landscape for patients with malignant ventricular tachyarrhythmias yet there are reservations. It is only in the highest risk patients that ICD is superior to amiodarone (see Table 8-6). In patients with a cardiac arrest in the setting of decompensated heart failure, an ICD may simply replace sudden cardiac death with delayed death due to heart failure. An important point is that the ICD should be selectively applied, specifically to patients at serious risk of sudden cardiac death yet otherwise having a reasonable expected overall cardiac prognosis.

REFERENCES

1. ACC/AHA Guidelines. ACC/AHA 2002 Guideline update for the management of patients with chronic stable angina—summary article. *Circulation* 2003;107:149–158.
2. Antithrombotic Trialists' Collaboration. Collaborative meta-analysis of randomized trials of antiplatelet therapy for prevention of death, myocardial infarction and stroke in high-risk patients. *Br Med J* 2002;324:71–86.
3. Meade T. Randomized trial of low-intensity oral anticoagulation with warfarin and low-dose aspirin in the primary prevention of ischaemic heart disease in men at increased risk. The medical TM Research Council General Practice Research Framework. *Lancet* 1998;351:233–241.
4. O'Connor C, et al. Azithromycin for the secondary prevention of coronary heart disease events. The WIZARD Study: a randomized control trial. *JAMA* 2003;290:1459–1466.
5. Heidenreich PA, et al. Meta-analysis of trials comparing β-blockers, calcium antagonists, and nitrates for stable angina. *JAMA* 1999;281:1927–1936.
6. Trialists BP. Effects of different blood-pressure lowering regimens on major cardiovascular events: results of prospectively-designed overviews of randomised trials. *Lancet* 2003;362:1527–1535.
7. Pitt B, et al. Effect of amlodipine on the progression of atherosclerosis and the occurrence of clinical events. *Circulation* 2000;102:1503–1510.
8. IONA Study Group. Effect of nicorandil on coronary events in patients with stable angina: the Impact Of Nicorandil in Angina (IONA) Randomized Trial. *Lancet* 2002;359:1269–1275.
9. Chaitman BR, et al. Effects of ranolazine with atenolol, amlodipine, or diltiazem on exercise tolerance and angina frequency in patients with severe chronic angina: a randomized controlled trial. *JAMA* 2004;291:309–316.
10. Borer J, et al. Antianginal and anti-ischemic effects of ivabradine, an If inhibitor, in stable angina. *Circulation* 2003;107:817–823.
11. Tardif J-C. *Presented at the Sessions of the European Society of Cardiology.* Vienna. 2003.
12. HOPE Investigators. Effects of an angiotensin-converting enzyme inhibitor, ramipril, on cardiovascular events in high-risk patients. *N Engl J Med* 2000;342:145–153.
13. HOPE Study Investigators. Effects of ramipril on cardiovascular and microvascular outcomes in people with diabetes mellitus. Results of the HOPE study and the MICRO-HOPE substudy. *Lancet* 2000;355:253–259.
14. Fox KN. European Trial On Reduction of Cardiac Events with Perindopril in Stable Coronary Artery Disease Investigators: efficacy of perindopril in reduction of cardiovascular events among patients with stable coronary artery disease: randomized, double-blind, placebo-controlled, multicentre trial (the EUROPA Study). *Lancet* 2003;362:782–788.
15. Kris-Etherton P, et al. Benefits of a mediterranean-style, National Cholesterol Education Program/American Heart Association Step I dietarypattern on cardiovascular disease. *Circulation* 2001;103:1823–1825.
16. Barsness G, et al. The International EECP Patient Registry (IEPR) design, methods, baseline characteristics, and acute results. *Clin Cardiol* 2001;24:435–442.
17. Mannheimer C, et al. The effects of transcutaneous electrical nerve stimulation in patients with severe angina pectoris. *Circulation* 1985;71:308–316.
18. de Jongste M, et al. Efficacy of spinal cord stimulation as adjuvant therapy for intractable angina pectoris: a prospective, randomized clinical study. Working Group on Neurocardiology. *J Am Coll Cardiol* 1994;23:1592–1597.
19. Frazier O, et al. Transmyocardial revascularization with a carbon dioxide laser in patients with end-stage coronary artery disease. *N Engl J Med* 1999;341:1021–1028.
20. Stone G, et al. A prospective, multicenter, randomized trial of percutaneous transmyocardial laser revascularization in patients with non-recannulizable chronic total occlusions. *J Am Coll Cardiol* 2002;39:1581–1587.
21. Losordo DW, et al. Gene therapy for myocardial angiogenesis: initial clinical results with direct myocardial injection of phVEGF165 as sole therapy for myocardial ischemia. *Circulation* 1998;98:2800–2804.
22. Caplice NM, et al. Stem cells to repair the heart: a clinical perspective. *Circ Res* 2003;92:6–8.
23. Rihal C, et al. Indications for coronary artery bypass surgery and percutaneous coronary intervention in chronic stable angina. *Circulation* 2003;108:2439–2445.
24. Corpus RA, et al. Optimal glycemic control is associated with a lower rate of target vessel revascularization in treated type II diabetic patients undergoing elective percutaneous coronary intervention. *J Am Coll Cardiol* 2004;43:8–14.
25. Eefting F, et al. Randomized comparison between stenting and off-pump bypass surgery in patients referred for angioplasty. *Circulation* 2003;108:2870–2876.
26. Khan NE, et al. A randomized comparison of off-pump and on-pump multivessel coronary-artery bypass surgery. *N Engl J Med* 2004;350:21–28.
27. Serruys PW, et al. A comparison of balloon-expandable stent implantation with balloon angioplasty in patients with coronary artery disease. *N Engl J Med* 1994;331:489–495.
28. Rankin JM, et al. Improved clinical outcome after widespread use of cornary artery stenting in Canada. *N Engl J Med* 1999;341:1957–1965.
29. Moses JW, et al. Sirolimus-eluting stents versus standard stents in patients with stenosis in a native coronary artery. *N Engl J Med* 2003;349:1315–1323.
30. Schofield P. Indications for percutaneous and surgical revascularisation: how far does the evidence base guide us? *Heart* 2003;89:565–570.

31. Morrison DA, et al. Percutaneous coronary intervention versus coronary artery bypass graft surgery for patients with medically refractory myocardial ischemia and risk factors for adverse outcomes with bypass: A multicenter, randomized trial. Investigators of the Department of Veterans Affairs Cooperative Study #385. The Angina With Extremely Serious Operative Mortality Evaluation (AWESOME). *J Am Coll Cardiol* 2001;38:143–149.

32. Sedlis SD, et al. Percutaneous coronary intervention versus coronary bypass graft surgery in diabetic patients with unstable angina and risk factors for adverse outcomes with bypass: an outcome of diabetic patients in the AWESOME Randomized Trial and Registry. *J Am Coll Cardiol* 2002;40:1555–1566.

33. Oler A, et al. Adding heparin to aspirin reduced the incidence of myocardial infarction and death in patients with unstable Angina. A meta-analysis. *JAMA* 1996;276:811–815.

34. Yusuf S, et al. Clopidogrel in Unstable Angina to Prevent Recurrent Events Trial Investigators: effects of clopidogrel in addition to aspirin in patients with acute coronary syndromes without ST-segment elevation. *N Engl J Med* 2001;345:494–502.

35. Mehta SR, et al. Clopidogrel in Unstable angina to prevent Recurrent Events trial (CURE) Investigators: effects of pretreatment with clopidogrel and aspirin followed by long-term therapy in patients undergoing percutaneous coronary intervention: the PCI-CURE study. *Lancet* 2001;358:527–533.

36. ISAR-COOL Trial. Evaluation of prolonged antithombotic pretreatment ("Cooling-Off" Strategy) before interventon in patients with unstable coronary syndromes. A randomized controlled trial. *JAMA* 2003;290:1593–1599.

37. Kastrati A, et al. A clinical trial of abciximab in elective percutaneous coronary intervention after pretreatment with clopidogrel. *N Engl J Med* 2004;350:232–238.

38. Cannon CP. Diagnosis and management of patients with unstable Angina. *Curr Probl Cardiol* 1999;24:681–744.

39. ESSENCE Study Group. A comparison of low-molecular-weight heprin with unfractionated heparin for unstable coronary artery disease. *N Engl J Med* 1997;337:447–452.

40. Antman E, et al. For the TIMI IIB Investigators. Enoxaparin prevents death and cardiac ischemic events in unstable angina-non-Q-wave myocardial infarction: results of the Thrombolysis in Myocardial Infarction (TIMI) 11B Trial. *Circulation* 1999;100:1593–1601.

41. Kline W, et al. Comparison of low-molecular-weight heparin with unfractionated heparin acutely and with placebo for six weeks in the management of unstable coronary artery disease. FRagmin In Unstable Coronary Artery Disease Study (FRIC). *Circulation* 1997;96:61–68.

42. FRAXIS Study Group. Comparison of two treatment durations (6 days and 14 days) of a low molecular weight heparin with a 6-day treatment of unfractionated heparin in the initial management of unstable angina or non-Q-wave myocardial infarction: FRAXIS (Fraxiparine in Ischaemic Syndrome). *Eur Heart J* 1999;20:1553–1562.

43. Collet J, et al. Percutaneous coronary intervention after subcutaneous enoxaparin pretreatment in patients with unstable angina pectoris. *Circulation* 2001;103: 658–663.

44. Kereiakes D, et al. Enoxaparin and abciximab adjunctive pharmacotherapy during percutaneous coronary intervention. *J Invas Cardiol* 2001;13:272–278.

45. RITA-3 Trial. For the Randomised Intervention Trial of unstable Angina (RITA) Investigators. Interventional versus conservative treatment for patients with unstable angina or non-ST-elevation myocardial infarction: the British Heart Foundation RITA-3 randomised trial. *Lancet* 2002;360:743–751.

46. SYNERGY Trial Investigators. Enoxaparin vs unfractionated heparin in high-risk patients with non-ST-segment elevation acute coronary syndromes managed with an intended early invasive strategy: primary results of the SYNERGY randomized trial. *JAMA* 2004;292:45–54.

47. OASIS-2 Investigators. Organisation to Assess Strategies for Ischemic Syndromes. Effects of recombinant hirudin (Lepirudin) compared with heparin on death, myocardial infarction, refractory angina, and revascularisation procedures in patients with acute myocardial ischaemia without ST elevation: a randomised trial. *Lancet* 1999;353:429–438.

48. Bittl J, et al. Bivalirudin versus heparin during coronary angioplasty for unstable or postinfarction angina: final report reanalysis of the Bivalirudin Angioplasty Study. *Am Heart J* 2001;142:952–959.

49. Lincoff AM, et al. REPLACE-2 Investigators. Bivalirudin and provisional glycoprotein IIb/IIIa blockade compared with heparin and planned glycoprotein IIb/IIIa blockade during percutaneous coronary intervention: REPLACE-2 randomized trial. (Erratum in: 2003;289:1638). *JAMA* 2003;289:853–863.

50. Boersma E, et al. Platelet glycoprotein IIb/IIIa inhibitors in acute coronary syndromes: a meta-analysis of all major randomized clinical trials. *Lancet* 2002;359:189–198.

51. CAPTURE Investigators. Randomized placebo-controlled trial of abciximab before and during coronary intervention in refractory unstable angina; The CAPTURE Study. *Lancet* 1997;349:1429–1435.

52. EPIC Investigators. Use of a monoclonal antibody directed against the platelet glycoprotein IIb-IIIa receptor and high risk angioplasty. *N Engl J Med* 1994; 330:956–961.

53. EPILOG Investigators. Platelet glycoprotein IIb-IIIa receptor blockade and low-dose heparin during percutaneous coronary revascularization. *N Engl J Med* 1997;336: 1689–1696.

54. PRISM-Plus Study. The Platelet Receptor Inhibition in Ischemic Syndrome Management in Patients Limited by Unstable Signs and Symptoms (PRISM-Plus) Study Investigators. Inhibition of the platelet glycoprotein IIb/IIIa receptor with tirofiban

in unstable angina and non-Q-wave myocardial infarction. *N Engl J Med* 1998;338:1488–1497.

55. PURSUIT Trial Investigators. Inhibition of platelet glycoprotein IIb/IIIa with eptifibatide in patients with acute coronary syndromes. *N Engl J Med* 1998;339:436–433.

56. HINT Study. Early treatment of unstable angina in the coronary care unit, a randomised, double-blind placebo controlled comparison of recurrent ischemia in patients treated with nifedipine or metoprolol or both. Holland Inter-university Nifedipine Trial. *Br Heart J* 1986;56:400–413.

57. Hohnloser SH, et al. For the European Esmolol Study Group. Usefulness of esmolol in unstable angina pectoris. *Am J Cardiol* 1991;67:1319–1323.

58. Göbel EJ, et al. Long-term follow-up after early intervention with intravenous diltiazem or intravenous nitroglycerin for unstable angina pectoris. *Eur Heart J* 1998;19:1208–1213.

59. FRISC II Prospective Randomized Multicenter Study. Long-term low-molecular-mass heparin in unstable coronary artery disease. Fragmin and fast revascularisation during instability in coronary artery disease investigators. FRISC II Prospective Randomized Multi-Center Study. *Lancet* 1999;354:708–715.

60. Cannon CP, et al. Comparison of early invasive and conservative strategies in patients with unstable coronary syndromes treated with a glycoprotein IIb/IIIa inhibitor tirofiban. *N Engl J Med* 2001;344:1879–1887.

61. Prasad A, et al. Current management of non-ST-segment elevation acute coronary syndrome. Reconciling the results of randomized control trials. *Eur Heart J* 2003;24:1544–1553.

62. Regar E, et al. Angiographic findings of the multicenter Randomised Study with the Sirolimus-Eluting Bx Velocity Balloon-Expandable Stent (RAVEL). *Circulation* 2002;106:1949–1956.

63. Heeschen C. Angiographic findings in patients with refractory unstable angina according to troponin status. *Circulation* 1999;100:1509–1514.

64. Cannon CP, et al. The electrocardiogram predicts one-year outcome of patients with unstable angina and non-Q-wave myocardial infarction; results of the TIMI III Registry ECG Ancillary Study. *J Am Coll Cardiol* 1997;30:133–140.

65. Foo K, et al. A single serum glucose measurement predicts adverse outcomes across the whole range of acute coronary syndromes. *Heart* 2003;89:512–516.

66. Sabatine MS, et al. Multimarker approach to risk stratification in non-ST-elevation acute coronary syndromes: simultaneous assessment of troponin I, C-reactive protein, and B-type natriuretic peptide. *Circulation* 2002;105:1760–1763.

67. Brennan M-L, et al. Prognostic value of myeloperoxidase in patients with chest pain. *N Engl J Med* 2003;349:1595–1604.

68. Farkouh ME, et al. A clinical trial of a chest-pain observation unit for patients with unstable angina, chest pain evaluation in the emergency room (CHEER) investigators. *N Engl J Med* 1998;334:1882–1888.

69. HPS Collaborative Group. MRC/BHF Heart Protection Study of cholesterol lowering with simvastatin in 20 536 high-risk individuals: a randomised placebo-controlled trial. *Lancet* 2002;360:7–22.

70. Albert CM, et al. Blood levels of long-chain n-3 fatty acids and the risk of sudden death. *N Engl J Med* 2002;346:1113–1118.

71. Braunwald E, et al. ACC/AHA 2002 Guideline update for the management of patients with unstable angina and non-ST-segment elevation myocardial infarction— summary article. A Report of the American College of Cardiology/American Heart Association Task Force on Practice Guidelines (Committee on the Management of Patients with Unstable Angina). *J Am Coll Cardiol* 2002;40:1366–1374.

72. Schomig A, et al. Therapy-dependent influence of time-to-treatment interval on myocardial salvage in patients with acute myocardial infarction treated with coronary artery stenting or thrombolysis. *Circulation* 2003;108:1084–1088.

73. Keeley E, et al. Primary angioplasty versus intravenous thrombolytic therapy for acute myocardial infarction: a quantitative review of 23 randomised trials. *Lancet* 2003;361:13–20.

74. Grines CL, et al. For the Stent Primary Angioplasty in Myocardial Infection Study Group. Coronary angioplasty with or without stent implantation for acute myocardial infarction. *N Engl J Med* 1999;341:1949–1956.

75. Dangas G. Interventional therapy for acute yycardial infarction: respect for microvasculature. *J Am Col Cardiol* 2003;42:1403–1405.

76. Wang F, et al. Distal myocardial protection during percutaneous coronary intervention with an intracoronary beta-blocker. *Circulation* 2003;107:2914–2919.

77. De Luca G, et al. Time delay to treatment and mortality in primary angioplasty for acute myocardial infarction: every minute of delay counts. *Circulation* 2004; 109:1223–1225.

78. Welsh RC, et al. Prehospital management of acute ST-elevation myocardial infarction: time for reappraisal in North America. *Am Heart J* 2003;145:1–8.

79. Gibler WV, et al. Persistence of delays in presentation and treatment for patients with acute myocardial infarction: the GUSTO-1 and GUSTO-3 experience. *Ann Intern Med* 2002;39:123–130.

80. Qasim A, et al. Safety and efficacy of nurse-initiated thrombolysis in patients with acute myocardial infarction. *Br Med J* 2002;324:1328–1331.

81. Loubeyre C, et al. Outcome after combined reperfusion therapy for acute myocardial infarction, combining pre-hospital thrombolysis with immediate percutaneous coronary intervention and stent. *Eur Heart J* 2001;22:1128–1135.

82. Scheller N, et al. For the SIAM-III Study Group. Beneficial effects of immediate stenting after thrombolysis in acute myocardial infarction. *J Am Coll Cardiol* 2003; 42:634–641.

83. Matetzky S, et al. Acute myocardial infarction with isolated ST-segment elevation in posterior chest leads V_{7-9}. Hidden ST segment elevations revealing acute posterior infarction. *J Am Coll Cardiol* 1999;34:748–753.

84. GUSTO Investigators. The effects of tissue plasminogen activator, streptokinase, or both on coronary artery patency, ventricular function, and survival after acute myocardial infarction (published erratum appears in N Engl J Med 1994; 350: 516). *N Engl J Med* 1993;329:1615–1622.

85. ACC/AHA/ACP-ASIM. Guidelines for the Management of Patients with Chronic Stable Angina. The Report of the ACC/AHA Task Force Practice Guidelines (Committee on the Management of Patients with Chronic Stable Angina). *J Am Coll Cardiol* 1999;33:2097–2197.

86. ASSENT-2 Investigators. Assessment of the Safety and Efficacy of a New Thrombolytic (ASSENT-2) Investigators. Single-bolus tenecteplase compared with front-loaded alteplase in acute myocardial infarction: the ASSENT-2 double-blinded randomised trial. *Lancet* 1999;354:716–722.

87. GUSTO-III Investigators. (The Global Use of Strategies to Open Occluded Coronary Arteries). A comparison of reteplase with alteplase for acute myocardial infarction. *N Engl J Med* 1997;337:1118–1123.

88. Eisenberg M, et al. Glycoprotein IIb/IIIa inhibition in the setting of acute ST-segment elevation myocardial infarction. *J Am Coll Cardiol* 2003;42:1–6.

89. Van de Werf F. Comparison of Lanetoplase (n-PA) with TPA demonstrated equivalence in the In Time-II Study. 48th Scientific Sessions of the American College of Cardiology 1999.

90. RAPPORT Investigators. Randomized, Placebo-Controlled Trial of Platelet Glycoprotein IIb-IIIa Blockade with Primary Angioplasty for Acute Myocardial Infarction. ReoPro and Primary PTCA Organization and Randomized Trial (RAPPORT) Investigators. *Circulation* 1998;98:734–741.

91. ISAR-2 Intracoronary Stenting and Antithrombotic Regime Trial. Effect of glycoprotein IIb/IIIa receptor blockade with abciximab on clinical and angiographic restenosis rate after the placement of coronary stents following acute myocardial infarction. *J Am Coll Cardiol* 2000;35:915–921.

92. ADMIRAL Investigators. Platelet glycoprotein IIb/IIIa inhibition with coronary stenting for acute myocardial infarction. *N Engl J Med* 2001;344:1895–1903.

93. CADILLAC Investigators. Comparison of angioplasty with stenting, with or without Abciximab in acute myocardial infarction. *N Engl J Med* 2002;346:957.

94. CADILLAC Investigators. Cost-Effectiveness of coronary stenting and abciximab for patients with acute myocardial infarction. *Circulation* 2003;108:2857–2863.

95. ACE Trial. ACE-randomized trial comparing primary infarct artery stenting with or without abciximab in acute myocardial infarction. *Lancet* 2003;357:1905–1914.

96. Wallentin L, et al. Oral ximelagatran for secondary prophylaxis after myocardial infarction: the ESTEEM randomised controlled trial. *Lancet* 2003;362:789–797.

97. Singh M, et al. Rationale for on-site cardiac surgery for primary angioplasty: a time for reappraisal. *J Am Coll Cardiol* 2002;39:1881–1889.

98. Gibson C, et al. Early and long-term clinical outcomes associated with reinfarction following fibrinolytic administration in the thrombolysis in myocardial infarction trials. *J Am Col Cardiol* 2003;42:7–16.

99. ASSENT-3 Investigators. Efficacy and safety of tenecteplase in combination with enoxaparin, abciximab or unfractionated heparin: the ASSENT-3 randomised trial in acute myocardial infarction. *Lancet* 2001;358:605–613.

100. ASSENT-3 PLUS. Efficacy and Safety of Tenecteplase in combination with the Low-Molecular-Weight Heparin Enoxaparin or Unfractionated Heparin in the Prehospital Setting. *Circulation* 2003;108:135–142.

101. Direct Thrombin Inhibitor Trialists' Collaborative Group. Direct thrombin inhibitors in acute coronary syndromes: principal results of a meta-analysis based on individual patients' data. *Lancet* 2002;359:294–302.

102. HERO-2 Trial Investigators. Thrombin-specific anticoagulation with bivalirudin versus heparin in patients receiving fibrinolytic therapy for acute myocardial infarction: the HERO-2 randomised trial. *Lancet* 2001;358:1855–1863.

103. PENTALYSE Study. A synthetic factor-Xa inhibitor (ORG31540/SR9017A) as an adjunct to fibrinolysis in acute myocardial infarction. *Eur Heart J* 2001;22:1716–1724.

104. Teo KK, et al. Effects of prophylactic antiarrhythmic drug therapy in acute myocardial infarction. An overview of results from randomized controlled trials. *JAMA* 1993;270:1589–1595.

105. Harjai K, et al. Effects of prior beta-blocker therapy on clinical outcomes after primary coronary angioplasty for acute myocardial infarction. *Am J Cardiol* 2003;91:655–660.

106. Ellis K, et al. Mortality benefit of beta blockade in patients with acute coronary syndromes undergoing coronary intervention: pooled results from the Epic, Epilog, Epistent, Capture and Rapport Trials. *J Interv Cardiol* 2003;16:299–305.

107. Barron HV, et al. Intracranial hemorrhage rates and effect of immediate beta-blocker use in patients with acute myocardial infarction treated with tissue plasminogen activator. *Am J Cardiol* 2000;85:294–298.

108. Pfisterer M, et al. Atenolol use and clinical outcomes after thrombolysis for acute myocardial infarction; the GUSTO-I Experience. Global Utilization of Streptokinase and TPA (Alteplase) for Occluded Coronary Arteries. *J Am Coll Cardiol* 1998;32:634–640.

109. Pfeffer MA, et al. Valsartan, captopril or both in myocardial infarction complicated by heart failure, left ventricular dysfunction or both. *N Engl J Med* 2003;349:1893–1906.

110. Diaz R, et al. On behalf of the ECLA (Estudios Cardiologicas Lantinoamerica) Collaborative Group. Metabolic Modulation of Acute Myocardial Infarction. The ECLA Glucose-Insulin-Potassium Pilot Trial. *Circulation* 1998;98:2227–2234.

111. van der Horst I, et al. Glucose-Insulin-Potassium infusion in patients treated with primary angioplasty for acute myocardial infarction. *J Am Coll Cardiol* 2003;42: 784–791.

112. Opie LH. Proof that glucose-insulin-potassium provides metabolic protection of ischaemic myocardium? (Editorial). *Lancet* 1999;353:768–769.

113. Bybee KA, et al. Effect of concomitant or very early statin administration on inhospital mortality and reinfarction in patients with acute myocardial infarction. *Am J Cardiol* 2001;87:771–774.

114. Saia F, et al. Early fluvastatin treatment reduces the long-term incidence of major adverse cardiovascular events following successful first percutaneous coronary intervention with or without the use of stent: the Lescol Intervention Prevention Study. *J Am Coll Cardiol* 2003;41:1010–1146.

115. MacMahon S, et al. Effects of prophylactic lidocaine in suspected acute myocardial infarction. An overview of results from the randomized, controlled trials. *JAMA* 1988;260:1910–1916.

116. Hochman JS, et al. Early revascularization in acute myocardial infarction complicated by cardiogenic shock. SHOCK investigators. Should we emergently revascularize occluded coronaries for cardiogenic shock? *N Engl J Med* 1999;341: 625–634.

117. Holmes DR Jr, et al. Cardiogenic shock in patients with acute ischemic syndromes with and without ST-segment elevation. *Circulation* 1999;100:2067–2073.

118. Hochman JS. Cardiogenic shock complicating acute myocardial infarction. Expanding the paradigm. *Circulation* 2003;107:2998–3002.

119. Cotter G, et al. L-NMMA (a nitric oxide synthase inhibitor) is effective in the treatment of cardiogenic shock. *Circulation* 2000;101:1358–1361.

120. Young-Xu Y, et al. Long-term statin use and psychological well-being. *J Am Coll Cardiol* 2003;42:690–697.

121. Bush D, et al. Even minimal symptoms of depression increase mortality risk after acute myocardial infarction. *Am J Cardiol* 2001;88:337–341.

122. Friedmann R, et al. Pet ownership, social support, and one-year survival after acute myocardial infarction in the Cardiac Arrhythmia Suppression Trial (CAST). *Am J Cardiol* 1995;76:1213–1217.

123. Hurt RD, et al. A comparison of sustain-release buprorion and placebo for smoking cessation. *N Engl J Med* 1997;337:1195–1202.

124. de Lorgeril M, et al. Mediterranean diet: traditional risk factors, and the rate of cardiovascular complications after myocardial infarction: final report of the Lyon Diet Heart Study. *Circulation* 1999;99:779–785.

125. Trichopoulou A, et al. Adherence to a Mediterranean diet and survival in a Greek population. *N Engl J Med* 2003;348:2599–2608.

126. Burr ML, et al. The effects of changes in fat, fish, and fibre intakes on death and myocardial infarction; Diet and Reinfarction Trial (DART). *Lancet* 1989;2:757–761.

127. GISSI-Prevenzione Trial. Dietary supplementation with n-3 polyunsaturated fatty acids and vitamin E after myocardial infarction: results of the GISSI-Prevenzione trial. *Lancet* 1999;354:447–455.

128. Kris-Etherton P, et al. AHA Science Advisory: Lyon Diet Heart Study. Benefits of a Mediterranean-style, National Cholesterol Education Program/American Heart Association Step I Dietary Pattern on Cardiovascular Disease. *Circulation* 2001;103: 1823–1825.

129. Singh R, et al. Effect of an Indo-Mediterranean diet on progression of coronary artery disease in high risk patients (Indo-Mediterranean Diet Heart Study): a randomised single blind trial. *Lancet* 2002;360:1455–1461.

130. Lip G, et al. More evidence on blocking the renin-angiotensin-aldosterone system in cardiovascular disease and the long-term treatment of hypertension: data from recent clinical trials (CHARM, EUROPA, ValHeFT, HOPE-TOO and SYST-EUR-2). *J Hum Hypertens* 2003;17:747–750.

131. von Birgelen C, et al. Relation between progression and regression of atherosclerotic left main coronary artery disease and serum cholesterol levels as assessed with serial long-term (>12 months) follow-up intravascular ultrasound. *Circulation* 2003;108: 2757–2762.

132. Gottlieb SS, et al. Effect of beta-blockade on mortality among high-risk and low-risk patients after myocardial infarction. *N Engl J Med* 1998;339:489–497.

133. Huikuri H, et al. Prediction of sudden cardiac death after myocardial infarction in the beta-blocking area. *J Am Coll Cardiol* 2003;42:652–658.

134. Dargie H. Effect of carvedilol on outcome after myocardial infarction in patients with left ventricular dysfunction: the CAPRICORN randomised trial. *Lancet* 2001;357:1385–1390.

135. Opie LH, et al. Current status of safety and efficacy of calcium channel blockers in cardiovascular diseases. A critical analysis based on 100 studies. *Prog Cardiovasc Dis* 2000;43:171–196.

136. APRICOT-2 Trial. Aspirin plus Coumarin versus Aspirin Alone in the Prevention of Reocculsion after Fibrinolysis for Acute Myocardial Infarction. Results of the Antithrombotics in the Prevention of Reocclusion in Coronary Thrombolysis. *Circulation* 2002:659–665.

137. ASPECT-2 Study. Aspirin and coumadin after acute coronary syndromes (the APECT-2 study: a randomised controlled trial. *Lancet* 2002;360:109–113.

138. CHAMP Study Group. Department of Veterans Affairs cooperative studies program clinical trial comparing combined warfarin and aspirin with aspirin alone in

survivors of acute myocardial infarction: primary results of the CHAMP study. *Circulation* 2002;105.

139. Hurlen M, et al. Warfarin, aspirin or both after myocardial infarction. *N Engl J Med* 2002;347:969–974.
140. PEACE Study. Prevention of Events with Angiotensin-Converting Enzyme Inhibition (The PEACE Study Design). *Am J Cardiol* 1998;82:25H–30H.
141. EUROPA Trial. The European trial on reduction of cardiac events with perindopril in stable coronary artery disease (EUROPA). *Eur Heart J* 1998;19:J52–J55.
142. Hurlen M, et al. Aspirin does not influence the effect of angiotensin-converting enzyme inhibition on left ventricular ejection fraction 3 months after acute myocardial infarction. *Eur J Heart Fail* 2001;3:203–207.
143. Amiodarone Trials-Meta-Analysis Investigators (ATMAI). Effect of prophylactic amiodarone on mortality after acute myocardial infarction and in congestive heart failure; meta-analysis of individual data from 6500 patients in randomized trials. *Lancet* 1997;350:1417–1424.
144. Bardy G. Sudden cardiac death in heart failure trial (SCD-HeFT). *www.theheart.org* 2004;March 8.
145. Buxton A, et al. Electrophysiologic testing to identify patients with coronary artery disease who are at risk for sudden death. *N Engl J Med* 2000;342:1937–1945.
146. Moss AJ, et al. For the Multicenter Automatic Defibrillator Implantation Trial (MADIT) Investigators. Improved survival with an implanted defibrillator in patients with coronary artery disease at high risk for ventricular arrhythmia. *N Engl J Med* 1996;335:1933–1940.
147. Tsang T, et al. The prevalence of atrial fibrillation in incident stroke cases and matched population controls in Rochester, Minnesota. Changes over three decades. *J Am Col Cardiol* 2003;42:93–100.
148. Cotter G, et al. Conversion of recent onset paroxysmal atrial fibrillation to normal sinus rhythm: the effect of no treatment and high-dose amiodarone. A randomized, placebo-controlled study. *Eur Heart J* 1999;20:1833–1842.
149. Podrid PJ. Redefining the role of antiarrhythmic drugs. *N Engl J Med* 1999;340:1910–1912.
150. Azpitarte J, et al. Value of single oral loading dose of propafenone in converting recent onset atrial fibrillation. Results of the randomized, double-blind, controlled study. *Eur Heart J* 1997;10:1649–1654.
151. ACC/AHA/ESC Guidelines. ACC/AHA/ESC Guidelines for the Management of Patients with Atrial Fibrillation: Executive Summary. *J Am Coll Cardiol* 2001;38:1231–1265.
152. De Simone A, et al. Pretreatment with verapamil in patients with persistent or chronic atrial fibrillation who underwent electrical cardioversion. *J Am Coll Cardiol* 1999;34:810–814.
153. Malouf J, et al. Critical appraisal of transesophageal echocardiography in cardioversion of atrial fibrillation. *Am J Med* 2002;113:587–595.
154. Klein A, et al. Role of transesophageal echocardiography-guided cardioversion of patients with atrial fibrillation. *J Am Coll Cardiol* 2001;37:691–704.
155. AFFIRM Investigators. The Atrial Fibrillation Follow-up Investigation of Rhythm Management. A comparison of rate control and rhythm control in patients with atrial fibrillation. *N Engl J Med* 2002;347:1825–1833.
156. Hohnloser S, et al. Rhythm of rate control in atrial fibrillation— Pharmacological Intervention in Atrial Fibrillation (PIAF): a randomised trial. *Lancet* 2000;356:1789–1794.
157. van Gelder IC, et al. For the Rate Control versus Electrical Cardioversion for Persistent Atrial Fibrillation Study Group. A comparison of rate control and rhythm control in patients with recurrent persistent atrial fibrillation. *N Engl J Med* 2002;347:1834–1840.
158. Falk R. Management of atrial fibrillation—radical reform or modest modification? *N Engl J Med* 2002;347:1883–1884.
159. Brignole M. Ablate and pace; a pragmatic approach to paroxysmal atrial fibrillation not controlled by antiarrhythmic drugs. *Heart* 1998;79:531–533.
160. Dries DL, et al. Atrial fibrillation is associated with increased risk for mortality and heart failure progression in patients with asymptomatic and symptomatic left ventricular systolic dysfunction. A retrospective analysis of the SOLVD trials. Studies of left ventricular dysfunction. *J Am Coll Cardiol* 1998;32:695–703.
161. Oral H, et al. Facilitating transthoracic cardioversion of atrial fibrillation with ibutilide pretreatment. *N Engl J Med* 1999;340:1849–1854.
162. Li H, et al. Usefulness of ibutilide in facilitating successful external cardioversion of refractory atrial fibrillation. *Am J Cardiol* 1999;84:1096–1098.
163. Madrid A, et al. Use of irbesartan to maintain sinus rhythm in patients with long-lasting persistent atrial fibrillation: a prospective and randomized study. *Circulation* 2002;106:331–336.
164. Vermes E, et al. Enalapril decreases the incidence of atrial fibrillation in patients with left ventricular dysfunction: insight from the Studies Of Left Ventricular Dysfunction (SOLVD) trials. *Circulation* 2003;107:2926–2931.
165. Torp-Pedersen C, et al. Dofetilide in patients with congestive heart failure and left ventricular dysfunction. *N Engl J Med* 1999;341:857–865.
166. Ezekowitz M, et al. Preventing stroke in patients with atrial fibrillation. *JAMA* 1999;281:1830–1835.
167. Olsson S. Executive Steering Committee, on behalf of the SPORTIF III Investigators. Stroke prevention with the oral direct thrombin inhibitor ximelagatran compared with warfarin in patients with non-valvular atrial fibrillation (SPORTIF III)l: randomised controlled trial. *Lancet* 2003;362:1691–1698.

168. Eikelboom J, et al. Ximelagatran or warfarin in atrial fibrillation? *Lancet* 2004;363:734; author reply 734, 736.

169. Cox J, et al. Successful surgical treatment of atrial fibrillation. Review and clinical update. *JAMA* 1991;266:1976–1980.

170. Haissaguerre M, et al. Spontaneous initiation of atrial fibrillation by ectopic beats originating in the pulmonary veins. *N Engl J Med* 1998;339:659–666.

171. Oral H, et al. Catheter ablation for paroxysmal atrial fibrillation: segmental pulmonary vein ostial ablation versus left atrial ablation. *Circulation* 2003;108:2355–2360.

172. Wazni O, et al. Randomized study comparing combined pulmonary vein—left atrial junction disconnection and cavotricuspid isthmus ablation versus pulmonary vein—left atrial junction disconnection alone in patients presenting with typical atrial flutter and atrial fibrillation. *Circulation* 2003;108:2479–2483.

173. McCord JK, et al. Usefulness of intravenous magnesium for multifocal atrial tachycardia in patients with chronic obstructive pulmonary disease. *Am J Cardiol* 1998;81:91–93.

174. Pappone C, et al. A randomized study of prophylactic catheter ablation in asymptomatic patients with the Wolff-Parkinson-White syndrome. *N Engl J Med* 2003;349:1787–1789.

175. CASH Study. Preliminary results of the Cardiac Arrest Study Hamburg (CASH). *Am J Cardiol* 1993;72:109–113.

176. Singer I, et al. Azimilide decreases recurrent ventricular tachyarrhythmias in patients with implantable cardioverter defibrillators. *J Am Coll Cardiol* 2004;43:39–43.

177. Morrison L, et al. Utility of a rapid B-natriuretic peptide assay in differentiating congestive heart failure from lung disease in patients presenting with dyspnea. *J Am Coll Cardiol* 2002;39:202–209.

178. de Lemos J, et al. B-type Natriuretic peptide in cardiovascular disease. *Lancet* 2003;362:316–322.

179. Pfeffer MA, et al. Effects of candesartan on mortality and morbidity in patients with chronic heart failure: the CHARM-overall programme. *Lancet* 2003;362:777–781.

180. Packer M, et al. Effect of carvedilol on the morbidity of patients with severe chronic heart failure: results of the Carvedilol Prospective Randomized Cumulative Survival (COPERNICUS) Study. *Circulation* 2002;106:2194–2199.

181. Pitt B, et al. For the Randomized Aldactone Evaluation Study Investigators. The effect of spironolactone on morbidity and mortality in patients with severe heart failure. *N Engl J Med* 1999;341:709–717.

182. Pitt B, et al. Eplerenone, a selective aldosterone blocker in patients with left ventricular dysfunction after myocardial infarction. *N Engl J Med* 2003;348:1309–1321.

183. Elkayam U, et al. Double-blind, placebo-controlled study to evaluate the effect of organic nitrates in patients with chronic heart failure treated with angiotensin-converting enzyme inhibition. *Circulation* 1999;99:2652–2657.

184. Stevenson WG, et al. Atrial fibrillation in heart failure (Editorial). *N Engl J Med* 1999;341:910–911.

185. Burger A, et al. Effect of nesiritide (B-type natriuretic peptide) and dobutamine on ventricular arrhythmias in the treatment of patients with acutely decompensated congestive heart failure: the PRECEDENT study. *Am Heart J* 2002;144:1102–1108.

186. Silver MA, et al. Effect of nesiritide versus dobutamine on short-term outcomes in the treatment of patients with acutely decompensated heart failure. *J Am Coll Cardiol* 2002;39:798–803.

187. VMAC Investigators. Intravenous nesiritide vs nitroglycerin for treatment of decompensated congestive heart failure. *JAMA* 2002;287:1531–1540.

188. Zafeiridis A, et al. Regression of cellular hypertrophy after left ventricular assist device support. *Circulation* 1998;98:623–624.

189. Katz AM. Regression of left ventricular hypertrophy. New hope for dying hearts (Editorial). *Circulation* 1998;98:623–624.

190. Gottdiener J, et al. Outcome of congestive heart failure in elderly persons: influence of left ventricular systolic function. The Cardiovascular Health Study. *Ann Intern Med* 2002;137:631–639.

191. Yusuf S, et al. Effects of candesartan in patients with chronic heart failure and preserved left-ventricular ejection fraction: the CHARM-Preserved Trial. *Lancet* 2003;362:777–781.

192. Westheim AS, et al. Hemodynamic and neuroendocrine effects for candoxatril and frusemide in mild stable chronic heart failure. *J Am Coll Cardiol* 1999;34:794–801.

193. Kasper EK, et al. A randomized trial of the efficacy of multidisciplinary care in heart failure outpatients at high risk of hospital readmission. *J Am Coll Cardiol* 2002;39:471–480.

194. Cotter G, et al. Randomized trial of high-dose isosorbide dinitrate plus low-dose furosemide versus high-dose furosemide plus low-dose Isosorbide dinitrate in severe pulmonary edema. *Lancet* 1998;351:389–393.

195. Annane D, et al. Placebo-controlled randomized double-blind study of intravenous enalaprilat of efficacy and safety in acute cardiogenic pulmonary edema. *Circulation* 1996;94:1360–1324.

196. Hamilton RJ, et al. Rapid improvement of acute pulmonary edema with sublingual captopril. *Acad Emerg Med* 1996;3:205–212.

197. Moritz F, et al. Boussignac continuous positive airway pressure device in the emergency care of acute cardiogenic pulmonary oedema: a randomized pilot study. *Eur J Emerg Med* 2003;10:204–208.

198. Mehta S, et al. Randomized, prospective trial of bilevel versus continuous positive airway pressure in acute pulmonary edema. *Crit Care Med* 1997;25:620–628.

199. Patel R, et al. Simvastatin induces regression of cardiac hypertrophy and fibrosis and improves cardiac function in a transgenic rabbit model of human hypertrophic cardiomyopathy. *Circulation* 2001;104:317–324.

200. Semsarian C, et al. The L-type calcium channel inhibitor diltiazem prevents cardiomyopathy in a mouse model. *J Clin Invest* 2002;109:1013–1020.
201. Matsubara H. Salutory effect of disopyramide on left ventricular diastolic function in hypertrophic obstructive cardiomyopathy. *J Am Coll Cardiol* 1995;26:768–775.
202. Betocchi S, et al. Effects of diltiazem on left ventricular systolic and diastolic function in hypertrophic cardiomyopathy. *Am J Cardiol* 1996;78:451–457.
203. Sherrid MV, et al. Mechanism of benefit of negative inotropes in obstructive hypertrophic cardiomyopathy. *Circulation* 1998;97:41–47.
204. Sitges M, et al. Comparison of left ventricular diastolic function in obstructive hypertrophic cardiomyopathy in patients undergoing percutaneous septal ablation versus surgical myotomy/myectomy. *Am J Cardiol* 2003;91:817–821.
205. Schwammenthal E, Levine RA. Dynamic subaortic obstruction: a disease of the mitral valve suitable for surgical repair? *J Am Coll Cardiol* 1996;28:203–206.
206. van der Lee C, et al. Sustained improvement after combined anterior mitral leaflet extension and myectomy in hypertrophic obstructive cardiomyopathy. *Circulation* 2003;108:2088–2092.
207. Maron BJ, et al. Efficacy of implantable cardioverter-defibrillators for the prevention of sudden death in patients with hypertrophic cardiomyopathy. *N Engl J Med* 2000;342:365–373.
208. Sorajja P, et al. Adverse prognosis of patients with hypertrophic cardiomyopathy who have epicardial coronary artery disease. *Circulation* 2003;108:2342–2348.
209. McNamara D, et al. Controlled trial of intravenous immune globulin in recent-onset dilated cardiomyopathy. *Circulation* 2001;103:2254–2259.
210. Cooper L, et al. Multicenter Giant-Cell Myocarditis Study Group Investigators. Idiopathyic Giant-Cell Myocarditis–Natural History and Treatment. *N Engl J Med* 1997;336:1860–1866.
211. Bradley DJ, et al. Cardiac resynchronization and death from progressive heart failure. *JAMA* 2003;289:730–740.
212. Stevenson L. The Points for Pacing. *J Am Coll Cardiol* 2003;42:1460–1462.
212a. Bristow MR, et al. Cardiac resynchronization therapy with or without an implantable defibrillator in advanced chronic heart failure. *N Engl J Med* 2004;350:2140–2150.
213. REMATCH Study Group. Long-term use of a left ventricular assist device for end-stage heart failure. *N Engl J Med* 2001;345:1435–1443.
214. Batista R. Partial left ventriculectomy—the Batista Procedure. *Eur J Cardiothoracic Surg* 1999;15:S12–S19.
215. Dajani A, et al. Treatment of acute streptococcal pharyngitis and prevention of rheumatic fever; a statement for health professionals. *Pediatrics* 1995;96:758–764.
216. Shapera RM, et al. Erythromycin therapy twice daily for streptococcal pharyngitis; a controlled comparison with erythromycin or penicillin phenoxymethyl four times daily or benicillin G benzathine. *JAMA* 1973;226:531–535.
217. Hein S, et al. Progression from compensated hypertrophy to failure in the pressure-overloaded human heart. Structural deterioration and compensatory mechanisms. *Circulation* 2003;107:984–991.
218. Pereira J, et al. Survival after aortic valve replacement for severe aortic stenosis with low transvalvular gradients and severe left ventricular dysfunction. *J Am Coll Cardiol* 2002;39:1356–1363.
219. Khot UN, et al. Nitroprusside in critically ill patients with left ventricular dysfunction and aortic stenosis. *N Engl J Med* 2003;348:1756–1763.
220. Rajamannan N, et al. Calcific aortic stenosis: from bench to the bedside—emerging clinical and cellular concepts. *Heart* 2003;89:801–805.
221. Bonow RO, et al. ACC/AHA Guidelines for the Management of Patients with Valvular Heart Disease; a report of the American College of Cardiology/AHA Task Force on Practice Guidelines (Committee on Management of Patients with Valvular Heart Disease). *J Am Coll Cardiol* 1998;32:1486–1588.
222. Vincentelli A, et al. Acquired von Willebrand syndrome in aortic stenosis. *N Engl J Med* 2003;349:343–349.
223. Cribier A, et al. Percutaneous transcatheter implantation of an aortic valve prosthesis for calcific aortic stenosis. *Circulation* 2002;106:3006–3008.
224. Prendergast BD, et al. Valvular heart disease; recommendations for investigation and management; summary of guidelines produced by a Working Group at the British Cardiac Society in the Research Unit of the Royal College of Physicians. *J Royal Coll Phys* 1995;30:309–315.
225. Galal O, et al. Follow-up results of balloon aortic valvuloplasty in children with special reference to causes of late aortic insufficiency. *Am Heart J* 1997;133:418–427.
226. Iung B, et al. Late results of percutaneous mitral commissurotomy in a series of 1024 patients. Analysis of late clinical deterioration, frequency, anatomic findings and predictive factors. *Circulation* 1999;99:3272–3278.
227. Borer J, et al. Contemporary approach to aortic and mitral regurgitation. *Circulation* 2003;108:2432–2438.
228. Scognamiglio R, et al. Nifedipine in asymptomatic patients with severe aortic regurgitation and normal left ventricular function. *N Engl J Med* 1994;331:689–694.
229. Runo J, et al. Primary pulmonary hypertension. *Lancet* 2003;361:1533–1544.
230. Fuster V, et al. Primary pulmonary hypertension: natural history and the importance of thrombosis. *Circulation* 1984;70:580–587.
231. Olschewski H, et al. Inhaled iloprost for severe pulmonary hypertension. *N Engl J Med* 2002;347:322–329.
232. Galie N, et al. Effects of beraprost sodium, an oral prostacyclin analogue in patients with pulmonary arterial hypertension: a randomized double-blind, placebo-controlled trial. *J Am Coll Cardiol* 2002;139:1496–1502.

233. Rubin L, et al. Bosentan therapy for pulmonary arterial hypertension. *N Engl J Med* 2002;346:896–903.
234. Michelakis E, et al. Long-Term treatment with oral sildenafil is safe and improves functional capacity and hemodynamics in patients with pulmonary arterial hypertension. *Circulation* 2003;108:2066–2069.
235. National Cholesterol Education Program Expert Panel. Detection, evaluation and treatment of high blood cholesterol in adults. (Adult Treatment Panel III). *Circulation* 2002;106:3143–3421.
236. Plutzky J. Peroxisome Proliferator-Activated Receptors as Therapeutic Targets in Inflammation. *J Am Coll Cardiol* 2003;42:1764–1766.
237. Sobel BE, et al. Burgeoning dilemmas in the management of diabetes and cardiovascular disease: rationale for the Bypass Angioplasty Revascularization Investigation 2 Diabetes (BARI 2D) trial. *Circulation* 2003;107:636–642.
238. UKPDS 38. UK Prospective Diabetes Study Group. Tight blood pressure control and risk of macrovascular and microvascular complications in type 2 diabetes: UKPDS 38. *Br Med J* 1998;317:703–713.
239. Williams K, et al. Comparison of the associations of apolipoprotein B and low-density lipoprotein cholesterol with other cardiovascular risk factors in the Insulin Resistance Atherosclerosis Study (IRAS). *Circulation* 2003;108:2312–1216.
240. Nesto R, et al. Thiazolidienone use, fluid retention, and congestive heart failure. *Circulation* 2003;108:2941–2948.
241. Detre KM, et al. The effect of previous coronary-artery bypass surgery on the prognosis of patients with diabetes who have acute myocardial infarction. *N Engl J Med* 2000;342:989–997.
242. MICRO-HOPE Study. Effects of ramipril on cardiovascular and microvascular outcomes in people with diabetes mellitus: results of the HOPE study and the MICRO-HOPE substudy. *Lancet* 2000;355:253–259.
243. Opie LH, et al. Diabetic nephropathy. Can renoprotection be extrapolated to cardiovascular protection? (Editorial). *Circulation* 2002;106:643–645.
244. Sattar N, et al. Metabolic syndrome with and without C-reactive protein as a predictor of coronary heart disease and diabetes in the West of Scotland Coronary Prevention Study. *Circulation* 2003;108:414–419.
245. Kahn H, et al. Metabolic risks identified by the combination of enlarged waist and elevated triacylglycerol concentration. *Am J Clin Nutr* 2003;78:902–903.
246. Tuomilehto J, et al. Prevention of Type-2 Diabetes Mellitus by Changes in Lifestyle among Subjects with Impaired Glucose Tolerance. *N Engl J Med* 2001;344:1343–1350.
247. Moreillon P, et al. Infective endocarditis. *Lancet* 2004;363:139–149.
248. Vikram HR, et al. Impact of valve surgery on 6-month mortality in adults with complicated, left-sided native valve endocarditis: a propensity analysis. *JAMA* 2003;290:3207–3214.
249. Dajani AS, et al. Prevention of bacterial endocarditis; recommendations by the American Heart Association. *Circulation* 1997;96:358–366.
250. Burns P, et al. Management of peripheral arterial disease in primary care. *Br Med J* 2003;326:584–588.
251. Meijer W, et al. Determinants of peripheral arterial disease in the elderly: the Rotterdam study. *Arch Intern Med* 2000;160:2493–2498.
252. CAPRIE Steering Committee. A randomized, blinded trial of clopidogrel versus aspirin in patients at risk of ischemic events (CAPRIE). *Lancet* 1996;348:1329–1339.
253. Dawson D, et al. A comparison of cilostazol and pentoxyfylline for treating intermittent claudication. *Am J Med* 2000;109:523–530.
254. Pittler M, et al. Ginkgo Biloba extract for the treatment of intermittent claudication: a meta-analysis of randomised trials. *Am J Med* 2000;108:276–281.
255. Radack K, et al. Beta-adrenergic blocker therapy does not worsen intermittent claudication in subjects with peripheral arterial disease. A meta-analysis of randomized controlled trials. *Arch Intern Med* 1991;151:1769–1776.
256. Bagger JP, et al. Effect of verapamil in intermittent claudication. A randomized, double-blind, placebo-controlled, cross-over study after individual dose-response assessment. *Circulation* 1997;95:411–414.
257. Coppock JS, et al. Objective relief of vasospasm by glycerol trinitrate in secondary Raynaud's phenomenon. *Postgrad Med J* 1986;62:15–18.
258. Mazer S, et al. Reverse CPR: a pilot study of CPR in the prone position. *Resuscitation* 2003;57:279–285.
259. Stiell I, et al. Health-related quality of life is better for cardiac arrest survivors who received citizen cardiopulmonary resuscitation. *Circulation* 2003;108:1939–1944.
260. Bunch T, et al. Long-term outcomes of out-of-hospital cardiac arrest after successful early defibrillation. *N Engl J Med* 2003;348.
261. AHA in Collaboration with the International Liaison Committee on Resuscitation (ILCOR). Guidelines 2000 for Cardiopulmonary Resuscitation and Emergency Cardiovascular Care. *Circulation* 2000;102:I-142–I-157.
262. Kudenchuk PJ, et al. Amiodarone for resuscitation after out-of-hospital cardiac arrest due to ventricular fibrillation. *N Engl J Med* 1999;341:871–878.
263. Dorian P, et al. Amiodarone as compared with lidocaine for shock-resistant ventricular fibrillation. *N Engl J Med* 2002;346:884–890.
264. Wenzel V, et al. A comparison of vasopressin and epinephrine for out-of-hospital cardiopulmonary resuscitation. *N Engl J Med* 2004;350:105–113.
265. Schneider T, et al. Multicenter randomized controlled trial of 150-J biphasic shocks compared with 200- to 30-J monophasic shocks in the resuscitation of out-of-hospital cardiac arrest victims. *Circulation* 2000;102:1780–1787.
266. Morley P. Vasopressin or epinephrine: which initial vasopressor for cardiac arrests? *Lancet* 2001;358:85–86.

267. McIntyre KM. Vasopressin in asystolic cardiac arrest. *N Engl J Med* 2004;350:
     179–181.
268. Brown C, et al. A comparison of standard-dose and high-dose epinephrine in cardiac
     arrest outside the hospital. *N Engl J Med* 1992;327:1051–1055.
269. Criley J, et al. Cough-induced cardiac compression. Self-administered from car-
     diopulmonary resuscitation. *JAMA* 1976;236:1246–1250.
270. Nolan J, et al. Therapeutic hypothermia after cardiac arrest. An advisory statement
     by the advanced life support task force of the International liaison committee on
     resuscitation. *Circulation* 2003;108:118–121.
271. Volgman AS, et al. Conversion efficacy and safety of intravenous ibutilide compared
     with intravenous procainamide in patients with atrial flutter or fibrillation. *J Am Coll
     Cardiol* 1998;31:1414–1419.
272. VanderLugt J, et al. Efficacy and safety of ibutilide fumarate for the conversion of
     atrial arrhythmias after cardiac surgery. *Circulation* 1999;100:369–375.

Index

Note: Page numbers followed by f refer to figures; page numbers followed by t refer to tables.

A

Abciximab, 286t, 288–289, 290
  acute coronary syndrome for, 364t
  during pregnancy, 401t
  vs. tirofiban, 291
Acebutolol, 2t, 22t, 27, 237. *See also* Beta-blockers.
  hepatic metabolism of, 20, 21f
  lipid effects of, 330t
  renal excretion of, 21, 21f
Acetazolamide, 95
N-Acetylcysteine, nitroglycerin with, 45
Acetylsalicylic acid. *See* Aspirin.
Activated charcoal, in digoxin toxicity, 161
Activated partial thromboplastin time, 293
Acute coronary syndromes, 9, 9f, 285f, 354–360, 354f, 355f, 359t. *See also* Angina pectoris; Myocardial infarction.
  antiplatelet agents in, 282, 285–286, 285f, 287, 355–357
  beta-blockers in, 9, 9f, 357–358
  calcium channel blockers in, 358
  clopidogrel in, 285, 287, 354f, 355, 355f
  conservative vs. invasive strategy in, 358
  glycoprotein IIb/IIIa receptor antagonists in, 285f, 286t, 288–291, 288t, 357
  heparin in, 294, 295, 356
  invasive strategy, 358
  nitroglycerin in, 357
  non-ST elevation, 359t
  phosphodiesterase-5 inhibitors and, 39
  ST elevation, 363t
  triage, 356
Acute myocardial infarction. *See* Myocardial infarction.
Adenosine, 220t, 221t, 248–250, 249f
  contraindications to, 250
  dipyridamole interaction with, 230t, 250
  dose of, 221t, 249
  drug interactions with, 230t, 250
  in heart failure, 175
  in paroxysmal supraventricular tachycardia, 221t, 249, 253–254

Adenosine *(Continued)*
  in Wolff-Parkinson-White syndrome, 249
  indications for, 249–250
  proarrhythmic effects of, 250
  side effects of, 250
A_1-Adenosine receptor antagonists, diuretic effect of, 95
Adrenocorticotropic hormone, furosemide interaction with, 84
African-American patients
  ACE inhibitors for, 125, 208
  beta-blockers for, 11, 208
  calcium channel blockers for, 12, 208
  hypertension in, 128–129, 203
Afterload reduction, in heart failure, 171–172
Alacepril, 113t. *See also* Angiotensin-converting enzyme (ACE) inhibitors.
Albuterol, in heart failure, 168
Alcohol septal ablation, in hypertrophic cardiomyopathy, 388
Alcohol use, 345–346
Aldactazide, 95
Aldosterone, 140–141, 141f
  excess of, 108f, 109
  in heart failure, 104, 109, 125
  inhibitors of. *See* Aldosterone antagonists; Angiotensin-converting enzyme (ACE) inhibitors.
Aldosterone antagonists
  in heart failure, 94, 94t, 120–121, 123, 140–142, 141f, 180–181
  in hypertension, 94, 196
  outcomes trials of, 114t
Alka-Seltzer, 283
Allopurinol, 92
Almonds, 346
Alpha-blockers, 186f, 186t, 205
  for elderly patients, 207
  lipid effects of, 206, 330t
Alteplase, 292f, 305t, 307–308, 310t
  prehospital, 306
  vs. streptokinase, 306–307
AMI. *See* Acute myocardial infarction.
Amiloride, 81t, 82f, 93, 94t, 196
Aminoglycosides, diuretic interaction with, 84, 90
Amiodarone, 220t, 224t, 237–243
  after myocardial infarction, 383

Amiodarone *(Continued)*
  beta-blocker interaction with, 240, 243
  cardiac arrest and, 265
  CNS side effects of, 242
  contraindications to, 240
  corneal side effects of, 242
  digoxin interaction with, 159, 243
  disopyramide interaction with, 229t
  dose of, 224t, 239, 242
  drug interactions with, 159, 229t, 240, 243
  during pregnancy, 401t
  electrophysiology of, 238
  flecainide interaction with, 229t
  gastrointestinal side effects of, 242
  in atrial fibrillation, 240, 258, 258t, 259, 260f
  in heart failure, 240, 242
  in paroxysmal supraventricular tachycardia, 254
  in ventricular arrhythmias, 224t, 239–240, 264–265, 383
  indications for, 239–240
  intravenous, 240
  low-dose, 240
  pharmacokinetics of, 239
  phenytoin interaction with, 243
  pigmentation with, 243
  pulmonary side effects of, 242
  quinidine interaction with, 229t
  side effects of, 228t, 240, 242–243
  sotalol interaction with, 229t, 243
  thyroid side effects of, 242
  torsades de pointes with, 240, 242
  toxicity screening with, 243
  trials with, 240, 241t
  visual side effects of, 242
  warfarin interaction with, 229t, 243
Amlodipine, 73–75
  cautions with, 74
  contraindications to, 71t, 74
  dose of, 71t, 74–75
  drug interactions with, 71t, 74
  for elderly patients, 207
  in coronary spasm, 58
  in effort angina, 74
  in hypertension, 60, 74, 76t, 186f
  in Prinzmetal's (variant) angina, 74
  lipid effects of, 330t, 331
  outcome trials of, 75, 76t
  pharmacokinetics of, 74
  side effects of, 66t, 71t, 74–75
  vascular protective effects of, 53
  vs. lisinopril, 59
Amrinone
  in beta-blocker overdose, 27
  in heart failure, 170f
Amyl nitrite, 36t. *See also* Nitrates.
Anemia, enalapril and, 125
Anesthetics
  lidocaine interaction with, 229t, 232
  nifedipine interaction with, 70, 72
Aneurysm, dissecting, beta-blockers in, 17
Angina pectoris, 350–354
  ACE inhibitors in, 352

Angina pectoris *(Continued)*
  antianginal drugs, 351f
  aspirin in, 282
  beta-blockers in, 2t, 7–8, 11, 351–352, 351f
    withdrawal of, 8
  calcium channel blockers in, 351–352, 351f
  cold intolerance and, 8
  cotherapy in, 8
  effort
    amlodipine in, 74
    beta-blockers in, 7, 8
    calcium channel blockers in, 56, 60, 64, 68, 69, 72–73, 74
    combination therapy for, 46–47
    diltiazem in, 68
    nifedipine in, 60
    nitrates in, 39
    nitroglycerin in, 39, 350–351
    revascularization for, 353–354
    step-care for, 42, 42t, 46
    triple therapy for, 47
    verapamil in, 64
  exercise in, 7
  glycoprotein IIb/IIIa receptor antagonists in, 289
  hypertension and, 206
  ivabradine in, 352
  long-term prophylaxis for, 358, 360
  management, 350
  mixed (double-component), 8
  nicorandil in, 352
  nitrates in, 9f, 33–34, 39–41, 42–43, 350–351, 351f. *See also* Nitrates.
  Prinzmetal's (variant), 8, 64, 68, 73, 74, 360
  ranolazine in, 352
  refractory, 353
  revascularization, 353
  risk factor modification in, 352
  trimetazidine in, 352
  triple therapy in, 8
  unstable, 9, 9f
    aspirin in, 9f
    beta-blockers in, 9, 9f, 11
    calcium channel blockers in, 9f, 58
    dalteparin in, 295
    diltiazem in, 9f, 58, 68
    enoxaparin in, 295
    glycoprotein IIb/IIIa receptor blockers in, 9f, 289
    heparin in, 9f, 292–293, 294
    lepirudin in, 297
    nifedipine in, 9f, 69, 73
    nitrates in, 9f, 39. *See also* Nitrates.
    verapamil in, 64
  vitamin E supplements and, 352
Angioedema, ACE inhibitors and, 117
Angioplasty. *See* Percutaneous coronary interventions.
Angiotensin-converting enzyme (ACE), 106
  gene polymorphism of, 111
Angiotensin-converting enzyme (ACE) inhibitors, 104–134

Angiotensin-converting enzyme
(ACE) inhibitors (*Continued*)
after myocardial infarction, 10,
126, 127f, 373–374
angioedema and, 117
angiotensin-II receptor blocker
with, 137
anti-ischemic effect of, 126–127
antiadrenergic effects of, 109
antialdosterone effect of, 94–95
antiarrhythmic effects of, 109, 261
aspirin interaction with, 283–284
beta-blockers with, 10, 119–120
bradykinin formation and, 110,
110t
calcium channel blockers with,
197t
cardiovascular protection with,
126–127
classes of, 112, 113t, 115f
cough and, 112, 116, 116f
creatinine level and, 117, 123, 124
diabetes mellitus and, 125–126
diuretics with, 196–197, 197t, 204
enzyme genotypes and, 111
eplerenone with, 123
for African-American patients, 208
for elderly patients, 207–208
hyperkalemia and, 116, 116f
hyponatremia and, 116, 124
hypotension and, 116, 116f
in acute pulmonary edema, 387
in angina pectoris, 352
in diabetes mellitus, 125–126,
127–128, 130, 135, 203, 209,
395
in early phase myocardial
infarction, 126
in heart failure, 16, 100, 117–125,
180, 384. *See also* Heart
failure, ACE inhibitors in.
in hypertension, 109, 121t,
125–126, 201
in postinfarct left ventricular
dysfunction, 126, 127f
in renal failure, 128–129
indications for, 112, 112t
lipid effects of, 330t
mechanisms of action of,
104–112, 104t, 105f, 106f
neurohumoral effects of, 119
neutropenia and, 117
nitrate with, 45
outcomes trials of, 112, 114
potassium retention with, 94–95
pregnancy contraindication to,
117, 204, 401t
renal side effects of, 116–117,
116f, 124
renin-angiotensin-aldosterone
system and, 108–109, 108f
renin secretion and, 109, 110
selection of, 134
side effects of, 112, 115t, 116–117,
116f
sodium status and, 109
spironolactone with, 123, 204
tissue renin-angiotensin systems
and, 110, 111f
vs. angiotensin-II receptor
blockers, 121t, 122t, 140

Angiotensin-converting enzyme
(ACE) inhibitors (*Continued*)
vs. calcium channel blockers, 59,
201
Angiotensin-I, 104, 106f
Angiotensin-II, 105t, 106, 106f, 107
ACE inhibitor effect on, 110, 110f
adrenergic activity of, 109
aldosterone stimulation by, 109
in renal failure, 128, 129f
renin inhibition by, 109
Angiotensin-II receptor, 107–108,
107f, 136f
Angiotensin-II receptor blockers,
104, 112, 134–140
ACE inhibitor with, 137
compared with ACE inhibition,
122t, 136f
contraindications to, 115t
diuretic with, 137, 139, 197t
in diabetes mellitus, 135, 209,
395
in heart failure, 16, 135–136,
136f, 178–179, 180–181,
384
in hypertension, 121t, 134, 137,
138t, 140, 204–205
in myocardial infarction, 368
lipid effects of, 330t
outcomes trials of, 114t
potassium retention with, 94–95
pregnancy contraindication to,
401t
vs. ACE inhibitors, 121t, 122t, 140
Angiotensinogen, 104
Antacids, rosuvastatin interaction
with, 63
Antiarrhythmic drugs, 219–270. *See
also specific arrthythmias.*
class IA, 219–220, 220t, 223t,
225–230, 225f, 228t,
235–236
class IB, 220t, 223t–224t,
230–233, 231f, 235
class IC, 220t, 224t, 233–235,
236, 241t
class II, 220t, 221t, 236–237, 241t
class III, 220t, 222t, 224t,
237–248, 241t
class IV, 220t, 221t, 222t,
248–250, 249f
class IV-like, 220t, 221t, 248–250
classification of, 219, 220t,
221t–222t, 223t–224t
combinations of, 250
digoxin interaction with, 159,
159t
proarrhythmic effects of, 234,
251–252, 252f, 260
QT-prolongation with, 244, 245f,
252
thiazide diuretic interaction with,
90
trials with, 240, 241t
Antibiotics
digoxin with, 154
diuretic interaction with, 84, 90
dofetilide interaction with, 248
in infective endocarditis,
397–398, 397t
warfarin interaction with, 299

Anticoagulants. See Heparin; Warfarin.
Antihistaminics, QT-prolongation with, 245f
Antihypertensive drugs, 185–215, 186f, 186t. See also Hypertension.
Antioxidants, 345
Antiplatelet agents, 284–291, 285f, 286t, 288t, 355–357. See also specific platelet inhibitors.
    warfarin interaction with, 299–300
Antipsychotics, QT-prolongation with, 245f
Antivirals, dofetilide interaction with, 248
Anuria, furosemide and, 83
Anxiety, beta-blockers in, 2t, 17
Aortic regurgitation, 392–393
Aortic stenosis, 391–392
Aortocoronary saphenous vein bypass graft, low-dose warfarin in, 304
Apolipoprotein B, in coronary artery disease, 327
Apoptosis
    beta-blockers and, 16
    catecholamines and, 165
L-Arginine, with nitrates, 46
Arrhythmias. See also Antiarrhythmic drugs and specific arrhythmias.
    drug-induced, 91–92, 159–161, 160f, 160t, 234, 251–252, 251f, 259
    therapy of, 375t
Arteriovenous shunt, aspirin with, 283
Aspirin, 281–284
    ACE inhibitors with, 123
    after coronary artery bypass surgery, 282–283
    after myocardial infarction, 373, 374
    anti-inflammatory effects of, 281, 282
    before coronary angioplasty, 283
    clinical use of, 282–284
    contraindications to, 283
    drug interactions with, 283–284
    during pregnancy, 401t
    gastrointestinal side effects of, 281, 283
    glycoprotein IIb/IIIa receptor antagonists with, 289–290
    in acute coronary syndromes, 282, 283, 354f, 355, 355f
    in arteriovenous shunt, 283
    in atrial fibrillation, 283, 379
    in renovascular hypertension, 283
    in stroke prevention, 283
    low-dose, 283
    platelet inhibition with, 281
    resistance to, 281–282
    side effects of, 283
    warfarin interaction with, 299–300
    with prosthetic heart valves, 283
Astemizole, QT-prolongation with, 245f

Asthma, beta-blocker contraindication in, 21, 25
Asystole, 400, 402, 403f
Atenolol, 2t, 23t, 27–28. See also Beta-blockers.
    after myocardial infarction, 10–11
    for African-American patients, 11
    in atrial fibrillation, 256t, 257
    in silent myocardial ischemia, 8, 11
    intellectual effects of, 211
    lipid effects of, 330t
    renal excretion of, 21, 21f
    side effects of, 24, 211
Atherosclerosis. See Coronary artery disease.
Atorvastatin, 333t, 335t, 338–339. See also Statins.
    clopidogrel interaction with, 287
    verapamil interaction with, 62
Atrial fibrillation, 255–262, 374–379, 375f, 376t
    acute onset, 375–377, 376t
    algorithm for, 260f
    amiodarone in, 240, 258, 258t, 259, 260f
    anticoagulation in, 262, 379
    aspirin in, 283, 379
    atenolol in, 256t, 257
    azimilide in, 378–379
    beta-blockers in, 2t, 13, 256t, 257
    cardioversion in, 258–259, 376t, 378
    carvedilol in, 257
    catheter ablation in, 379
    chronic, 377–379
    digoxin in, 156, 256t, 257
    diltiazem in, 68, 256t, 257
    disopyramide in, 258t
    dofetilide in, 246–247, 258, 258t, 259, 260f, 378–379
    drug selection algorithm for, 259, 260f
    esmolol in, 256t, 257
    flecainide in, 258–259, 258t, 260, 260f
    guidelines for, 261
    ibutilide in, 245–246, 258, 258t
    in heart failure, 181, 385
    in hypertension, 210, 211
    in hypertrophic cardiomyopathy, 389
    in myocardial infarction, 369
    intermittent, 302
    "lone," 302
    low-dose warfarin in, 304
    magnesium in, 248
    maze operation in, 379
    metoprolol in, 256t, 257
    nadolol in, 256t, 257
    pacemaker in, 257
    paroxysmal, 260f
    persistent, 260f
    pharmacological conversion of, 258–259, 258t
    pindolol in, 256t, 257
    postoperative, 260
    presentation of, 256
    procainamide in, 258, 258t
    propafenone in, 235, 258–259, 258t, 260, 260f

Atrial fibrillation *(Continued)*
  propranolol in, 256t, 257
  quinidine in, 258t
  radiofrequency catheter ablation
    in, 261–262
  rate control in, 256–257, 256t,
    261, 377–378
  recurrent, 378
  renin-angiotensin inhibition in,
    259
  sinus rhythm maintenance in,
    258–262, 260f, 378–379
  sinus rhythm restoration in,
    258–262, 258t, 260f
  sotalol in, 244, 258t, 260, 260f
  stroke and, 260, 261, 262, 283,
    298, 302–303
  transesophageal echocardiography
    in, 377
  ventricular preexcitation with, 257
  verapamil in, 64, 256t, 257
  warfarin in, 262, 301–303, 379
  Wolff-Parkinson-White syndrome
    with, 158
  ximelagatran in, 298, 379
Atrial flutter, 262–263, 379. *See also*
    Atrial fibrillation.
  amiodarone in, 240
  diltiazem in, 68
  dofetilide in, 246–247, 263
  ibutilide in, 245–246, 263
  verapamil and, 64
Atrial septal defect, anticoagulation
    in, 302
Atrial stunning, 377
Atrial tachycardia, 253f, 254
Atrioventricular block with syncope,
    381
Atrioventricular nodal heart block,
    158
Atrioventricular nodal reentrant
    tachycardia, 252–255, 253f
Atrioventricular nodal reentry, 226f
Atrioventricular reentrant
    tachycardia, 252–255, 253f
Atropine, in bradyarrhythmias, 27
Azimilide, 248
  in atrial fibrillation, 378–379
  in paroxysmal supraventricular
    tachycardia, 254

B

Bed rest, in heart failure, 179–180
Benazepril, 113t, 115f, 133. *See also*
    Angiotensin-converting enzyme
    (ACE) inhibitors.
Bendrofluazide, 88t, 196. *See also*
    Thiazide diuretics.
Benecol margarine, 345
Benthiazide, 88t. *See also* Thiazide
    diuretics.
Benznidazole, in Chagas' disease,
    390
Beraprost, in pulmonary
    hypertension, 394
Beri-beri heart disease, 399–400
Beta$_1$-adrenergic receptor, 1, 3f
  blockade of, 3, 4f. *See also* Beta-
    blockers.

Beta$_1$-adrenergic receptor
    (Continued)
  downregulation of, 4–5
  in heart failure, 13, 14–15, 14f,
    15f, 162, 162f, 164, 164f
  upregulation of, 5
Beta$_2$-adrenergic receptor, 1, 3, 3f
  in heart failure, 14–15, 14f, 15f,
    16, 162, 164, 164f
Beta$_3$-adrenergic receptor, 3
Beta$_1$-adrenergic receptor kinase, 5,
    14, 14f
Beta-blockers, 1–30, 2t, 220t
  ACE inhibitors with, 10, 119–120
  after myocardial infarction, 2t,
    10–11, 13, 372
  amiodarone interaction with, 240,
    243
  apoptosis and, 16
  bradycardia and, 15, 27
  calcium channel blockers with,
    7–8, 72, 72f, 352
  cardiac contraindications to, 26t
  cardiovascular effects of, 5–7, 6f
  cautions with, 26t–27t
  central nervous system side effects
    of, 24, 26t
  cimetidine interaction with, 21
  concomitant disease and, 21, 24
  contraindications to, 10, 25, 25f,
    26t–27t, 63t, 237, 352
  coronary blood flow and, 5–7, 6f
  digoxin with, 16–17
  disopyramide interaction with,
    229t
  diuretics with, 12, 92, 197t
  drug interactions with, 21, 62,
    229t, 232, 240, 243, 248
  during pregnancy, 26t, 401t
  during surgery, 17, 26t
  elimination of, 20–21, 21f
  flecainide interaction with, 229t
  for African-American patients, 11
  for diabetic hypertensive patient,
    11–12
  for elderly patient, 11, 27t
  half-life of, 20, 22t–23t
  heart rate and, 7, 15, 25, 27
  hepatic metabolism of, 20, 21f
  ideal kinetics of, 21
  in acute coronary syndromes, 9,
    9f, 357–358
  in angina pectoris, 2t, 7–8,
    351–352, 351f
  in anxiety, 2t, 17
  in arrhythmias, 12–13, 13f, 20,
    29, 236–237
  in atrial fibrillation, 2t, 13, 256t,
    257
  in congenital QT-prolongation, 17
  in diabetes mellitus, 11, 24, 26t
  in dissecting aneurysm, 17
  in Fallot's tetralogy, 17
  in glaucoma, 17
  in heart failure, 2t, 10, 13–16, 14f,
    15f, 16t, 178f, 180, 384
  in hypertension, 12, 29, 191t,
    197t, 198–199, 198f, 201
  in hypertrophic cardiomyopathy,
    2t, 16, 388
  in Marfan's syndrome, 17

Beta-blockers *(Continued)*
  in migraine, 2t, 18
  in mitral stenosis, 16–17
  in mitral valve prolapse, 17
  in myocardial infarction, 10–11,
    367–368
  in neurocardiogenic syncope, 17
  in paroxysmal supraventricular
    tachycardia, 254
  in perioperative hypertension, 29
  in peripheral vascular disease, 399
  in silent myocardial ischemia, 8,
    11
  in supraventricular tachycardia, 2t,
    13, 29, 254
  in surgical patient, 17, 26t, 29
  in thyrotoxicosis, 17
  in ventricular arrhythmias, 13,
    266
  intravenous, 28–29
  lidocaine interaction with, 21,
    229t, 232
  lipid effects of, 27t, 206, 330–331,
    330t
  liver effects of, 26t
  membrane stabilizing activity of,
    20
  mexiletine interaction with,
    229t
  nifedipine with, 72
  nitrates with, 7–8, 46, 47
  nonresponse to, 7
  nonselective, 18f, 19, 22t, 23t. *See
    also* Propranolol.
  overdose of, 25, 27
  oxygen-conserving properties of, 3
  peripheral vascular
    contraindications to, 26t
  pharmacokinetic properties of,
    20–21, 21f
  pharmacologic properties of,
    18–20, 18f, 19f
  physiologic effects of, 3, 4f
  protein binding of, 20
  pulmonary contraindications to,
    26t
  quality of life and, 25
  quinidine interaction with, 229t
  Raynaud's phenomenon and, 21
  renal disease and, 24, 26t
  renal metabolism of, 21, 21f
  respiratory disease and, 21
  selective, 18f, 19–20, 22t–23t
  sexual function and, 25
  sick sinus syndrome and, 21
  side effects of, 24–25, 26t–27t,
    211
  systemic circulation and, 7
  ultra-short–acting, 28–29
  verapamil interaction with, 21, 62,
    248
  vs. calcium channel blockers, 50,
    52–53, 53f, 54f, 201
  weight gain and, 25
  withdrawal of, 8
Betaxolol, 23t
  in glaucoma, 17
Bezafibrate, 342–343
Bile acid sequestrants, 332f, 340,
    344
  statin with, 344

Bisoprolol, 2t, 23t, 28. *See also* Beta-
    blockers.
  hepatic metabolism of, 20, 21f
  in heart failure, 16, 16t
  in hypertension, 12
  in surgical patient, 17
Bivalirudin, 292f, 297
  in acute coronary syndromes,
    357
  in myocardial infarction, 367
  streptokinase with, 309
Bleeding
  aspirin and, 283, 284
  glycoprotein IIb/IIIa receptor
    antagonists and, 288
  heparin and, 293
  streptokinase and, 309
  warfarin and, 300
Blood pressure, 185, 187–189, 188t
  ambulatory monitoring of, 187
  early morning, 210
  elevation of, 187, 188t, 189. *See
    also* Hypertension.
  epinephrine effects on, 164
  ideal level of, 187
  in diabetic patient, 394–395
  norepinephrine effects on, 164
  prehypertensive, 187
  sildenafil effects on, 38
Bone, thiazide effects on, 99
Bosentan, in pulmonary
    hypertension, 394
Bradyarrhythmias, 381–382
Bradycardia, 381
  amiodarone and, 242
  atropine in, 361
  beta-blockers and, 15, 25, 27
  nitrates and, 41t
Bradykinin, 110, 110t
Bretylium tosylate, 224t
Bronchospasm
  beta-blockers and, 21, 24, 25
  in acute pulmonary edema, 387
Bumetanide, 84–85
  dose of, 84, 85t
  in heart failure, 84
  in renal edema, 84
  side effects of, 85
Bypass tract. See Wolff-Parkinson-
    White.

C

C-reactive protein, 281, 327
Caffeine, adenosine interaction with,
    230t, 250
Calcium antagonists. See Calcium
    channel blockers.
Calcium, excess of
  diuretics in, 98
  thiazide-related, 92–93
Calcium channel, 50, 52f, 54f
Calcium channel blockers, 50–77,
    51t
  ACE inhibitors with, 197t, 204
  after myocardial infarction, 59,
    372–373
  anti-ischemic effects of, 55, 56f
  beta-blockers with, 7–8, 12, 72,
    72f, 352

Calcium channel blockers
(*Continued*)
classification of, 50, 51t, 53–56,
54f, 55f
dihydropyridine, 50, 51t, 53–55,
54f, 63t, 69–76. *See also*
Amlodipine; Nifedipine.
diuretic effect of, 95
during pregnancy, 401t
efficacy of, 59–60
for African-American patients, 208
for elderly patients, 207
in acute coronary syndromes, 358
in angina pectoris, 9f, 56, 58, 60,
64, 68, 69, 72–73, 74,
351–352, 351f
in atrial fibrillation, 256t, 257
in coronary spasm, 58
in diabetes mellitus, 60
in hypertension, 58–59, 60, 64,
68, 74, 75, 191t, 199–201,
200f, 204
in hypertrophic cardiomyopathy,
388
in ischemic heart disease, 60
in paroxysmal supraventricular
tachycardia, 254
in Prinzmetal's (variant) angina, 8
in pulmonary hypertension,
393–394
in supraventricular tachycardia,
56, 59, 64
indications for, 56–59
lipid effects of, 330t, 331
nitrates with, 46
non-dihydropyridine, 50, 51t,
55–56, 55f. *See also*
Diltiazem; Verapamil.
outcome trials of, 75, 76t
pharmacologic properties of, 50,
52–53
safety of, 59–60, 75
side effects of, 56, 66t
vascular effects of, 52–53, 53f,
59
vs. ACE inhibitors, 59
vs. beta-blockers, 50, 52–53, 53f,
54f, 201
Calcium sensitizers, in heart failure,
168–169
Calmodulin, calcium interaction
with, 52
Candesartan, 114t, 137–138, 138t.
See also Angiotensin-II receptor
blockers.
Candoxatril, 176
Canrenone, 142
Captopril. *See also* Angiotensin-
converting enzyme (ACE)
inhibitors.
after myocardial infarction, 130
contraindications to, 130
dose for, 113t, 124, 129–130
in acute pulmonary edema, 387
in acute severe hypertension, 203,
212, 213t
in diabetic nephropathy, 130
in heart failure, 113t, 114t, 120t,
130
in hypertension, 129–130, 212,
213t

Captopril (*Continued*)
in hypertensive emergency, 212,
213t
in renovascular hypertension,
203
indications for, 129–130
neutropenia and, 117, 130
precautions with, 130–131
proteinuria and, 130
side effects of, 130
sublingual, 203
vs. furosemide, 119
Carbamazepine, verapamil
interaction with, 63
Carbonic anhydrase inhibitors, 82f,
95
Cardiac arrest, 400, 402–403, 402f,
403f
amiodarone and, 265
long-term care after, 403
prevention of, 266–268, 268f
shock after, 403
Cardiac edema, indapamide in, 91
Cardiac output, 185
digoxin effect on, 154
in myocardial infarction, 370
Cardiac resynchronization therapy,
182, 268, 268f
Cardiac tamponade, nitrates and,
41t
Cardiogenic shock, 150, 151–152,
369–371
Cardiomyopathy
dilated, 389–390
anticoagulation in, 302
implantable cardioverter-
defibrillator in, 267,
389–390
left ventricular assist device in,
390
transplantation in, 390
hypertrophic, 387–389
alcohol septal ablation in, 388
arrhythmias in, 389
beta-blockers in, 2t, 16, 388
digoxin and, 158
disopyramide in, 388
dual chamber pacing in, 388
nitrates and, 41t
surgery in, 388–389
verapamil in, 64–65, 388
restrictive, 390–391
Cardiopulmonary resuscitation, 400,
402–403, 402f, 403f
Cardioversion
in atrial fibrillation, 258t, 259,
376t, 378
in atrial flutter, 263
Carotid artery disease, verapamil in,
65
Carteolol, 2t, 22t
in glaucoma, 17
renal excretion of, 21, 21f
Carvedilol, 2t, 23t, 28. *See also* Beta-
blockers.
hepatic metabolism of, 20, 21f
in angina pectoris, 7
in atrial fibrillation, 257
in heart failure, 16, 16t, 179–180
lipid effects of, 330t
postinfarct, 10–11

Catheter ablation
   in atrial fibrillation, 261–262, 379
   in paroxysmal supraventricular
      tachycardia, 254–255, 255f,
      381
   in ventricular tachycardia, 383
Celiprolol, 28. *See also* Beta-
      blockers.
Cerebral ischemia
   atrial fibrillation and, 260, 261,
      262, 283, 298, 302–303
   low-dose warfarin in, 304
Cerivastatin, 334
Chagas' disease, 390
Chaotic multifocal atrial tachycardia,
      379–380
Charcoal, activated, in digoxin
      toxicity, 161
Chlorothiazide, 88t. *See also*
      Thiazide diuretics.
Chlorthalidone, 88t, 89. *See also*
      Thiazide diuretics.
   for African-American patients, 208
   impotence and, 93
   in hypertension, 89, 195
   lipid effects of, 92
Cholelithiasis, fibrates and, 341–342
Cholesterol, 323, 325t, 326f. *See also*
      Lipid(s); Lipoproteins; Statins.
   in diabetes mellitus, 328
   non-HDL, 327
   thiazide diuretic effects on, 92
Cholesterol absorption inhibitors,
      343–344
Cholestyramine, 340, 344
   in digoxin toxicity, 161
Cigarette smoking
   beta-blockers and, 27t
   hypertension and, 208
Cilazapril, 113t, 115f, 133. *See also*
      Angiotensin-converting enzyme
      (ACE) inhibitors.
Cilostazol, in peripheral vascular
      disease, 399
Cimetidine
   beta-blocker interaction with, 21
   dofetilide interaction with, 230t
   lidocaine interaction with, 229t,
      232
   nifedipine interaction with, 70
   procainamide interaction with, 229t
   quinidine interaction with, 229t
   verapamil interaction with, 63
   warfarin interaction with, 299
Cirrhosis, torsemide in, 86
Claudication, 398–399
   beta-blockers and, 24
   verapamil in, 65
Clonidine
   in hypertension, 186f, 186t, 206
   intellectual effects of, 211
Clopidogrel, 285, 287
   after myocardial infarction, 373
   clinical trials of, 285, 287
   dose of, 287
   in acute coronary syndromes, 285,
      287, 354f, 355, 355f
   pharmacokinetics of, 287
   side effects of, 287
   warfarin interaction with,
      299–300

Coagulation, 279–280, 280f, 291,
      292f
Cognition, antihypertensive drugs
      and, 211
Cold intolerance, angina pectoris
      and, 8
Colesevelam, 340
Colestipol, 340
Congestive heart failure. *See* Heart
      failure.
Continuous positive airway pressure,
      in pulmonary edema, 387
Contraceptives, lipid effects of, 331
Contrast-dye nephropathy, 167
Cor pulmonale, 393
   digoxin and, 159
   nitrates and, 41t
Cornea, amiodarone effects on, 242
Coronary angioplasty
   aspirin with, 283
   vs. fibrinolysis, 311–312
Coronary artery bypass surgery,
      353–354
   aspirin after, 282–283
Coronary artery disease. *See also*
      Angina pectoris; Myocardial
      infarction.
   apolipoprotein B in, 327
   atheroma volume in, 323
   bile acid sequestrants in, 340
   C-reactive protein in, 327
   cholesterol absorption inhibitors
      in, 343–344
   combination therapy in, 344–345
   diet in, 328 330, 329t, 345, 360
   endothelium in, 322–323, 323f
   estrogen and, 345
   fibrates in, 341–343
   hypertension and, 187, 189f, 190,
      202–203
   in women, 328
   inflammation in, 322–323, 323f
   life style changes in, 328–329,
      345–346
   Lipid Clinic referral in, 345
   lipid profile in, 323–328, 325t
   long-term prophylaxis for, 358,
      360
   metabolic syndrome and, 326
   nicotinic acid in, 341
   nondrug therapy in, 328–330,
      329t
   nonlipid risk factors for, 327
   pregnancy and, 345
   prevention of, 321–322, 322t,
      322t
   risk evaluation for, 321–322, 322t,
      322t
   statins in, 331–340, 332f, 333t,
      335t
   treatment goals in, 327
Coronary spasm, calcium channel
      blockers in, 58, 67
Cotrimoxazole, warfarin interaction
      with, 299
Coughing
   ACE inhibitors and, 112, 116,
      116f
   in heart attack, 402
Creatine kinase, before statin
      therapy, 334

Creatinine
    ACE inhibitors and, 117, 123, 124
    digoxin and, 158–159
Cyanide toxicity, 172–173
Cyclo-oxygenase, aspirin effects on, 278f, 281
Cyclopenthiazide, 88t, 89. See also Thiazide diuretics.
Cyclosporin
    rosuvastatin interaction with, 63
    verapamil interaction with, 63
Cyclothiazide, 88t. See also Thiazide diuretics.

D

Dalteparin, 295
Danaparoid, 293
Defibrillation, 402f
Delapril, 113t, 115f. See also Angiotensin-converting enzyme (ACE) inhibitors.
Diabetes insipidus, thiazide diuretics in, 99
Diabetes mellitus, 394–395
    abciximab in, 289
    ACE inhibitors in, 125–126, 127–128, 203, 395
    angiotensin-II receptor blockers in, 135, 395
    beta-blockers in, 11–12, 24, 26t
    blood pressure in, 127–128, 394–395
    calcium channel blockers in, 60
    cholesterol levels in, 328
    diuretics and, 92, 192, 192f
    heart failure in, 395
    hypertension in, 11–12, 60, 127–128, 192, 192f, 203, 209
    lipids in, 328, 395
    microalbuminuria in, 128
    myocardial infarction in, 362t, 395
    nephropathy in. See Diabetic nephropathy.
    new, 125
    percutaneous coronary intervention in, 289
    secondary prevention, 332f
    thiazide diuretics and, 92
Diabetic nephropathy
    ACE inhibitors in, 128, 130, 135, 203, 209
    angiotensin II receptor blockers in, 135, 209
    beta-blockers in, 24
    captopril in, 130
    irbesartan in, 139
    losartan in, 137
    verapamil in, 65
Diabetic retinopathy, 308
Diastolic dysfunction, 124, 385
Diet
    after myocardial infarction, 372
    in coronary artery disease, 328–330, 329t, 345, 360
    in heart failure, 124, 386
    Mediterranean, 329
    potassium in, 96
    sodium in, 185
Digibind, 161

Digoxin, 152–161, 153f, 181
    administration of, 157
    amiodarone interaction with, 229t, 243
    antibiotics with, 154
    arrhythmias with, 157f, 159–161, 160f, 160t, 233
    atorvastatin interaction with, 339
    autonomic effects of, 153–154
    beta-blockers with, 16–17
    blood levels of, 156–157, 157f
    contraindications to, 158
    dose for, 156–157, 158
    drug interactions with, 61, 62, 70, 159, 159t, 229t
    during pregnancy, 401t
    hemodynamic effects of, 154
    in acute pulmonary edema, 387
    in atrial fibrillation, 156, 256t, 257
    in elderly patient, 158
    in myocardial infarction, 159, 370
    indications for, 154, 156
    nifedipine interaction with, 70
    outmoded indications for, 156
    pharmacokinetics of, 154, 154t, 155t
    pharmacologic properties of, 153–154
    proarrhythmic effect of, 157f, 159–161, 160f, 160t, 233
    propafenone interaction with, 229t
    pulmonary heart disease and, 159
    quinidine interaction with, 229t
    relative contraindications to, 158
    renal function and, 158–159
    renin-angiotensin effects of, 153–154
    sodium pump inhibition with, 153, 153f
    toxicity of, 157f, 159–161, 160f, 160t, 233
    verapamil interaction with, 61, 62
Dihydropyridines, 50, 51t, 53–55, 54f, 63t, 69–76. See also Amlodipine; Nifedipine.
Diltiazem, 51t, 54f, 55–56, 55f, 57t, 58f, 65–69. See also Calcium channel blockers.
    after cardiac transplantation, 68
    after myocardial infarction, 59
    contraindications to, 62f, 63t, 67
    dose of, 57t, 67
    drug interactions with, 67, 230t
    for African-American patients, 11
    in acute coronary syndromes, 358
    in angina pectoris, 60, 68
    in arrhythmias, 68, 220t, 222t, 248
    in atrial fibrillation, 256t, 257
    in cardiac transplantation, 68
    in hypertension, 58–59, 60, 68, 74, 76t, 186f, 191t, 199–201, 200f, 204
    in ischemic heart disease, 68
    in paroxysmal supraventricular tachycardia, 222t, 253–254
    in Prinzmetal's (variant) angina, 68

Diltiazem *(Continued)*
  in supraventricular tachycardia,
    56, 59, 68
  in unstable angina pectoris, 9f,
    58, 68
  intravenous, 67
  outcome trials of, 75, 76t
  pharmacokinetics of, 67
  side effects of, 56, 66t, 67
  vs. adenosine, 250
Diphenylhydantoin. *See* Phenytoin.
Dipyridamole, 288
  adenosine interaction with, 230t,
    250
Direct thrombin inhibitors, 292f,
  296–298
  in acute coronary syndromes, 357
  in myocardial infarction, 367
Disopyramide, 220t, 223t, 235–236
  drug interactions with, 62, 229t
  in atrial fibrillation, 258t
  in hypertrophic cardiomyopathy,
    388
  in ventricular tachycardia, 223t,
    264
  side effects of, 228t
  verapamil interaction with, 62
Dissecting aneurysm, beta-blockers
  in, 17
Diuretics, 80–101, 81t
  ACE inhibitors with
    in heart failure, 119–120,
      122–123, 124
    in hypertension, 196–197,
      197t, 204
  allopurinol interaction with, 92
  angiotensin-II receptor blockers
    with, 137, 139, 197t
  aspirin interaction with, 284
  beta-blockers with, 12, 197t, 199
  braking with, 97
  combination, 94t, 95
  diabetes mellitus and, 92, 192,
    192f
  digoxin interaction with, 159
  dofetilide interaction with, 248
  drug interactions with, 92, 159,
    229t, 248, 284
  during pregnancy, 401t
  fluid challenge for, 97
  for African-American patients, 208
  for elderly patients, 207
  high-ceiling, 87, 87f
  hyponatremia and, 98
  in acute pulmonary edema, 387
  in heart failure, 80–82, 99–100,
    180, 384
  in hypercalcemia, 98
  in hypertension, 80–82, 191t,
    193–198, 193f, 194f,
    200–201
  in malignant hypertension, 98
  in refractory hypertension, 212
  in renal failure, 98
  incorrect use of, 97
  lipid effects of, 84, 86, 91, 92,
    206, 330t, 331
  loop, 82–87, 82f, 85t. *See also*
    Furosemide.
  losartan with, 92
  low-ceiling, 87, 87f

Diuretics *(Continued)*
  minor, 95
  overdiuresis with, 96–97
  patient management of, 97
  potassium-sparing, 81t, 82f,
    93–95, 94t, 196
  proarrhythmic effects of, 91–92
  prodiabetic effects of, 12
  quinidine interaction with, 229t
  resistance, 98f, 99t
  sequential nephron blockade
    with, 87, 100
  site of action, 82f
  sotalol interaction with, 229t
  thiazide, 87–90, 88t, 89t. *See also*
    Thiazide diuretics.
  tolerance to, 84, 97, 98f, 99t
  vs. calcium channel blockers,
    200–201
Dobutamine, 163t, 164f, 165–166
  in beta-blocker overdose, 27
  vs. dopamine, 167
Dofetilide, 220t, 222t, 246–247
  adverse effects of, 248
  dose of, 222t, 247
  drug interactions with, 230t, 248
  in atrial fibrillation, 246–247, 258,
    258t, 259, 260f, 378–379
  in atrial flutter, 246–247, 263
  in paroxysmal supraventricular
    tachycardia, 254
  indications for, 247
Dopamine, 163t, 164f, 166–167
  diuretic effect of, 82f, 95, 97, 167
  vs. dobutamine, 167
Dopamine-receptor stimulators, in
  heart failure, 176
Doxazosin
  in hypertension, 186f, 186t, 205
  lipid effects of, 330t
Dronedarone, 248
Dual chamber pacing, in
  hypertrophic cardiomyopathy,
  388
Dyazide, 94t, 95

E

Edema
  ankle, 70, 71t, 74
  cardiac, 91
  pulmonary, 83, 387
Elderly patients
  ACE inhibitors for, 207–208
  alpha-blockers for, 207
  beta-blockers for, 11, 27t
  calcium channel blockers for, 207
  cholesterol levels in, 328
  digoxin for, 158
  diuretics for, 207
  hypertension in, 203, 207–208
Electromechanical dissociation, 402
Enalapril, 113t, 114t, 115f, 120t,
  131–132. *See also* Angiotensin-
  converting enzyme (ACE)
  inhibitors.
  anemia and, 125
  contraindications to, 132
  dose for, 113t, 124, 131–132
  in early heart failure, 119, 120t

Enalapril (Continued)
  indications for, 131–132, 134
  lipid effects of, 330t
Enalaprilat
  in acute pulmonary edema, 387
  in acute severe hypertension, 175,
      212, 213t, 214t
  in heart failure, 176
  in hypertensive emergency, 212,
      213t, 214t
Endocarditis, infective, 396–398
  antibiotics in, 397–398, 397t
  anticoagulation in, 396–397
Endothelin receptor antagonists, in
      pulmonary hypertension, 394
Endothelium
  impairment of
    in coronary artery disease, 233f,
        322–323
    quinapril in, 132
  nitrate effects on, 34
Enoxaparin, 295–296
  during pregnancy, 401t
Enoximone, 170f, 171
Enterococci, in endocarditis, 396
Epilepsy, 233
Epinephrine, 163t, 164f, 167–168
Eplerenone
  ACE inhibitors with, 123
  in heart failure, 94, 114t,
      120–121, 123, 142, 181, 384
  in hypertension, 94, 94t, 196
Epoprostenol sodium, in pulmonary
      hypertension, 394
Eprosartan, 140
Eptifibatide, 286t, 288–289, 288t,
      291
  during pregnancy, 401t
Erectile dysfunction, 210–211
  beta-blockers and, 25, 211
  diuretics and, 93, 211
  drug treatment of, 38, 38f
  nitrates and, 38, 38f, 39
Erythromycin
  atorvastatin interaction with, 339
  QT-prolongation with, 245f
Esmolol, 2t, 28–29, 221t. See also
      Beta-blockers.
  half-life of, 20
  in acute severe hypertension, 212,
      213t, 214t
  in arrhythmias, 237
  in atrial fibrillation, 256t, 257
  in hypertensive emergency, 214t
  in perioperative hypertension, 29
  in supraventricular tachycardia,
      13, 29, 221t
Esophageal varices, beta-blockers in,
      2t
Estrogen, antiatherosclerotic effects
      of, 345
Etanercept, 181
Ethacrynic acid, 86
Exercise
  antidiabetic effect of, 346
  beta-blockers and, 25
  in angina pectoris, 7
  in hypertension, 209
Ezetimibe, 332f, 343–344
  statin with, 344

F

Factor VIIa, 280, 280f
Factor Xa, 279–280, 280f
  inhibitors of, 367
Fallot's tetralogy, beta-blockers in,
      17
Fatigue, beta-blockers and, 24
Felodipine
  in hypertension, 71t, 75
  side effects of, 66t, 71t
Fenofibrate, 341–342, 343
Fenoldopam
  in acute severe hypertension, 176,
      212, 213t, 214t
  in hypertensive emergency, 212,
      213t, 214t
Fibrates, 332f, 341–343, 344
  statin with, 334, 344
Fibrinolytic (thrombolytic) therapy,
      304–312, 305t
  adjunctive therapy with, 306
  alteplase for, 292f, 305t, 307–308,
      308t
  blood pressure reduction before,
      361–362
  contraindications to, 308, 308t,
      309, 310t, 357
  goals of, 304–305
  monteplase for, 310
  prehospital, 306
  reperfusion indicators in, 306
  reteplase for, 292f, 305t, 309
  saruplase for, 310
  staphylokinase for, 310
  streptokinase for, 292f, 305t,
      306–307, 309, 310t
  tenecteplase for, 292f, 305t, 308,
      308t, 310t
  timing of, 305–306, 307f
  trials of, 306–307, 308t
  vs. percutaneous coronary
      intervention, 306, 307f,
      311–312, 363t–364t, 365
Flecainide, 220t, 224t, 228t,
      233–234
  amiodarone interaction with,
      229t
  drug interactions with, 229t
  in atrial fibrillation, 258–259,
      258t, 260f
  in paroxysmal supraventricular
      tachycardia, 254
  in ventricular tachycardia, 224t,
      234, 264
  proarrhythmic effects of, 228t,
      234
  side effects of, 228t, 234
  verapamil interaction with, 62
Fluid challenge, 97
Fluvastatin, 333t, 338
Folic acid, 345
  with nitrates, 46
Fondaparinux, 297
Fosinopril, 113t, 115f. See also
      Angiotensin-converting enzyme
      (ACE) inhibitors.
Free radicals, in nitrate tolerance,
      44–45
Fruit juices, 346
Frumil, 94t

Furosemide, 81t, 82–84, 94t, 95
    ACE inhibitor with, 124
    braking with, 84
    contraindications to, 83
    dose of, 83, 85t
    drug interactions with, 84
    during pregnancy, 401t
    hyperglycemia with, 84
    hypersensitivity to, 83, 86
    hyperuricemia with, 84
    hypokalemia with, 83–84, 86
    hypovolemia with, 84
    in heart failure, 83, 98, 100, 180
    in hypercalcemia, 98
    in hypertension, 83, 98, 196
    in pulmonary edema, 83
    in renal failure, 98
    intravenous, 83
    ototoxicity of, 84
    pharmacokinetics of, 82–83
    pharmacologic effects of, 82–83,
        82f
    side effects of, 83–84
    tolerance to, 84
    vs. captopril, 119

G

Ganglion blockers, in hypertension,
    186f, 186t, 212
Gastrointestinal tract
    amiodarone effects on, 242
    aspirin effects on, 281, 283, 284
Gemfibrozil, 342
    during pregnancy, 401t
    statin with, 334, 340
Gentamicin sensitivity, 308
Glaucoma
    beta-blockers in, 2t, 17
    carbonic anhydrase inhibitors in,
        95
    nitrates and, 41t
Glomerular injury, 129f
Glucagon, in beta-blocker overdose,
    27
Glucose, diuretic effects on, 84, 86, 92
Glucose-insulin-potassium, in
    myocardial infarction, 368
Glycoprotein IIb/IIIa receptor
    antagonists, 285f, 286t,
        288–291, 288t, 357
Gout, 92
Grapefruit juice, nifedipine
    interaction with, 70
Guanabenz, 186f, 186t, 206
Guanadrel, 186f, 186t, 212
Guanethidine, 186f, 186t, 212
Guanfacine, 186f, 186t, 206

H

Haloperidol, QT-prolongation with,
    245f
Halothane, lidocaine interaction
    with, 229t, 232
HDL. *See* Lipoproteins.
Headache
    migraine, 2t, 18
    nifedipine and, 70
    nitrates and, 41–42, 41t

Heart
    surgery on, 182, 353–354. *See also*
        Percutaneous coronary
        interventions.
    transplantation of, 68, 182, 390
Heart failure, 150–183, 162f,
    369–371, 383–386
    ACE inhibitors in, 100, 117–125,
        126, 127f, 178f, 180, 384
        aldosterone antagonists with,
            123
        anemia and, 125
        angiotensin-II receptor blocker
            with, 137
        aspirin with, 123
        beta-blockers with, 119–120
        diastolic dysfunction and, 124
        diuretics with, 122–123, 124
        dose for, 123, 124
        for African-American patients,
            125
        hyponatremia and, 124
        hypotension and, 123, 124
        nonsteroidal anti-inflammatory
            drugs with, 123
        outcome trials of, 119, 120t,
            121t
        patient assessment for, 123–124
        preventive use of, 119, 120t
        renal failure and, 123–124
        skeletal muscle myopathy and,
            124–125
        vs. angiotensin-II receptor
            blockers, 122t, 179
        vs. diuretics, 119
    acute, 150, 151, 162f, 176, 177f
    adenosine in, 175
    afterload reduction in, 171–172
    albuterol in, 168
    aldosterone antagonists in, 94,
        94t, 120–121, 140–142, 141f,
        180–181, 384
        ACE inhibitors with, 123
    aldosterone in, 125
    Alka-Seltzer contraindication in,
        283
    amiodarone in, 240, 242
    amrinone in, 170f
    angiotensin-II receptor blockers
        in, 135–136, 136f, 178–179,
        178f, 181, 384
        ACE inhibitor with, 137
        vs. ACE inhibitors, 122t, 179
    antiarrhythmics in, 181
    aspirin in, ACE inhibitors with,
        123
    atrial fibrillation in, 385
    atriopeptidase inhibition in, 386
    beta$_1$-adrenergic receptors in,
        14–15, 14f, 15f
    beta$_2$-adrenergic receptors in,
        14–15, 14f, 15f, 162, 164,
        164f
    beta-blockers in, 2t, 10, 13–16,
        14f, 16t, 178f, 180, 384
        ACE inhibitors with, 119–120
        mechanisms of action of,
            14–16, 15f
        principles of, 16, 16t
    bumetanide in, 84
    calcium sensitizers in, 168–169

Heart failure *(Continued)*
  candesartan in, 137
  captopril in, 130
  carvedilol in, 16, 16t, 179–180
  chronic, 150–152, 152f, 176–182,
    178f, 179t
  congestive, 178f
  cough in, 112
  diagnosis of, 150–152, 151f
  diastolic dysfunction in, 124,
    385–386
  diet in, 386
  digoxin in, 152–161, 153f, 181.
    See also Digoxin.
  diuretics in, 80–82, 83, 98, 178f,
    180, 384
    ACE inhibitors with, 100,
      119–120, 122–123, 124
    combination of, 95
    step-care, 99–100
  dobutamine in, 163t, 164f,
    165–166
  dopamine in, 163t, 164f,
    166–167
  dopamine-receptor stimulators in,
    176
  Dyazide in, 94t, 95
  enalapril in, 131, 134
  enoximone in, 170f, 171
  epinephrine in, 163t, 164f,
    167–168
  eplerenone in, 142, 181
  experimental, arrhythmias in, 15
  furosemide in, 83, 98, 100, 180
  heart rate in, 15
  hydralazine in, 39, 44, 174–175
  hydrochlorothiazide in, 89
  hyperphosphorylation in, 14, 15f
  hypertension and, 203–204
  hyponatremia in, 98
  hypotension in, 116
  in diabetes mellitus, 395
  inodilators in, 169–171, 169f, 170f
  intractable, 385
  isoproterenol in, 168
  left ventricular wall stress in,
    118–119
  levosimendan in, 386
  lifestyle measures in, 179–180
  load reduction in, 171–176
  losartan in, 137
  maximum treatment of, 179–182
  Maxzide in, 94t, 95
  methoxamine in, 165
  milrinone in, 165, 170–171, 170f,
    181
  Moduretic in, 94t, 95
  nesiritide in, 174, 386
  neurohumoral effects of, 117–119,
    118f
  neutral endopeptidase inhibitors
    in, 176
  nitrates in, 39, 44, 172–174
  nonsteroidal anti-inflammatory
    drugs in, 123
  norepinephrine in, 162, 163t,
    164, 164f, 165, 168
  omapatrilat in, 176, 386
  perindopril in, 132
  peripheral vascular resistance in,
    118

Heart failure *(Continued)*
  phenylephrine in, 165
  phosphodiesterase-III
    inhibitors in, 169–171,
    169f, 170f
  preload reduction in, 171, 172
  quadruple therapy in, 122
  quinapril in, 132
  ramipril in, 132–133, 134
  renin-angiotensin-aldosterone
    system in, 117–118, 118f
  skeletal muscle myopathy and,
    124–125
  spironolactone in, 94, 140–142,
    180–181
  statins in, 334
  terbutaline in, 168
  thiazide diuretics in, 89
  torsemide in, 85
  trandolapril in, 133
  valsartan in, 139
  vasodilators in, 171–176, 178f,
    181, 384–385
  ventricular arrhythmias in, 385
Heart rate
  beta-blockers and, 7, 15, 25, 27
  calcium channel blockers and,
    55–56, 57t
  in heart failure, 15
Heart transplantation, 182
  diltiazem after, 68
  in dilated cardiomyopathy, 390
Heparin, 291–296
  during pregnancy, 294, 401t
  glycoprotein IIb/IIIa receptor
    antagonists with, 289–290,
    291
  in acute coronary syndromes, 294,
    295, 356
  in myocardial infarction, 294,
    296, 366–367
  in percutaneous coronary
    interventions, 294, 295–296
  in unstable angina pectoris, 9f,
    292–293, 294
  indications for, 294
  intravenous, 292–293
  low-molecular-weight, 294–296
    glycoprotein IIb/IIIa receptor
      antagonists with, 289–290
    in acute coronary syndromes,
      295, 356
    in myocardial infarction, 296,
      367
  mechanism of action of, 291–292,
    292f
  nitrate interaction with, 39
  precautions with, 293
  side effects with, 293
  streptokinase with, 309
  subcutaneous, 293
  thrombocytopenia (HIT), 293–294
  thrombosis syndrome with,
    293–294
  unfractionated, 296
    glycoprotein IIb/IIIa receptor
      antagonists with, 289–290,
      291
    intravenous, 292–293
    subcutaneous, 293
Heparin resistance, 39, 41t

Hirudin, 296–297
  in acute coronary syndromes, 357
  in myocardial infarction, 367
HMG CoA reductase inhibitors. *See* Statins.
Home nursing, in heart failure, 180
Homocysteine, 345
Homozygous familial hypercholesterolemia, statins in, 334
Hormone replacement therapy, 372
Hydralazine
  in heart failure, 39, 44, 174–175
  in hypertension, 186f, 186t, 205, 212, 213t
  in hypertensive emergency, 212, 213t
  nitrate interaction with, 39
Hydrochlorothiazide, 88t, 89–90, 94t. *See also* Thiazide diuretics.
  bisoprolol with, 12
  diabetogenic effect of, 92
  dose of, 87, 89
  in heart failure, 89
  in hypertension, 88t, 89–90, 94t, 195, 196
  lipid effects of, 92
Hydroflumethiazide, 88t. *See also* Thiazide diuretics.
3-Hydroxy-3-methyl-glutaryl-coenzyme A reductase inhibitors. *See* Statins.
Hypercalcemia
  diuretics in, 98
  thiazide-related, 92–93
Hypercalciuria, idiopathic, thiazide diuretics in, 99
Hyperglycemia, loop diuretics and, 84, 86
Hyperkalemia
  ACE inhibitors and, 94–95, 116, 116f
  potassium-sparing diuretics and, 94–95
Hyperphosphorylation, in heart failure, 14, 15f
Hypertension, 185–215, 186f, 186t
  ACE inhibitors in, 109, 121t, 125–126, 191t, 201–204, 202f
    calcium channel blockers with, 197t, 204
    coronary artery disease and, 202–203
    diuretics with, 204
    for elderly patients, 203
    heart failure and, 203–204
    renal disease and, 203
    vs. angiotensin-II receptor blockers, 121t
    vs. calcium channel blockers, 201
  after myocardial infarction, 206–207
  aldosterone antagonists in, 196
  alpha-blockers in, 186f, 186t, 205
  amiloride in, 81t, 82f, 93, 94t, 196
  amlodipine in, 60, 74, 76t, 186f
  angiotensin-II receptor blockers in, 121t, 134–135, 137, 138t, 140, 191t, 204–205

Hypertension (*Continued*)
  diuretics with, 137, 139, 197t
    vs. ACE inhibitors, 121t, 140
  anticoagulation in, 302
  atrial fibrillation in, 210, 211
  benazepril in, 133
  bendrofluazide in, 88t, 196
  beta-blockers in, 2t, 11–13, 29, 191t, 198–199, 198f, 201
    anti-hypertensive effects of, 11
    diuretics with, 12, 197t, 199
    dosage for, 199
    in African-American patients, 11
    in diabetic patients, 11
    in elderly patients, 11
    indications for, 11
    pharmacokinetics of, 199
    quality of life and, 25
    side effects of, 199
    vs. calcium channel blockers, 201
  bisoprolol in, 12
  blood pressure in, 187, 188t, 189
  C-reactive protein in, 187
  calcium channel blockers in, 58–59, 90t, 199–201, 200f, 204
    ACE inhibitors with, 197t, 204
    outcomes with, 60, 64, 68, 74, 75, 76t
    safety of, 60, 75, 76t, 200, 201
    vs. ACE inhibitors, 201
    vs. beta-blockers, 201
    vs. diuretics, 200–201
  candesartan in, 137
  captopril in, 129–130, 203, 212, 213t
  central adrenergic inhibitors in, 206
  chlorthalidone in, 89, 195
  clonidine in, 206
  combination diuretics in, 95
  complications of, 187, 189f
  coronary artery disease and, 187, 189f, 190, 202–203
  diabetes mellitus in, 12, 60, 127–128, 192, 192f, 203, 209
  diltiazem in, 58–59, 60, 68, 74, 76t, 191t, 199–201, 200f, 204
  diuretics in, 80–82, 83, 191t, 193–198, 193f, 194f, 200–201
    ACE inhibitors with, 196–197, 197t, 204
    angiotensin-II receptor blockers with, 197t
    beta-blockers with, 12, 197t
    complications of, 194–195
    thiazide, 87, 89–90, 89t
    vs. calcium channel blockers, 200–201
  doxazosin in, 186f, 186t, 205
  drug treatment of, 189–193, 191t, 193f
    angina and, 206
    combination, 197f
    cost-effectiveness of, 211
    efficacy of, 192–194, 194t
    erectile dysfunction and, 210–211
    goals of, 210–211

Hypertension (*Continued*)
guidelines for, 191
in African-American patients,
128–129, 203, 208
in cigarette smokers, 208
in diabetic patient, 209
in elderly patient, 203, 207–208
in exercising patient, 209
in obese patient, 208
in pregnant patient, 209
in resistant disease, 212, 214
in urgency, 211–212, 213t, 214t
initial drug, 190
intellectual effects of, 211
lipidemia and, 206
metabolic considerations in,
192, 192f
myocardial infarction and,
206–207, 361–362
patient profiling for, 206–210
quality of life with, 211
selection of, 190, 191t, 192,
193f
during pregnancy, 203, 209, 210,
401t
Dyazide in, 94t, 95
enalapril in, 131
enalaprilat in, 175, 212, 213t, 214t
eplerenone in, 94, 94t, 196
eprosartan in, 140
exercise in, 209
felodipine in, 71t, 75
fenoldopam in, 176, 212, 213t,
214t
fosinopril in, 132
furosemide in, 83, 98, 196
guanabenz in, 186f, 186t, 206
guanadrel in, 186f, 186t, 212
guanethidine in, 186f, 186t, 212
guanfacine in, 186f, 186t, 206
guidelines for drugs, 191t
heart failure and, 203–204
hydralazine in, 186f, 186t, 205,
212, 213t
hydrochlorothiazide in, 88t,
89–90, 94t, 195, 196
hyponatremia in, 98
imidazole receptor blockers in, 206
in African-American patients,
128–129, 203, 208
in elderly patient, 203, 207–208
indapamide in, 88t, 90–91, 196
insulin-resistance in, 192, 192f
irbesartan in, 139
lacidipine in, 76t
left ventricular hypertrophy with,
210
lipids in, 206
lisinopril in, 133
losartan in, 137
management of, 193f
Maxzide in, 94t, 95
methyldopa in, 186f, 186t, 206
metolazone in, 88t, 90, 196
minoxidil in, 186f, 186t, 205, 212
Moduretic in, 94t, 95
morning blood pressure in, 210
mykrox in, 90
nifedipine in, 69, 73, 76t, 95,
186f, 212

Hypertension (*Continued*)
nondrug treatment of, 185,
187–189
olmesartan in, 140
perindopril in, 132
prazosin in, 186f, 186t, 205
pulmonary, 393–394
anticoagulation and, 303
quinapril in, 132
ramipril in, 129, 132–133,
202–203
renovascular, 203, 283
reserpine in, 206
resistant, 212, 214
risk factors for, 187
severe, acute, 211–212, 213t, 214t
telmisartan in, 139
terazosin in, 186f, 186t, 205
thiazide diuretics in, 12, 87,
89–90, 89t
torsemide in, 85, 86, 196
trandolapril in, 133
triamterene in, 81t, 93, 94t, 196
vasodilators in, 186f, 186t, 205
ventricular arrhythmias with, 210
verapamil in, 58–59, 60, 64, 74,
76t, 191t, 199–201, 200f, 204
weight loss in, 187, 208
Hypertensive emergency, 211–212,
213t, 214t
Hypertensive urgency, 211–212, 213t
Hyperthyroidism, amiodarone and,
242
Hypertrophic cardiomyopathy. *See*
Cardiomyopathy.
Hyperuricemia, furosemide and, 84
Hypokalemia
loop diuretics and, 83–84, 86
thiazide diuretics and, 91–92, 93
Hypomagnesemia, thiazide diuretics
and, 92
Hyponatremia
ACE inhibitors and, 116, 124
in heart failure, 98
in hypertension, 98
thiazide diuretics and, 91
Hypoproteinemia, beta-blockers
and, 20
Hypotension
ACE inhibitors and, 116, 116f,
123, 124
nitrates and, 41t
Hypothyroidism, amiodarone and,
242
Hypovolemia, furosemide and, 84

I

Ibopamine, 176
Ibuprofen, aspirin interaction with,
283
Ibutilide, 220t, 222t, 245–246
dose of, 222t, 246
drug interactions with, 229t
in atrial fibrillation, 245–246,
258, 258t
in atrial flutter, 245–246, 263
QT-prolongation with, 245f, 246
torsades de pointes with, 246
Imidazole receptor blockers, in

hypertension, 206
Implantable cardioverter
defibrillator, 182
after myocardial infarction,
266–268, 268f, 374
antiarrhythmic drugs with, 266
cardiac resynchronization therapy
with, 268, 268f
in dilated cardiomyopathy, 267,
389–390
in ventricular arrhythmias, 240,
241t, 383
vs. amiodarone, 240
Impotence. *See* Erectile dysfunction.
Indapamide. *See also* Thiazide
diuretics.
antiarrhythmic effect of, 90–91
during pregnancy, 401t
in cardiac edema, 91
in hypertension, 88t, 90–91, 196
lipid effects of, 330t
Indolol, lipid effects of, 330t
Indomethacin, diuretic interaction
with, 84, 90
Infective endocarditis, 396–398
antibiotics in, 397–398, 397t
anticoagulation in, 396–397
Inodilators, 169–171, 169f, 170f
Inositol trisphosphate, 107
Inotropes, sympathomimetic, 163t
Insulin-resistance
in hypertension, 192, 192f
obesity and, 208
Intermittent claudication, 65,
398–399
Intubation, in acute pulmonary
edema, 387
Irbesartan, 114t, 139, 138t, 140. *See
also* Angiotensin-II receptor
blockers.
atrial fibrillation and, 259
Isoproterenol, in heart failure, 163t,
168
Isosorbide dinitrate, 37t, 40, 40t. *See
also* Nitrates.
in heart failure, 44
intravenous, 37t, 43
pharmacokinetics of, 35
prophylactic, 40, 40t
sublingual, 37t, 39
sublingual nitroglycerin with, 46
Isosorbide mononitrate, 37t, 40,
40t. *See also* Nitrates.
Isradipine, 75
Ivabradine, 47, 352

J

Juices, 346
nifedipine interaction with, 70

K

Kallikrein-kinin system, 110
Ketoconazole
dofetilide interaction with, 230t,
248
QT-prolongation with, 245f

verapamil interaction with, 63
Kidneys
ACE inhibitor effects on, 116–117,
116f
beta-blocker elimination by, 21, 21f
bradykinin synthesis in, 110
carcinoma of, thiazide diuretics
and, 93
failure
ACE inhibitors and, 116–117,
123–124, 128–129
angiotensin-II and, 128, 129f
beta-blockers and, 24, 26t
bumetanide and, 85
captopril and, 130
digoxin and, 154, 158–159
diuretics in, 98
furosemide in, 98
torsemide and, 85–86
trandolapril in, 133, 137
in diabetes mellitus, 128

L

Labetalol, 2t, 23t, 28. *See also* Beta-
blockers.
in hypertensive emergency, 212,
213t, 214t
lipid effects of, 330t
Lacidipine, 75, 76t
vascular protective effects of, 53
Left ventricular assist devices, in
dilated cardiomyopathy, 390
Left ventricular hypertrophy,
118–119. *See also* Heart failure.
diastolic dysfunction and, 124
eplerenone in, 94
in hypertension, 189f, 210
indapamide in, 91
Lepirudin, 296–297
Lercanidipine, 75
Levobunolol, in glaucoma, 17
Levocarnitine, 399
Levosimendan, 168–169, 176, 386
Lidocaine, 220t, 223t, 231–233
beta-blocker interaction with, 21,
229t, 232
clinical use of, 223t, 232
dose for, 223t, 232
drug interactions with, 21, 229t,
232
failure of, 232–233
in digoxin toxicity, 161
in myocardial infarction, 232, 369
in ventricular tachycardia, 223t,
231–233, 264
pharmacokinetics of, 231–232,
231f
side effects of, 228t, 232
Lipid(s), 323–328, 325t
alpha-blocker effects on, 206, 330t
beta-blocker effects on, 27t, 206,
330–331, 330t
diuretic effects on, 84, 86, 91, 92,
206, 330t, 331
drug-related changes in, 330–331,
330t
guidelines, 322t
in diabetes mellitus, 328, 395
oral contraceptive effects on, 331

Lipid-lowering drugs, 331–345, 332f
cholesterol absorption inhibitors
as, 343–344
combination of, 344
fibrates as, 332f, 334, 341–343,
344
levels, ideal, 322t
nicotinic acid as, 332f, 341, 344
pregnancy contraindication and,
345
resins as, 332f, 340, 344
statins as, 331–340, 332f, 333t,
335t. *See also* Statins.
Lipoproteins, 323–327, 325t, 326f
high-density, 323–325, 325t, 326f
low-density, 322t, 323, 325t, 326f,
327, 332f
Lisinopril, 113t, 114t, 133. *See also*
Angiotensin-converting enzyme
(ACE) inhibitors.
for African-American patients,
208
vs. amlodipine, 59
Lithium
diuretic interaction with, 84, 90
verapamil interaction with, 63
Liver
beta-blocker metabolism in, 20,
21f
disease of
beta-blockers and, 26t
fibrates and, 341–342
statins and, 334
torsemide in, 86
Long-QT syndrome. *See also*
Torsades de pointes.
beta-blockers in, 17
congenital, 233, 252, 266
drug-induced, 244, 245f, 246,
248, 252
Loop diuretics, 82–87, 82f, 85t. *See
also* Furosemide.
side effects of, 86–87
Losartan, 114t, 137, 138t, 204–205.
See also Angiotensin-II receptor
blockers.
diuretic with, 92
lipid effects of, 330t, 331
Lovastatin, 333t, 335t, 336. *See also*
Statins.
verapamil interaction with, 62
Lungs, amiodarone effects on, 242
LVH. *See* Left ventricular
hypertrophy.

M

Magnesium, intravenous, 248,
368–369
Malignant hypertension, 98
Marfan's syndrome, beta-blockers in,
17
Margarine, 345
Maxzide, 94t, 95
Maze operation, 379
Mediterranean-type diet, 329, 345,
360
Melagatran, 292f, 298
Metabolic syndrome, 192, 193t,
326, 395

Methemoglobinemia, nitrates and,
41t, 42
Methoxamine, in heart failure, 165
Methyldopa
during pregnancy, 401t
in hypertension, 186f, 186t, 206
Methylxanthines, adenosine
interaction with, 230t, 250
Metipranolol, in glaucoma, 17
Metolazone, 88t, 90, 196. *See also*
Thiazide diuretics.
Metoprolol, 2t, 23t, 28. *See also*
Beta-blockers.
half-life of, 20
hepatic metabolism of, 20, 21f
in atrial fibrillation, 256t, 257
in heart failure, 16, 16t
in ventricular tachyarrhythmia, 13
lipid effects of, 330t
postinfarct, 10–11
side effects of, 24
verapamil interaction with, 21
Metronidazole, warfarin interaction
with, 299
Mexiletine, 220t, 223t, 235
drug interactions with, 229t
side effects of, 228t
Micro-K, 96
Microalbuminuria, in diabetes
mellitus, 128
Migraine, beta-blockers in, 2t, 18
Milrinone, 163t, 165, 169–171,
170f, 181
in beta-blocker overdose, 27
Minoxidil, in hypertension, 186f,
186t, 205, 212
Mitral regurgitation, 302, 393
Mitral stenosis, 392
atrial fibrillation and, 302
beta-blockers in, 16–17
Mitral valve, in hypertrophic
cardiomyopathy, 388–389
Mitral valve prolapse
anticoagulation and, 303
beta-blockers in, 17
Moduretic, 94t, 95
Monteplase, 310
Moricizine, 224t, 236
Morphine, in myocardial infarction,
360
Muscle, statin effects on, 334
Myalgia, bumetanide and, 85
Myectomy, in hypertrophic
cardiomyopathy, 388
Mykrox, 90
Myocardial infarction, 360–374
ACE inhibitors in, 10, 126, 127f,
368, 370, 373–374
angiotensin-II receptor blockers
in, 368
antiplatelet therapy in, 312
arrhythmias after, 361, 369, 374,
383
aspirin in, 281, 282, 304, 373, 374
atropine in, 361
beta-blockers in, 2t, 10–11, 13,
367–368, 372
bivalirudin in, 367
bradyarrhythmias in, 361
calcium channel blockers in, 59,
372–373

Myocardial infarction (*Continued*)
  captopril in, 130
  cardiac output in, 370
  cardiac remodeling after, 126,
    127f
  chronic phase, 361f
  clopidogrel in, 373
  diet in, 372
  digoxin in, 159, 370
  diltiazem in, 68
  direct thrombin inhibitors in, 367
  early phase, 360–371, 361f, 362t,
    363t–364t
    ACE inhibitors in, 126, 368
    beta-blockers in, 10, 367–368
    digoxin contraindication in,
      159
    diltiazem in, 68
    fibrinolytic therapy in,
      363t–364t, 365–366. *See
      also* Fibrinolytic
      (thrombolytic) therapy.
    glucose-insulin-potassium in,
      368
    glycoprotein IIb/IIIa receptor
      antagonists in, 366
    heparin in, 366–367
    magnesium in, 368–369
    nitrates in, 370
    percutaneous coronary
      intervention in, 361f,
      362–367, 363t–364t
    statins in, 369
  enalapril in, 131–132
  facilitated reperfusion, 366
  factor Xa inhibitors in, 367
  fibrinolytic therapy in, 365–366.
    See also Fibrinolytic
    (thrombolytic) therapy.
  follow-up management in,
    371–374, 371t
  glucose-insulin-potassium in, 368
  glycoprotein IIb/IIIa receptor
    antagonists in, 288–291,
    288t, 312, 366
  heparin in, 292–293, 294, 296,
    366–367
  hormone replacement therapy
    and, 372
  hypertension and, 206–207,
    361–362
  implantable cardioverter
    defibrillator in, 266–268,
    268f, 374
  intravenous magnesium in,
    368–369
  left ventricular failure in, 126,
    130, 369–371
  lidocaine in, 232, 369
  lisinopril in, 133
  low-molecular-weight heparin in,
    296, 367
  management after, 371–374, 371t
  metabolic support in, 368–369
  microvascular dysfunction in,
    366
  morphine in, 360
  nitrates in, 41t, 43–44, 370
  norepinephrine in, 165
  oxygen in, 360
  pentasaccharide in, 367

Myocardial infarction (*Continued*)
  percutaneous coronary
    intervention in, 361f,
    362–367, 363t–364t
  postinfarct management, 371
  preload reduction in, 370
  prevention of
    aspirin in, 281, 282, 304
    pravastatin in, 336
    warfarin in, 304
  prognosis after, 371–372
  ramipril in, 132–133
  remodeling, 127f
  reocclusion after, 366–367
  reperfusion injury in, 366
  revascularization for, 362
  shock in, 369–371
  sinus tachycardia in, 361
  size of, 360
  statins in, 369, 372
  sudden death prevention after,
    266–267
  supraventricular arrhythmias in,
    369
  trandolapril in, 133
  trials in, 363t–364t, 365
  ventricular arrhythmias after, 369,
    383
  verapamil in, 65
  warfarin in, 300–301, 303–304,
    373
  ximelagatran in, 298, 373
  zofenopril in, 133
Myocardial ischemia
  exercise induced. *See* Angina
    pectoris, effort.
  silent, beta-blockers in, 8, 11
Myocardial malperfusion, 311
Myopathy
  in heart failure, 124–125
  statins and, 334
Myotomy, in hypertrophic
  cardiomyopathy, 388

N

Nadolol, 2t, 22t, 28. *See also*
  Beta-blockers.
  in atrial fibrillation, 256t, 257
  renal excretion of, 21, 21f
Nebivolol, 23t, 28. *See also*
  Beta-blockers.
Nephron
  diuretic action on, 82f
  function of, 80, 81f
Nephropathy. *See also* Diabetic
  nephropathy.
  contrast-dye, 167
  ramipril in, 128, 132–133, 203
Nesiritide, in heart failure, 174
Neuromuscular blocking agents,
  verapamil interaction with, 63
Neutral endopeptidase inhibitors, in
  heart failure, 176
Neutropenia
  ACE inhibitors and, 117
  captopril and, 117, 130
  clopidogrel and, 287
  ticlopidine and, 284
Niaspan, 341

Nicardipine, 75
  in acute pulmonary edema, 387
  in acute severe hypertension, 212,
    213t, 214t
  in hypertensive emergency, 214t
Nicorandil, 47, 352
Nicotinic acid, 332f, 341, 344
  during pregnancy, 401t
  statin with, 344
Nifedipine, 51t, 54f, 55, 55f, 69–73
  ankle edema with, 70
  beta-blockers with, 72
  cautions with, 70, 71t
  cessation of, 72
  contraindications to, 69, 70, 70f,
    71t
  dose of, 69, 71t
  drug interactions with, 70, 71t,
    229t
  for elderly patients, 207
  headache with, 70
  in acute coronary syndromes,
    357–358
  in acute severe hypertension, 212
  in angina pectoris, 9f, 60, 69,
    72–73
  in hypertension, 69, 73, 76t, 95,
    186f, 212
  in Prinzmetal's (variant) angina,
    8, 73
  in unstable angina pectoris, 9f,
    69, 73
  long-acting, 69–73
  nitrates with, 72
  off-license uses of, 73
  outcome trials of, 75, 76t
  pharmacokinetics of, 69
  poisoning with, 72
  proischemic effects of, 55
  quinidine interaction with, 229t
  rebound after, 72
  short-acting, 69
  side effects of, 66t, 70, 71t
  vascular protective effects of, 53, 73
Nisoldipine, 75
Nitrates, 33–48, 37t–38t, 40t, 174
  ACE inhibitor with, 45
  antiplatelet effect of, 34
  beta-blockers with, 7–8, 46, 47
  bioavailability of, 34–35
  calcium channel blockers with, 46
  combinations of, 46
  contraindications to, 41–42, 41t,
    43–44
  drug interactions with, 35, 38–39,
    38f
  during pregnancy, 401t
  endothelial effects of, 34
  erectile dysfunction and, 38, 38f,
    39
  failure of, 42
  headache with, 41–42, 41t
  heparin interaction with, 39
  hydralazine interaction with, 39
  in acute pulmonary edema, 44,
    387
  in angina pectoris, 9f, 33–34,
    39–41, 42–43, 350–351, 351f
  in heart failure, 39, 44, 174
  in myocardial infarction, 43–44,
    370

Nitrates (Continued)
  in percutaneous transluminal
    coronary angioplasty, 43
  in unstable angina pectoris, 9f,
    39, 42–43
  intravenous, 36t, 43, 357
    in hypertensive emergency, 212,
      213t
    in pulmonary edema, 44
  long-acting, 40–41, 40t
  methemoglobinemia with, 41t, 42
  nifedipine with, 72
  on/off strategy for, 35
  oxygen demand in, 33
  pharmacokinetics of, 34–35
  precautions with, 41–42, 41t
  prophylactic, 40–41, 40t
  safety of, 47
  short-acting, 39
  side effects of, 41–42, 41t
  sildenafil interaction with, 38,
    38f, 39
  stepped-care with, 42, 42t, 46
  tadalafil interaction with, 38, 38f,
    39
  tolerance to, 41t, 42, 44–46, 45f
    prevention of, 45–46
  transdermal, 36t, 40–41, 40t, 43
  vardenafil interaction with, 38,
    38f, 39
  vasodilatory effects of, 33–34, 34f,
    35f
  withdrawal from, 41t
Nitrendipine, for elderly patients,
  207
Nitroglycerin, 36t. *See also* Nitrates.
  heparin interaction with, 39
  in acute coronary syndromes, 357
  in acute severe hypertension, 212,
    213t, 214t
  in angina pectoris, 39, 40–42, 43,
    350–351, 351f
  in hypertensive emergency, 212,
    213t, 214t
  in myocardial infarction, 43–44,
    370
  in percutaneous transluminal
    coronary angioplasty, 43
  in pulmonary edema, 44
  intravenous, 36t, 43, 357
    in hypertensive emergency, 212,
      213t
    in pulmonary edema, 44
  N-acetylcysteine with, 45
  pharmacokinetics of, 35
  prophylactic, 40–41, 40t
  spray formulation of, 36t, 39
  sublingual, 36t, 39, 350–351
    in pulmonary edema, 44
    isosorbide dinitrate with, 46
  transdermal, 36t, 40–41, 40t, 43
  verapamil with, 46
Nitroprusside, 172–174
  contraindications to, 173
  dose for, 173
  in acute pulmonary edema, 387
  in acute severe hypertension, 212,
    213t, 214t
  indications for, 173
  side effects of, 173
  toxicity of, 172–173, 174

Nodal. *See* Atrioventricular nodal.
Nondihydropyridine calcium
    channel blockers, 51t, 55–56,
    55f
Nonsteroidal anti-inflammatory
    drugs
    ACE inhibitors with, in heart
        failure, 123
    loop diuretic interaction with, 84
    thiazide diuretic interaction with,
        90
Norepinephrine, in heart failure, 15,
    162, 163t, 164, 164f, 165, 168
Norverapamil, 61

O

Obesity, hypertension and, 208
Olmesartan, 140
Omapatrilat, 176, 386
Omega-3 fatty fish oils, 329, 372
Oral contraceptives
    atorvastatin interaction with, 339
    blood lipids with, 331
Ototoxicity, of furosemide, 84
Overdiuresis, 96–97
Oxygen, in myocardial infarction,
    360

P

Pacemaker, in atrial fibrillation, 257
Paroxysmal supraventricular
    tachycardia, 252–255, 253f,
    380–381, 380t
    adenosine in, 221t, 249, 253–254
    diltiazem in, 222t, 253–254
    flecainide in, 234
    in myocardial infarction, 369
    prevention of, 381
    propafenone in, 234, 235, 254
    radiofrequency catheter ablation
        in, 254–255, 255f
    recurrent, 254
    refractory, 381
    verapamil in, 254
Penbutolol, 22t, 28. *See also* Beta-
    blockers.
Pentaerythritol tetranitrate, 37t. *See
    also* Nitrates.
Pentoxifylline, 181, 399
Percutaneous coronary interventions
    abciximab in, 289, 290, 294
    aspirin in, 283
    bivalirudin in, 297
    facilitated, 355f
    glycoprotein IIb/IIIa receptor
        antagonists in, 288–291, 288t
    heparin in, 294, 295–296
    in effort angina, 353–354
    nitroglycerin in, 43
    rescue, 306, 311
    ticlopidine in, 284
    vs. fibrinolysis, 306, 307f,
        311–312, 363t–364t, 365
Perindopril, 113t, 114t, 115f, 124,
    126–127, 132, 134, 203. *See
    also* Angiotensin-converting
    enzyme (ACE) inhibitors.

Peripheral vascular disease, 21,
    398–399
Peripheral vascular resistance, 185
Phenobarbital
    aspirin interaction with, 284
    nifedipine interaction with, 70
    verapamil interaction with, 63
Phenothiazines, QT-prolongation
    with, 243, 245f
Phentolamine
    in acute severe hypertension, 212,
        213t
    in hypertensive emergency, 212,
        213t
Phenylephrine, in heart failure, 163t,
    165
Phenytoin, 220t, 224t, 228t, 233
    amiodarone interaction with,
        229t, 243
    aspirin interaction with, 284
    in digoxin toxicity, 161, 233
    in ventricular arrhythmias, 220t,
        224t, 233
    nifedipine interaction with, 70
    side effects of, 228t
    verapamil interaction with, 63
Pheochromocytoma, 2t, 213t
Phosphodiesterase-III inhibitors, in
    heart failure, 169–171, 169f,
    170f
Pill in the pocket, 235, 258–259,
    258t
Pindolol, 2t, 23t
    hepatic metabolism of, 20, 21f
    in atrial fibrillation, 256t, 257
    lipid effects of, 330t
Plant sterols, 345
Platelet(s), 279
    activation of, 278f, 279
    adhesion of, 277f, 279
    aggregation of, 278f, 279
    aspirin effects on, 278f, 281
    nitrate effects on, 34
    secretory products of, 280–281
Platelet inhibitors, 278f, 281–291,
    285f, 286t, 288t. *See also specific
    inhibitors.*
Pneumonitis, amiodarone and,
    242
Polythiazide, 88t. *See also* Thiazide
    diuretics.
Potassium
    deficiency of
        loop diuretics and, 83–84,
            86
        thiazide diuretics and, 91–92,
            93
    excess of
        ACE inhibitors and, 94–95, 116,
            116f
        potassium-sparing diuretics
            and, 94–95
Potassium chloride, 96
    in digoxin toxicity, 161
Potassium-sparing diuretics, 81t, 82f,
    93–95, 94t, 196
    hyperkalemia with, 94–95
Potassium supplements, 95–96
Pravastatin, 328, 333t, 335t,
    336–337
Prazosin, 186f, 186t, 205

Pregnancy, 400, 401t
ACE inhibitor contraindication during, 117, 204, 401t
beta-blockers during, 26t, 401t
coronary artery disease and, 345
heparin during, 294, 401t
hypertension during, 203, 209, 210, 401t
methyldopa during, 210
statin contraindication during, 334, 336, 345, 401t
torsemide during, 86, 401t
warfarin during, 300, 401t
Preload reduction
in heart failure, 171, 172
in myocardial infarction, 170
Proarrhythmic effects, 251–252, 251f, 259
of adenosine, 250
of digoxin, 159–161, 160f, 160t
of diuretics, 91–92
of flecainide, 228t, 234
of quinidine, 225–227
Probenecid
aspirin interaction with, 284
diuretic interaction with, 84, 90
Procainamide, 220t, 223t, 227, 228t, 230
amiodarone interaction with, 243
compared with lidocaine, 264
contraindications to, 230t
dose of, 223t, 227, 230
drug interactions with, 229t
in atrial fibrillation, 257, 258t
in ventricular tachycardia, 223t, 227, 264
side effects of, 228t, 230
Propafenone, 220t, 224t, 228t, 234–235
digoxin interaction with, 159
drug interactions with, 159, 229t
in atrial fibrillation, 235, 258, 258t, 259, 260f
in paroxysmal supraventricular tachycardia, 234, 254
in supraventricular tachycardia, 234, 235, 254
in ventricular arrhythmias, 235
side effects of, 228t
l-Propionyl-carnitine, in peripheral vascular disease, 399
Propranolol, 2t, 22t, 27. *See also* Beta-blockers.
antiarrhythmic therapy with, 237
cimetidine interaction with, 21
diltiazem interaction with, 67
half-life of, 20, 22t
hepatic metabolism of, 20, 21f
in anxiety, 17
in atrial fibrillation, 256t, 257
in hypertrophic cardiomyopathy, 16
in migraine, 18
in paroxysmal supraventricular tachycardia, 253
in Prinzmetal's (variant) angina, 8
in thyroid storm, 17
intellectual effects of, 211
lidocaine interaction with, 232
lipid effects of, 330t

Propranolol *(Continued)*
membrane stabilizing activity of, 20
postinfarct, 10–11
side effects of, 24, 211
verapamil interaction with, 21
Prostacyclin analogs, in pulmonary hypertension, 394
Prostaglandins, bradykinin effects on, 110
Prosthetic cardiac valves
aspirin and, 283
warfarin and, 303
Protamine sulfate, 293
Protein, beta-blocker binding to, 20
Protein-C deficiency, warfarin and, 300
Protein kinase C, 107
Proteinuria
captopril and, 130
rosuvastatin and, 340
Prothrombin, 280, 280f
Pulmonary edema, 44, 83, 177f, 387
Pulmonary embolism, 301
Pulmonary heart disease, digoxin and, 159
Pulmonary hypertension, 393–394
Pulseless electrical activity, 402
Pyridostigmine, disopyramide interaction with, 229t

Q

QT-prolongation. *See also* Torsades de pointes.
beta-blockers in, 17
congenital, 17, 252, 266
drug-induced, 244, 245f, 246, 248, 252
Quality of life, 211
Quinapril, 113t, 115f, 132. *See also* Angiotensin-converting enzyme (ACE) inhibitors.
Quinidine, 220, 220t, 223t, 225–227, 228t
amiodarone interaction with, 243
contraindications to, 227
digoxin interaction with, 159
doses for, 223t, 225
drug interactions with, 159, 229t
electrophysiology with, 220, 226f, 228t
flecainide interaction with, 229t
hypersensitivity reactions to, 227
in atrial fibrillation, 258t
indications for, 220, 225
precautions for, 225–227
proarrhythmic effects of, 225–227
QRS duration with, 226
side effects of, 227, 228t
toxicity of, 225–227, 245f
Quinine, digoxin interaction with, 159

R

Radiofrequency catheter ablation
in atrial fibrillation, 262

Radiofrequency catheter ablation
(*Continued*)
  in paroxysmal supraventricular
    tachycardia, 255, 255f
  in ventricular tachycardia, 383
Ramipril, 113t, 114f, 115t, 120t,
    126–127. *See also* Angiotensin-
    converting enzyme (ACE)
    inhibitors.
  after myocardial infarction, 133,
    134
  in hypertension, 129, 133,
    202–203
  in nephropathy, 128, 133, 203
  in renal failure, 128
Ranolazine, 47, 352
Rauwolfia root, 186f, 186t
Raynaud's phenomenon, 21, 26t,
    399
Red wine, 345–346
Remodeling, 127f
Renal artery stenosis, ACE inhibitors
    and, 117
Renal cell carcinoma, thiazide
    diuretics and, 93
Renal failure. *See* Kidneys, failure
    of.
Renin, 104, 106
  digoxin effect on, 154
  release of, 108–109, 108f
Renin-angiotensin-aldosterone
    system, 104, 108–109, 108f,
    140–141, 141f
  beta-blocker effect on, 53
  in heart failure, 16, 117–118,
    118f
Reperfusion injury, 311
Reserpine, in hypertension, 186f,
    186t, 192, 206
Resins, 332f, 340, 344
Resuscitation. *See*
    Cardiopulmonary.
Reteplase, 292f, 305t, 309, 310t
Retinopathy, diabetic, 308
Rhabdomyolysis, statins and, 334
Rifampin
  aspirin interaction with, 284
  nifedipine interaction with, 70
  verapamil interaction with, 63
Risk stratification
  coronary disease in, 321, 322t
  hypertension in, 188
Rosuvastatin, 333t, 339–340

S

Salicylates
  furosemide interaction with, 84
  poisoning with, carbonic
    anhydrase inhibitors in, 95
Salt restriction, 124, 179–180, 185
Salt sensitivity, 109
Saruplase, 310
Septic shock, 165
Sexual dysfunction, 210–211
  beta-blockers and, 25, 211
  diuretics and, 93, 211
  drug treatment of, 38, 38f
  nitrates and, 38, 38f, 39
Shock

cardiogenic, 150, 151–152,
    369–371
  septic, 165
  therapy of, 177f
  warm, 168
Sick-sinus syndrome, 21, 381
Signal transduction, in beta-
    adrenoreceptors, 1, 3, 3f, 4f
Sildenafil
  in pulmonary hypertension, 394
  nitrate interaction with, 38, 38f,
    39
  verapamil interaction with, 63
Silent myocardial ischemia, beta-
    blockers in, 8, 11
Simvastatin, 333t, 335t, 337–338.
    See also Statins.
  verapamil interaction with, 62
Sinus bradycardia, 381
Sinus rhythm, heart failure with,
    156
Sinus tachycardia, 2t, 361
Sirolimus, 354f
Skin
  amiodarone effects on, 242
  warfarin effects on, 300
Sodium, dietary, 109, 124, 179–180,
    185
Sodium pump, digoxin effect on,
    153, 154f
Sotalol, 2t, 22t, 28, 220t, 224t,
    243–245. *See also*
    Beta-blockers.
  antiarrhythmic therapy with, 237
  contraindications to, 244
  disopyramide interaction with,
    229t
  dose of, 224t, 244
  drug interactions with, 229t, 243
  during pregnancy, 401t
  electrophysiology of, 243–244
  in atrial fibrillation, 244, 258t,
    259, 260f
  in paroxysmal supraventricular
    tachycardia, 254
  in ventricular arrhythmias, 13,
    224t, 244, 264
  indications for, 244
  quinidine interaction with, 229t
  renal excretion of, 21, 21f
  side effects of, 228t, 244
  torsades de pointes with, 244,
    245f
Spirapril, 113t, 115f. *See also*
    Angiotensin-converting enzyme
    (ACE) inhibitors.
Spironolactone, 82f, 94, 94t
  ACE inhibitors with, 123, 204
  blood lipids with, 330t
  in heart failure, 94, 114t,
    120–121, 123, 140–141,
    180–181
  lipid effects of, 330t
Stanol margarines, 345
Staphylococcus, in endocarditis, 396
Staphylokinase, 310
Statins, 331–340, 332f, 333t, 335t
  after myocardial infarction, 336,
    372
  bile acid sequestrants with, 344
  clopidogrel interaction with, 287

Statins (*Continued*)
  contraindications to, 334
  drug interactions with, 62, 339,
      340
  ezetimibe with, 344
  fibrates with, 334, 344
  in myocardial infarction, 369
  indications for, 331, 334
  liver damage with, 334
  myopathy with, 334
  nicotinic acid with, 344
  non-lipid effects, 331
  pregnancy contraindication to,
      334, 336, 345, 401t
  trials of, 335t, 338–339
  verapamil interaction with, 62
Stents, 354
Step diet, 329
Steroids
  loop diuretic interaction with, 84
  thiazide diuretic interaction with,
      90
Streptococcus viridans, in endocarditis,
      396
Streptokinase, 292f, 305t, 306–307,
      309, 310t
Stroke
  atrial fibrillation and, 260, 261,
      262, 283, 298, 302–303
  calcium channel blockers and, 59
  hypertension and, 212
  prevention of, 122t, 133, 283,
      284, 304
Sudden cardiac death
  in hypertrophic cardiomyopathy,
      389
  prevention of, 266–267
Sulfinpyrazone, 288
  aspirin interaction with, 284
  warfarin interaction with,
      299–300
Sulfonamide sensitivity, 86
Supraventricular arrhythmias,
      374–381. *See also* Atrial
      fibrillation; Atrial flutter;
      Supraventricular tachycardias.
Supraventricular tachycardias,
      252–255, 253f, 380–381, 380t
  adenosine in, 221t, 249, 253–254
  beta-blockers in, 2t, 13, 29
  calcium channel blockers in, 56,
      59, 64, 68, 222t, 253–254
  diltiazem in, 59, 222t, 253–254
  dofetilide in, 222t, 254
  esmolol in, 13, 29, 221t
  flecainide in, 234
  in myocardial infarction, 369
  prevention of, 381
  propafenone in, 234, 235, 254
  radiofrequency catheter ablation
      in, 254–255, 255f
  recurrent, 254
  refractory, 381
  verapamil in, 56, 59, 64, 221t,
      254
Syncope
  atrioventricular block with, 381
  neurocardiogenic, beta-blockers
      in, 17
  nitrates and, 41t

T

Tachycardia/bradycardia syndrome,
      302, 381
Tadalafil, nitrate interaction with,
      38, 38f, 39
Tamponade, nitrates and, 41t
Tandolapril, 115f
Telmisartan, 138t, 139
Tenecteplase, 292f, 305t, 308, 308t,
      310t
Terazosin, 186f, 186t, 205
Terbutaline, in heart failure, 168
Terfenadine, QT-prolongation with,
      245f
Testes, amiodarone effects on, 242
Theophylline
  adenosine interaction with, 230t,
      250
  mexiletine interaction with, 229t
  verapamil interaction with, 63
Thiamine, in beri-beri heart disease,
      399–400
Thiazide diuretics, 81t, 82f, 87–90,
      88t, 89t
  aspirin interaction with, 284
  beta-blockers with, 12, 92
  contraindications to, 90
  diabetogenic effects of, 92
  dose of, 87–89, 88t
  drug interactions with, 90
  hypercalcemia with, 92–93
  hypokalemia with, 91–92, 93
  hypomagnesemia with, 92
  hyponatremia with, 91
  impotence and, 93
  in diabetes insipidus, 99
  in heart failure, 89
  in hypertension, 12, 87, 89–90,
      89t
  in idiopathic hypercalciuria, 99
  lipid effects of, 91, 92, 330t
  pharmacokinetics of, 82f, 87,
      87f
  pharmacologic action of, 87,
      87f
  renal cancer and, 93
  side effects of, 90, 91–93
  urate excretion with, 92
  ventricular arrhythmias with, 91
Thrombin, 280, 280f
Thrombin inhibitors, 296
Thrombocytopenia
  abciximab and, 290
  heparin and, 293–294
  ticlopidine and, 290
Thrombolysis. *See* Fibrinolytic
      (thrombolytic) therapy.
Thrombosis, 276–281, 277f, 278f
  antiplatelet agents in, 281–291,
      285f, 286t, 288t
  aspirin in, 278f, 281–284
  direct thrombin inhibitors in,
      296–297
  fibrinolytic therapy in, 304–312,
      305t, 307f, 308t, 310t
  fondaparinux in, 297–298
  glycoprotein IIb/IIIa receptor
      antagonists in, 278f, 285f,
      288–291, 288t
  heparin in, 291–296, 292f

Thrombosis *(Continued)*
  heparin-induced, 293–294
  low-dose warfarin in, 304
  warfarin in, 301, 304
  ximelagatran in, 298
Thromboxane A2, aspirin effects on, 278f, 281
Thyroid gland, amiodarone effects on, 242
Thyroid storm, beta-blockers in, 17
Thyrotoxicosis
  anticoagulation in, 302
  beta-blockers in, 2t, 17
Ticlopidine, 284
Timolol, 2t, 22t, 28. *See also* Beta-blockers.
  hepatic metabolism of, 20, 21f
  in glaucoma, 17
  postinfarct, 10–11
Tirofiban, 286t, 288–289, 288t, 290
  during pregnancy, 401t
  vs. abciximab, 291
Tissue factor, 279–280, 280f
Tissue plasminogen activator, 292f, 305t, 307–308, 308t
Tocainide, 220t, 223t
  drug interactions with, 229t
  side effects of, 228t
Tolerance
  to diuretics, 84, 97, 98f, 99t
  to nitrates, 41t, 42, 44–46, 45f
Torsades de pointes, 245f, 252
  amiodarone and, 240, 242
  dofetilide and, 248
  ibutilide and, 246
  sotalol and, 244
Torsemide, 85–86
  dose of, 85, 85t
  during pregnancy, 401t
  hypokalemia and, 86
  in cirrhosis, 86
  in heart failure, 85
  in hypertension, 85, 196
  in renal failure, 85–86
  side effects of, 86
Trandolapril, 113t, 114t, 115f, 120t, 133, 352. *See also* Angiotensin-converting enzyme (ACE) inhibitors.
  atrial fibrillation and, 259
Transesophageal echocardiography, in atrial fibrillation, 377
Transient ischemic attack
  ticlopidine in, 284
  warfarin in, 303
Treprostinil, in pulmonary hypertension, 394
Triamterene, in hypertension, 81t, 93, 94t, 196
Trichlormethiazide, 88t. *See also* Thiazide diuretics.
Tricyclic antidepressants
  QT-prolongation with, 243, 245f
  sotalol interaction with, 229t
Triglycerides
  blood, 325–326, 325t
  resin effects on, 340
Trimetazidine, 47, 352
Trimethoprim, dofetilide interaction with, 230t

V

Valsartan, 114t, 138t, 139. *See also* Angiotensin-II receptor blockers.
Valvular heart disease, 16–17, 302, 391–393
Valvuloplasty, 392
Vardenafil, nitrate interaction with, 38, 38f, 39
Vasodilators. *See also specific vasodilators.*
  in acute pulmonary edema, 387
  in heart failure, 169f, 171–176, 181, 384–385
  in hypertension, 186f, 186t, 205
  in refractory hypertension, 212
Ventricular arrhythmias, 2t, 223t 224t, 241t, 263–266, 382–383
  amiodarone in, 224t, 239–240, 264–265, 383
  beta-blockers in, 13, 266, 383
  drug selection for, 265–266, 382
  electrophysiological testing in, 265–266
  flecainide in, 224t, 234, 264
  hemodynamic status in, 264
  ibutilide and, 246
  in heart failure, 385
  in hypertension, 210
  in myocardial infarction, 369
  lidocaine in, 223t, 231–233, 264
  mexiletine in, 223t, 235
  moricizine in, 224t, 236
  phenytoin in, 220t, 224t, 233
  procainamide in, 223t, 227, 264
  propafenone in, 235
  sotalol in, 224t, 244, 264
  thiazide diuretics and, 91
  tocainide in, 223t, 235
  verapamil in, 65, 248, 266
  without heart disease, 266
Ventricular pacing, in digoxin toxicity, 161
Ventricular preexcitation, atrial fibrillation with, 257
Verapamil, 51t, 54f, 55–56, 55f, 58f, 60–65. *See also* Calcium channel blockers.
  after myocardial infarction, 59, 65
  beta-blocker interaction with, 21, 62, 248
  contraindications to, 61–62, 62f, 63t
  digoxin interaction with, 61, 62, 159
  disopyramide interaction with, 62, 229t
  dofetilide interaction with, 230t
  dose for, 57t, 61
  drug interactions with, 61, 62–63, 159, 229t, 230t
  electrophysiology of, 60
  flecainide interaction with, 62
  in arrhythmias, 220t, 221t, 248
  in atrial fibrillation, 64, 256t, 257
  in atypical ventricular tachycardia, 65
  in carotid atherosclerosis, 65
  in coronary spasm, 58

Verapamil *(Continued)*
  in diabetes mellitus, 65
  in effort angina, 56, 57t, 64
  in hypertension, 58–59, 60, 64,
    74, 76t, 186f, 191t, 199–201,
    200f, 204
  in hypertrophic cardiomyopathy,
    64–65, 388
  in intermittent claudication, 65
  in paroxysmal supraventricular
    tachycardia, 254
  in supraventricular tachycardias,
    56, 59, 64, 221t
  in unstable angina, 58, 64
  in ventricular arrhythmias, 65,
    248, 266
  indications for, 64–65
  nitroglycerin with, 46
  outcome trials of, 75, 76t
  pharmacokinetics of, 60–61
  quinidine interaction with, 229t
  side effects of, 56, 61, 66t
  slow-release, 61
  statin interaction with, 62
  toxicity of, 63
  vs. adenosine, 250
Vitamin C, with nitrates, 46
Vitamin E, angina pectoris and, 352

W

Warfarin, 292f, 298–304
  after myocardial infarction, 301,
    303–304, 373
  amiodarone interaction with,
    229t, 243
  aspirin interaction with, 283
  bleeding with, 300
  complications of, 300
  contraindications to, 300
  dose of, 298–299
    reduction of, 299
  drug interactions with, 283,
    299–300, 342

Warfarin *(Continued)*
  during pregnancy, 300, 401t
  fibrate interaction with, 342
  in atrial fibrillation, 262,
    301–303, 379
  in atrial flutter, 263
  in low ejection fraction, 301
  in myocardial infarction,
    300–301
  in venous thromboembolism,
    301, 304
  indications for, 300–303
  INR range of, 299
  ischemia prevention with, 304
  low-dose, 303–304
  mechanism of action of, 298
  overdose of, 300
  pharmacokinetics of, 298
  propafenone interaction with,
    229t
  quinidine interaction with, 229t
  self-monitoring of, 299
  skin necrosis with, 300
  vs. ximelagatran, 298
Weight gain, beta-blockers and, 25
Weight loss, in hypertension, 187,
  208
Wide-complex tachycardia,
  adenosine in, 249
Wine, 345–346
Wolff-Parkinson-White syndrome,
  61, 158, 220, 226f, 249, 381

X

Ximelagatran, 292f, 298, 373
Xipamide, 88t. *See also* Thiazide
  diuretics.

Z

Ziac, 12, 28
Zofenopril, 133